Fiberoptic Endoscopy and the Difficult Airway

Second Edition

Fiberoptic Endoscopy and the Difficult Airway

Second Edition

Andranik Ovassapian, M.D.
Professor and Associate Chairman
Department of Anesthesiology
Northwestern University Medical School and
Chief, Anesthesiology Service
Veterans Affairs
Lakeside Medical Center
Chicago, Illinois

Lippincott - Raven
PUBLISHERS
Philadelphia • New York

Lippincott-Raven Publishers, 227 East Washington Square, Philadelphia, Pennsylvania 19106-3780

Printed in Hong Kong

Library of Congress Cataloging-in-Publication Data

Fiberoptic endoscopy and the difficult airway / [edited by] Andranik Ovassapian. — 2nd ed.
p. cm.
Rev. ed. of: Fiberoptic airway endoscopy in anesthesia and critical care / Andranik Ovassapian. 1990.
Includes bibliographical references and index.
ISBN 0-7817-0272-0
1. Trachea—Intubation. 2. Endoscopy. 3. Airway (Medicine) I. Ovassapian, Andranik. II. Ovassapian, Andranik Fiberoptic airway endoscopy in anesthesia and critical care.
[DNLM: 1. Airway Obstruction—therapy. 2. Endoscopy—methods. 3. Fiber Optics. 4. Intubation, Intratracheal—methods. WO 280 F443 1996]
RF517.093 1996
617.9′6—dc20
DNLM/DLC
for Library of Congress 96-4639
CIP

The material contained in this volume was submitted as previously unpublished material, except in the instances in which credit has been given to the source from which some of the illustrative material was derived.

Great care has been taken to maintain the accuracy of the information contained in the volume. However, neither Lippincott-Raven Publishers nor the author can be held responsible for errors or for any consequences arising from the use of the information contained herein.

9 8 7 6 5 4 3 2 1

To
my loving wife Ashkhen
and
our children and their families

Contents

Contributors

Andranik Ovassapian, M.D.
Professor and Associate Chairman, Department of Anesthesiology, Northwestern University Medical School and Chief, Anesthesiology Service, V.A. Lakeside Medical Center, 333 East Huron Street, Chicago, Illinois 60611

Tom C. Krejcie, M.D.
Associate Professor of Anesthesiology, Northwestern University Medical School, 303 East Superior Street, Chicago, Illinois 60611

Paul S. Mesnick, M.D., M.J.
Assistant Professor of Anesthesiology, Northwestern Unversity Medical School, 303 East Superior Street, Chicago, Illinois 60611

Lee Sider, M.D.
Associate Professor of Radiology, Northwestern University Medical School, 710 North Fairbanks, Chicago, Illinois 60611

Tod B. Sloan, M.D., Ph.D.
Professor and Director of Neuroanesthesia, University of Texas Health Science Center, 7703 Floyd Curl Drive, San Antonio, Texas 78284

Melissa Wheeler, M.D.
Assistant Professor of Anesthesiology, Northwestern University Medical School, Attending Anesthesiologist, Children's Memorial Hospital, 2300 Children's Plaza, Chicago, Illinois 60614

Foreword

One of life's pleasures is derived from observing the positive effect of a close colleague's efforts in the discipline in which he works. One can be excused for feeling proud of friends' accomplishments and thankful for the improvements in patient care that they have achieved. I am thankful that Dr. Ovassapian and I have been colleagues and I am proud of the advances in patient care that he has made as a member of our faculty. I have observed the growth of his influence on the standards of clinical practice, not only in the field of anesthesiology, but also in other disciplines of medicine, in which airway management is a primary concern.

Errors in airway management in patients unconscious from any cause have, in the past, often led to life-threatening disasters or death. These problems captured Dr. Ovassapian's interest early in his career. When he first saw the flexible fiberoptic bronchoscope, he readily recognized the potential it offered to help improve airway management. He mastered its use and taught all the trainees in the Northwestern residency program the techniques of fiberoptic management of the difficult airway. He established a series of workshops and sponsored by this department and offered three or four times a year, to teach colleagues from other institutions.

Eventually he took his workshop to other academic centers, and to state, regional, national, and international meetings. As Andy's efforts spread beyond the local scene, he met others with similar interests who were attempting to introduce techniques that master the difficult airway. He brought special airways into our department and even designed one of his own. He introduced us to the laryngeal mask airway, which is now part of the didactic curriculum for each of the trainees in this program. One of Dr. Ovassapian's strengths is the gentle way in which he mentors his young colleagues. Many of his trainees are now engaged in carrying forth his gospel. His interests have served as a focal point that has allowed us to recruit faculty candidates.

Dr. Ovassapian's networking with a group of physicians of like mind has led to the development of a program for registry of patients who have had prior difficulty with airway management, and with a means for their identification to future health care providers.

Five years have passed since the First Edition of *Fiberoptic Airway Endoscopy in Anesthesia and Critical Care* was published. An update is needed to include the many advances made in the intervening period. The change in the title of the current edition, *Fiberoptic Endoscopy and the Difficult Airway*, reflects a broader focus. In addition to presenting the fiberscope as an airway managment tool, Dr. Ovassapian and his colleagues describe other techniques of airway management such as the laryngeal mask airway and the combitube, an esophageal device. Two new chapters will prove to be especially valuable and useful to clinicians involved in airway management. The chapter on conscious sedation will provide information on drugs commonly used and techniques for sedation during awake intubation. Extubation of the difficult airway has been recognized as fraught with danger and a sizable literature over the past five years dealing with this aspect of airway management has been summarized in its own chapter.

Dr. Ovassapian, in this Second Edition of his monograph, has updated and integrated an enormous literature, much of which has been published in the last five years. This book will be useful to both experienced clinicians and trainees in those specialties dealing with airway management.

Edward A. Brunner, M.D., Ph.D.

Preface

Since publication of the First Edition in 1990, much has been written about airway management. New devices have been developed, and new techniques have been described. The title change of the Second Edition is intended to reflect more accurately the content and goal of the new edition.

The book contains five new chapters. In addition, eight chapters are rewritten and substantially expanded. The book reflects twenty years of combined experience of the members of the anesthesia department at Northwestern University and Veterans Affairs Lakeside Medical Center in the use of fiberoptic endoscopes in airway management.

The goal of this book is to encourage airway specialists in the use of fiberoptic bronchoscopy to its fullest extent, and not merely limiting its use to tracheal intubation. Plenty of drawings and color pictures are included to help make the techniques described simple and understandable. The pertinent literature is reviewed and updated.

In the field of anesthesia, the use of the fiberoptic bronchoscope in airway management has substantially expanded the value of this instrument in critically-ill patients. I have no doubt that the proliferation of fiberoptic airway management has contributed to the safety of anesthesia and decreased the incidence of airway-related trauma, mortality, and delay, or cancellation of surgical cases.

The book is aimed at all physicians involved in critical patient care wherever airway management, oxygenation, and ventilation are imporatnt factors. Anesthesiologists, emergency medicine physicians, critical care specialists, otolaryngologists, and trauma surgeons will particularly find this text useful. The nurse anesthetist, as well as technicians dealing with fiberoptic endoscopes, will also benefit from this new edition.

The first critical element of difficult airway management is the knowledge and understanding of the pathophysiology of disease, the degree of airway compromise, ventilation/oxygenation impairment, and the urgency of the situation. The second critical element is the knowledge and skill of the physician in drugs used in airway management and the techniques applied to secure the airway. Deficiency in any area may result in a poor judgement or selection of a less than ideal approach for the particular patient.

In my view, the airway is related to major patient morbidity and mortality far more frequently than is believed or stated in the anesthesia literature. Many planned and emergency tracheostomies can be avoided if expert help is available. Airway-related disasters are far more common outside of the operating room and in trauma patients because of the emergency nature of the circumstances surrounding the incident and the frequent lack of adequate help and expertise. Many patients who lose their lives because of airway emergencies might otherwise survive, with many years of productive life ahead of them, if the acute airway problem is managed appropriately.

I hope that this book will contribute to the general knowledge and safety of airway management inside and outside of the operating room and hospital.

Acknowledgments

I gratefully acknowledge the help of my colleagues at the Veterans Affairs Lakeside Medical Center, and the anesthesia residents at the McGaw Medical Center, Northwestern University for their willingness to participate in the teaching and learning of fiberoptic airway management, and for completing a questionnaire on every fiberoptic intubation during the last 17 years.

I am grateful to Edward A. Brunner, M.D., Ph.D., Chairman of the Department of Anesthesia, Northwestern University Medical School, who has always supported and encouraged my commitment to education and to the writing of this book. He has also contributed to this book with his gracious foreword.

I am particularly indebted to Paul Mesnick, M.D., for reviewing eight book chapters, providing me with valuable suggestions, and co-authoring two chapters. My sincere thanks to Tod B. Sloan, M.D., Ph.D., Lee Sider, M.D., and Mellisa Wheeler, M.D., for contributing the first, second, and seventh chapters respectively. My gratitude to Tom Krejcie, M.D., for reviewing two chapters and co-authoring Chapter 6.

Appreciation is acknowledged to the editorial and production teams of Lippincott-Raven Publishers and Lesley Poliner, Senior Production Editor, for their excellent and timely completion of this book. Elizabeth Greenspan and Craig Percy deserve special thanks for their support and advice.

The support of Mr. Gene Eldridge, Senior Product Manager, and Olympus America Inc., Medical Instrument Division, in providing photographs and the loan of fiberscopes (BF 6C30 and 3C30), for taking the fiberoptic pictures shown in this book is highly appreciated.

The Pentax Precision Instrument Corporation also provided photographs for use in this text. Their support is gratefully acknowledged.

Fiberoptic Endoscopy and the Difficult Airway

Second Edition

CHAPTER 1

The Principles of Fiberoptic Endoscopes

Tod B. Sloan, M.D., Ph.D. and Andranik Ovassapian, M.D.

In 1954, Hopkins and Kapany (1) developed an optically arranged glass fiber bundle, named it the fiberscope, and suggested its use as a flexible instrument for investigating the stomach. Such a device was first used in 1957 when Hirschewitz used a gastroscope to examine a duodenal ulcer (1). In 1966, the first fiberoptic bronchoscope was constructed, based on specifications and characteristics that were proposed by Ikeda (2). He demonstrated the use and application of the instrument and named it the flexible bronchofiberscope. During the past 30 years there have been numerous improvements in fiberoptic technology and a wider range of application for these instruments.

THE PHYSICS OF FLEXIBLE FIBEROPTIC ENDOSCOPES

A beam of light entering one end of an ordinary glass rod is trapped by repeated internal reflections off the walls until it emerges at the other end. It is this trapping of light within the glass rod that forms the basis for the use of fiberoptics to transmit images (1).

If a glass rod is heated and stretched, strands less than 25 μ in diameter can be formed. These strands become flexible and are more properly termed fibers (Fig. 1). The light entering such a fiber is trapped and, after many reflections off the walls (up to 10,000 reflections/meter), emerges uniformly distributed over the exit face of the fiber. Not all the light striking the entry face of the fiber actually enters the fiber. Part of the light is reflected back, depending on the angle of impact. Most of the light striking perpendicular to the entry surface of the fiber is able to pass through, while beyond a "critical angle," all light is reflected off the surface. The amount reflected will depend on the refractive index (RI) of the glass, and the amount of reflection increases as the angle increases from perpendicular toward the critical angle. A specific or detailed image cannot be transmitted in a recognizable form over a single fiber, since the image is completely blurred on transmission down each fiber. Therefore, the image must be formed as a composite of many such fibers.

A large number of glass fibers fastened together with both ends tightly fixed makes a flexible bundle. How-

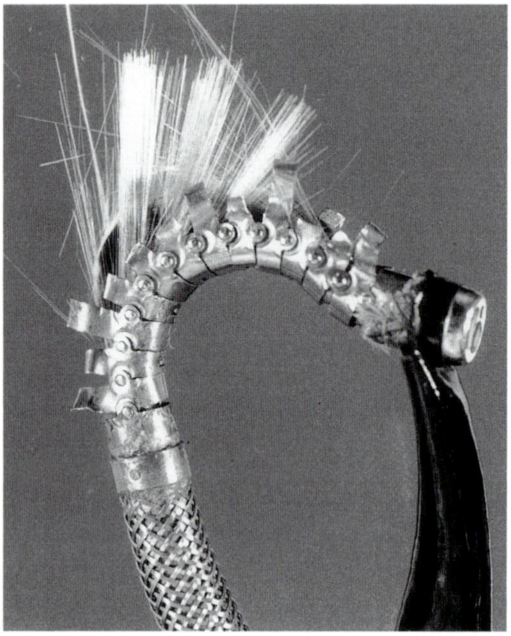

FIG. 1. Glass fibers at the distal end of the insertion cord of an old Olympus fiberscope. Each light-carrying (incoherent) and image-carrying (coherent) glass fiber bundle is enclosed in a plastic tube and is separated from the other (see Fig. 3). The plastic tube is opened to expose the glass fibers. Dissected bending section shows cut metal rings joined by hinges to metal wires to provide maximum bending at the distal tip.

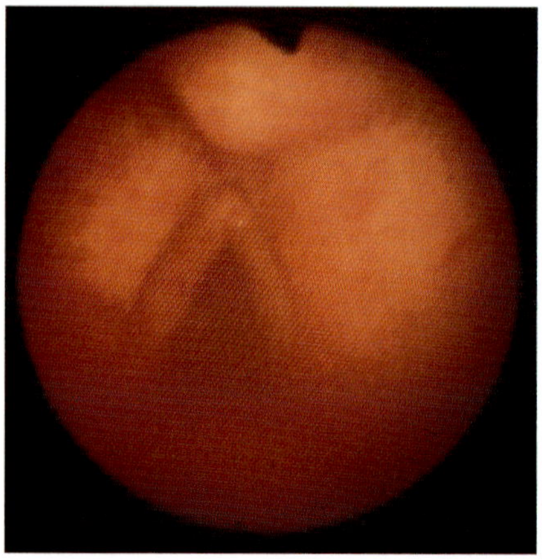

FIG. 2. Magnified endoscopic picture. Each dot represents one fiber.

ever, in order for an optical image to be transmitted through the bundle and subsequently identified, it is essential that the arrangement of fibers at each end of the bundle be precisely the same. This type of organized bundle is called a coherent bundle. In such a bundle, complete optical insulation of each fiber in the bundle is essential. This is accomplished by coating each glass fiber with a 1-μ-thick layer of another type of glass, which has a lower RI (a process called cladding). This helps maintain total internal reflection of light and aids in image transmission along the fiber, even though the fiber may be bent or twisted.

The resolution of an image formed by the composite of individual fibers in a coherent bundle is related to the diameter of the individual fibers. Resolution is improved by increasing the number of fibers in the bundle and using smaller diameter fibers. Glass fibers of 8 μ or less are not suitable for this purpose; as light is not transmitted well in such a narrow channel.

Light from the subject strikes the distal end of the bundle, is transmitted through the individual fibers in the bundle, and is reconstructed at the proximal end. The proximal image (at the eyepiece) consists of a lattice or raster of small spots of light, each with uniform intensity and color. This is similar to a television picture, which, in like manner, is composed of discrete picture elements or pixels. A typical fiberoptic image bundle has a diameter of 1.5 mm and contains about 10,000 fibers of 10–12 μ in diameter. As a consequence, there are only 100 fibers or picture elements at any given diameter of the bundle, giving rise to the graininess seen in magnified endoscopy images (Fig. 2). An objective lens is placed at the distal end of the image transmission bundle to focus the object being transmitted by the fibers. An eyepiece, consisting of several lenses, is placed in the handle to focus the proximal image from the bundle onto the viewer's retina and to provide image magnification. Except at the ends where fibers are fused for strength, the bundle is flexible. However, these fibers are delicate, and breakage may occur. When broken, a fiber will no longer pass its image, and the viewer will view a black dot in that fiber's location.

A fiberoptic bundle is also used to conduct light from an external source to the distal end of an endoscope. This light transmission bundle is subjected to fewer constraints, since no discernible image need be identified. Fiber size can be larger (typically 25 μ), and the fibers do not need to be arranged in a precise manner (incoherent bundle) (1).

The two remaining factors in endoscope design include controls to maneuver the tip and a means for providing a coordinated rotation. Small wires are used to bend the tip via a control lever, and the coordinated rotation is inherent in the basic construction (Fig. 3). Coordinated rotation means that the tip rotates to the same degree as the handle when the latter is turned. Thus, the tip can be bent in any direction by a combination of rotation and bending.

BASIC ANATOMY OF A BRONCHOFIBERSCOPE

The basic structure of a bronchofiberscope is shown in Fig. 4. The major components are the handle, insertion cord, and universal cord. Each of these is designed

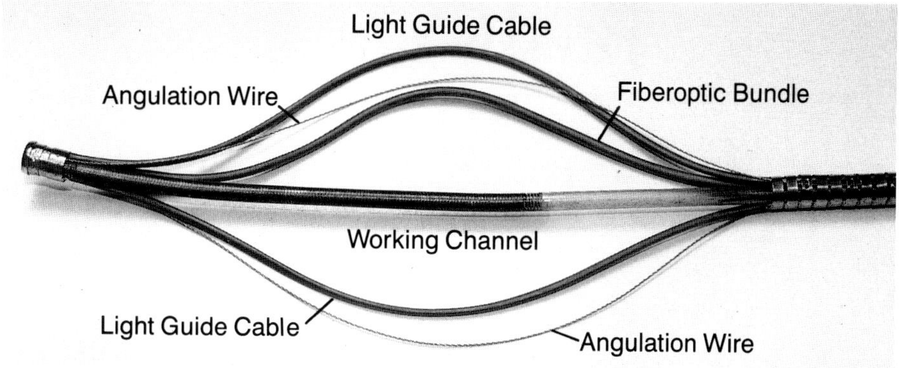

FIG. 3. Inside of a fiberoptic bronchoscope insertion tube. Two angulation wires control the bending of the tip of the fiberscope. Two light guide cables contain fiberoptic bundles (incoherent), which bring light to the tip of the fiberscope. The fiberoptic bundle contains the coherent bundle, which transmits images from the objective lens at the tip of the fiberscope to the eyepiece of the fiberscope. The working or suction channel is used for suctioning of secretions and instillation of local anesthetics. (Courtesy of Pentax Precision Instrument Corp., Orangeburg, New York 10963-2699.)

to contribute to the overall functioning of the endoscope and may come in several varieties, depending on the particular manufacturer and model. However, several basic generalizations exist across all instruments (3–5).

The Handle

The handle is held by either the right or the left hand and contains the eyepiece for viewing, the lever for controlling the bending motion of the tip, and access to the working (suction or injection) channel. Many fiberscopes will have a tip-locking lever to lock the bending tip at a desired position. This lock is used during bronchoscopic biopsy or photography and is not usually used during airway examination and intubation. Most handles are made to be held comfortably in one hand in such a way that the thumb can maneuver the bending lever and the index finger can regulate the suction. This allows the operator's other hand to be free to manipulate the insertion cord or endotracheal tube. The bending lever, which is located on the back of the handle, controls movement of the insertion cord tip in one plane of motion. This plane is along the vertical axis when the fiberscope is oriented in the usual fashion; some fiberscopes have a notch that can be seen along the margin of the picture. This notch defines the plane of rotation and is at the 12 o'clock position. Usually, the connection of the handle to the insertion cord is tapered, such that an endotracheal tube may be held there by being pushed onto the taper. The eyepiece contains a diopter adjustment ring to focus and adjust the eyepiece to fit each viewer's eye. The handle is also used to allow coordinated rotation of the scope by rotation of the handle along the axis of the insertion cord by flexion or extension of the wrist. Hence, to look to the right, the bending lever is moved to bend the viewing end upward and then the handle is rotated clockwise so that the actual view is to the right (alternatively the bending lever could be adjusted to look downward and the handle rotated counterclockwise).

Insertion Cord

The insertion cord or tube is the long portion of the fiberscope that is inserted into the patient and over which endotracheal tubes are passed during fiberoptic intubation. It contains the light guide and image transmission bundles, the working channel, and the tip-bending control wires. These are wrapped with a water-impermeable coating (typically polyurethane) whose outside diameter determines the size of the smallest endotracheal tube that can be used. The insertion cord is flexible, such that it will tolerate gentle bending to accommodate the bends of the airways and patient anatomy. The only portion of the insertion cord that is designed for maximum bending is the distal tip. This tip is made more flexible by enclosing the contents within a series of metal rings, which are joined by hinges to metal wires along two sides (Fig. 1). The tip is then able to bend up and down at right angles to these hinges according to the tension in two control wires. The coating on the tip is made of thin rubber, so that it remains sealed yet flexible. The delicate nature of the rings, wires, bundles, and coating makes this a very easily damaged region.

In new videobronchoscopes the image-transmitting fiber bundle is omitted. Alternatively, a small camera chip (CCD) is positioned at distal end of the insertion cord behind the objective lens. The digitalized signal of the videobronchoscope provides the opportunity to capture images electronically.

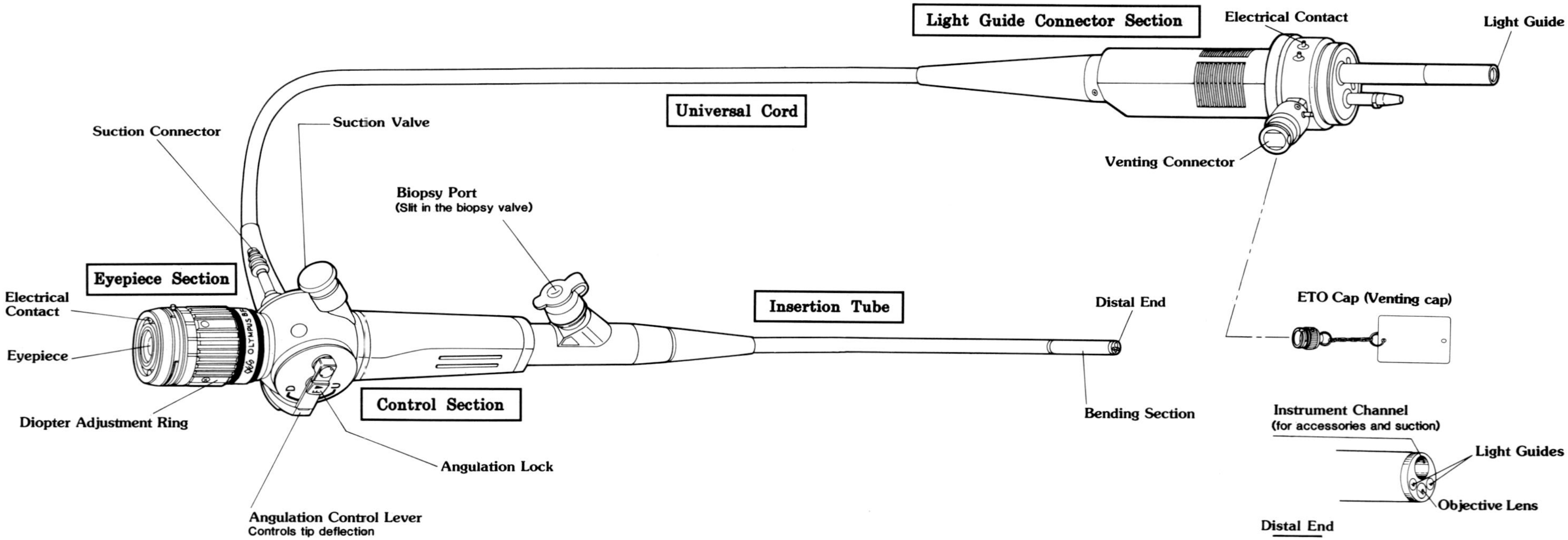

FIG. 4. Components of a bronchofiberscope. Olympus BF-20 D series. The BF-30 series fiberscopes are similar in design to BF-20 series. Changes include improved optics and introduction of disposable suction valve and connector system.

With these units there is no eyepiece and, therefore, no option to view the airway directly. Rather, the digital image is processed and colorized by a computerized video system and displayed on a color TV monitor. The image can also be archived on any of several hard copy image storage media.

Light Guide Bundles

The light to illuminate the image is transmitted through one or two light guide bundles to the tip of the fiberscope. These glass fibers extend to the light guide bundle of the universal cord, which is connected to the external light source.

Image Transmission Bundle

The basic optical construction of the viewing portion of the fiberscope involves the objective lens, image transmission bundle, and eyepiece. Since the distal tip is sealed to eliminate patient secretions and cleaning solutions from damaging the insertion cord contents or interfering with optical isolation between individual fibers of the viewing bundle, focusing by movement of the objective lens is not possible. Thus, the fiberscope is "fixed focus" at the distal tip. Light reflected off the object is focused by the objective lens onto the distal end of the image transmission bundle (object face). This image is then transmitted to the proximal end of the image transmission bundle to the face near the eyepiece (image face). Because the glass fibers in the image transmission bundle are placed so that each fiber is in the same relative location on the image face as the object face, the image seen will faithfully represent that object.

The depth of view field is the range of distances from the tip of the fiberscope within which objects can be located and appear with the same degree of clarity to the viewer. The exact range depends on the fiber size and the effective aperture of the objective lens; however, most fiberscopes have a depth of view field of 3–5 mm.

The field of view is the cone-shaped visual field given in degrees (°) afforded by the design of a particular fiberscope (Fig. 5). The field of view of the fiberscope is governed by the number of fibers and the amount of field allocated to each fiber. A wider field of view can be accomplished by increasing the number of fibers while maintaining detail, or by sacrificing detail with a smaller number of fibers and allocating more visual field per fiber. Most endoscopes have a field of view of 55–120°.

The upper limit of magnification is practically limited by the illumination of the field as well as the design and construction of the small optical system, which must be enclosed at the tip of the fiberscope (Figs. 6A–D).

Working Channel

This channel extends from the handle of the fiberscope to the tip of the insertion cord and can be used to suction secretions, inject drugs, insufflate oxygen, or pass various biopsy and brush instruments. The working channel is lined with plastic tubing to prevent liquids from entering the insertion cord, which would fog the field of vision by contaminating the light bundle.

Since the overall diameter of the fiberscope is dependent on the component parts, the size of the working channel is sacrificed for smaller diameter scopes to maintain reasonable image clarity. Scopes with outer diameters less than 2 mm do not have a working channel, and scopes with outer diameters less than 3.6 mm have working channels of 1.5 mm or less. For adequate suctioning of secretions, it is recommended that a working channel be at least 2 mm in diameter. The smaller channels may still be useful for insufflating ox-

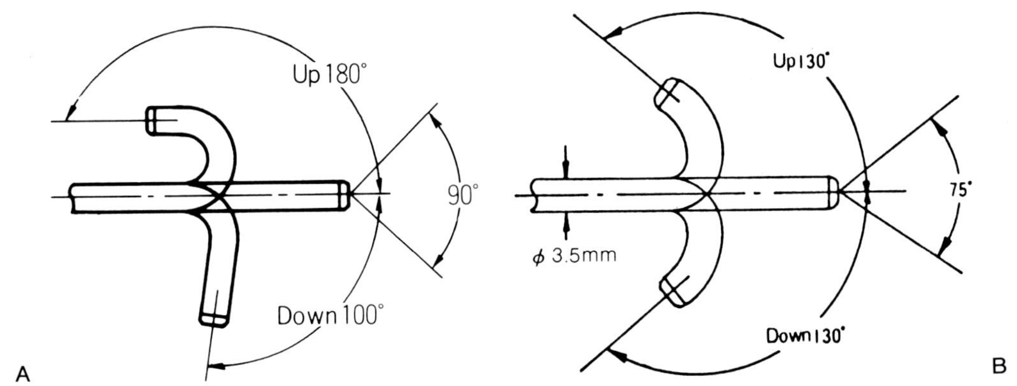

FIG. 5. A, B: Bending section of two fiberscopes with different degrees of up and down bending capability and different degrees of depth of field of view.

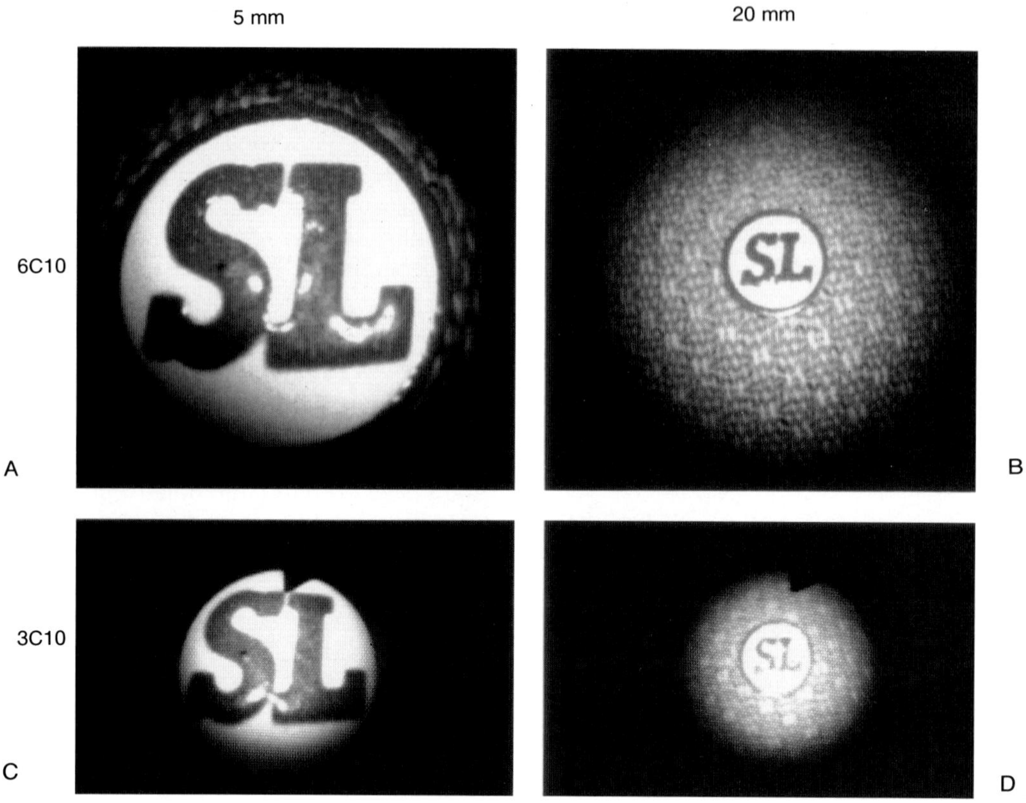

FIG. 6. A–D: Endoscopic view of letters from 5 and 20 mm distances as seen through two different fiberscopes: (**A, B**) Olympus 6C10 adult bronchofiberscope and (**C, D**) Olympus 3C10 pediatric bronchofiberscope. (Please refer to Tables 1 and 2 for comparison and characteristics of fiberscopes.)

ygen or injecting medications (such as local anesthetic).

Tip-Bending Lever

The bending of the distal section of the insertion tube is achieved by movement of the bending lever located at the handle. Two separate small wires travel from the bending lever to the tip of the fiberscope (Fig. 3). When the lever is moved downward, the wire that controls the anterior deflection of the tip is tightened, and the tip of the fiberscope bends upward or anteriorly. When the lever is moved upward, the tip of the fiberscope bends downward or posteriorly. Care should be exercised not to put excessive pressure on the lever when the tip of the fiberscope is against resistance. This will result in breakage of the delicate wires, with loss of bending control. With substantial usage, and especially with improper handling, loss of distal tip flexion is common.

Distal Tip

All fiberscopes are "frontal view" instruments, i.e., the objective lens is perpendicular to the longitudinal axis of the instrument. A drawing of two types of tips and bending sections is shown in Fig. 5.

Universal Cord

The universal cord contains the light guide fiber bundle and electrical wiring for the automatic photography exposure system. The universal cord ends at the light guide connector. The light guide connector contains the plug, air vent connector, and electrical contacts and is plugged into the light source prior to use of the fiberscope. The air vent connector accepts the ethylene oxide (ETO) sterilization venting cap and leakage tester (Fig. 4). When the ETO cap is installed, it provides venting of the fiberscope interior to equalize internal and external pressures. The ETO cap must be installed for ETO gas sterilization and aeration, otherwise the vacuum phase of sterilization will cause the rubber coating on the flexible tip to balloon and explode. The ETO cap should also be applied in the event of transportation. It must be removed prior to immersion of the fiberscope into water or disinfectant solutions, or when the fiberscope is in use.

TABLE 1. *Adult bronchofiberscopes*

	Insertion cord				
	Diameter (mm)	Length (mm)	Working channel (mm)	Tip deflection (degrees)	Field of view (degrees)
Olympus					
LF-2	4.0	600	1.5	up 120 down 120	90
BF-P30	5.0	550	2.2	up 180 down 130	120
BF-30	6.0	550	2.2	up 180 down 130	120
BF-1T30	6.0	550	2.8	up 180 down 130	120
BF-XT30D	6.1	550	3.2	up 180 down 130	120
BF-6C20	6.0	550	1.5	up 160 down 100	120
Pentax					
FB-15P	4.9	600	2.2	up 180 down 130	100
FB-18P	6.0	600	2.8	up 180 down 90	100
FB-19H2	6.3	550	2.0	up 160 down 100	100
FB-19H3	6.3	550	1.7	up 160 down 100	120

The depth of field is 3–50 mm with all models. The bending mechanism is lever type with all models. Universal cord (light guide cable) length is 5 ft in all models except Olympus LF-2, which is 7 ft.

COMPARISON OF AVAILABLE FIBERSCOPES

A common but important question that is often asked is which fiberscope is best for each application. Ideally, the endoscopist should make such a decision based on personal experience. However, to gain experience in a wide variety of clinical situations is difficult, except in teaching environments. It is also difficult to compare fiberscopes from different manufacturers, as institutions are usually reluctant to purchase several different expensive fiberscopes. Further, changes in instrument design are a continuous process, such that newer fiberscopes may incorporate new features or eliminate older, less practical designs.

Several excellent fiberscopes are currently available (Tables 1–4). These fiberscopes can be used for a variety of purposes, from upper airway examination and intubation of the trachea to diagnostic and therapeutic

TABLE 2. *Pediatric bronchofiberscopes/laryngoscopes*

	Insertion cord				
	Diameter (mm)	Length (mm)	Working channel (mm)	Tip deflection (degrees)	Field of view (degrees)
Olympus					
BF-3C30	3.6	550	1.2	up 180 down 130	120
LF-2	4.0	600	1.5	up 120 down 120	90
LF-P	2.2	600	0.0	up 120 down 120	75
Pentax					
FB-10X	3.5	600	1.2	up 180 down 130	95
FI-10P	3.5	600	1.2	up 130 down 130	90

The depth of field is 3–50 mm in all models. The bending mechanism is lever type in all models. Universal cord (light guide cable) length is 5 ft in all models except Olympus LF-2, which is 7 ft.

TABLE 3. *Rhino-Laryngofiberscopes*

	Insertion cord Diameter (mm)	Insertion cord Length (mm)	Working channel (mm)	Tip deflection (degrees)	Field of view (degrees)
Olympus					
ENF-P3	3.6	255	0	up 130 down 130	85
ENF-L3	4.3	365	0	up 130 down 130	85
ENF-T3[b]	5.0	365	2.2	up 130 down 130	85
Pentax					
FNL-10P2/10Rp2	3.5	300	0	up 130 down 130	75
FNL-13S/13H[a]/13RS	4.2	300(350 13H)	0	up 130 down 130	85
FNL-15P2/15RP2[b]	4.9	300	2.2	up 130 down 130	75

[a] Designed for still photography and video documentation with larger superior images.
[b] Therapeutic nasopharyngolaryngoscope with large suction channel.
The depth of field is 3–50 mm with all models. The bending mechanism is lever type with all models.
The light guide cable is 5 ft in all models.

bronchoscopy. These fiberscopes can be characterized by several important design criteria that are useful for comparison.

Diameter of Insertion Cord

The diameter of the insertion cord determines the size of the endotracheal tube or airway with which the fiberscope can be used. The inside diameter of the endotracheal tube should generally be 1 mm larger than the outside diameter of the insertion cord. Thus, a fiberscope of small diameter will be necessary for pediatric applications or for use in a double-lumen tube. A small fiberscope, however, has several disadvantages when it is used with larger tubes. These include reduced working channel size, small objective image, excessive flexibility (reducing its effectiveness as a "stylette"), and increased susceptibility to damage. Stiffer insertion cords will partially overcome the greater flexibility of the small fiberscopes; however, this stiffness obviously reduces the flexibility that is helpful during airway endoscopy and bronchoscopy. Very small fiberscopes (<2.7 mm) may not have guide

TABLE 4. *Videobronchofiberscopes*

	Insertion cord Diameter (mm)	Insertion cord Length (mm)	Working channel (mm)	Tip deflection (degrees)	Field of view (degrees)
Olympus Endoscopic Video Information System (EVIS 200 series)					
BF-P200	5.3	550	2.0	up 180 down 130	100
BF-1T200	6.0	550	2.6	up 180 down 130	100
BF-200	6.3	550	2.0	up 180 down 130	120
OCV-200: video converter					
Pentax Video Endoscopic System					
EB/VB-1910	6.8	600	1.2	up 180 down 130	120
EB/VB-2000	7.5	600	2.0	up 180 down 130	120
EB/VB-1530	5.5	600	1.2	up 180 down 130	120
EB/VB-1830	6.3	600	2.0	up 180 down 130	120
PVA-1010: video module used with bronchofiberscope and Pentax video processor to create color images.					

wires for easy scope manipulation. In some cases the manipulation may be done by a long guide wire with a gentle curve on the end. In some cases these wires can protrude beyond the scope tip and cause tracheal damage or perforation (6).

Length of Insertion Cord

The length of the insertion cord defines the usable length of the fiberscope. To allow for easy placement of double-lumen endobronchial tubes and nasotracheal intubation with the endotracheal tube fitted on the insertion cord, the length of the insertion cord should be greater than the length of the tube and the airway (optimally, 60 cm). The average length of the nasotracheal tubes used in adults is 28–30 cm. Considering that the distance from the nares to midtrachea is 22–25 cm, it means that the endotracheal tube must enter the nasal passage before the tip of a 55-cm fiberscope reaches the midtrachea. For orotracheal intubation in adults, a 55-cm insertion cord is needed for most circumstances.

The Size of the Working Channel

The presence and size of the working channel should be considered. Secretions and blood obscuring the view is a major cause of failure during fiberoptic intubation. The working channel can be used to suction these secretions during viewing and to assist exposure of the epiglottis and vocal cords. Small channels are inefficient for suctioning, can easily be clogged with secretions, and must be meticulously cleaned each time they are used. As discussed above, channels smaller than 2 mm may be used for insufflation of oxygen or injection of local anesthetics. In some cases oxygen sufflation may assist in removing secretions from the viewing tip.

If suctioning is required and the suction channel is of insufficient size, one clever technique is the use of a wire through the channel to hold a suction catheter along the outside of the fiberscope, the so-called bronchoscopic shuttle (7). Since the channel increases insertion cord diameter, some small-diameter fiberscopes have eliminated the channel to achieve a smaller overall diameter. With small channels, insufflation of oxygen or injection of fluids (e.g., sterile saline) may clean the viewing tip and therefore serve as an alternative to suctioning to improve the view.

The Field of View

The field-of-view angle defines the overall picture available to the viewer. A wide field of view will give a good perspective on the anatomy; however, this may sacrifice the resolution or image quality. Fortunately, most of the presently available fiberscopes combine a wide depth of field coupled with a reasonable field of view and image resolution. These qualities, as well as the durability and arrangement of the handle controls, are best evaluated individually.

The Bending Radius of the Distal Tip

The bending characteristics of the distal tip of the insertion cord should be evaluated. Sufficient bending must be available to allow maneuvering in the airway, especially in the presence of pathology or a compromised airway. In general, for intubation of the trachea, the upward flexibility is most important, since the most difficult angle of the airway is usually the upward bend from the posterior pharynx behind the epiglottis into the trachea. However, for evaluation of the bronchial tree and management of the airway in the presence of mass or tumor, both upward and downward bends become critical. Upward bending of 160° or more and downward bending of 120° or more are needed for successful airway management under different circumstances.

The Control Mechanisms of the Bending Tip

The control mechanism of the bending section of the insertion cord is important. The thumb control lever system, which is placed on the back section of the body of the fiberscope, is considered superior by many operators. The maneuverability of the instrument is greatly improved, and the fiberscope can be handled by either the left or right hand without difficulty (Figs. 4 and 7).

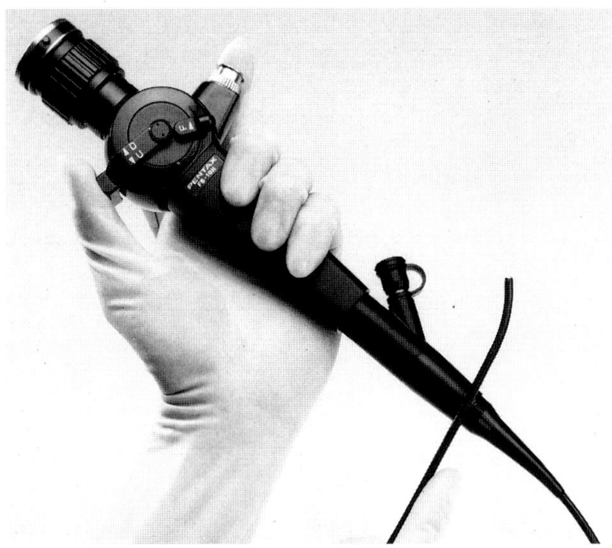

FIG. 7. Holding the fiberscope. (Courtesy of Pentax Precision Instrument Corp., Orangeburg, New York 10963-2699.)

Other factors that should also be considered when purchasing a fiberscope are the need for taking pictures, the use of video systems, and the compatibility with existing fiberscopes and light sources. Extremely important are the quality and speed of service provided by the manufacturer. Even with careful handling, fiberscopes will eventually need repair and servicing. A convenient service provided by the company is the loan of an instrument while repairs are being conducted.

VIDEOBRONCHOSCOPES

Both Olympus and Pentax videobronchoscopes utilize the single-plate red, green, and blue (RGB) surface-scanning method and a newly developed charge coupled device (CCD) (camera chip). The triple color coding function is carried out sequentially by a single picture element housed within the CCD. This is an advanced electronic signal processing system. The image-transmitting fiber bundle (coherent bundle) of regular bronchofiberscope is omitted, and, alternatively, a small CCD image sensor is positioned behind the objective lens at distal end of the videobronchoscope insertion cord. The digitalized signal of the videobronchoscope provides the opportunity to capture and transmit images electronically. The electronic signals provide a clearer image on the monitor than that produced by a conventional bronchofiberscope.

The use of an ultra compact CCD allows the fiberscope's working channel and light guide fibers to be incorporated within the housing of an insertion cord less than 6 mm in diameter.

The light colors red, green, and blue are transmitted sequentially from the light source to the object. The resultant images illuminated by these colors are received in sequence by the CCD, which transmits multiple black-and-white images in the same sequence to the computerized image processor, and are stored in

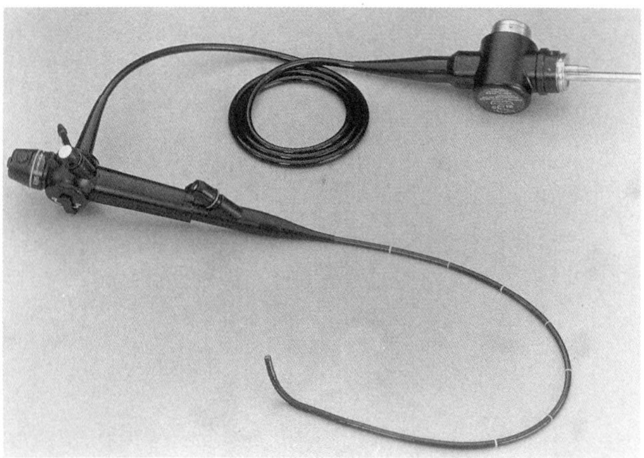

FIG. 8. Olympus videobronchoscope BF-P200.

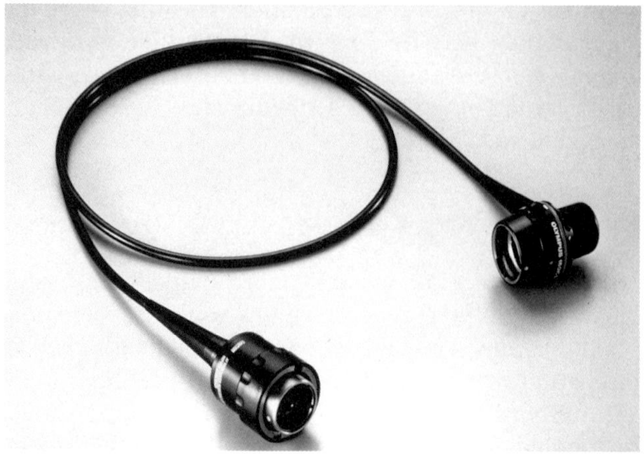

FIG. 9. The Olympus OCV-200 Video Converter is used to connect regular bronchofiberscopes to the videosystem. One end of the video converter is connected to the scope, the other end is connected to the CV-200 system.

the memory. All three color signals are then transmitted simultaneously from the memory to the monitor to be reproduced.

The Olympus videobronchoscope is lightweight and easy to handle. It has the widest-angle optical system possible for bronchoscopes with a small insertion cord. The videobronchoscope has four fingertip-controlled remote switches. These switches activate the Release, Freeze, Iris, Zoom, and video tape recorder functions without interrupting the procedure.

The Olympus P3 bronchofiberscopes and videobronchoscopes have disposable suction valves and connectors to reduce the risk of cross-contamination (Fig. 8). The biopsy port is located at the base of the handle section of the fiberscope. A disposable cap is provided for the biopsy port for easy cleaning.

If the water-resistant cap is attached, the entire instrument is fully immersible, which simplifies the process of cleaning and disinfecting the instrument.

Figure 9 illustrates the video converter used to connect regular bronchofiberscopes to the video system.

ACCESSORY INSTRUMENTS

A variety of accessories and attachments are available for the fiberscope. Some of these accessories are an integral part of the fiberscope necessary for viewing, cleaning, or testing. Most of the remaining attachments are used either for teaching or for photography.

Light Sources

The ability to distinguish the object depends on adequate illumination; thus, the light source is an integral

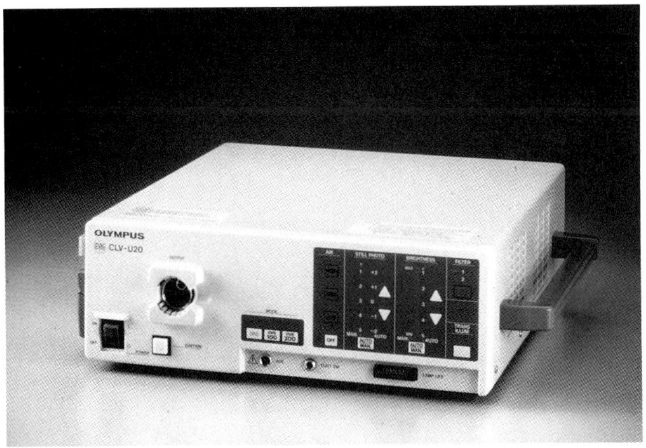

FIG. 10. Olympus CLV-U20 universal light source. A xenon light source compatible with both videobronchoscopes and bronchofiberscopes. Uses a 300 W xenon semiflash system. The light intensity for still photography increases to 1.5 times the viewing illumination, producing sharp and bright images. (Courtesy of Olympus Corporation, Medical Instrument Division, Lake Success, New York 11042.)

part of the fiberoptic endoscope system. Various light sources are available, which provide adequate illumination not only for viewing but also for taking pictures or videotapes (Fig. 10). An intense light is generated and is focused on the proximal end of the light guide cable by a source lens or a spherical reflecting mirror. A heat filter or reflecting mirror is used to reduce the amount of heat focused on the light guide cable. The powerful light source needed for videotaping is more expensive, but it will provide adequate light for viewing when the fiberscope has sustained damage and part of the light-carrying fibers are broken. It is important to note that proper attachment of the universal cord to the light source is made. Should the cord be inserted too close to the light source (such as by using an improper adapter or connector), the heat can melt the glass fibers or damage the cord coating.

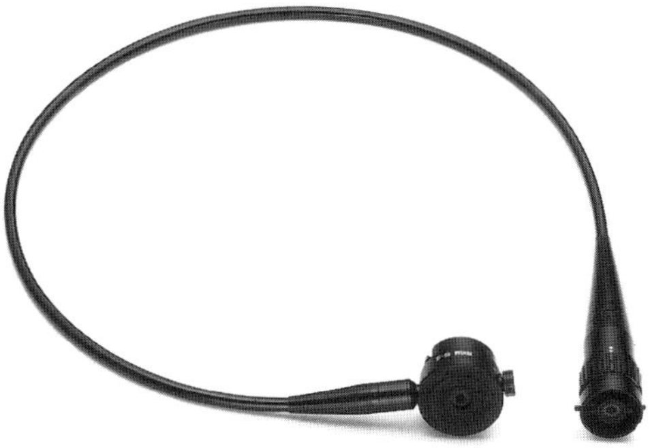

FIG. 11. Pentax teaching attachment, model FO-T2, allows assistant to take pictures. The camera is attached to the teaching attachment eyepiece. The brightness control knob is turned on to increase the ratio of the light passing through the eyepiece. (Courtesy of Pentax Precision Instrument Corp., Orangeburg, New York 10963-2699.)

Teaching Attachments

Teaching attachments are available that allow a second viewer to observe as the endoscopist carries out the procedure. They are attached to the eyepiece of the fiberscope and provide an invaluable teaching aid. The teaching attachment allows splitting of the beam, so that an observer has the same view as the endoscopist. This is usually done by a beam-splitting mirror or prism. Generally, the endoscopist receives 35% of the original light, the observer 35%, and 30% is lost by the inefficiency of the beam-splitting process. In addition, image degradation occurs due to diffusion via the finite size of the teaching attachment bundles. This usually results in a 30% reduction in resolution seen by the observer. Newer designs of the teaching attachment (Fig. 11) have a greater number of fibers, so that the image is clear and sharp, even through the assistant's eyepiece. The photographic camera can be attached to

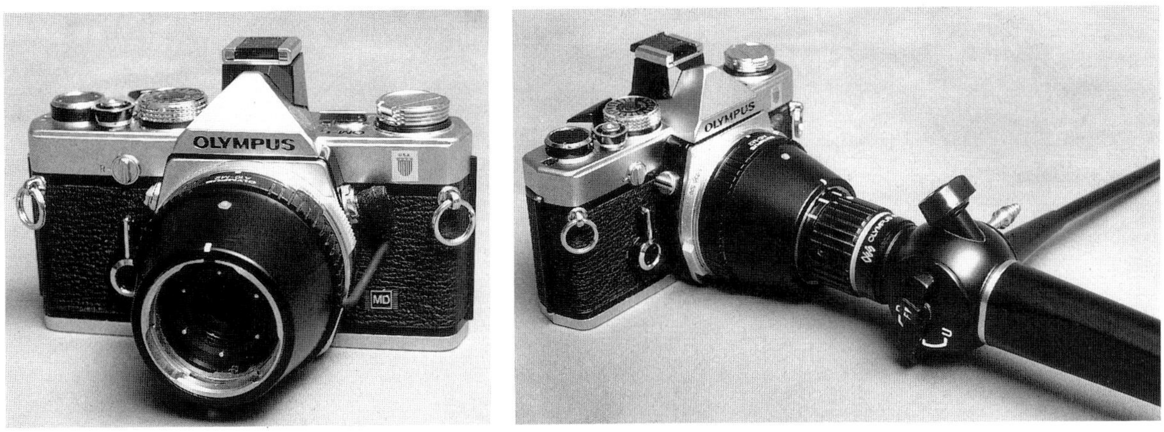

A B

FIG. 12. A: Olympus OM-IN 35-mm camera mounted with a special adapter for still endoscopic photography. **B:** Olympus camera mounted on bronchofiberscope.

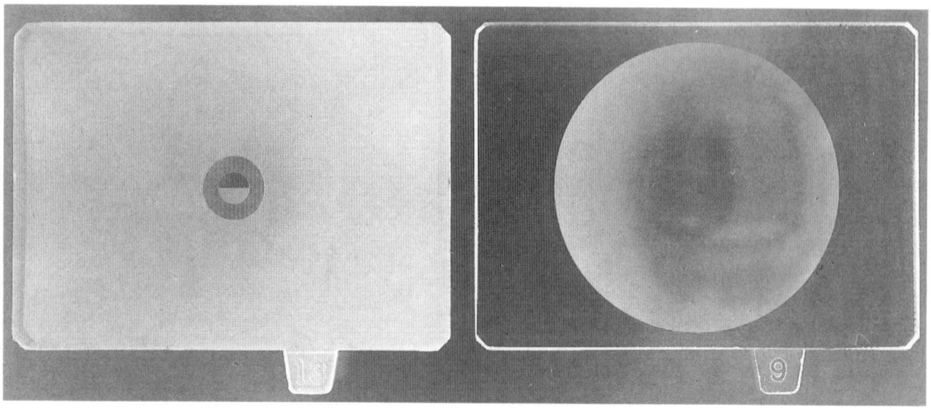

FIG. 13. **Left:** Regular focusing screen. **Right:** 1–9 endoscopic focusing screen.

the assistant's eyepiece, and photographs can be taken by the assistant simply by turning the brightness control knob to change the brightness ratio from 6:4 to 1:9 (primary observer:assistant).

Photography Instruments

Still-camera photography, cine photography, or television recording can be accomplished through fiberscopes both for documentation purposes and for demonstration and teaching.

For taking color slides, a light source with flash capability is needed. Basically, light sources produce either halogen flash light or xenon flash light. Halogen sources are useful for Kodak ISO (ASA) 160 tungsten-type film and xenon sources for Kodak ISO (ASA) 200 (Ektachrome) daylight-type film.

To make color slides through a fiberscope, specially designed, fully automatic compact endoscopic cameras or a regular 35-mm photographic camera can be used (Fig. 12). The Pentax MF 35-mm camera with automatic exposure control should be used with Pentax fiberscopes. For Olympus fiberscopes, an Olympus OM-IN regular 35-mm photographic camera can be used with some modification. First, the existing focusing screen in the camera viewfinder is replaced with a 1–9 endoscopic focusing screen (Fig. 13). Second, the camera lens is removed and is replaced by a special adapter, which makes it possible to mount the camera on the fiberscope (Fig. 14). Before taking a picture, the photo diopter setting and visual diopter setting (white dots) must be aligned. The diopter adjusting ring should be rotated counterclockwise on the eyepiece to align the white dots. This will automatically correct the diopter to the diopter position and ensure optimal focus for picture taking. Once the camera is attached to the fiberscope, no attempts should be made to focus the image to the user's eye using the diopter adjustment, as this will result in improperly focused photographs. After completion of picture taking, the camera is removed and the diopter adjusting ring is rotated clockwise to adjust to the individual user's eyesight for direct vision. The syncro-cord plug of the adapter is plugged into the camera X/FP terminal. The shutter speed is set at ¼ sec ("4"). The syncro-switch is set at "X" for xenon light and at "FP" for halogen flash light. For bigger, brighter pictures, a xenon light source should be used with an A10-M2 Olympus adapter. Dur-

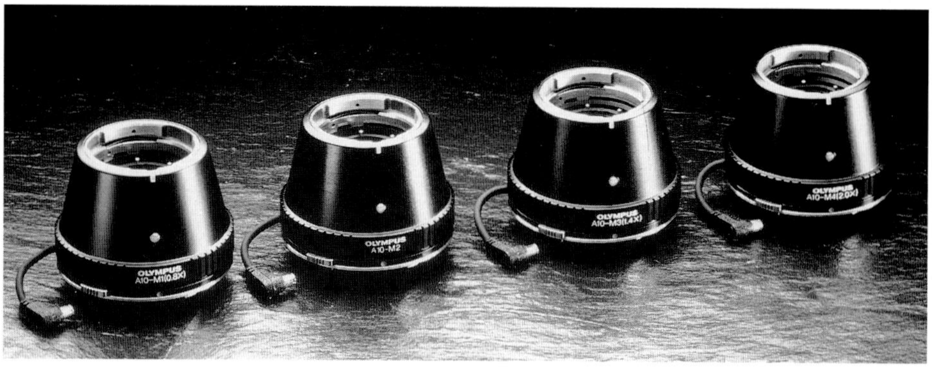

FIG. 14. A wide selection of OES (Olympus endoscopy system) adapters allows choice of optimum image size. With halogen light, adapter A10-M1 is recommended; with xenon light, adapter A10-M2 is recommended. For larger images, adapters A10-M3 and A10-M4 may be used.

ing endoscopy, the operator's view through the camera is the same as that through the fiberscope. When a picture is taken, the automatic flash system is activated to deliver the light necessary for proper exposure of the film. The flash is not observed by the endoscopist when he is looking through the fiberscope. However, with each flash, the light source "clicks" when the flash system is activated. If the clicks are not heard, all electrical contacts in the fiberscope eyepiece, camera, and light guide connector should be examined and cleaned. Undesirable blurs on the picture can be avoided by using a method known as pushing. This is accomplished by setting the ISO of the camera at twice the ISO of the film. However, once set, the entire roll must be exposed at the "pushed" setting, and the developer must be informed prior to development that the film was pushed. Various photographic and videotaping cameras are available for use with fiberscopes from different manufacturers. For further information on the proper selection of photographic adapters, the different light sources, and the proper use of cameras, the reader should refer to companies' instruction books.

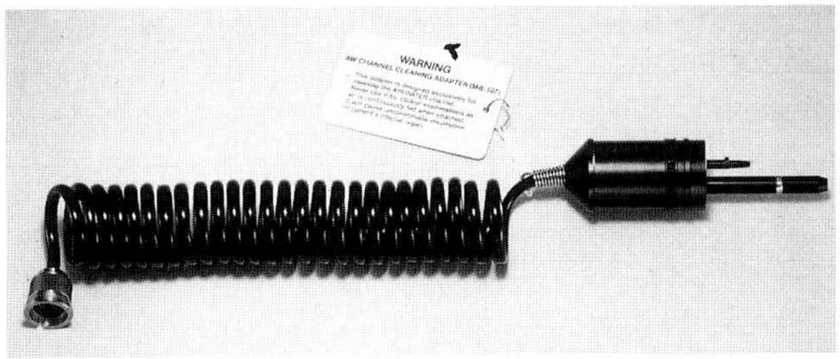

FIG. 15. Air leak tester. The cap is attached to the fiberscope venting connector. The adapter is attached to the light source. The air pumped by the light source pressurizes the fiberscope. Any air leak from the fiberscope indicates that the waterproof system is damaged and needs to be repaired before it can be soaked in solution. (Courtesy of Olympus Corp., Medical Instrument Division, Lake Success, New York 11042.)

Forceps and Brushes

Different size brushes are available, as well as a variety of forceps for tissue biopsy and removal of foreign bodies. Anesthesiologists are rarely faced with situations requiring accessories other than the cleaning brush. When inserting these devices it is important to use caution so that they do not damage the plastic lining of the working channel.

CLEANING AND STERILIZATION

After each use, the fiberscope should be cleaned and disinfected to prevent damage to the fiberscope by dried secretions and transmission of disease. Specific recommendations for sterilization or disinfection made by the manufacturer and by each health care facility should be followed. As a general rule, the insertion cord of all fiberscopes is immersible. However, the handle and the universal cord of some instruments may be damaged by immersion in solutions, although most modern fiberscopes are designed to withstand complete immersion in disinfected solutions.

The fiberscope should be washed immediately after use, and the working channel should be flushed with water to remove secretions before they dry. Prior to soaking in disinfecting solution, all portions of the fiberscope to be immersed should be inspected for defects that might allow liquids to enter into the sealed portions. The rubber covering of the distal portion of the insertion cord should be carefully examined, as frequent use of the fiberscope may cause tears and defects in this covering. Although the integrity of the plastic lining of the working channel cannot be checked, unexplained fogging of the images or suspected damage to the channel from using guide wires may prompt evaluation of its integrity prior to immersion. Totally immersible fiberscopes should be tested for leaks using a leakage tester and pressurized air prior to immersion in the solution (Fig. 15). Since solutions will cause extensive damage to the optical system, the fiberscope should promptly be sent to the manufacturer for appropriate repair when defects are identified.

After inspection, the suction port assembly should be removed, and the immersible portions of the fiberscope should be soaked in disinfectant solution. Solutions recommended vary with individual manufacturers and include 0.5% povidone-iodine; 2% glutaraldehyde; mild, nonabrasive soap solutions; and 0.016% iodophor. Recommended immersion times after use in noninfected patients vary from 10 min for glutaraldehyde, to 20 min for the iodine-containing solutions, to 30 min for the soap solutions. Each solution is potentially caustic to the materials in the fiberscope; thus, the manufacturers' recommendations for disinfectant concentration and maximum soaking time should be carefully observed. Prolonged contact with disinfectant solutions can cause premature aging of the coating due to chemical reactions. When povidone-iodine (Betadine) is used, the viewing tip should be gently wiped with nonabrasive cloth to prevent permanent yellowish discoloration of the viewing lens (9).

The working channel should be filled with disinfectant solution using a syringe. The use of a cleaning brush may be needed for removal of secretions from the working channel. The brush should only be inserted at the handle end to avoid kinking of the brush in the fiberscope and subsequent difficulty removing it. Finally, the fiberscope should be washed and the working channel suctioned with water to remove all traces of the disinfectant solution. The portions of the fiberscope that cannot be immersed are wiped with a cloth containing 70% alcohol; however, the contact time with the alcohol should be limited, as it can destroy the rubber coating on the fiberscope.

If the patient has tuberculosis or other transmissible illness, the entire fiberscope should be sterilized. Fiberscope sterilization is also important prior to use on patients with immune deficiencies. The fiberscope should not be autoclaved or placed in boiling water, but complete sterilization can be accomplished by ethylene oxide gas sterilization. Generally, maximally tolerated conditions for ETO sterilization include: temperature of 55°C, pressure of 24 PSI, time of 4 hr, humidity of 50% and gas concentration of 10% (10).

Manufacturers' recommendations should be followed so that damage does not occur. The ethylene oxide cap must be securely attached to the venting connector on the light guide connector and must remain in place throughout the sterilization and aeration process. This is necessary to avoid pressure buildup inside the fiberscope during gas sterilization. This cap must be removed prior to immersion and clinical examination. It is important to recognize that the gas sterilization procedure is lengthy, and it may take as long as 24 hr before the fiberscope is ready for use.

In order to reduce contamination from *Mycobacterium tuberculosis,* one author recommends cleaning prior to disinfection when the fiberscopes are heavily contaminated by patients (11). The cleaning process involves neutral detergents with particular attention to the working channel. The authors stress the need for freshly activated glutaraldehyde disinfectant since older, weaker (diluted by use) glutaraldehyde may be ineffective (12). Studies of contamination of fiberscopes suggest that *Mycobacterium chilonae* can occur from tap water (12). After cleaning, the fiberscope should be dried thoroughly and stored for subsequent use. The ideal container allows the insertion cord to remain straight. Carrying cases or small sterilization trays, in which the insertion cord is bent, are less desirable for storage, as the bending stresses the insertion cord and will ultimately damage fibers; carrying cases should only be used for shipping. The storage location must be clean, dry, well-ventilated, and maintained at room temperature. Direct sunlight, high temperature, high humidity, and X-ray exposure may cause fiberscope damage.

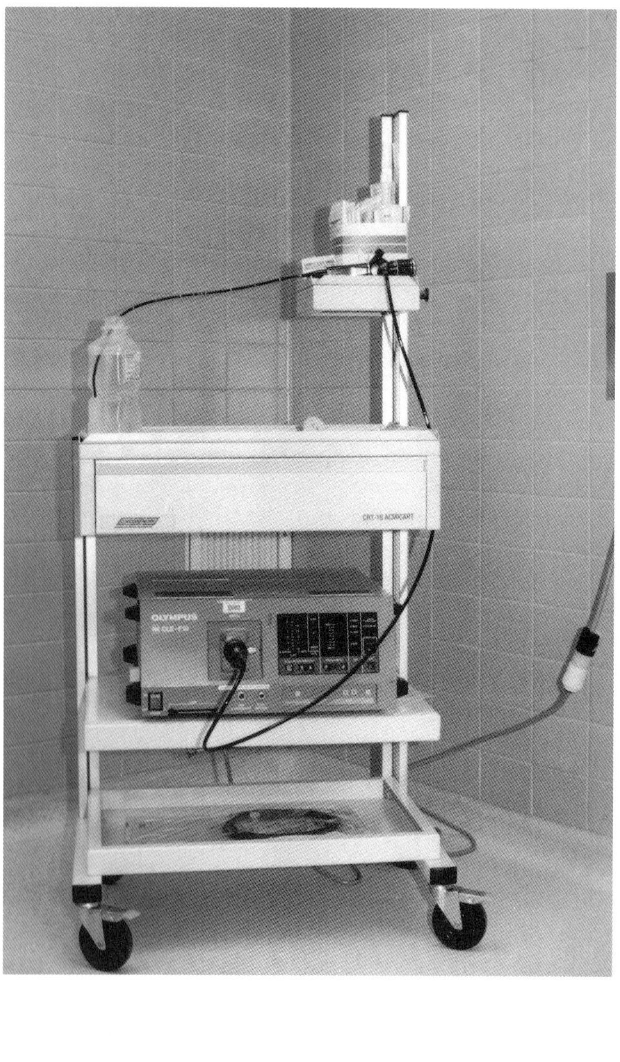

A

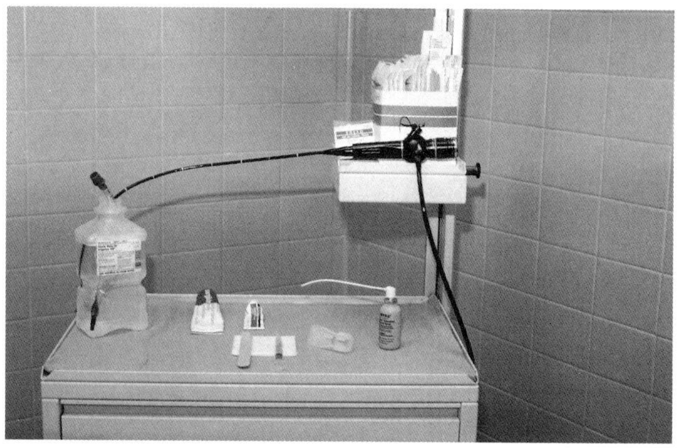

B

FIG. 16. A: One example of a simple fiberoptic cart arrangement. The top surface of the cart is cleaned with disinfectant solution after each use and is covered with a clean towel. The fiberscope is placed on the top of the cart and is covered with clean towels ready for next use. Special carts are available at much higher cost. **B:** Closer view of the top of the cart prepared for awake tracheal intubation.

THE FIBEROPTIC CART

The immediate availability of a fiberscope, light source, ancillary equipment, and routinely used supplies is critical for effective application of the fiberscope in airway management. A properly equipped fiberoptic cart with large wheels is ideal. The cart can be moved to the operating room or to the bedside at short notice to allow convenient access to all the accessories used for airway endoscopy and intubation (Fig. 16).

SUGGESTIONS FOR FIBERSCOPE USAGE

A variety of do's and don'ts have been suggested to improve the usage, avoid the complications, and increase the life expectancy of the flexible fiberscope (2–5). The following is an expanded list of do's and don'ts, which, if carefully applied, will avoid unnecessary and untimely instrument damage.

Do's

1. Do clean, prepare, and check all the necessary equipment and supplies before each use to be certain they function satisfactorily.
2. Do adjust the brightness of the light to a comfortable but minimum effective level to avoid thermal mucosal injury as well as to protect the user's eye.
3. Do lubricate the insertion cord with a sterile water-soluble lubricant (petroleum lubricants may damage the rubber coating).
4. Do adjust the tip of insertion cord to the neutral position before insertion into the endotracheal tube and before withdrawal from the tube.
5. Do advance the fiberscope gently and small distances at a time.
6. Do operate the tip-bending lever gently.
7. Do clean the fiberscope and the suction channel immediately after each use (particularly to prevent dried secretions in the channel).
8. Do dry the fiberscope thoroughly, including all lenses and electrical contacts, prior to storing.
9. Do store the fiberscope with the insertion cord as straight as possible.
10. Do use the correct light source adapter to prevent damage to the universal cord fibers.
11. Do follow hospital and manufacturers' recommendations for cleaning and disinfecting.
12. Do use a bite block to protect the fiberscope if intubating orally on an awake patient.
13. Do send a fiberscope for repair if damage to the outer coating is recognized. Using this scope before repair risks expensive damage to the optical fibers.
14. Do bend the scope with gentle angles. Sharp angulation of the insertion cord can damage the optical fibers.

Don'ts

1. Do not drop the fiberscope or bang the tip against a hard object, as it may break and be extensively damaged.
2. Do not sharply bend the insertion cord, as this will break the delicate glass fibers.
3. Do not strike the distal end of the insertion cord on a hard surface, as this may crack the objective lens.
4. Do not squeeze or bend the distal bending section by hand, as this will damage the bending mechanism.
5. Do not tort or twist the insertion cord by hand, as this will change the shape and damage the cord. (Rotate the handle by bending the wrist of the hand holding the handle).
6. Do not leave the fiberscope plugged into the light source with the lamp on when not in use. This will increase the risk of thermal injury and will reduce the life of the light bulb.
7. Do not scratch the electrical contacts with sharp tools. This will cause damage and improper contact.
8. Do not spill liquids on the head of the fiberscope (nonimmersible), light source, or photographic and videotaping systems, for this may cause equipment damage and electrical hazards.
9. Do not use abrasive cleaners on lens surfaces, for surfaces may be scratched.
10. Do not withdraw the fiberscope with the angle lock lever in the "engaged" position or while the distal tip is bent. This will cause extensive damage to the bending section and bending control wires and may cause trauma to the airway.
11. Do not twist the fiberscope with force when the tip is in a narrow orifice or tube. This will damage the insertion cord and may cause tissue damage.
12. Do not apply force when bending the tip of the fiberscope, as rupture of the bending wires and loss of bending of the tip may occur.
13. Do not expose the fiberscope to direct sunlight, dust, high humidity, and high temperature, so as to prevent instrument damage.
14. Do not store the fiberscope in the carrying case. It is airtight and may predispose to organism growth and contamination.
15. Do not expose the fiberscope to excessive X-ray radiation. This will result in a yellow discoloration and darkening of the glass fibers.
16. Do not try to introduce the fiberscope with force in any case.
17. Do not immerse a fiberscope with a venting cap on, or gas sterilize a fiberscope without a venting cap on, if the fiberscope has such a cap.

18. Do not exceed 1 hr of immersion for cold sterilization.

REFERENCES

1. Hopkins HH. The physics of the fiberoptic endoscope. In: Berci G, ed. *Endoscopy*. New York: Appleton-Century-Crofts, 1976; 27–63.
2. Ikeda S. *Atlas of flexible bronchofiberscopy*. Baltimore and London: University Park Press, 1974.
3. Ono R. *Bronchoscopy. Practical methods and case reports by videobronchoscopy*. Tokyo: Nakayama-Shoten, 1994.
4. Prakash UBS. *Bronchoscopy*. New York: Raven Press, 1994.
5. Stradling P. *Diagnostic bronchoscopy*. 4th ed. Edinburgh: Churchill-Livingstone, 1981.
6. Finkelhor BK, Healy GB. Disposable flexible fiberoptic mini-bronchoscope for evaluating the pediatric airway. *Otolaryngology Head and Neck Surgery* 1989;101:511–512.
7. Haruno MM, Williams JH Jr. The flexible fiberoptic bronchoscopic shuttle. *Chest* 1992;102:944–945.
8. Riff EJ, Mitra S, Baker MC. Pediatric fiberoptic video bronchoscopy: the use of computer interfacing. *Comput Biol Med* 1993; 23:345–347.
9. Mehta AC, Curtis PS, Scalzitti ML, Meeker DP. The high price of bronchoscopy—maintenance and repair of the flexible fiberoptic bronchoscope. *Chest* 1990;98:448–454.
10. Elford B. Care and cleansing of the fiberoptic bronchoscope. *Chest* 1978;3:62–68.
11. Hanson PJV, Chadwick MV, Gaya H, Collins JV. A study of glutaraldehyde disinfection of fibreoptic bronchoscopes experimentally contaminated with Myobacterium tuberculosis. *J Hosp Infection* 1992;22:137–142.
12. Fraser VJ, Jones M, Murray PR, Medoff G, Zhang Y, Wallace Jr RJ. Contamination of flexible fiberoptic bronchoscopes with myobacterium chelonae linked to an automated bronchoscope disinfection machine. *Am Rev Respir Dis* 1992;145:853–855.

CHAPTER 2

Anatomy of the Airway

Andranik Ovassapian, M.D.

For the safe management of the airway and conduct of tracheal and bronchial intubation, a basic knowledge of airway anatomy is essential. The purpose of this chapter is to present briefly the anatomic factors that are important for airway management.

THE MOUTH

The mouth extends from the lips anteriorly to the palatoglossal folds posteriorly. The anterior two-thirds of the tongue forms the floor of the mouth, and the hard and soft palates constitute its roof. Important anatomic structures for the endoscopist are: teeth, tongue, uvula, and soft palate. The shape and status of the patient's dentition are important factors to be considered during rigid laryngoscopy. The tongue is the largest organ in the mouth, is composed of intrinsic and extrinsic muscles, and fills most of the oral cavity. Because of its size, mobility, and attachments to the mandible, hyoid bone, and epiglottis, the tongue plays a major role in maintaining an open airway. The extrinsic muscles of the tongue originate from structures above and below it and insert into it (Table 1). Contraction of the extrinsic muscles of the tongue is important during deglutition, swallowing, and speech, as well as for maintenance of an open airway. The mucous membrane of the tongue connects the tongue laterally to the pharyngeal wall and posteriorly to the epiglottis through the glossoepiglottic folds.

THE NOSE

The nose extends from its external openings (external nares or nostrils), through the nasal cavity and its posterior openings (choanae), into the nasopharynx. The hard palate constitutes the floor of the nose and separates the nasal cavity from the mouth. The nasal cavity is divided into two chambers by the nasal septum, which constitutes their medial wall. The lateral wall has three bony projections called turbinates or conchae. The inferior turbinate is the longest and broadest; the superior turbinate is the smallest. The area below each turbinate is called a meatus, into which the paranasal sinuses open. A single paranasal sinus opening exists in each of the superior and inferior meati; the middle meatus receives all other paranasal sinus openings.

The sensory nerve supply of the nasal mucosa is from the first (ophthalmic) and second (maxillary) divisions of the trigeminal nerve (Fig. 1). The sympathetic innervation is from the superior cervical ganglion. Any increase in sympathetic activity will result in vascular spasm and shrinkage of the mucous membrane. General anesthesia depresses nervous system activity, including sympathetic activity, therefore causing vasodilatation and engorgement of the mucous membrane. This increases the incidence of nasal bleeding during nasotracheal intubation. In our series, nasotracheal intubation of conscious patients has caused less bleeding when compared with nasotracheal intubation performed under general anesthesia. This may be attrib-

TABLE 1. *Extrinsic muscles of the tongue*

Muscle	Origin	Insertion	Innervation	Action
Genioglossus	Superior genial tubercle of mandible	Inferior aspect of tongue and body of hyoid bone		Depresses tongue; posterior part protrudes tongue
Hyoglossus	Greater horn and body of hyoid bone	Side and inferior aspect of tongue	Hypoglossal nerve	Retracts tongue
Styloglossus	Styloid process	Side and inferior aspect of tongue		Retracts tongue
Palatoglossus	Palatine aponeurosis	Side of tongue	Pharyngeal plexus (11th cranial nerve)	Approximates palatoglossal folds

From O'Rahilly R. *Basic human anatomy*. Philadelphia: W.B. Saunders, 1983.

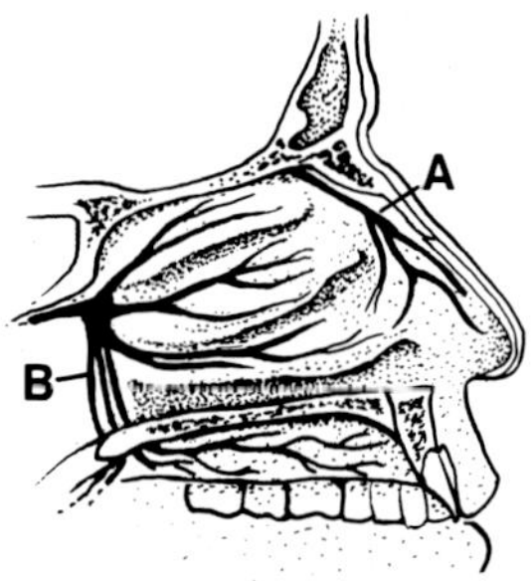

FIG. 1. Diagram of the lateral wall of the nasal cavity illustrating its sensory nerve supply. Anterior ethmoidal nerve, a branch of the ophthalmic division of the trigeminal nerve, supplies the anterior third of both the septum and the lateral wall (**A**). The maxillary division of the trigeminal nerve via the sphenopalatine ganglion supplies the posterior two-thirds of the septum and the lateral wall (**B**).

uted to the higher sympathetic tone and vasospasm of the vessels of the nasal mucosa in the conscious patient, as well as the gentle manner in which the endotracheal tube is advanced through the nose. The blood supply to the nasal mucosa is generous and is provided by the sphenopalatine artery, a branch of the maxillary artery, and the septal branch of the facial artery. Those two arteries anastomose with each other, forming Kisselbach's network at the anterior medial wall of the nose, which is a common site of nasal bleeding. Application of cocaine and vasoconstrictors is helpful in shrinking the mucous membrane, increasing the diameter of nasal passages, and decreasing the incidence of bleeding.

The nasotracheal tube should be passed directly backward along the floor of the nose and beneath the inferior turbinate. The adult male will accept 7- to 8-mm internal diameter (ID) and the adult female 6.5- to 7.5-mm ID nasotracheal tubes. The nasal passages may become blocked from swelling of the mucous membrane, deformity of the septum, hypertrophy of the turbinates, or polyps occupying the nasal cavities.

THE PHARYNX

The pharynx is 12–15 cm long and extends from the base of the skull to the level of the cricoid cartilage, where it becomes continuous with the esophagus. The pharyngeal muscles include the superior, middle, and inferior constrictors. During swallowing, these muscles contract and push the bolus of food downward. The lower part of the inferior constrictor muscle originates from the cricoid cartilage and is called cricopharyngeous muscle. This acts as a sphincter at the entrance of the esophagus. The cricopharyngeous muscle is considered the last barrier to regurgitation of gastric contents; however, with the onset of unconsciousness, the muscle loses its tone, and any fluid in the esophagus may enter the oropharynx, increasing the chance of aspiration. The pharynx communicates anteriorly with the nasal cavity (nasopharynx), the oral cavity (oropharynx), and the larynx (hypopharynx or laryngopharynx) (Fig. 2) (1).

Nasopharynx

The nasopharynx is bounded superiorly by the base of the skull, inferiorly by the soft palate, posteriorly by the body of the 1st cervical vertebra, and anteriorly by the nasal choanae and nasal septum. The opening of the eustachian tube lies in the lateral wall of the nasopharynx below the inferior turbinate. The normal soft tissue prominence surrounding the entrance of the eustachian tube is called the torus tubarius. Lateral to the torus tubarius is the fossa of Rosenmüller or pharyngeal recess. The adenoids or nasopharyngeal tonsils lie in the mucous membrane of the posterior wall of the nasopharynx. The enlarged adenoids can cause partial airway obstruction and prevent passage of a nasotracheal tube. The tip of a nasotracheal tube may also enter the pharyngeal recess, and, if force is used to advance it, the tube may penetrate the mucosa and create a false passage.

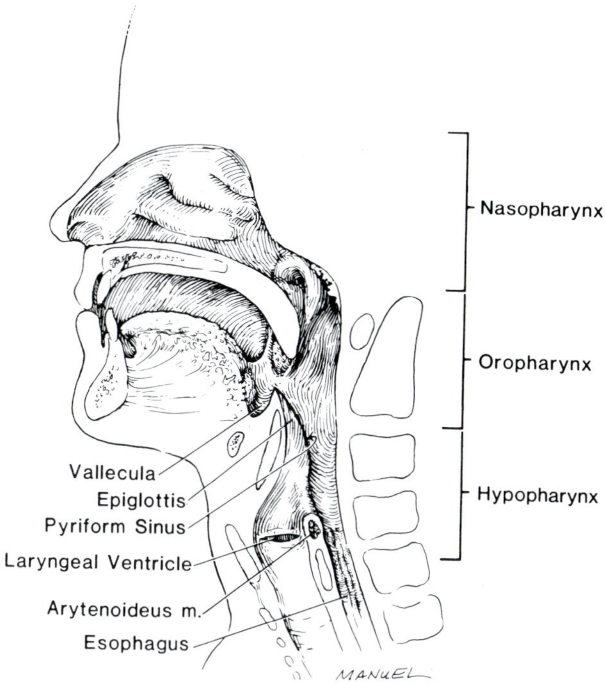

FIG. 2. Diagram of sagittal section of the pharynx to illustrate the subdivisions of the pharynx. (From ref. 1.)

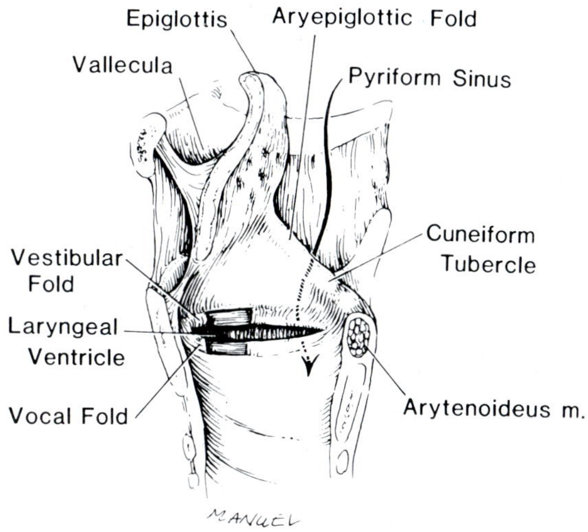

FIG. 3. Sagittal aspect of the laryngeal anatomy to illustrate the pyriform sinus and laryngeal ventricle. (From ref. 1.)

Oropharynx

The oropharynx is bounded superiorly by the soft palate, anteriorly by the posterior third of the tongue, inferiorly by the epiglottis, and posteriorly by the bodies of the 2nd and 3rd cervical vertebrae. On the lateral wall of the oropharynx is the tonsillar fossa with its anterior (palatoglossal) and posterior (palatopharyngeal) folds. The oropharyngeal walls are not rigid and are subject to collapse if negative transmural pressure develops. During regular inspiratory efforts, the negative transmural pressure in the oropharynx is minimal and does not cause collapse of the walls and airway obstruction. However, in the presence of partial airway obstruction and increased inspiratory efforts, the negative transmural pressure increases and may cause collapse of the soft tissues to exaggerate or cause a complete airway obstruction (2).

During the involuntary phase of swallowing, the pharyngeal wall muscles contract and push the food downward into the esophagus. Meanwhile, the soft palate moves up to prevent food from entering the nasopharynx, and the larynx is moved up to the base of the tongue and is sealed off by the epiglottis to prevent food from entering the larynx.

Hypopharynx

The hypopharynx lies at the level of the 4th to the 6th cervical vertebrae, between the superior border of the epiglottis and the inferior border of the cricoid cartilage. The pyriform fossae or sinuses constitute the lowest part of the hypopharynx and lie lateral to the larynx (Figs. 3 and 4).

The sensory innervation of the mucous membrane of the nasopharynx is the maxillary nerve, and that of the oropharynx is the glossopharyngeal nerve. The mucous membrane near the entrance of the larynx is innervated by the internal laryngeal branch of the vagus nerve.

THE LARYNX

In the adult male, the larynx is about 5–7 cm in length and lies opposite the 4th, 5th, and 6th cervical

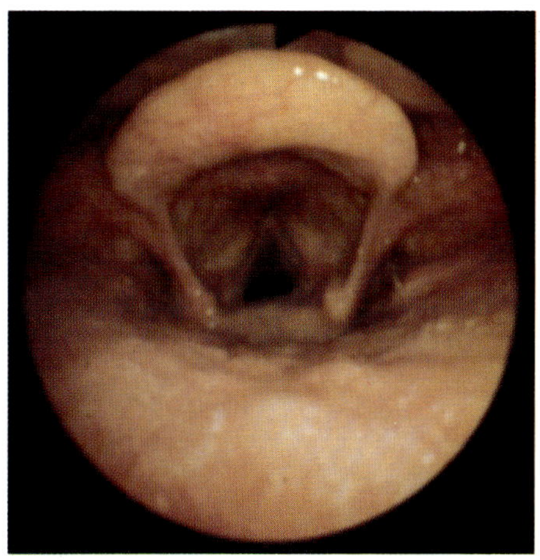

FIG. 4. Endoscopic view of the larynx. Pyriform sinuses represented by deepest part of the hypopharynx lateral to aryepiglottic folds bilaterally.

vertebrae. The larynx is shorter in women and children and is situated higher in the neck. The larynx is composed of cartilages, ligaments, and muscles.

Cartilages

The cartilages of the larynx include three single: thyroid, cricoid, and epiglottic; and three paired: arytenoid, corniculate, and cuneiform (Figs. 5 and 6). The thyroid cartilage is shield-shaped and is the largest. It has two laminae, 3 cm long, which are fused anteriorly to form the laryngeal prominence. The free posterior borders project into superior and inferior horns.

The cricoid cartilage is shaped like a signet ring; its narrow arch in front measures 5–7 mm in height, while the higher posterior segment, the lamina, measures 20–30 mm. The inferior margin of the cricoid cartilage, which is at the level of the 6th cervical vertebra, represents the inferior border of the larynx. The complete ring of the cricoid cartilage is about 15 mm below the true vocal cords, and it can occlude the esophagus when compressed posteriorly against the vertebral bodies.

The two arytenoid cartilages are pyramid-shaped and articulate with the superior aspect of the cricoid cartilage (Figs. 5 and 6). The two corniculate cartilages are located at the apex of each arytenoid cartilage (Fig. 6). The corniculate and cuneiform cartilages are embedded in the aryepiglottic fold to form two prominences on the posterior part of the rima glottidis. The true vocal cords (vocal folds or vocal ligaments) are attached posteriorly to the bases of the arytenoid cartilages. The false vocal cords (vestibular folds or vestibular ligaments) are attached slightly higher on the vertical parts of the arytenoids (Figs. 5 and 6). Both true and false vocal cords are attached anteriorly on the posterior aspect of the thyroid cartilage (Fig. 6).

The epiglottic cartilage is a single, leaf-shaped cartilage, lying behind the base of the tongue and the hyoid bone. The free upper margin of the epiglottis extends

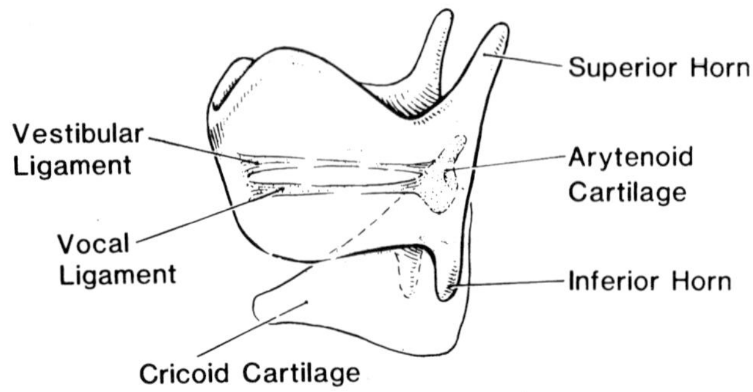

FIG. 6. Demonstrates thyroid, cricoid, and arytenoid cartilages and position of the vocal (true cords) and vestibular (false cords) ligaments. Laryngeal ventricle represents the space between the vocal and vestibular ligaments. (From ref. 1.)

backward into the lumen of the pharynx. In children and some adults, it is markedly curved and is called an omega, or infantile, epiglottis (Fig. 7). Its narrow lower margin is attached by the thyroepiglottic ligament to the back of the thyroid cartilage. The epiglottis is also attached to the tongue by a median and two lateral glossoepiglottic folds. The depressions between the two lateral and the median fold are called the valleculae.

Ligaments

The cricothyroid membrane stretches between the thyroid and cricoid cartilages (Fig. 8). Transtracheal oxygenation and ventilation, retrograde intubation, and cricothyrotomy to create an emergency airway are established through this membrane. Translaryngeal injection of local anesthetic is also performed through this ligament to produce topical anesthesia of the larynx and trachea. The thyrohyoid membrane stretches between the superior margin of the thyroid cartilage and the hyoid bone. This membrane is pierced by the internal branch of the superior laryngeal nerve and by

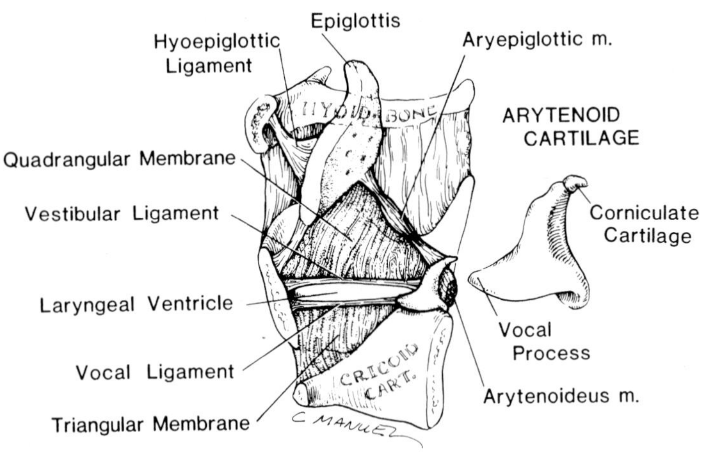

FIG. 5. Laryngeal cartilages. Thyroid cartilage is omitted to show internal relationship of laryngeal cartilages and position of the vocal (true cords) and vestibular (false cords) ligaments. (From ref. 1.)

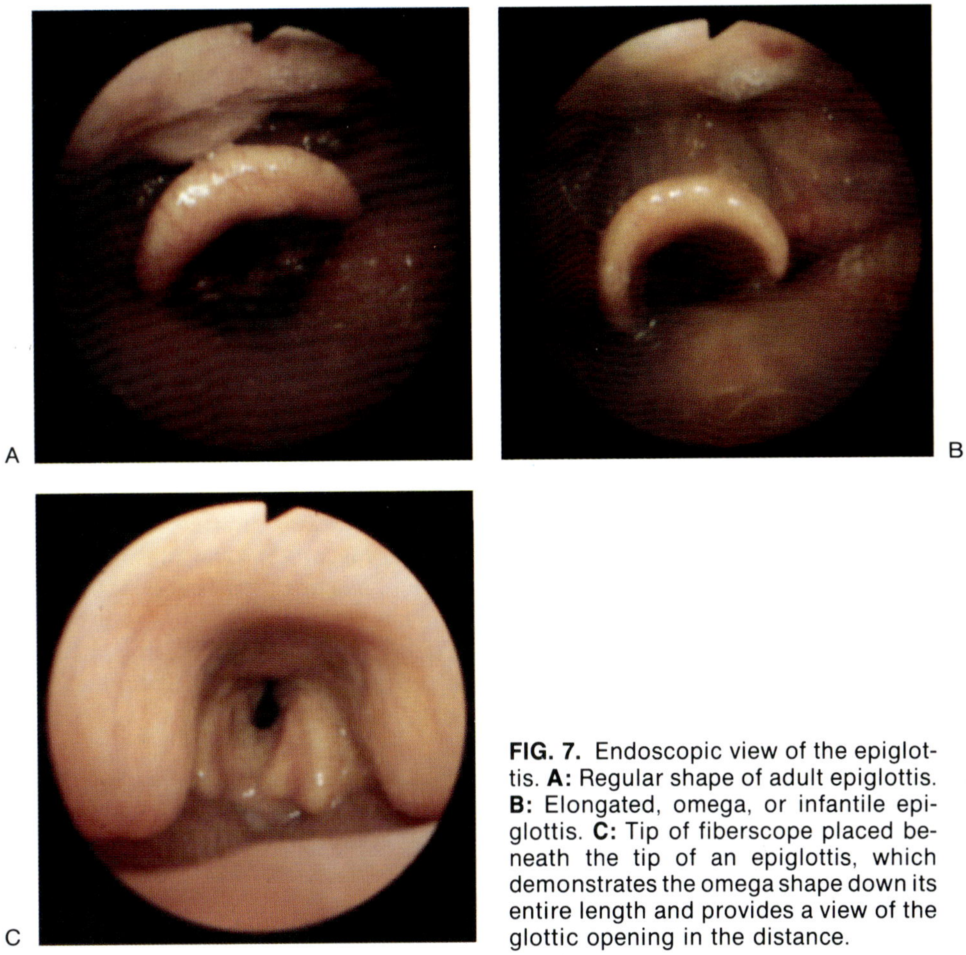

FIG. 7. Endoscopic view of the epiglottis. **A:** Regular shape of adult epiglottis. **B:** Elongated, omega, or infantile epiglottis. **C:** Tip of fiberscope placed beneath the tip of an epiglottis, which demonstrates the omega shape down its entire length and provides a view of the glottic opening in the distance.

the superior laryngeal vessels (Fig. 9). The hyoepiglottic ligament connects the anterior surface of the epiglottis to the posterior surface of the body of the hyoid bone.

The U-shaped hyoid bone is located between the mandible and the larynx at the level of the 3rd cervical vertebra (Figs. 5, 8, and 9). The hyoid bone is not part of the larynx, but it serves to maintain the larynx in position in the neck and to elevate the larynx during deglutition and phonation.

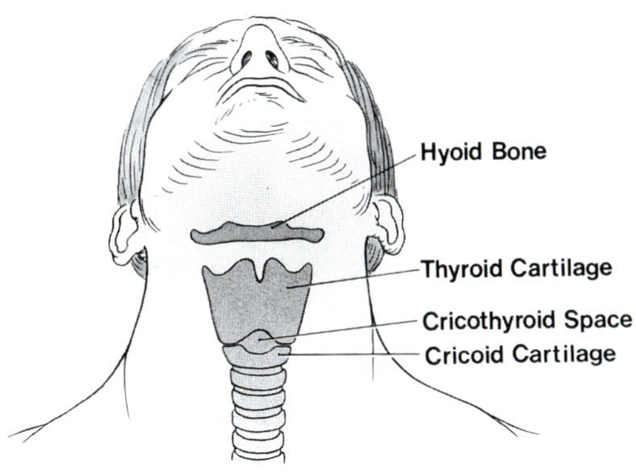

FIG. 8. Front view of the neck. Demonstrates the position of the hyoid bone and cricothyroid membrane in relation to the thyroid cartilage.

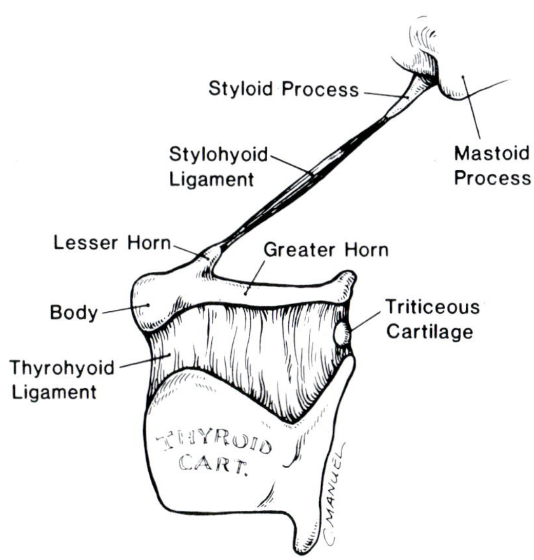

FIG. 9. The attachment of hyoid bone to larynx and styloid process of the base of the skull. (From ref. 1.)

Muscles

Muscles of the larynx are divided into the intrinsic and extrinsic groups. The intrinsic muscles have both their origin and insertion inside the larynx and cause movement of laryngeal structures. They are all paired, except for the interarytenoid muscle, and consist of two separate groups: those that open and close the laryngeal inlet and those that regulate the degree of tension of the vocal cords (Table 2).

During normal inspiration, the vocal cords are abducted, and the rima glottidis becomes triangular in shape. On deep inspiration, the vocal cords are maximally abducted, and the triangular shape of the glottis is converted into a diamond shape. On expiration, the vocal cords are adducted, leaving a small opening between them (Fig. 10).

The sensory innervation of the anterior surface of the epiglottis is by the glossopharyngeal nerve, and of the posterior surface of the epiglottis down to the vocal cords by the superior laryngeal nerve. The recurrent laryngeal nerve supplies the mucous membrane below the vocal cords. The superior and recurrent laryngeal nerves are branches of the vagus nerve.

The extrinsic muscles of the larynx move the larynx up and down during swallowing and originate from other structures in the neck. The suprahyoid group of muscles that elevate the larynx extend from the hyoid bone up to the mandible, tongue, and styloid process of the skull and include the digastric, stylohyoid, mylohyoid, and geniohyoid muscles. The depressor muscles of the larynx, the infrahyoid group, originate inferiorly and extend up to the hyoid bone and include the sternohyoid, sternothyroid, thyrohyoid, and omohyoid muscles. Calcification of the stylohyoid ligament has been blamed for poor exposure of the larynx during rigid laryngoscopy and tracheal intubation (3).

Vestibule

Vestibule is the portion of the cavity of the larynx above the vocal cords and is bounded anteriorly by the epiglottis, posteriorly by the arytenoid cartilages and interarytenoid muscle, and on either side by the aryepiglottic folds (Fig. 11).

For surgical purposes, the endolarynx is divided into three compartments. The area superior to the inferior margins of the false vocal cords is referred to as the supraglottis, and includes the epiglottis, aryepiglottic folds, arytenoids, and false vocal cords. The middle laryngeal compartment includes the ventricle or sinus, true vocal cords, anterior and posterior commissure, and tissue within 1 cm below the laryngeal ventricle (Fig. 3). The space between the free margins of the false cords and the free margins of the true cords is the laryngeal ventricle or sinus. The lower compartment, the subglottic space, extends from 1 cm below the laryngeal ventricle to the lower margin of the cricoid cartilage. This portion is a favorable site for the development of edema, because it consists of loose connective tissue.

Rima Glottidis

The anterior two-thirds of the rima glottidis or glottis is bounded by the vocal cords and the posterior one-third by the arytenoids. The rima glottidis is wider during inspiration and narrower during expiration. The average sagittal diameter of the glottis is 23 mm in adult men and 17 mm in adult women. The distance between the vocal processes when the cords are widely abducted is about 19 mm in males and 12 mm in females. In adults, the rima glottidis is the narrowest part of the larynx, but in children, the narrowest part of the larynx

TABLE 2. *Intrinsic muscles of the larynx*

Muscle	Origin	Insertion	Innervation	Action
Cricothyroid	Arch of cricoid cartilage laterally	Lamina and anterior horn of thyroid cartilage	External laryngeal	Lengthens, tenses, and adducts vocal fold
Posterior cricoarytenoid	Lamina of cricoid cartilage posteriorly	Muscular process of arytenoid cartilage		Abducts vocal fold
Lateral cricoarytenoid	Arch of cricoid cartilage	Muscular process of arytenoid cartilage		
Transverse and oblique arytenoid	One arytenoid cartilage	Opposite arytenoid cartilage	Recurrent laryngeal	Adducts vocal fold
Aryepiglottic	Continuation of oblique arytenoid muscle into aryepiglottic fold			Adducts aryepiglottic fold
Thyroarytenoid	Lamina of thyroid cartilage medially	Muscular process of arytenoid cartilage		Probably relaxes vocal fold
Vocalis	Angle between laminae of thyroid cartilage	Vocal process of arytenoid cartilage		Alters vocal fold in phonation

From O'Rahilly R. *Basic human anatomy*. Philadelphia: W.B. Saunders, 1983.

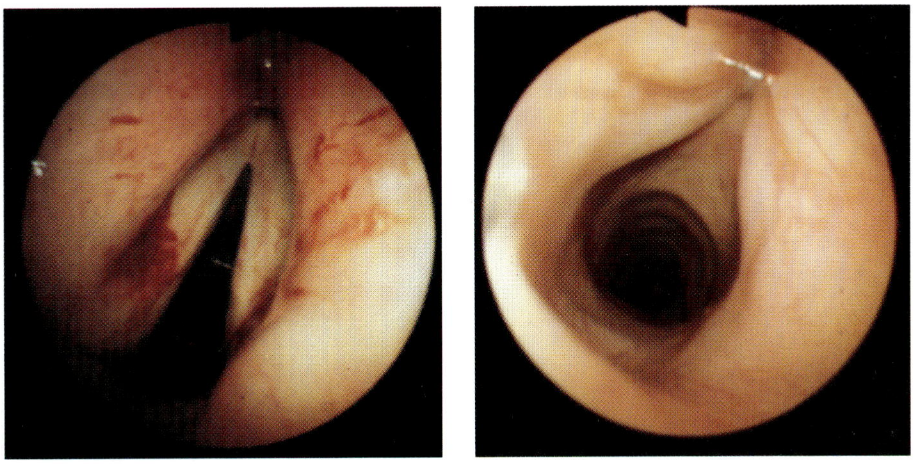

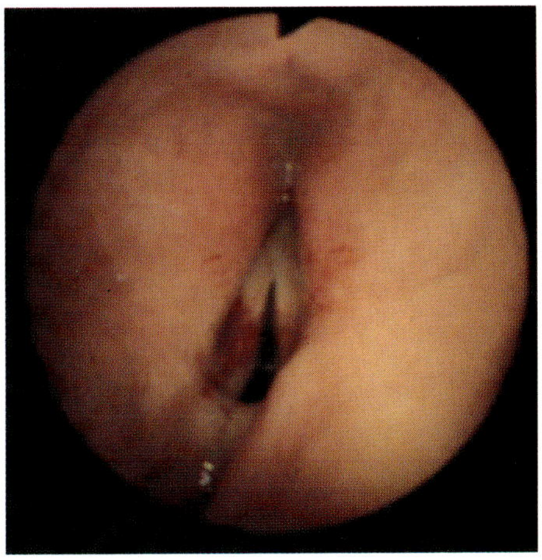

FIG. 10. Endoscopic view of rima glottidis during (**A**) normal inspiration, (**B**) deep inspiration, and (**C**) expiration.

is at the level of the cricoid ring (4). The anterior two-thirds of the rima glottidis is triangular in shape, and the posterior one-third is rectangular in shape, due to the anatomy of the arytenoid cartilages (Fig. 10). A round endotracheal tube does not use the entire anteroposterior dimension of the glottis but will often stretch the glottic opening in the transverse dimension (5). Be-

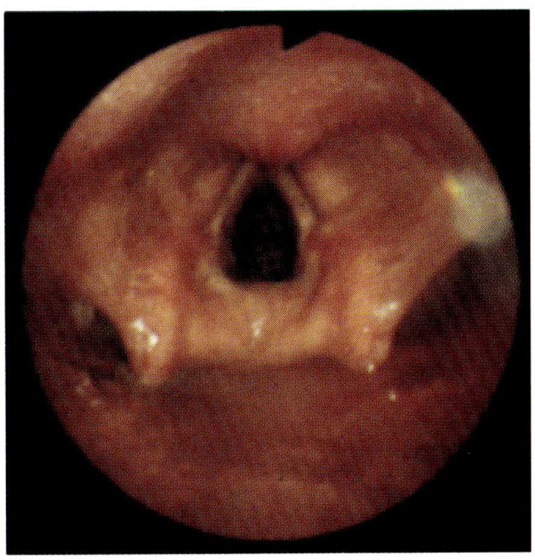

FIG. 11. Endoscopic view of the laryngeal vestibule showing the aryepiglottic folds with elevations produced by the corniculate cartilages. The interarytenoid ligament, the vestibular folds (false cords), vocal folds (true cords), and the tubercle of epiglottis are clearly seen. The vestibular folds are reddish and do not move with respiration; the vocal folds are white and move with respiration.

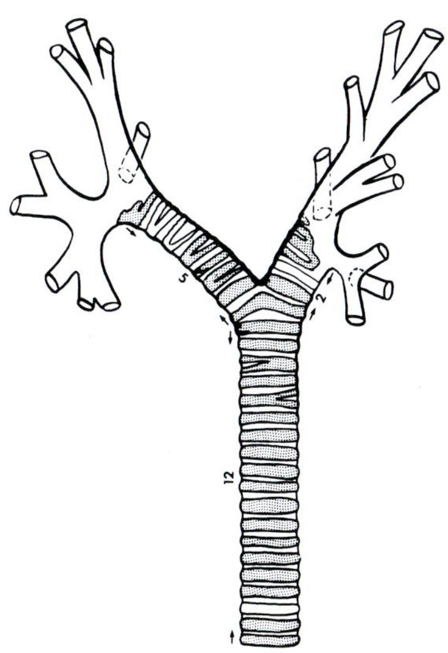

FIG. 12. The anatomy of the tracheobronchial tree with approximate dimensions (in centimeters) of an adult male.

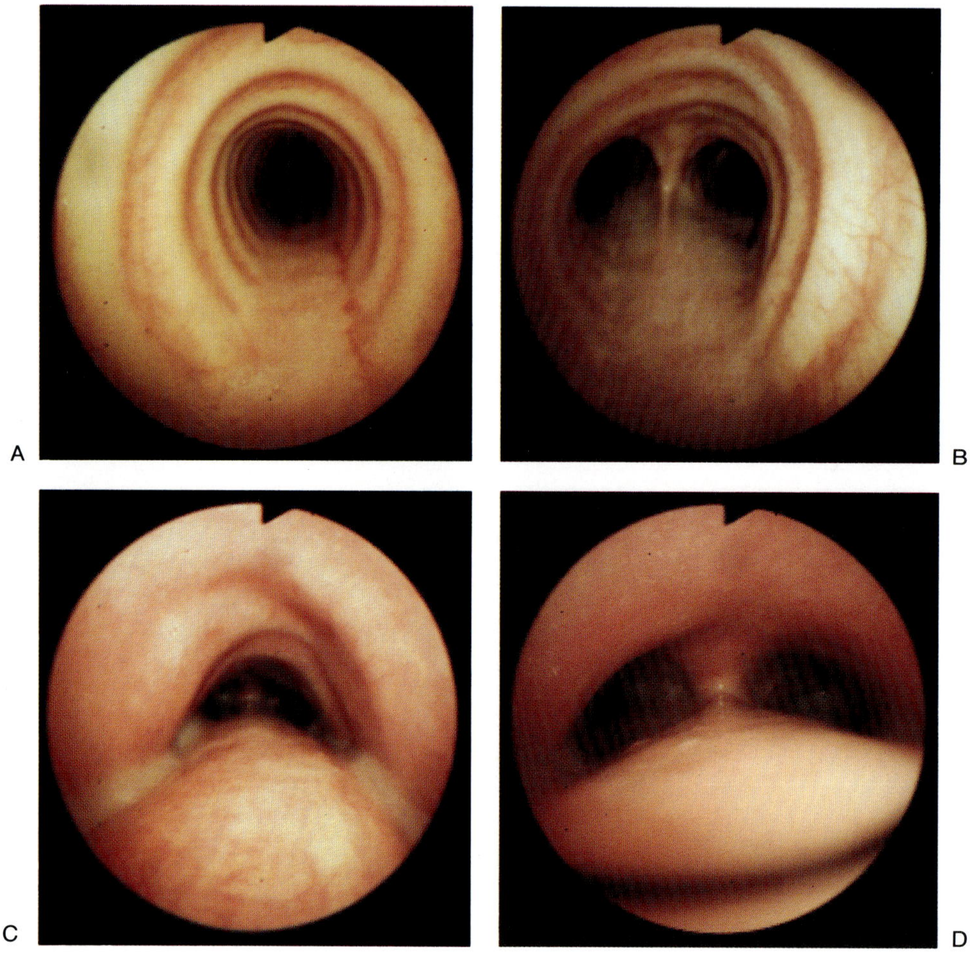

FIG. 13. Endoscopic view of the trachea and carina. **A, B:** High-domed trachea and carina. **C, D:** Lunate trachea and carina.

cause of the configuration of the upper airway and the shape of the endotracheal tube, the area of contact of the endotracheal tube will be the left and right vocal processes of the arytenoid cartilages and the cricoid cartilage. Constant pressure at these sites will lead to ischemia and ulceration, with the danger of subglottic stenosis developing. The use of low-pressure cuffs has reduced the tracheal injury due to intubation, but the incidence of laryngeal injury remains unchanged (5). Kaufman and associates (6) have suggested that the use of large-sized endotracheal tubes is responsible for subglottic injuries and stenosis.

LEFT LUNG

UPPER LOBE	UPPER DIVISION	1 & 2	Apical posterior
		3	Anterior
	LINGULA	4	Superior
		5	Inferior
LOWER LOBE		6	Superior
		7 & 8	Antero-medial basal
		9	Lateral basal
		10	Posterior basal

RIGHT LUNG

UPPER LOBE	1 Apical
	2 Posterior
	3 Anterior
MIDDLE LOBE	4 Lateral
	5 Medial
LOWER LOBE	6 Superior
	7 Medial basal
	8 Anterior basal
	9 Lateral basal
	10 Posterior basal

FIG. 14. Diagram of the trachea and main divisions of the bronchial tree as visualized by the endoscopist standing at the head of the table. Endoscopic views of the trachea and carina (**A**); right upper (**B**); right middle and lower (**C**); left upper and lower (**D**); and left lower bronchial orifices (**E**) are presented in color.

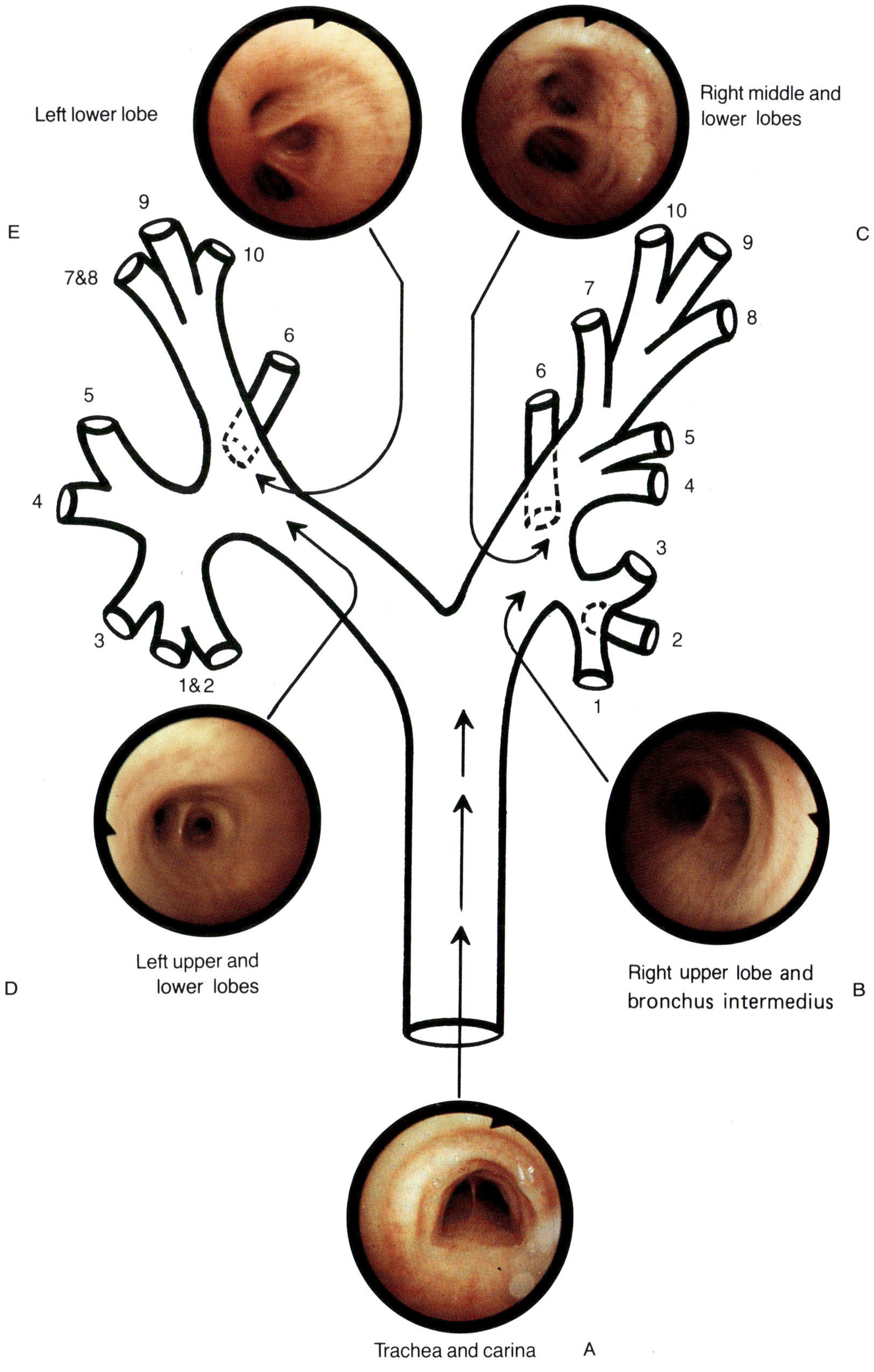
Left lower lobe
Right middle and lower lobes
E
C
9
10
7&8
6
5
4
3
1&2
10
9
7
8
6
5
4
3
2
1
Left upper and lower lobes
D
Right upper lobe and bronchus intermedius
B
Trachea and carina
A

THE TRACHEA AND BRONCHI

The trachea begins at the lower border of the cricoid cartilage and ends at the carina, where it divides into the right and left main bronchi at the level of the 5th thoracic vertebra. Approximately one-third of the trachea is above and two-thirds below the suprasternal notch. In the adult, the trachea is approximately 10–14 cm long and approximately 2.5 cm in diameter and is composed of 18–24 incomplete horseshoe-shaped cartilages connected posteriorly by the trachealis muscle (Fig. 12). The adult trachea varies in shape from high-domed, with a width/depth ratio of 0.6, to lunate, with a width/depth ratio of 3.0 (Fig. 13) (7). The trachea occupies a midline position in the neck, but the lower part of it is displaced to the right by the aortic arch. Lymph nodes are found on either side of the tracheobronchial tree and below the carina. A prominent aortic arch and enlarged paratracheal and bronchial lymph nodes can cause compression narrowing and displacement of the trachea and main bronchi. This can interfere with proper placement of endotracheal and endobronchial tubes (8).

The right mainstem bronchus leaves the trachea at an angle of 25–30°. Its lumen is about 16 mm, and its length averages 18 mm (range, 8–32 mm) (Fig. 14) (9,10). The right upper lobe bronchus arises from the lateral aspect (3 o'clock) of the main bronchus. The diameter of the right upper lobe bronchial orifice is 10.7 mm (range, 6–18 mm), and it is 1 cm long and branches into three segmental bronchi: the apical, posterior, and anterior. The intermediate bronchus extends from the lower end of the orifice of the right upper lobe bronchus to the level of the middle lobe orifice. The middle lobe bronchus is 1–2 cm long and arises from the anterior wall of the intermediate bronchus (12 o'clock). It divides into two segmental bronchi, the lateral and medial. The right lower lobe bronchus is the continuation of the intermediate bronchus and gives off five branches. The superior (apical) bronchus of the inferior lobe comes off at 6 o'clock just below and opposite the origin of the middle lobe bronchus. About 1.5 cm farther down, the medial basal bronchus arises from the medial side (9 o'clock) of the lower lobe bronchus, which then divides into the anterior, lateral, and posterior basal bronchi.

The left mainstem bronchus leaves the trachea at an angle of about 45°. It is slightly narrower but substantially longer than the right mainstem bronchus, with an average length of 5 cm (range, 3–7 cm). The primary division is into the left upper lobe and left lower lobe bronchi. The axis of this primary division commonly lies obliquely between 8 o'clock and 2 o'clock, but may also lie anywhere between the horizontal and vertical axes. The upper lobe bronchus is 8–9 mm in diameter, 0.5–1 cm in length, and divides into the upper division and lingular bronchi. The upper division or upper lobe bronchus divides into the apical posterior and anterior segments. The lingular division divides into the superior and inferior lingular segments. The superior bronchus of the left lower lobe arises from the posterior wall (6 o'clock) of the left lower lobe bronchus. The latter then divides into the anterior, lateral, and posterior basal bronchi. The posterior basal bronchus is the largest of the three and appears to be the continuation of the mainstem bronchus.

The tracheobronchial tree receives sympathetic innervation from the first to fifth thoracic ganglia. The vagus nerve supplies the parasympathetic fibers. Bronchomotor tone is a continuous and variable state of contraction of the bronchial musculature, which is present during both phases of respiration, but constriction of the bronchioles is greater during expiration than inspiration.

REFERENCES

1. Smith C, Ramsey RG. Xeroradiography of the lateral neck. *RadioGraphics* 1982;2:306–327.
2. Rodenstein DO, Stanescu DC. State of the art—the soft palate and breathing. *Am Rev Respir Dis* 1986;134:311–325.
3. Sharwood-Smith GH. Difficulty in intubation—calcified stylohyoid ligament. *Anaesthesia* 1976;31:508–510.
4. Eckenhoff JE. Some anatomic considerations of the infant larynx influencing endotracheal anesthesia. *Anesthesiology* 1951; 12:401–410.
5. Bishop MJ, Weymuller EA Jr, Fink BR. Laryngeal effects of prolonged intubation. *Anesth Analg* 1984;63:335–342.
6. Kaufman JA, Fortsor JK, Strong MS. Predictive factors of cricoid ring size in adults in relation to acquired subglottic stenosis. *Otol Head Neck Surg* 1983;91:177–182.
7. Campbell AH, Liddelow AG. Significant variations in the shape of the trachea and large bronchi. *Med J Austral* 1967;20: 1017–1020.
8. MacGillivray RG. Tracheal compression caused by aneurysm of the aortic arch. Implications for the anaesthetist. *Anaesthesia* 1985;40:270–277.
9. Merendino KA, KiriLuk LB. Human measurements involved in tracheobronchial resection and reconstruction procedures. *Surgery* 1954;35:590–597.
10. Benumof JL, Partridge BL, Salvatierra C, Keating J. Margin of safety in positioning modern double-lumen endotracheal tubes. *Anesthesiology* 1987;67:729–738.

BIBLIOGRAPHY

1. Myerson MC. *The human larynx*. Springfield: Charles C Thomas, 1964.
2. Moore KL. *Clinical oriented anatomy,* 2nd ed. Baltimore: Williams & Wilkins, 1985.
3. Ellis H, Feldman S. *Anatomy for anaesthetists,* 3rd ed. Oxford: Blackwell Scientific, 1977.
4. Meschan I. *An atlas of anatomy basic to radiology,* 1st ed. Philadelphia: W.B. Saunders, 1975.
5. O'Rahilly R. *Basic human anatomy: a regional study of human structure*. Philadelphia: W.B. Saunders, 1983.
6. Gray H. *Anatomy of the human body,* 13th American ed. Philadelphia: Lea & Febiger, 1985.

CHAPTER 3

Radiology of the Airway

Lee Sider, M.D.

The purpose of this chapter is to review the normal radiographic findings of the airway as they appear on conventional and xeroradiography of the neck, conventional tomography of the trachea and bronchi, and computed tomography (CT) of the entire airway. Some of the pathologic processes that compromise the airway and make instrumentation difficult are illustrated. Radiology of the cervical spine is included, as some changes in the bony cervical spine may contribute to the difficulty of airway management. In addition, fractures of the cervical spine must be recognized, as there is then danger of cervical cord trauma during tracheal intubation and artificial ventilation. I hope that this will help physicians involved in airway management to better comprehend the reports of X-ray examinations and to be able to interpret simple radiologic findings for safer airway management.

Radiographic evaluation of the soft tissues of the neck and chest had always been less than an exact imaging system until the advent of high resolution CT and, most recently, magnetic resonance imaging (MRI). The airway and surrounding soft tissues can be divided into their superficial component (mucosa) and the surrounding deep soft tissues for discussion. Conventional X-ray examinations are only successful in detecting masses that either involve the mucosa or are large enough to distort the airway. CT allows views of the surrounding soft tissues of the neck and chest, thus allowing the detection of smaller masses that do not involve the mucosal surface. A combination of fiberoptic laryngeal examination and CT is proving to be valuable in completely evaluating and staging processes involving the nasopharynx, oropharynx, larynx, and their surrounding soft tissues. The role of MRI is becoming increasingly important and may prove superior to CT with its further refinement.

RADIOLOGY OF THE UPPER AIRWAY

The use of X-rays to examine the upper airway involves plain films, conventional tomography, and xerography.

Plain Endolateral View of the Neck

The endolateral view of the neck demonstrates the vallecula, tongue, epiglottis, aryepiglottic folds, tonsils, arytenoids, air in the laryngeal ventricles, subglottic trachea, the bony hyoid, calcified thyroid cartilage, and bones of the cervical spine (Fig. 1). The vallecular recess is an air-containing space between the posterior aspect of the base of the tongue and the epiglottis. Any lesion that involves the base of the tongue such as thyroglossal cyst, lymphoid tissue, tumors, or enlargement of the epiglottis can produce obliteration of this recess (1). The epiglottis is normally outlined with a sharply pointed superior tip and a smooth anterior surface. The lower prevertebral or retropharyngeal space is identified between the air column and cervical spine on the lateral film. In adults, the maximum normal distance of this area is less than 7 mm at the C3-C4 level equal to approximately one-third to one-half times the AP diameter of the C4 vertebral body. The distance from a lower cervical vertebral body to the trachea, the retrotracheal space, is normally 5–22 mm (2). Any distance greater than 7 mm or 22 mm, depending on the level, should alert the physician to the presence of pathology, such as abscess, hematoma, or tumor.

Xerography

Xerography provides greater detail of the mucosal surface and bony structures than do plain film views (Fig. 2). Instead of exposing X-ray film, the beam exposes a special xerographic plate. The image is then transferred to paper, appearing blue in color. Xerogra-

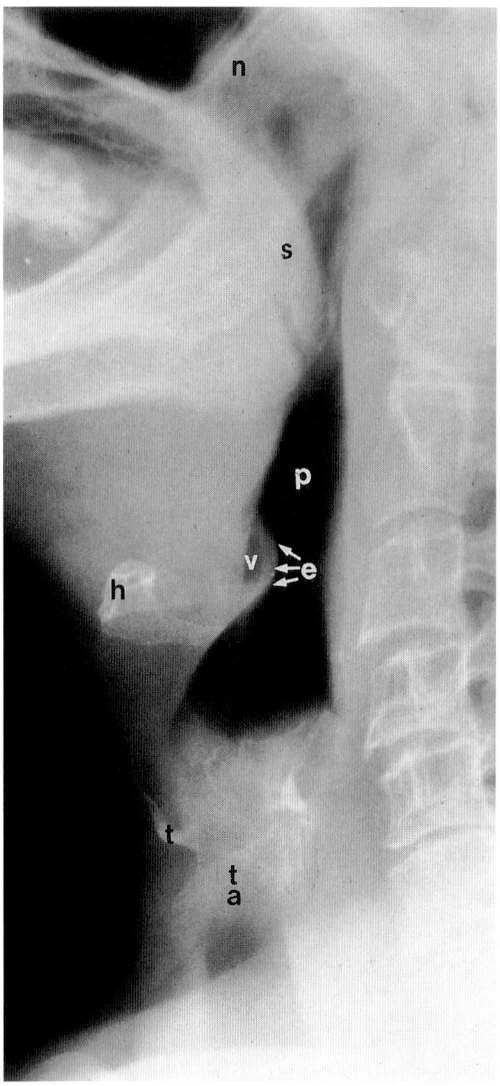

FIG. 1. Normal endolateral neck. n, nasopharynx; s, soft palate; p, pharynx; v, vallecula; e, epiglottis; h, hyoid bone; t, thyroid cartilage; ta, trachea.

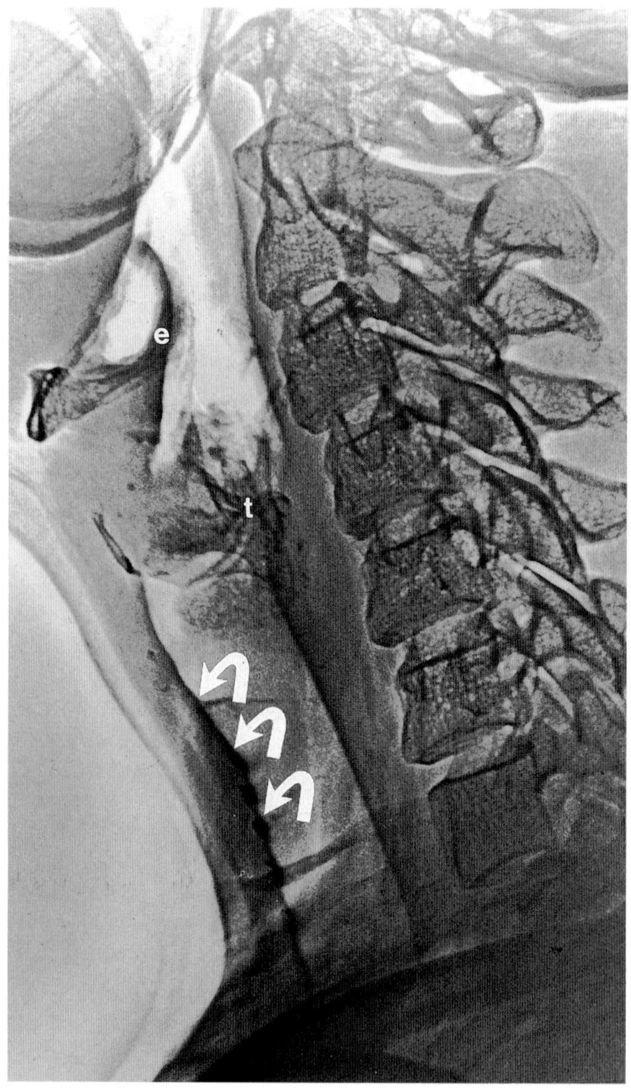

FIG. 2. Normal endolateral xerogram. The epiglottis (e), mucosal surface of the airway (*curved arrows*), and calcified thyroid cartilage (t) are sharply imaged.

phy is more costly and exposes the patient to more radiation than plain films do (3,4).

Tomography

Before the advent of CT, plain film tomography allowed the clearest views of the airway and its mucosal surface. By a photographic "trick" of moving the X-ray tube in one direction and the film in the opposite direction, one plane, a fulcrum plane, appears in focus where all structures above and below this plane appear blurred. This reveals soft tissue detail otherwise hidden by superimposed anatomy such as the cervical spine. On the frontal tomogram, one can identify the pyriform sinuses, false and true cords, and laryngeal ventricle, along with sharp outlines of the mucosal surface (Fig. 3A). In addition, with quiet breathing and phonation, cord movement can be documented (Fig. 3B).

Tomography of the airway is now enjoying new popularity as a preoperative guide in the application of laser surgery for the treatment of tracheal narrowing or stenosis. It provides a longitudinal view of the airway as the surgeon will see it at the time of surgery. The extent and severity of tracheal narrowing can be easily appreciated preoperatively.

PATHOLOGIC PROCESSES

Enlarged Adenoids and Tonsils

Perhaps the most frequent cause of compromise of the nasopharyngeal and oropharyngeal airway in chil-

A 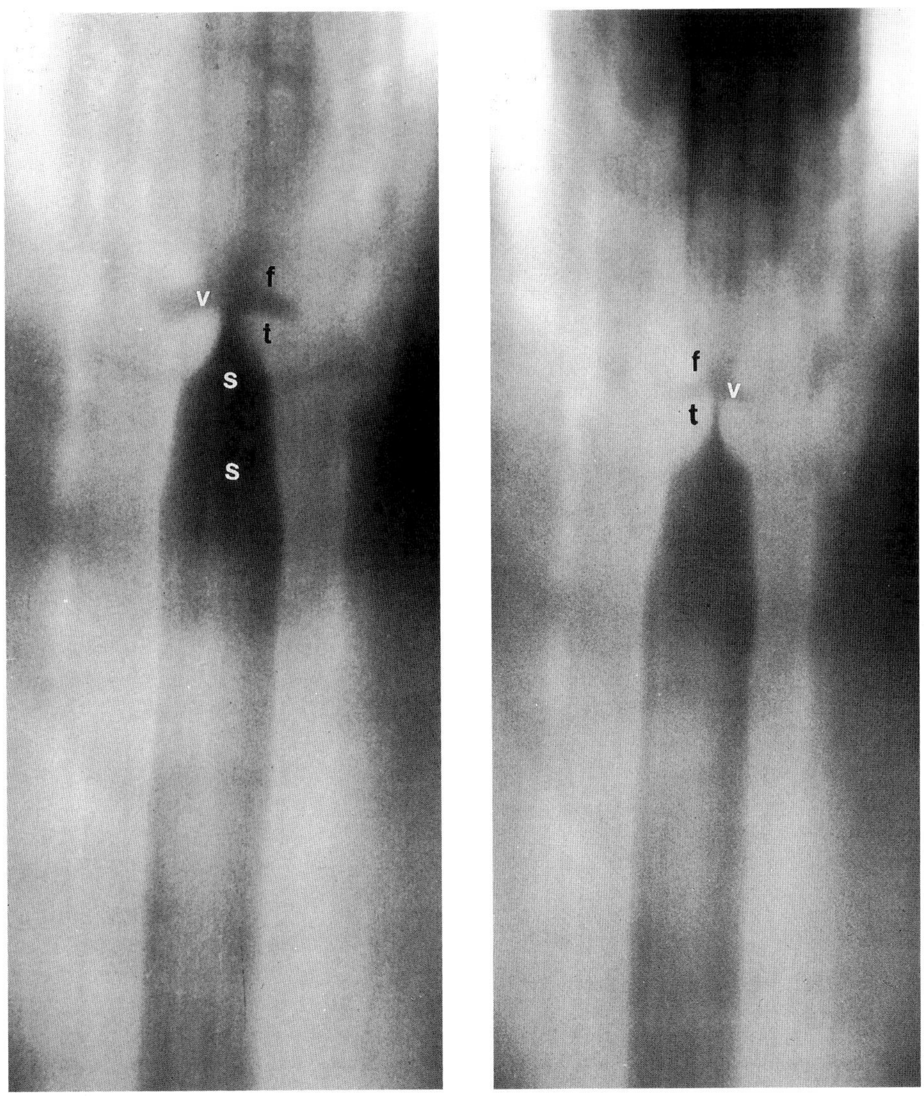 B

FIG. 3. Normal laryngeal tomogram. **A:** The cords are abducted during quiet breathing. f, false cords; v, laryngeal ventricle; t, true cords; s, infraglottic airway. **B:** With phonation ("EE"), the cords move together or are adducted. f, false cords; v, laryngeal ventricle; t, true cords.

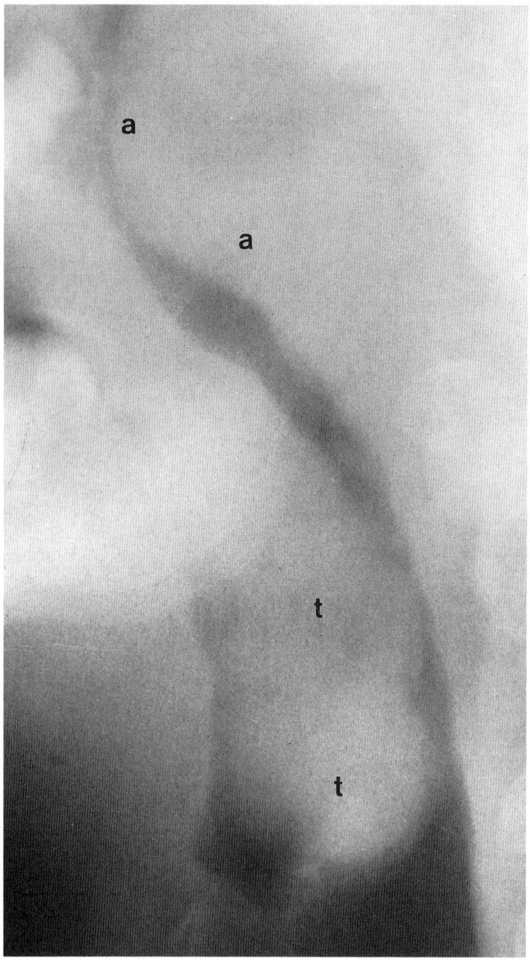

FIG. 4. Enlarged adenoids and tonsil. There is obvious enlargement of the adenoids (a) compromising the airway. The tonsils are also very enlarged and bulky (t).

dren is a simple enlargement of the adenoids and tonsils. They are easily identified on the endolateral view of the neck. The airway is smoothly and gradually narrowed at these expected levels (Fig. 4). Chronic airway obstruction due to enlarged adenoids can lead to chronic hypoxia, pulmonary hypertension, and right ventricular failure (5). Vascular tumors and various neoplasms may also involve the posterior wall of the pharynx and are among the differential diagnostic considerations.

Laryngotracheobronchitis

In croup (laryngotracheobronchitis), the subglottic portion of the trachea is narrowed from inflammatory edema. As a result of this narrowing, the superiorly placed hypopharynx dilates. Croup is easily diagnosed on a plain frontal X-ray of the neck. The subglottic trachea rapidly tapers on the frontal film and has been likened to the appearance of a church steeple (Fig. 5).

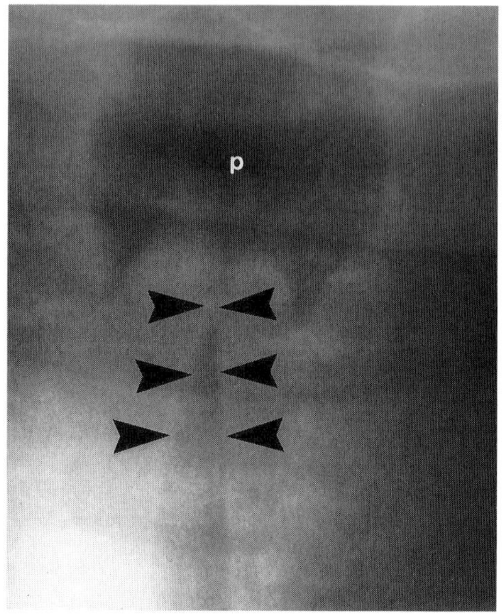

FIG. 5. Croup. The airway is smoothly narrowed or tapered (*arrowheads*). As a result, the hypopharynx is dilated (p).

Epiglottitis

Epiglottitis, which may occur at any age but is most common in young children, may lead to severe respiratory obstruction with dilatation of the hypopharynx. In epiglottitis, the lateral radiograph of the neck is the most helpful for showing the swollen-thumb appearance of the inflamed and edematous epiglottis and often-dilated hypopharynx (Fig. 6). Smooth, symmetric enlargement of the epiglottis may also be seen after smoke inhalation, trauma, and angioneurotic edema (6,7).

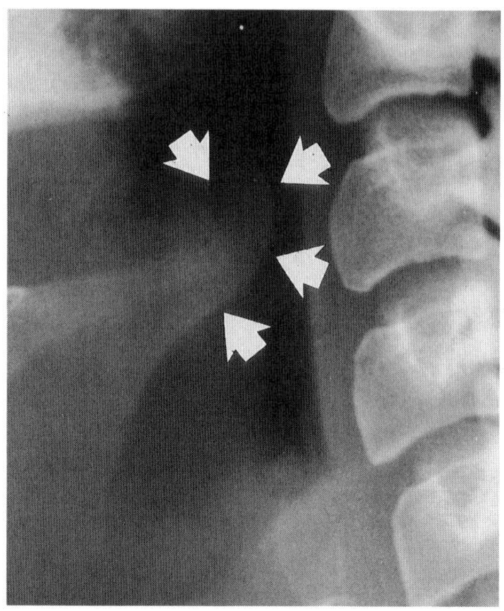

FIG. 6. Epiglottitis. The epiglottis is markedly swollen (*arrows*), compromising the airway.

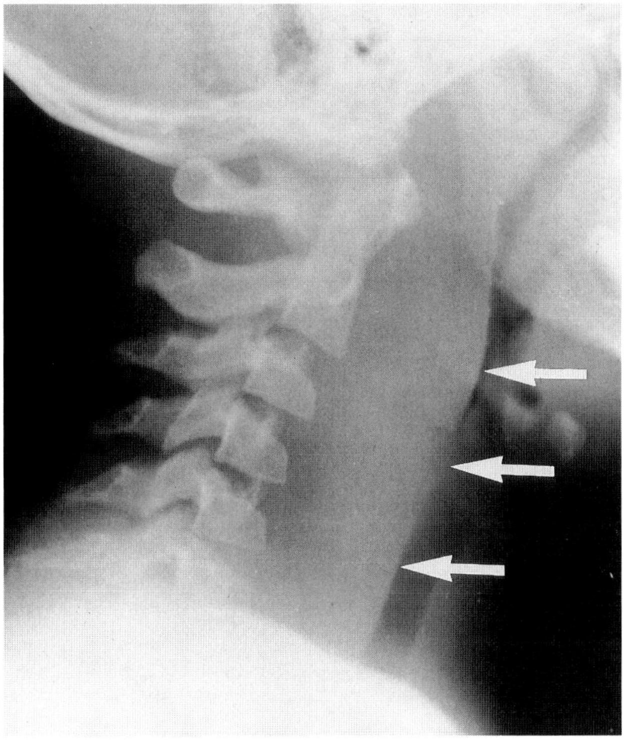

FIG. 7. Retropharyngeal/prevertebral abscess. There is obvious swelling of the prevertebral space with displacement of the airway anteriorly (*arrows*).

Retropharyngeal Abscess

Swelling or prominence of the retropharyngeal soft tissue may be produced by a variety of causes. The endolateral view of the neck shows a widening of the soft tissues in front of the spine accompanied by anterior displacement and compression of the airway (Fig. 7). In children, the swelling is frequently due to cellulitis or abscess formation. Following trauma, with or without cervical fracture, hemorrhage can fill in this space. Finally, in adults, tumor must always be a consideration.

Tumors

Tumors of the upper airway usually present in a more localized fashion. In an adult, prominence of the tonsils with filling in of the vallecular space should be viewed as potentially due to carcinoma or lymphoma. Tomography of the pharynx and larynx may also be helpful in detecting a mass lesion arising from within the pyriform sinus or on the vocal cords. Tomography reveals an irregular surface typical for tumor if it is superficial enough to involve the mucosa. Often the tomogram demonstrates only asymmetry of the airway, as the deeper portions of the tumor deform the airway but do not extend through into the airway. It is with these deep tumors that CT has made its greatest impact.

COMPUTED TOMOGRAPHY OF THE UPPER AIRWAY

CT provides a noninvasive imaging technique capable of a unique three-dimensional anatomic display of the airway. The advantages of CT over conventional radiography include elimination of superimposed structures and superior image quality. It is the radiologic procedure of choice to supplement the findings of laryngoscopy when additional diagnostic information is required to determine the feasibility of conservative surgery (8).

CT scans are obtained by shaping the three-dimensional X-ray beam (likened to a cone) into a fan beam of certain thickness (1.5–10 mm). The thickness of the beam determines scan section thickness and, for neck imaging, is usually 5 mm. The X-ray tube moves in a circular path about the patient. The beam is transmitted through the patient, then it exposes special X-ray detectors instead of X-ray film. Through computer assistance, an image is presented. The image is likened to an X-ray of a slice of salami of predetermined thickness (Fig. 8).

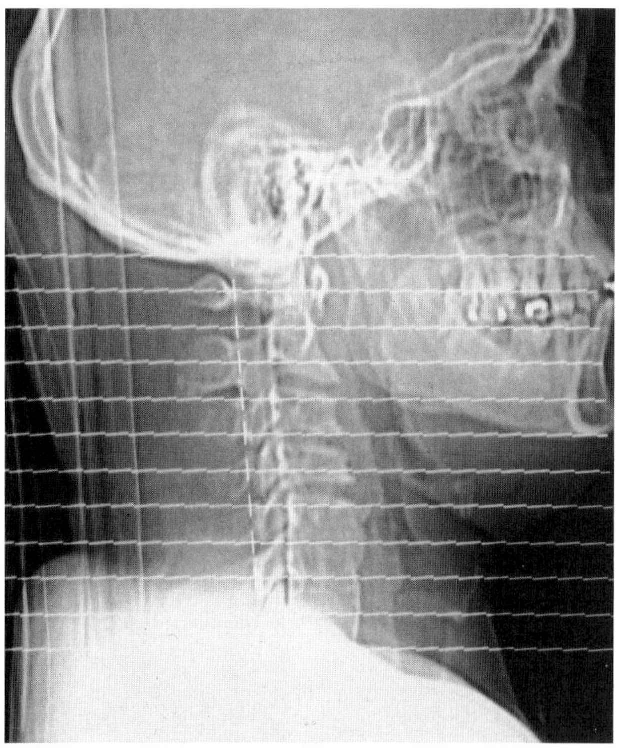

FIG. 8. CT of the upper airway. Scout of neck.

The Nasopharynx

On the CT scan, the soft tissues of the neck are fairly symmetric from side to side, and a careful inventory of the contents of the superficial and deep compartments allows early detection of pathology. CT landmarks of the superficial compartments at the level of the nasopharynx include the torus tubarius (eustachian cushion) and the neighboring fossa of Rosenmüller. The fossa of Rosenmüller is an air space and may be normally slightly asymmetric as it inflates with air to different degrees (Fig. 9). An important landmark of the deep soft tissue of the nasopharynx is the fat-containing parapharyngeal space. Fat has a distinctive low attenuation or black appearance on CT; thus, it is easily identified. The parapharyngeal space lies lateral to the torus tubarius. Inflammatory and neoplastic processes originating on the mucosal surface can break through the fascia surrounding the airway to "fill in" or obliterate this fat space. This results in asymmetry of the soft tissues. The carotid artery and vein are imaged as distinct tubular structures defined by the surrounding fat. Loss of their definition should alert one to the presence of a mass.

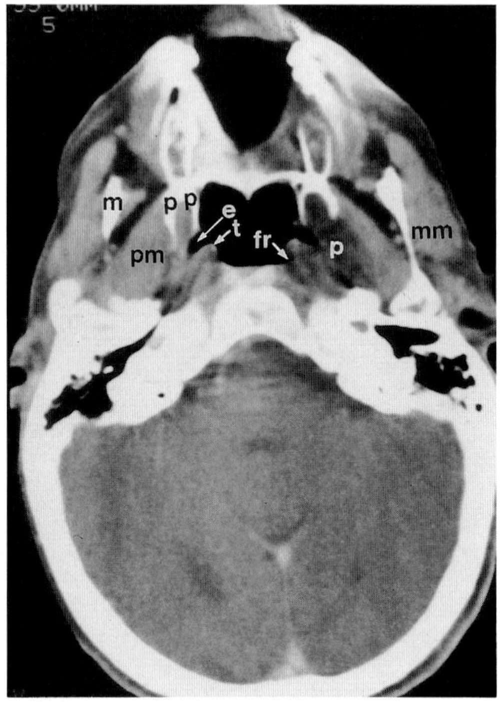

FIG. 9. Normal CT—nasopharynx. t, torus tubarius; e, eustachian orifice; fr, fossa of Rosenmüller; p, parapharyngeal space; pp, pterygoid plates; pm, lateral pterygoid muscle; mm, masseter muscle; m, mandible.

The Oropharynx

The airway at the level of the oropharynx appears flattened and is often asymmetric due to variations in lymphatic tissue content and position of the tongue. The soft tissues of the tonsils, soft palate, and surrounding muscles of the floor of the mouth blend to form the superficial boundaries of the oropharynx (Fig. 10). The intrinsic muscles of the tongue can be identified somewhat lower, followed by the arched epiglottis and anteriorly placed valleculae. The valleculae may normally be somewhat asymmetric (Fig. 11). At this level, the hyoid bone can also be identified. The deeper structures again include the carotid sheath and parapharyngeal fat space contiguous with the nasopharynx. The parotid and submandibular glands, mandible, and styloid processes should also be identified and compared for symmetry (Fig. 10).

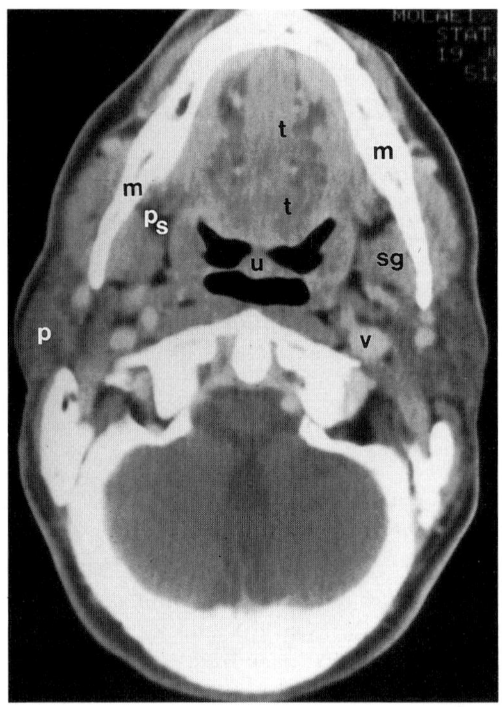

FIG. 10. Normal CT—oropharynx. Section through the base of the tongue. u, uvula; t, tongue; ps, fat-filled parapharyngeal space; v, vascular bundle; m, mandible; p, parotid gland; sg, submandibular gland.

The Larynx

CT has revolutionized the evaluation of the larynx. Symmetry of most of the laryngeal structures assists in the diagnosis of abnormalities. The larynx is divided into supraglottic, glottic, and subglottic levels for descriptive purposes. The area superior to the inferior margins of the false vocal cords including the epiglottis is referred to as supraglottic. The superficial anatomy of the supraglottic area includes the epiglottis and ary-

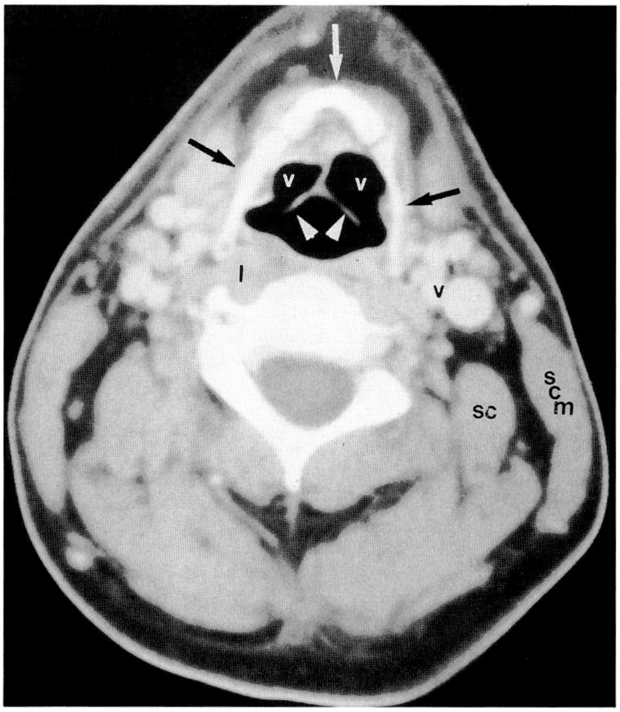

FIG. 11. Normal CT—oropharynx/supraglottic. The three parts of the hyoid bone (*arrows*) and thin arched epiglottis (*arrowheads*) identify the level. The valleculae (white v) are anterior and lateral to the epiglottis. v, vascular bundle; scm, sternocleidomastoid muscle; sc, scalene muscle; l, longus colli muscles.

epiglottic folds, which separate the laryngeal vestibule from the pyriform sinuses (Fig. 11). Asymmetry in the size and caudal extent of the pyriform sinuses, like the valleculae, is common. At this level, the hyoid bone and top of the partially calcified thyroid cartilage can be identified (Fig. 12). Within the deeper soft tissues of the supraglottic airway, the fat planes should be identified. The first is anterior to the epiglottis and is called the preepiglottic space. The fat of the preepiglottic space is contiguous with the paralaryngeal space laterally and inferiorly (Fig. 12). More posteriorly, the carotid artery, internal jugular vein, and sternocleidomastoid muscles should be identified as distinct structures defined by the surrounding fat. Calcified atherosclerotic plaques are frequently identified within the carotid artery, making identification of the arteries easy.

The glottic level is identified by the presence of the V-shaped body of the thyroid cartilage anteriorly and the arytenoid and cricoid cartilages posteriorly. With quiet breathing, the airway is dilated and symmetric, and the arytenoids are abducted (Fig. 13). With phonation, the aryepiglottic folds draw the arytenoid cartilage medially along with maximum dilatation of the pyriform sinuses. The false cords are symmetric, laterally placed soft tissue strips situated just above the level of the cricoid cartilage (Fig. 13). The symmetric soft tissue of the true cords can be identified when

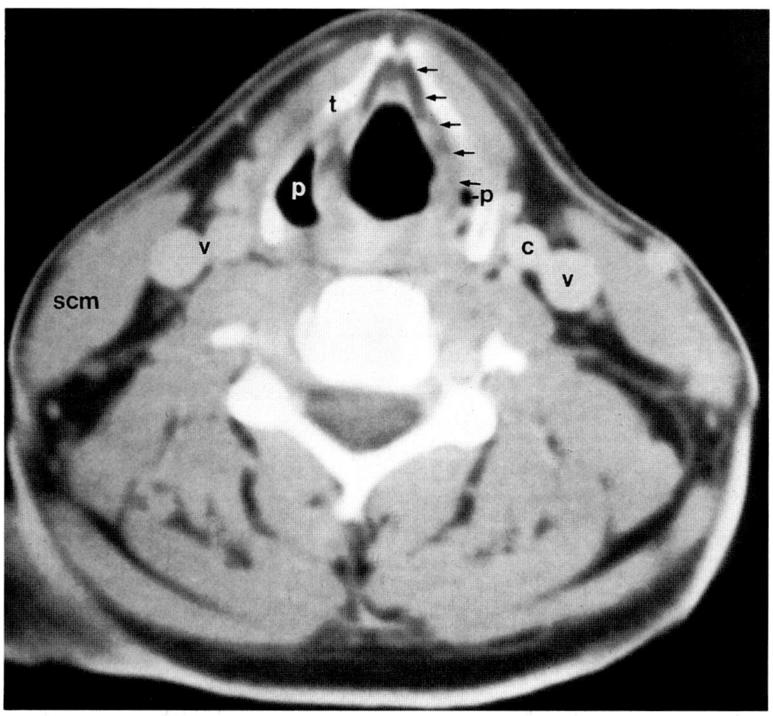

FIG. 12. Normal CT—aryepiglottic folds. White p, right pyriform sinus, and black p, left pyriform sinus demonstrate normal asymmetry of the pyriform sinuses. *Arrows,* fat of the parapharyngeal space; t, thyroid cartilage; scm, sternocleidomastoid muscle; v, jugular vein; c, carotid artery.

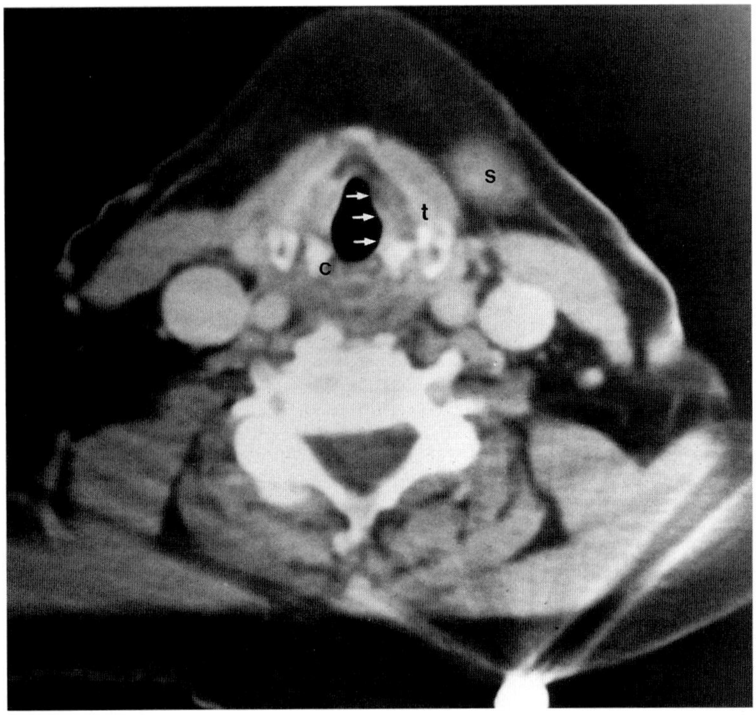

FIG. 13. Normal CT—false cords. The false cords barely can be imaged as tissue stripes on either side of the airway (*arrows*). c, cricoid cartilage; t, thyroid cartilage; s, left submandibular gland.

the body of the cricoid forms the lateral and posterior borders of the airway (Fig. 14). The empty space of the anterior commissure between the true cords should always be identified, as any tissue in this space signifies an abnormal mass crossing the midline, an important prognostic sign.

The immediate infraglottic area is marked by the now U shape of the thyroid cartilage. The cricoid cartilage is still present posteriorly. The airway is now round or oval and remains symmetric. The cartilaginous rings of the airway are incomplete in the infraglottic portion (Fig. 15).

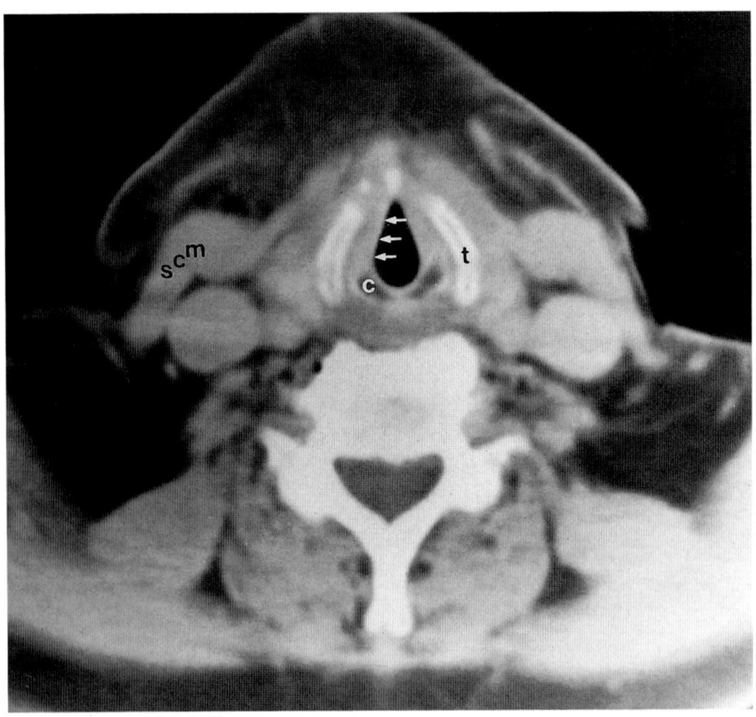

FIG. 14. Normal CT—true cords. The true cords are the lateral slips of soft tissue (*arrows*) on either side of the airway. c, cricoid cartilage; t, thyroid cartilage; scm, sternocleidomastoid muscle.

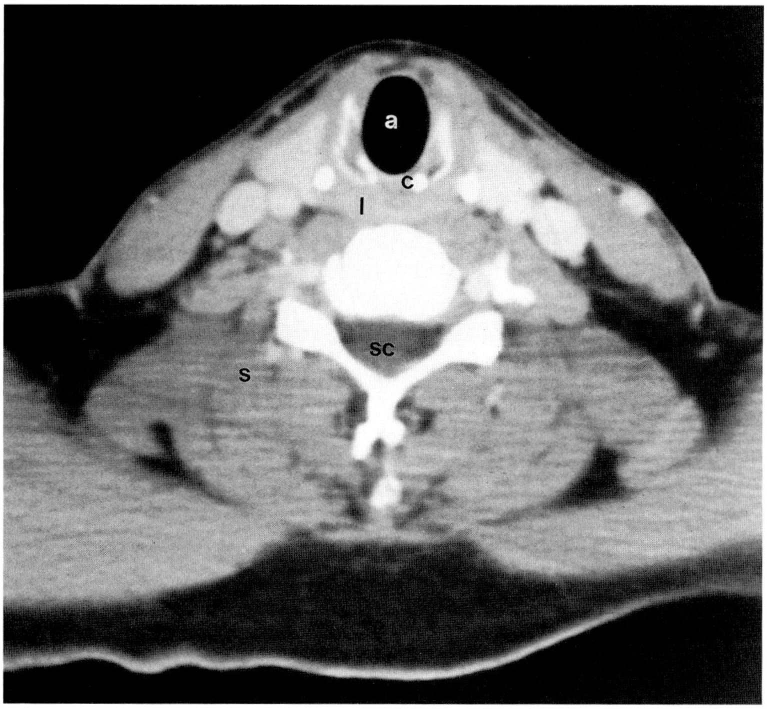

FIG. 15. Normal CT—infraglottic. The airway is oval (a) and remaining cricoid cartilage is seen posteriorly (c). l, longus colli muscles; s, scalene muscles; sc, spinal cord.

The thyroid is easily identified in lower CT sections of the neck, especially when intravenous contrast material is given. The thyroid often appears enlarged in Graves' disease or multinodular goiter along with deviation or narrowing of the airway (Figs. 16A and B).

MAGNETIC RESONANCE IMAGING OF THE UPPER AIRWAY

MRI may present images much like CT. The images are created with the use of a strong external magnet.

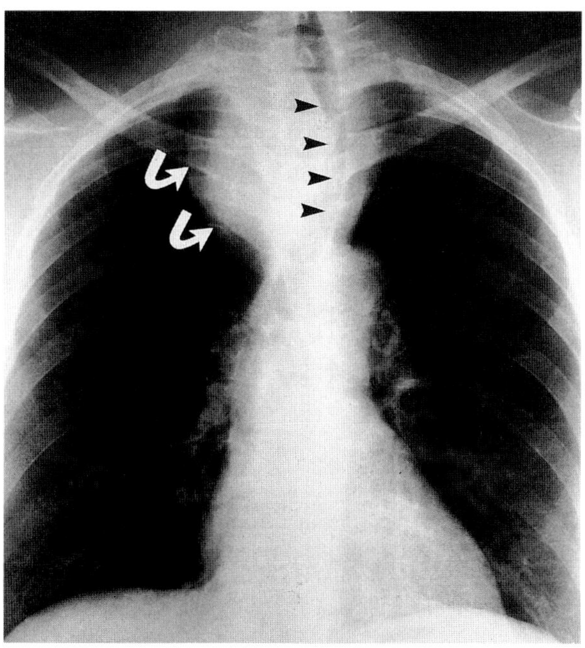
A

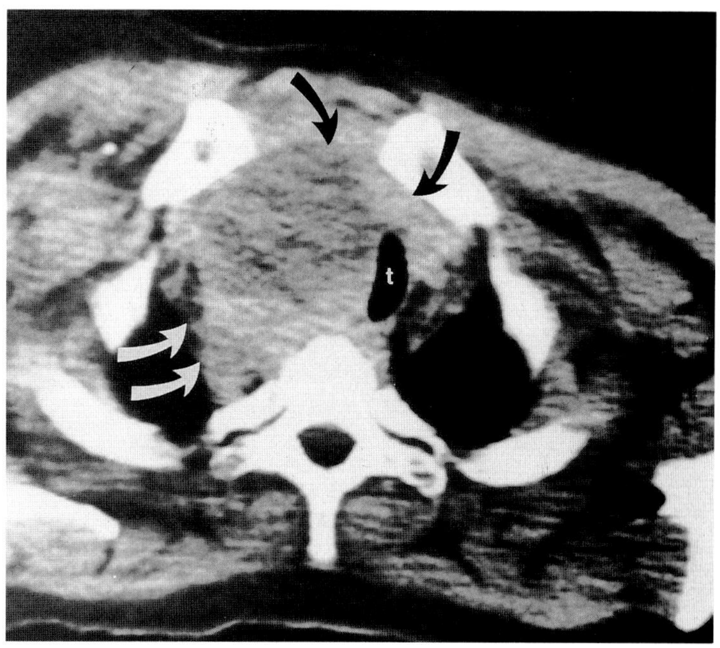

B

FIG. 16. Substernal goiter. **A:** A huge soft tissue mass projects from either side of the mediastinum (*curved arrows*). The trachea is both deviated and narrowed (*arrowheads*). **B:** Corresponding CT demonstrates the enlarged substernal thyroid as a mixed density (*curved arrows*). Again, note the distorted trachea (t).

The advantages of MRI over CT include use of no ionizing radiation, which is important if follow-up scans are needed after surgery. MRI presents images not only in the axial orientation like those of CT (Figs. 17A and B), but in midsagittal and coronal planes as well. This may help to define further the soft tissue extent of a tumor that, some claim, affords more accurate staging of a malignancy (Figs. 18A and B). The disadvantages of MRI include its inability to recognize bone or calcification, making it difficult to detect the cartilaginous or bony involvement of glottic tumors, which are important in staging. In addition, MRI is more expensive and usually less available than CT.

Pathologic Process

Most tumors of the pharynx and floor of the mouth are malignant (9). CT gives important staging information such as whether the tumor is restricted to the superficial mucosa or has extended into the deep soft tissues. It also reveals whether the deep infiltrating

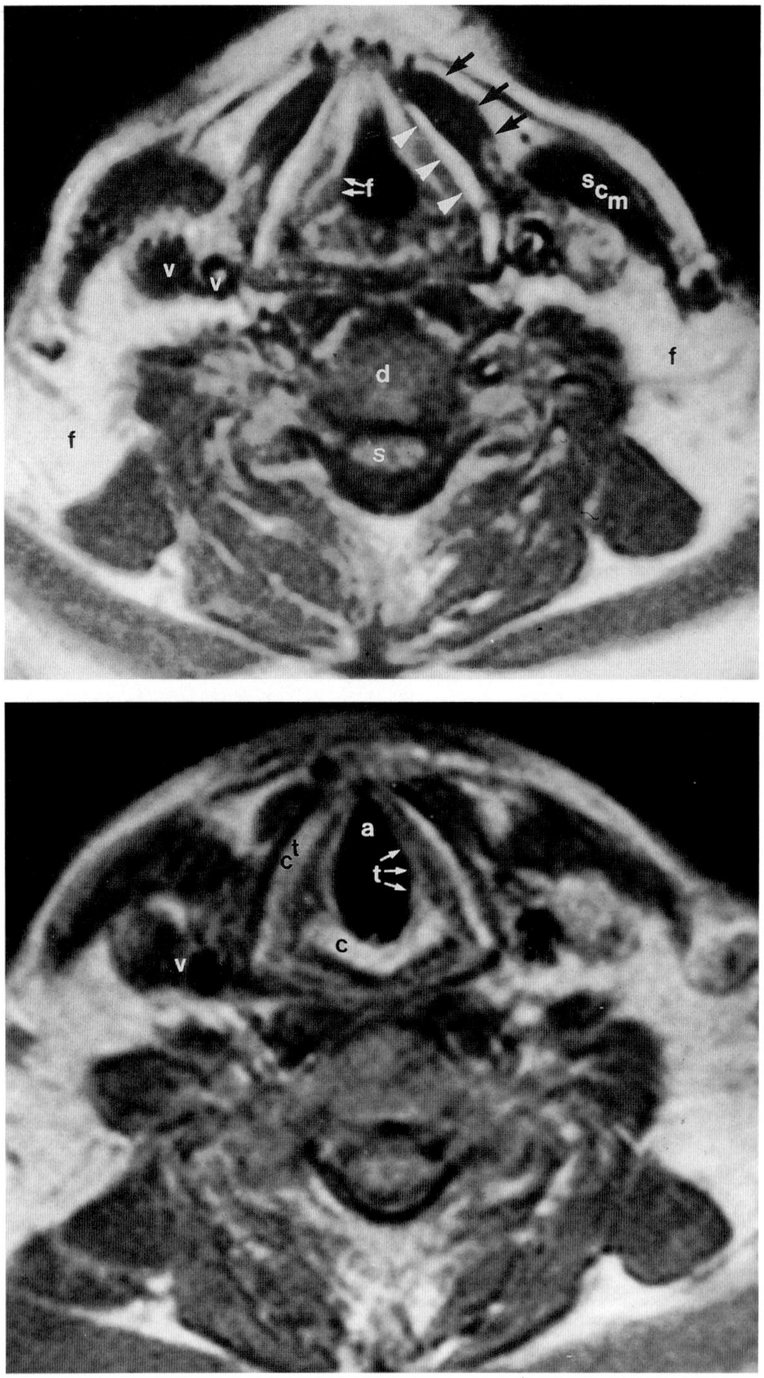

A

B

FIG. 17. Normal MRI. **A:** False cords. Same level on MRI shows the fat-filled centers of the thyroid cartilage are brightly imaged (*arrowheads*), but the cartilage itself appears as a black space (*black arrows*). White f, false cords; v, vascular bundle; d, disk material; s, spinal cord; black f, fat of the neck; scm, sternocleidomastoid muscle. **B:** True cords. Corresponding MRI shows the true cords. tc, fat of the thyroid cartilage; c, fat of the cricoid cartilage; t, true cords; a, airway; v, vascular bundle.

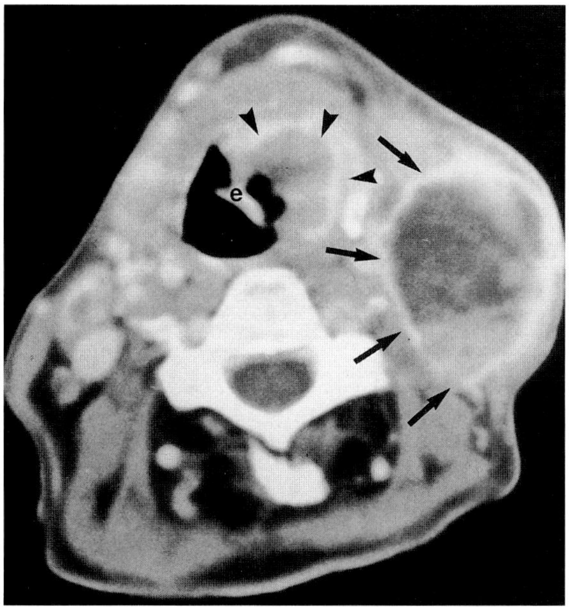

A

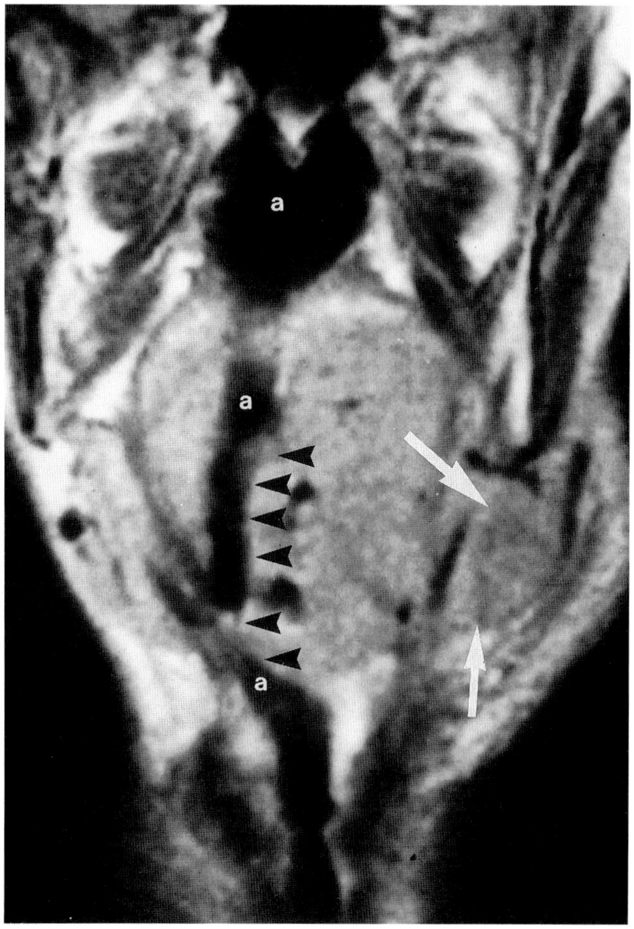

B

FIG. 18. Squamous cell carcinoma. **A:** CT scan demonstrates that the mucosal extent of the tumor results in a marked asymmetry and irregularity of the airway, with the epiglottis (e) shifted to the right. The tumor mass extends across the midline to the right side (*arrowheads*). In addition, there is a huge metastatic lymph node mass with an enhancing rim and low density center (*arrows*). **B:** Coronal MR images demonstrate the masses encircling the airway (a), resulting in its deviation to the right (*arrowheads*). The anteriormost portion of the lymph node mass is also identified (*arrows*).

portion of the tumor has crossed the midline or involves the carotid artery or jugular vein, and it detects the presence of surrounding lymph node metastasis.

Tumors of the larynx are most commonly malignant. CT and MRI have greatly improved the preoperative staging by defining the extent in the cephalocaudal and ventral dorsal directions (Figs. 18A and B). They can help the surgeon determine if a partial or complete laryngectomy will be needed (10).

CT most recently has been helpful in confirming that the airway in patients with sleep apnea is indeed anatomically narrower than in normal control patients. It is postulated that this anatomic narrowing predisposes to airway obstruction during sleep when neural compensation may be stifled (11). Sleep apnea occurs from pharyngeal obstruction that is probably both physiologic and anatomic in its origin. The obstruction is at the level of the soft palate as the tongue falls back to meet the posterior pharynx. The pharynx just below this level collapses as a result of the more superior obstruction (12,13). Marked hypertrophy of the adenoids and tonsils may produce the same obstructive pattern during sleep.

THE CERVICAL SPINE

Normal Presentation

The cervical spine consists of seven vertebrae articulating with the occiput above and the T1 vertebral body

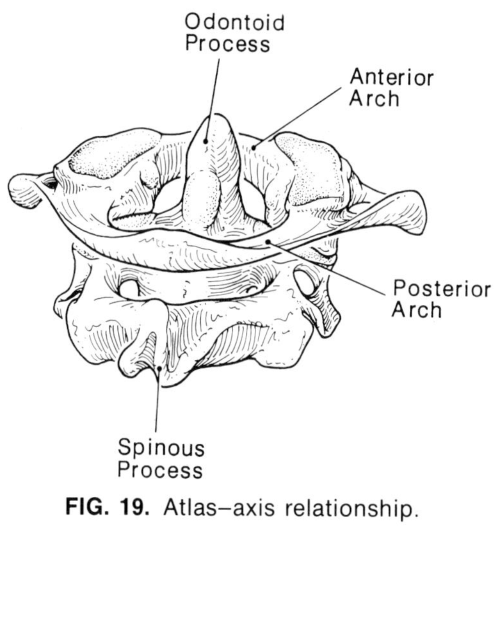

FIG. 19. Atlas–axis relationship.

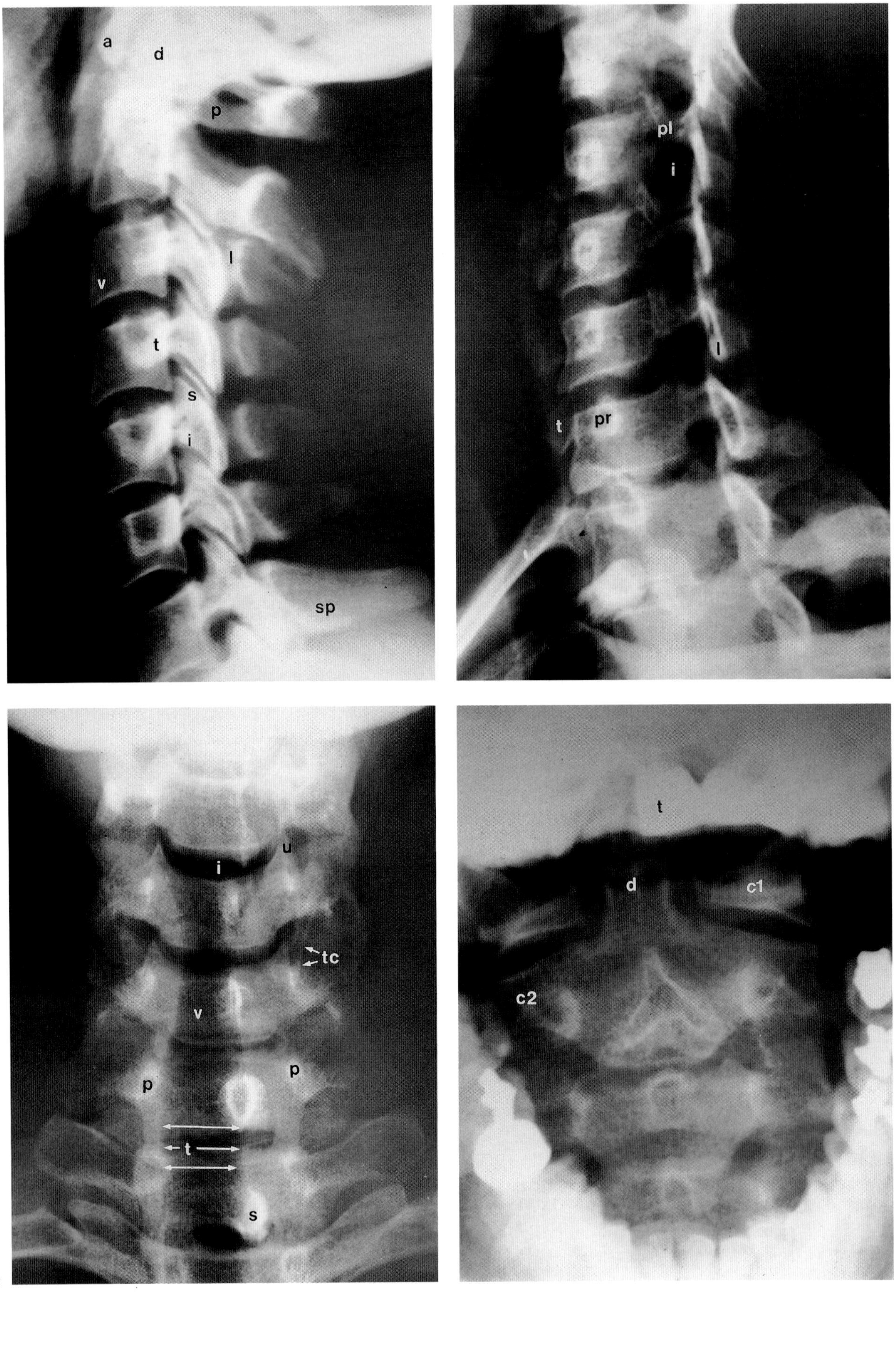

A B C D

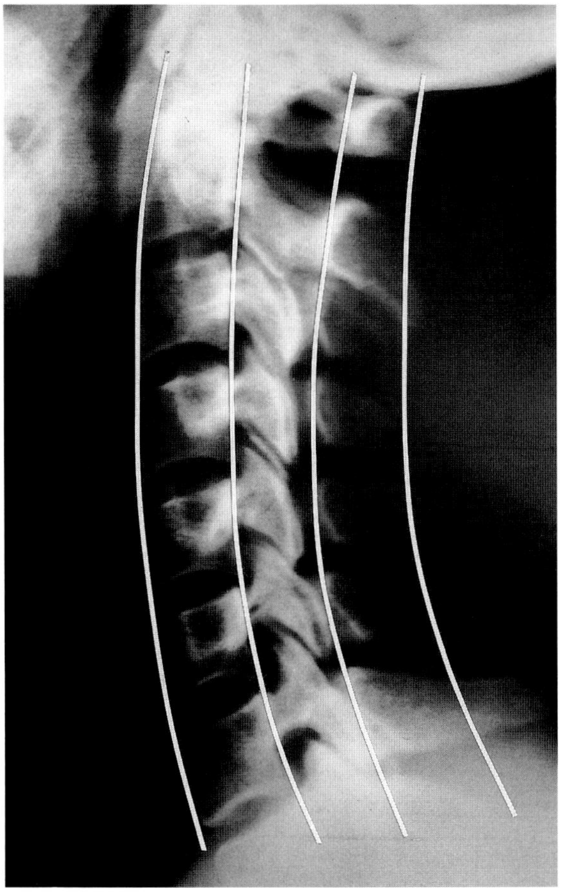

FIG. 21. Four lines of alignment of the lateral cervical spine.

below. The bony anatomy of the cervical spine is somewhat complicated by the unique structure of C1 (atlas) and C2 (axis). The atlas is unique in that it lacks a true vertebral body or spinous process and is basically ring shaped. The anterior portion of the ring contains a groove for the dens or odontoid process of the axis. The dens is a unique feature of the axis (Fig. 19). The dens appears as a toothlike projection from the superior surface of the vertebral body of the axis for its articulation with the anterior arch of the atlas. The bony spinal canal of C2 and the remainder of the cervical vertebrae (C3–C7) is formed by the pedicles and lamina, and conforms to a more consistent shape with similar bony landmarks. The vertebral bodies articulate with one another anteriorly by the intervertebral discs, and posteriorly by the facets. The routine cervical spine exam consists of a lateral film demonstrating all seven cervical bodies, along with right and left 30° oblique views, an anteroposterior (AP) view, and an open mouth view to demonstrate the relationship of the odontoid process to the atlas (Figs. 20A–D).

Flexion and extension occur between the atlas and the base of the skull, while rotation takes place between the axis and the atlas. The gap between the occiput and posterior tubercle of the atlas varies greatly among individuals (14). Reduction of this gap, and, to a lesser extent, the C1-C2 interspinous gap, will decrease the degree of extension of the head and has been suggested as a cause of difficult rigid laryngoscopy and tracheal intubation (14,15).

Many different ligaments stabilize the spine. These ligaments are the supraspinous ligament, the interspinous ligament, the anterior and posterior longitudinal ligaments, the capsule of the interfacetal joints, and the ligamentum flavum. Four "lines" can be traced joining the different vertebral levels. These lines consist of points adjoining the anterior surface of the vertebral bodies, the posterior surface of the vertebral bodies, and points adjoining the anteriormost portion and posteriormost portion of the spinous processes (Fig. 21). Any disruption in these lines signifies ligamentous injury (subluxation/dislocation) with shift of the vertebral bodies.

Cervical Trauma

Soft tissue swelling of the prevertebral space of greater than 7 mm at C3 or C4 is often the first clue to significant trauma and should be sought out. A simple sprain or "whiplash" injury consists of stretching of the ligaments beyond their normal limits, with surrounding hemorrhage. The cervical spine films are usually normal. More severe trauma may result in a tear of the spinous ligaments. Bony fracture usually occurs in association with ligamentous injury, but ligamentous injury can occur without significant bony trauma. Fractures of the bony elements of the cervical spine are classified as stable or unstable. The stable injury is one in which the patient initially has no, or perhaps

FIG. 20. Normal cervical spine—plain film. **A:** Lateral view. d, dens of axis (C2); a, anterior arch of C1; p, posterior arch of C1; v, vertebral body of C3; l, lamina of C3; t, transverse process of C4; s, superior articulating facet of C5; i, inferior articulating facet of C5; sp, spinous process of C7. **B:** Oblique view. pr, pedicle of C7 (*right*); l, lamina of C6; i, intervertebral foramen of C4-5; pl, pedicle of C4 (*left*); t, transverse process of C7. **C:** Frontal view. i, intervertebral disc space of C3-4; u, uncinate process of C4; tc, thyroid cartilage; v, vertebral body of C5; p, pedicle of C6; s, spinous process of C7; t, trachea (*arrows*). **D:** Open mouth view. d, dens of axis (C2); cl, anterior arch of C1; c2, body of C2; t, teeth.

minimal, neurologic symptoms, and movement results in no critical changes. The unstable injury is one in which the patient does indeed have neurologic symptoms and movement might produce further injury (Fig. 22).

If the lateral radiography of the cervical spine shows questionable or unclear findings or is normal but the patient has neurologic changes, conventional tomography may be performed to obtain clear visualization of the bony spine without the details being obscured by overlying bone. This is performed before the patient is allowed to move freely.

CT is now being used more commonly to study the cervical spine in suspected fractures. The cross-sectional or axial format allows easy recognition of fractures, the location of fracture fragments, and bony impingement on the spinal cord. Subtle displacement of facet surfaces or lucent lines through bony structures may be the most subtle findings of significant spinal injury that may be seen on the CT scan but go unnoticed on the plain film (Fig. 23).

Fractures of the dens present a special problem, as they may be difficult to differentiate from the many normal anatomic variations. The open mouth view is helpful in demonstrating a fracture through the base of the dens (Fig. 24). The lateral film will show soft tissue swelling produced anterior to C1 by fractures.

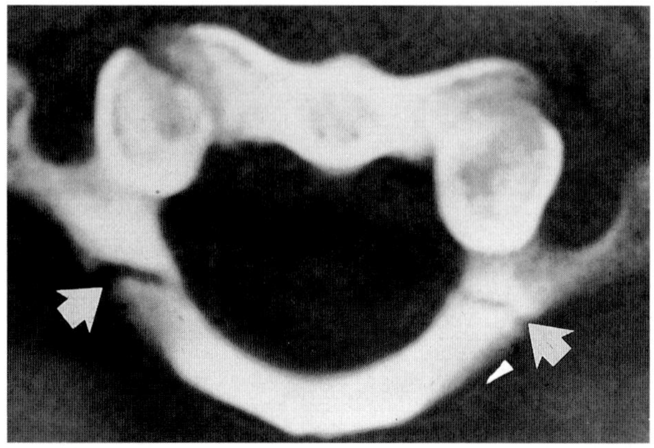

FIG. 23. CT scan of C1. Fractures are present interrupting the posterior arch of C1 (*arrows*).

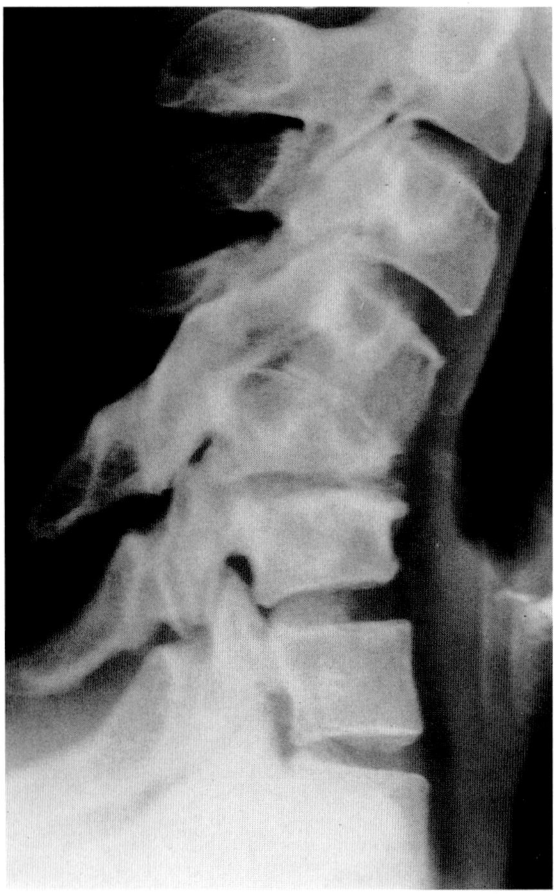

FIG. 22. Tear drop fracture. There is fracture along with compression and subluxation of C5 that resulted in total paralysis of the patient.

Inflammatory Lesions of the Cervical Spine

In an adult, the normal space between the posterior surface of the anterior arch of C1 and anterior surface of the dens is 3 mm. Any increased width in this space may suggest disruption of the transverse ligament that holds the dens in place. This occurs either acutely from trauma or chronically from various inflammatory etiologies, including suppurative pharyngitis, ankylosing spondylitis, and, perhaps the most common, rheumatoid arthritis. Rheumatoid arthritis is the result of

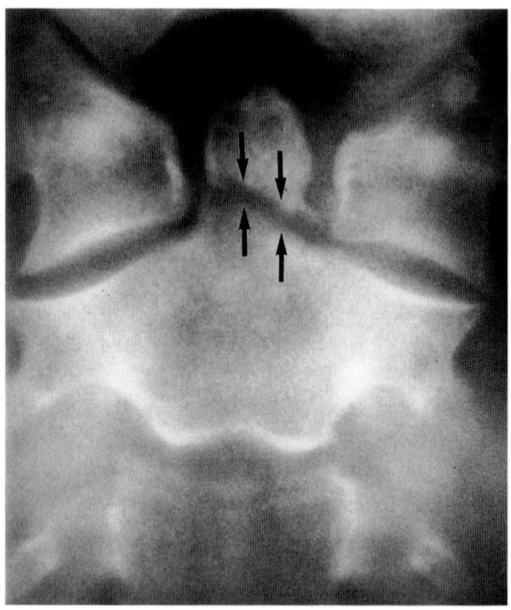

FIG. 24. Fracture of the dens. Frontal tomogram confirms oblique fracture involving the dens (*arrows*).

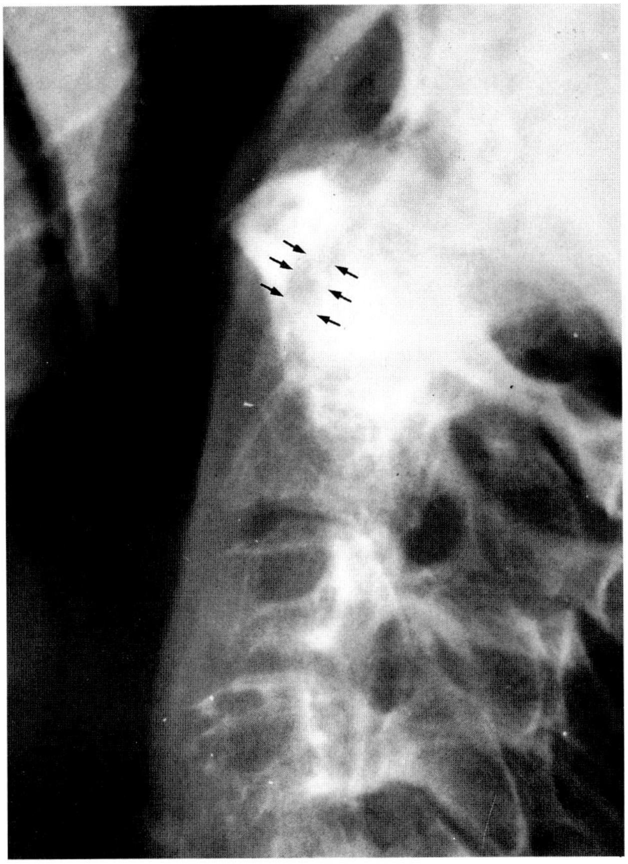

FIG. 25. Rheumatoid arthritis. There is a 5-mm separation between the anterior margin of the dens and the posterior margin of C1 (*arrows*).

chronic inflammation of synovial joints, most commonly affecting the hands. In the spine, this chronic synovitis most commonly involves the transverse ligament about the dens. After long periods of inflammation, the transverse ligament becomes lax, leading to a potential gap between the dens and atlas. This space can be markedly widened, causing atlantoaxial instability, and may be exaggerated when flexion and extension views of the cervical spine are performed (Fig. 25). The inflammation of rheumatoid arthritis also may involve other cervical vertebrae, leading to subaxial instability. The third, but least common, pattern of rheumatoid involvement of the cervical spine is superior migration of the odontoid process resulting from a severe degree of bone erosion (16,17). Superior migration of the dens causes triplane deviation of the larynx and caudal displacement. This makes tracheal intubation extremely difficult. The measurement of the perpendicular distance between the arch of C1 and the pedicle of C2 has been used to document superior migration of the dens. In men this distance is 17 mm and in women 15 mm, with a standard deviation of 2 mm. This space or interval should never measure less than 13 mm (18). Findings of osteoporosis with normal spaces between vertebral bodies suggest that the superior migration of the dens is indeed from rheumatoid arthritis.

Degenerative Arthritis

The most common arthritis to involve the cervical spine is that of simple degenerative arthritis. The degenerative process affects two portions of the spine, the facet joints and the intervertebral disk spaces. The disk material degenerates with age, causing joint space narrowing between the vertebral bodies and secondary osteophyte formation. Osteophytes may project anteriorly, posteriorly, or laterally. A large anterior osteophyte may project toward the airway, causing difficulty in intubation as well as swallowing (Fig. 26). A lateral osteophyte may compress an existing nerve root, leading to a neuropathy. Facet involvement also leads to joint space narrowing along with minimal shift or subluxation of involved vertebral bodies.

THE THORACIC AIRWAY

Plain Chest Radiography

Extension of the airway into the thoracic cavity is easily seen on the plain chest radiograph. If a more detailed view of the airway is required, then conventional tomography or CT may be of value.

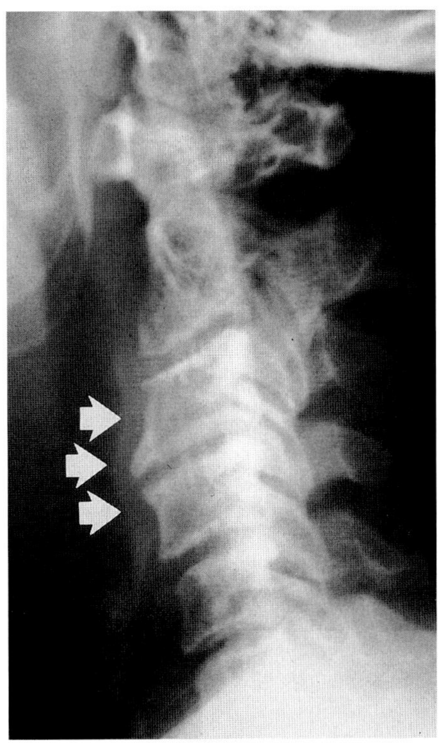

FIG. 26. Degenerative joint disease. Obvious osteophytes project anteriorly from C3 and C4 and indent the airway (*arrows*).

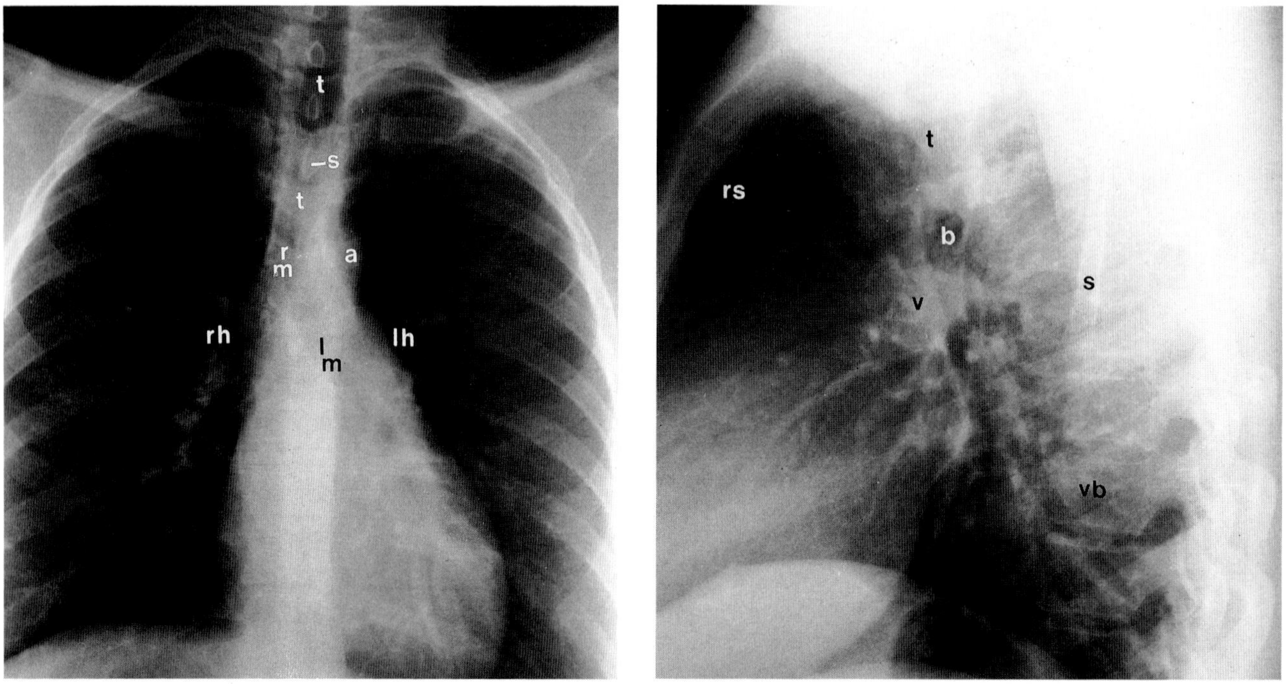

FIG. 27. Normal chest radiograph. **A:** t, trachea; lm, left mainstem bronchus; rm, right mainstem bronchus; a, aortic knob; lh, left hilus; rh, right hilus; s, spinous process. **B:** t, trachea; b, right upper lobe bronchus; v, pulmonary vessels; s, scapula; rs, retrosternal space; vb, vertebral body.

Chest films are usually obtained in the PA (frontal) and lateral directions to ensure an undistorted two-dimensional view of the mediastinum and lungs (Figs. 27A and B). The trachea usually takes a straight course and should be centered over the spinous processes, but on occasion it may make a slight curve to the right if displaced by the aortic arch. In older patients, the arch may be ectatic, and the prominent arch causes the trachea to be shifted to the right even more than expected (Fig. 28). The trachea bifurcates to form the carina at about the T5–T7 level. Normally, the carina forms a 40–70° angle as it splits to form the right and left mainstem bronchi (18).

Computed Tomography of the Chest

On CT scan, the thoracic portion of the trachea is round in cross section. It is important to identify the surrounding anatomy, which includes the thyroid, great vessels of the aortic arch, and esophagus (Fig. 29A). The pretracheal, paratracheal, and subcarinal spaces are normally fat-filled areas that contain important lymph nodes. Nodes under 1 cm in size are considered normal (Figs. 29B and C).

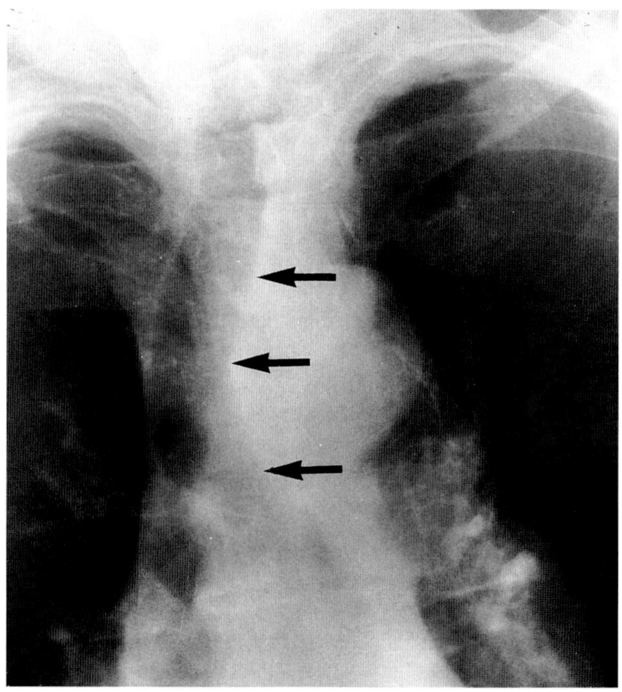

FIG. 28. Airway shift secondary to ectatic aorta. The trachea is shifted far to the right by the ectatic aorta (*arrows*).

FIG. 29. Normal CT of the chest. **A:** a, airway; t, thyroid; l, apex of left lung; r, ribs; s, scapula. **B:** a, airway; l, lung fields; v, great vessels; rp, right paratracheal space, fat-filled. **C:** c, carina; pt, pretracheal space; aa, ascending aorta; da, descending aorta; pa, pulmonary arteries.

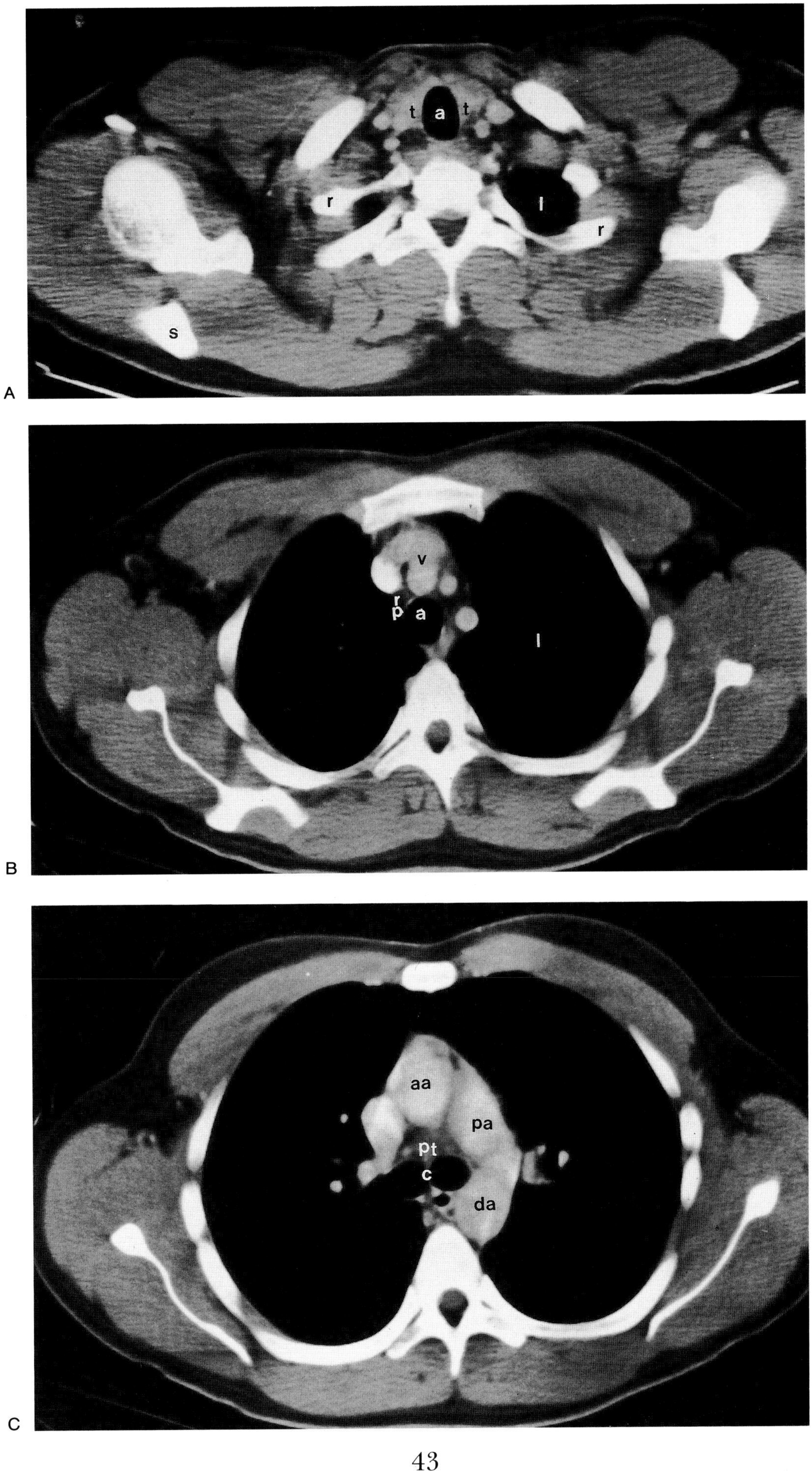
t
a
t
r
l
r
s
A
v
r
p
a
l
B
aa
pa
pt
c
da
C

The right and left mainstem bronchi and their more peripheral branches can be seen on either plain film or CT. Careful inspection of the bronchial lumen for endobronchial tumors must always be made. Secondary atelectasis or collapse may be the only sign of an endobronchial mass on chest radiograph or CT scan.

PATHOLOGIC PROCESS

One potential problem in intubation may be a shift of normal tracheal position from various causes including atelectasis, extrinsic compression, pneumonectomy, lobectomy, and pneumothorax. Atelectasis leading to volume loss is probably the most common cause of mediastinal shift. The mediastinum, along with the trachea, moves to the collapsed side. While the causes of atelectasis are many (endobronchial tumor, mucous plug, etc.), the appearance is consistent. First, the collapsed segment or lobe is identified as an airless radiopaque, often triangular, density. Because this is frequently mistaken for an infiltrate on a single view of the chest, both frontal and lateral films may be needed to identify the collapse.

Tumors

The trachea or bronchi may be narrowed or deformed by enlargement of the various neighboring structures, making intubation difficult. Benign or malignant processes of the thyroid or esophagus may secondarily encase or impinge on the trachea (Fig. 16A). More commonly, enlarged lymph nodes of the mediastinum deform or flatten the trachea. The adenopathy may be the result of sarcoidosis or an infectious etiology, but metastatic carcinoma and/or lymphoma are the more important etiologies (19). Adenopathy frequently results in focal deformity of the airway but may encase entire segments of the trachea or bronchi (Fig. 30).

Postpneumonectomy or Lobectomy

Pneumonectomy or lobectomy may also result in alterations of alignment of the airway. With pneumonectomy, the mainstem bronchus of that side is obviously absent. The empty hemithorax fills with fluid, and the contralateral lung overinflates to help fill the void. The mediastinum and trachea shift to the pneumonectomy side as a result of the loss of volume (Fig. 31). With lobectomy, this shift of the airway is less pronounced, as the remaining lobes on the operative side also hyperinflate to help fill the newly created space. Also with a lobectomy, there is a shift of second-order bronchi, as the remaining lobes shift position within the hemithorax.

Pneumothorax

A pneumothorax can result in a shift of the mediastinum to the side of the contralateral lung, resulting in

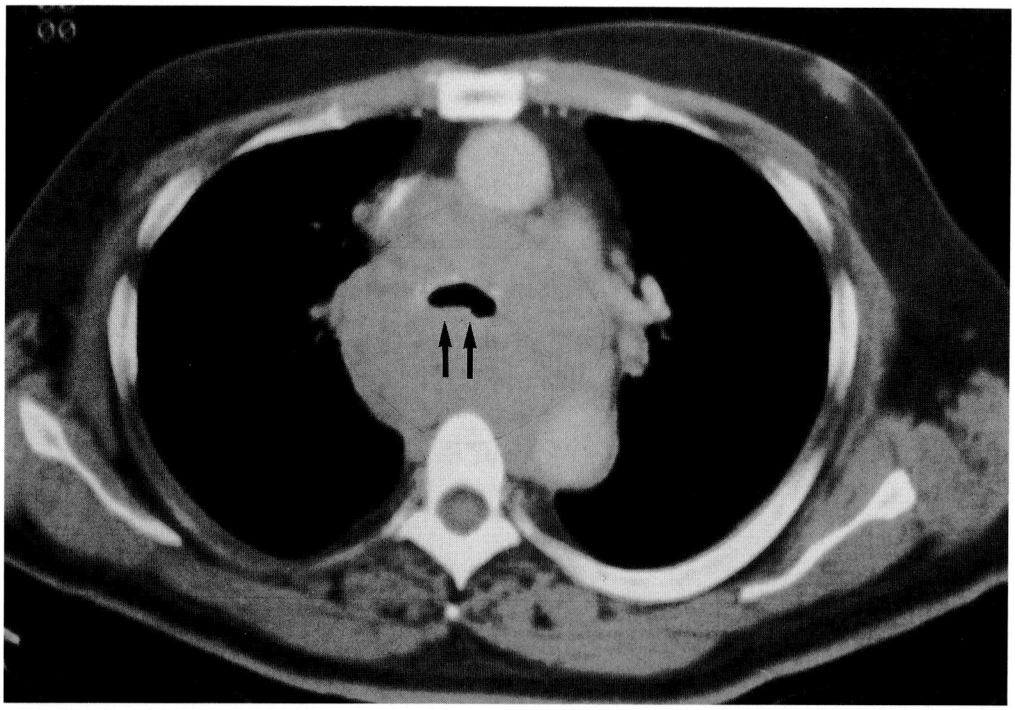

FIG. 30. Adenopathy compressing the airway. A large mass of adenopathy from lymphoma elevates and compresses the airway at the carina (*arrows*).

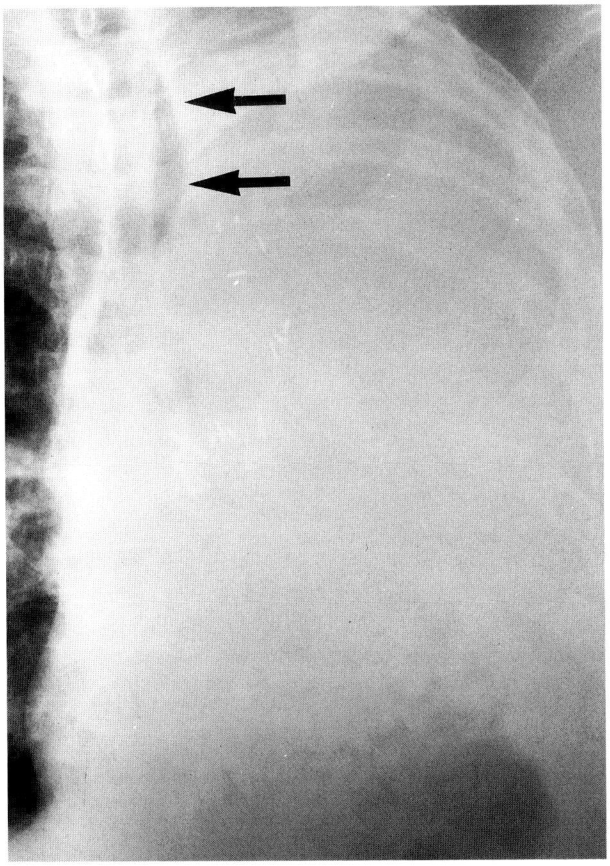

FIG. 31. Pneumonectomy. There is complete opacification of the left hemithorax. There is volume loss on the left, evidenced by shift of the airway (*arrows*) and heart to the left and elevation of the stomach bubble.

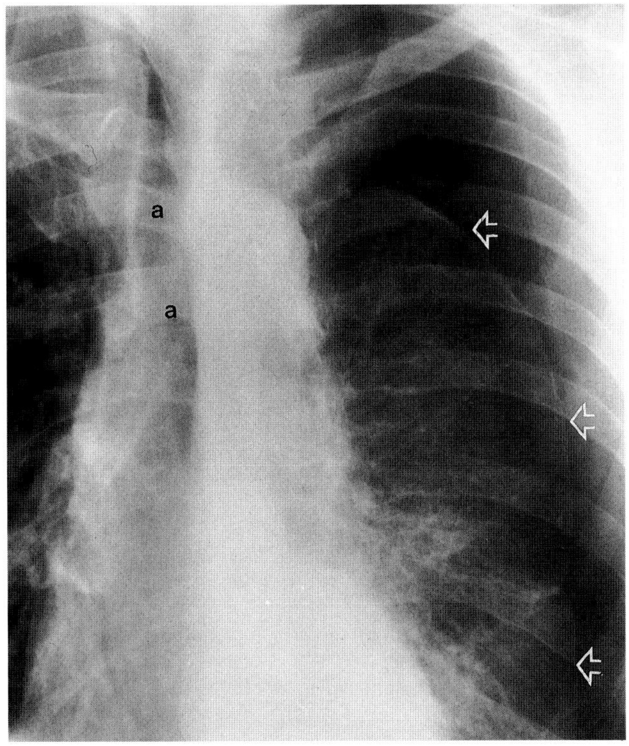

FIG. 32. Pneumothorax. The heart and airway are shifted to the right. The thin white line of the visceral pleura is identified (*open arrows*). a, airway.

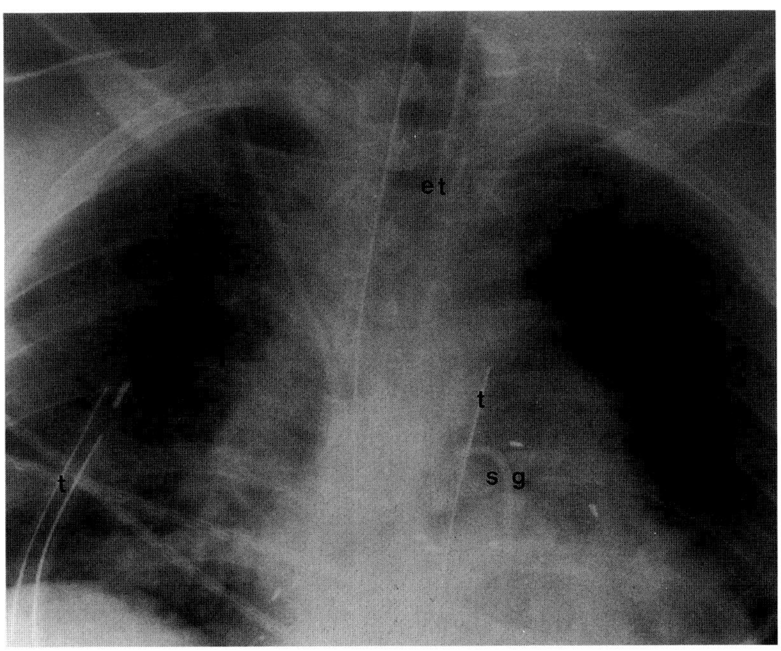

FIG. 33. Postcoronary artery bypass radiograph. An endotracheal tube (et) is in place in the midthoracic along with a Swan-Ganz catheter (sg) and chest tubes (t). Some infiltrate is present in both lower lobes, signifying some postoperative congestive heart failure.

a finding similar to that seen in atelectasis or after pneumonectomy. In addition, with a pneumothorax, the thin white line of the visceral pleural is visible along with loss of the more distal lung markings, which secure the diagnosis. If a tension pneumothorax develops, the airway will be shifted away from the collapsed lung by the increased intrathoracic pressure (Fig. 32).

Tracheal Tube Position

Finally, the chest film is important for detecting the position of various tubes and lines placed in a critically ill patient. A chest radiograph is often obtained after an endotracheal tube is inserted. Ideally, the tip of the tube should be about 3 to 5 cm from the carina (Fig. 33). This distance is chosen because, with flexion of the head, the tip of the tube often moves distally and may enter the right mainstem bronchus with secondary collapse of the nonaerated left lung (20).

REFERENCES

1. Lawson VG, Leleiever WC, Makerewich LA, et al. Unusual parapharyngeal lesions. *J. Otolaryngol* 1979;8:241–249.
2. Gehweiler JA, Osborne RL, Becker RF. *The radiology of vertebral trauma.* Philadelphia: W. B. Saunders, 1980.
3. Holinger PH, Lutterbeck EF, Bulger R. Xeroradiography of the larynx. *Ann Otol* 1972;81:806–808.
4. Moorthy SS, LoSasso AM, King H, Franken E. Evaluation of larynx and trachea by xeroradiography. *Anesth Analg* 1976;55: 598–600.
5. Levy AM, Tabakin BS, Hanson JS, Narkewicz RM. Hypertrophied adenoids causing pulmonary hypertension and severe congestive heart failure. *N Engl J Med* 1967;277:506–511.
6. Diaz JH, Lockhart CH. Early diagnosis and airway management of acute epiglottitis in children. *South Med J* 1982;75:399–403.
7. Watts FB Jr, Slovis TL. The enlarged epiglottis. *Pediatr Radiol* 1977;5:133.
8. Mancuso AA, Hansberger HR, Muraki A, Stevens MH. Computed tomography of cervical and retropharyngeal lymph nodes: normal anatomy, variance of normal, and applications in staging head and neck cancer. *Radiology* 1983;148:709–723.
9. Batsakis JG. *Tumors of the head and neck: clinical and pathological considerations,* 2nd ed. Baltimore: Williams & Wilkins, 1979.
10. Mancuso AA, Hanafee WN, Juillard GJF, et al. The role of computed tomography in the management of cancer of the larynx. *Radiology* 1977;24:243–244.
11. Haponik EF, Smith PL, Bohlman ME, et al. Computerized tomography in obstructive sleep apnea. Correlation of airway size with physiology during sleep and wakefulness. *Am Rev Respir Dis* 1983;127:221–226.
12. Suratt PM, Dee P, Atkinson RL, et al. Fluoroscopic and computed tomographic features of the pharyngeal airway in obstructive sleep apnea. *Am Rev Respir Dis* 1983;127:487–492.
13. Weitzman E, Pollack CP, Borowiecki B, et al. The hypersomnia-sleep apnea syndrome: site and mechanism of upper airway obstruction. In: Guilleminault C, Dement WC, eds. *Sleep apnea syndromes.* New York: Alan R. Liss, 1978;235–246.
14. Nichol HC, Zuck D. Difficult laryngoscopy—the "anterior" larynx and the atlanto-occipital gap. *Br J Anaesth* 1983;55:141–143.
15. White A, Kander PL. Anatomical factors in difficult direct laryngoscopy. *Br J Anaesth* 1975;47:468–473.
16. Keenan MA, Stiles CM, Kaufman RL. Acquired laryngeal deviation associated with cervical spine disease in erosive polyarticular arthritis. Use of the fiberoptic bronchoscope in rheumatoid disease. *Anesthesiology* 1983;58:441–449.
17. Ranawat CS, O'Leary P, Pellici P, et al. Cervical spine fusion in rheumatoid arthritis. *J Bone Joint Surg* 1979;61:1003–1010.
18. Pare JA, Fraser RG. *Diagnosis of diseases of the chest.* Philadelphia: W. B. Saunders, 1977;56.
19. Baron RL, Levitt RG, Sagel SS, et al. Computed tomography in the preoperative evaluation of bronchogenic carcinoma. *Radiology* 1982;145:727–732.
20. Goodman LR, Putman CE. *Intensive care radiology: imaging of the critically ill.* Philadelphia: W. B. Saunders, 1983;19–22.

CHAPTER 4

Topical Anesthesia of the Airway

Andranik Ovassapian, M.D.

The most essential step in performing a smooth awake tracheal intubation requires establishing good topical anesthesia of the respiratory tract (1). This is important to prevent coughing, undue swallowing, laryngeal spasm, and excessive salivation. All of these factors may contribute to increasing the difficulty of completing an awake fiberoptic intubation.

Awake airway instrumentation must be made painless and nonstressful, especially in those who may need repeated operations. Topical anesthetization of the mucous membranes of the respiratory tract is simple and effective and eliminates pharyngeal, laryngeal, and tracheobronchial reflexes. Despite widespread use, topical anesthetics are too often used without careful consideration of their pharmacologic properties, resulting in both inadequate anesthesia and excessive quantities of the drug being used. The respiratory tract mucous membranes rapidly absorb these agents, making overdose a likelihood under these circumstances.

For stress-free instrumentation of the airway one should be familiar with the physiology of airway reflexes, the effect of age and various medications on airway reflexes, and different methods of achieving topical anesthesia of the airway.

AIRWAY REFLEXES

The presence of airway reflexes is important in protection of the airway. However, to accomplish a stress-free tracheal intubation or fiberoptic airway endoscopy in an awake patient, airway reflexes must be suppressed (1).

Mechanical and chemical irritation of the laryngeal and nasal mucosa to produce reflex glottic closure was first demonstrated by Kratschmer in 1870 (Kratschmer reflex) (2). The reflex is mediated through stimulation of receptors located in the hypopharynx and the larynx (3). The afferent nerve pathways travel in the parasympathetic and sympathetic nervous system producing a motor response, causing temporary closure of the larynx (4).

It was demonstrated later that the laryngeal motor response to inhaled ammonia vapor was abolished by sectioning the superior laryngeal nerve (5). Vocal cord adduction takes place before a given noxious stimulus is strong enough to elicit a cough response (6).

The protective laryngeal reflexes decrease with advancing age (7,8) and also in patients following tracheal intubation (3). The reflexes may remain depressed up to 4 hr after intravenous injection of 15 mg diazepam (9). A significant depression of upper airway reflex sensitivity from 30–150 min occurs after administration of 20 mg of diazepam taken orally (10). Such patients are therefore at increased risk of aspirating despite the appearance of recovery from its sedative effects.

Topical anesthesia of the larynx does not impair voluntary motor function of the vocal cords, such as coughing on request (12). This may have important clinical implications for patients at high risk for aspiration, such as those undergoing tracheal intubation under topical anesthesia with light sedation. These patients are able to close their vocal cords voluntarily if instructed to do so, or if aware of the presence of food or liquids in the mouth.

LOCAL ANESTHETICS USED FOR TOPICAL ANESTHESIA

The judicious use of local anesthetics requires a sound knowledge of their pharmacology as well as of their proper application. The local anesthetic drugs block nerve conduction by preventing depolarization of the nerve membrane that follows influx of sodium ions through the fast sodium channels. Local anesthetic molecules interfere with the conformational changes needed for fast channels to open (13), thereby preventing the influx of sodium.

Most local anesthetics used today are tertiary amines, with an ester or amide linkage separating the hydrophilic amine from the lipophilic aromatic portion. They are usually weak bases, their dissociation constants (pK_a) being on the basic side. The pK_a is defined as the pH at which 50% of the drug is an uncharged base (un-ionized) and 50% an ionized salt. In this form, they are poorly soluble in water and rather unstable when exposed to air (13,14).

To be useful clinically, local anesthetics are prepared as water-soluble salts, usually of hydrochloric acid; therefore they are acidic and stable. When injected or topically applied, they are buffered within the tissues that release free base, which, being lipid-soluble, penetrates nerve tissues to cause anesthesia. The potency and delay of onset of the agents are related to their lipid solubility and pK_a, respectively. At lower pK_a's, more drug is present as un-ionized base at normal body pH; therefore, the onset of nerve block is quicker. When the pH of tissue and its buffering capacity are decreased, the release of free base is slowed. Infection lowers tissue pH to 6.0 or less, decreases release of active free base, and delays onset of action of the drug.

Topical local anesthetics are less effective because of the diminished buffering capacity of the mucous membranes, which limits release of the anesthetic base. To compensate for this, a higher concentration of drug must be used. Also, cilia and secretions are present, both barriers to the penetration of drugs. Although any local anesthetic agent can be used topically, the high concentrations needed for some to be effective make their use dangerous and impractical (15% mepivacaine and 20% procaine) (13,14).

The principles and guidelines for the safe use of local anesthetic agents for producing topical anesthesia have been summarized by Adriani and associates (15). It is essential to know the optimum effective concentration of each drug, the rapidity of onset of action, the recommended maximum safe dose, the rate of absorption from mucous membranes, and the appropriate techniques for application. The onset time shortens and the duration of anesthesia lengthens as the concentration of drug is increased (15). However, the maximally effective concentration is not necessarily either safe or recommended. For example, cocaine is maximally effective at 15–20% concentration, far in excess of the 4–10% recommended clinically. Combining two local anesthetics at their maximally effective concentrations neither improves nor prolongs the duration of topical anesthesia. However, systemic effects of the two drugs are additive and increase the possibility of systemic toxicity (16). In a mixture of short- and long-acting drugs, the duration of anesthesia will be that of the longer acting drug. Benzocaine, with its rapid onset, and tetracaine, with its prolonged action, complement each other.

The rate and amount of topical anesthetic absorbed vary according to the site of application, the dose of the drug, and individual variation (17,18). Absorption is more rapid from alveoli than from the tracheobronchial tree, and more rapid from the tracheobronchial tree than from the pharynx. Vasoconstrictors added to local anesthetics used for topical anesthesia neither slow the absorption nor prolong the duration of anesthesia (15). Plasma levels rise more rapidly after topical application to the respiratory tract than after injection into tissue; therefore, recommended doses of topical anesthetics for use within the respiratory tract are approximately one-half of the same drug injected into tissue.

The four most commonly used local anesthetics for topical anesthesia are lidocaine, cocaine, tetracaine, and benzocaine.

Lidocaine

Lidocaine, the first amide local anesthetic introduced into clinical practice (1940s), is the most widely used local anesthetic. Lidocaine is used extensively for topical anesthesia of the respiratory tract during fiberoptic bronchoscopy and awake tracheal intuba-

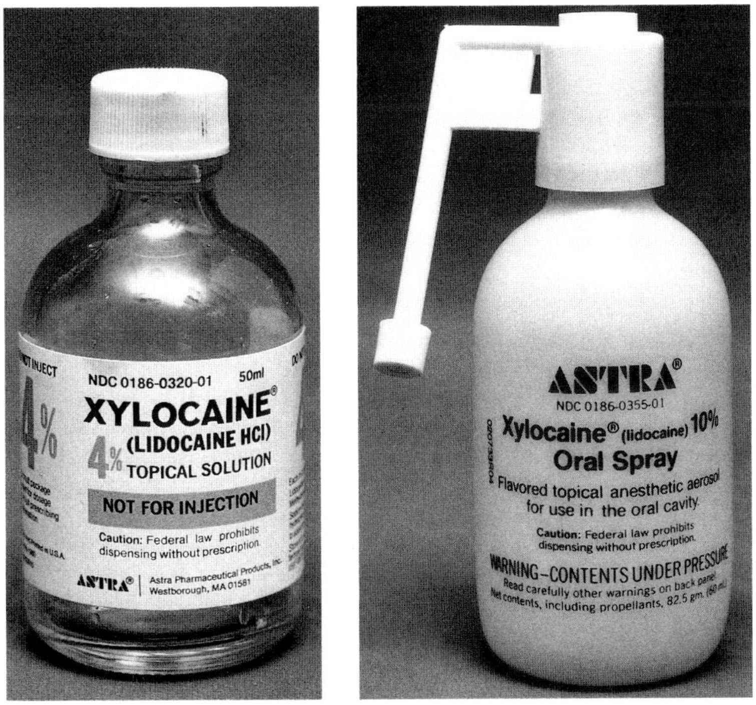

A,B

FIG. 1. Lidocaine preparations. **A:** Lidocaine 4% topical solution. **B:** Lidocaine 10% aerosol for nasal and oropharyngeal use.

tion. The drug can be delivered to the upper and lower airway by several methods in various preparations.

It is less toxic than tetracaine and cocaine and has shorter duration of action. Lidocaine is available in 0.5, 1, 2, and 4% solutions, 2% viscous solution, 10% aerosol preparation, and 2.5 and 5% ointment (Fig. 1). The 4% solution provides 15–20 min of topical anesthesia and is frequently applied to the larynx and trachea prior to tracheal intubation. While the 2% solution provides topical anesthesia, it is much less reliable than the 4% solution yet is useful in the distal bronchial tree and in children to avoid overdosage. Ten percent aerosol is available for spraying the oro- and nasopharynx; each depression of the release button delivers 0.1 ml (10 mg) of lidocaine. Two percent viscous solutions are used as gargles to induce topical anesthesia of the oropharynx.

Lidocaine is absorbed by the mucous membranes of the respiratory tract, gastrointestinal tract (19,20), rectum (21), and bladder (22,23). It is also absorbed through open and burned skin (24).

The rate and extent of lidocaine absorption from the respiratory tract depends on the area and method of application, and whether the patient is breathing spontanously or is anesthetized and on controlled ventilation. Peak plasma concentration levels are reached within 40–90 min with nasopharyngeal application, and 5–30 min following oropharyngeal, laryngeal and tracheal spraying (25). Intranasally applied lidocaine gel has the lowest absorption rate (26–28), and patients prefer lidocaine gel for nasopharyngeal anesthesia over that of aerosol or lidocaine solution (27).

The upper respiratory tract has a smaller surface area, and is less vascular than the lower airway. A fraction of lidocaine sprayed in the oropharynx is removed when suctioning secretions (28). In addition, some of the lidocaine sprayed into the oropharynx is swallowed, undergoing first pass metabolism in the liver with 70% being metabolized (29). The plasma level of lidocaine is therefore lower with upper airway application compared to that of lower airway application (30). Laryngotracheal application of lidocaine results in a lower plasma concentration of lidocaine than intravenous administration (31–33).

The maximum dose of lidocaine recommended for topical application to the respiratory tract is between 200–250 mg (3–4 mg/kg). Efthimiou reports that a lidicaine dose of 9.3 mg/kg produced mean plasma levels of 2.9 mg/l in 41 patients undergoing fiberoptic bronchoscopy. In two patients receiving a total of 12mg/kg of lidocaine (27), plasma lidocaine levels exceeded 5 mg/l with no clinical signs of toxicity developing.

After absorption, lidocaine is rapidly distributed into vessel-rich tissues, followed by redistribution into tissues with slower equilibration (19). The blood concentration is related to the total dose used, regardless of concentration of the solution (34,35). In conscious subjects, toxic symptoms may appear at plasma levels exceeding 5 μg/ml (36). Lidocaine, like most amide local anesthetics, is almost exclusively metabolized by hepatic microsomes; less than 10% of lidocaine is excreted unchanged in the urine, and a small amount is excreted in bile. About 70% of lidocaine is removed from blood in one passage through the liver. Patients with poor liver function or low hepatic blood flow will develop high lidocaine plasma levels, whereas those with a low cardiac output not only will have a higher plasma level, but also a similar level in the brain and myocardium, as these organs receive a disproportionally larger amount of the cardiac output under these circumstances (37,38). The half-life of lidocaine is approximately 90 min; therefore, a second dose given 90 min after the initial one should be reduced by at least one-half to avoid development of a toxic blood level (37). In patients with chronic liver disease the half-life increases to 300 min. Metabolism of lidocaine is rapid, except in the presence of heart failure and serious hepatic dysfunction. Allergic reactions to lidocaine are rare; therefore, it is a good substitute for ester compounds from which a reaction has occurred.

Cocaine

Cocaine is a natural alkaloid obtained from the leaves of *Erythroxylon coca*. It was the first local anesthetic to be discovered and is the only one that produces both topical anesthesia and vasoconstriction when applied to mucous membranes. As a result, cocaine has been widely used topically for intranasal operations and for nasotracheal intubations (39). Cocaine's vasoconstrictive action results from interference with the reuptake of circulating catecholamines by adrenergic nerve endings (40), the delay elevating blood catecholamine levels. Cocaine should be used cautiously in patients with hypertension, coronary disease, and thyrotoxicosis, and in those taking medications that augment the action of catecholamines, such as monoamine oxidase inhibitors. Cocaine used in conjunction with halothane, an agent that sensitizes the myocardium to catecholamines, may precipitate ventricular arrhythmias. In one study, patients given 150 mg of cocaine topically for laryngoscopy had an increased incidence of cardiac dysrhythmia, tachycardia, and hypertension (41). In another controlled investigation, 1–1.5 mg/kg cocaine applied topically to the nasal mucosa during nitrous oxide and halothane anesthesia did not produce a significant sympathomimetic effect (40).

Cocaine is available in variable strengths; however, 4–5% concentrations are recommended for topical use, allowing 3–5 min for optimal effect; the maximum dose should be 200 mg. While time of onset is shortened if a 10% solution is used, this strength increases the risk of toxicity; thus, it should be avoided. Because cocaine is addictive, some prefer to add phenylephrine to other local anesthetics. A 3 to 1 mixture of 4% lidocaine and 1% phenylephrine (produces 3% and 0.25%) provides both topical anesthesia and vasoconstriction of the nasal mucosa for nasotracheal intubation, thus eliminating the need for cocaine (42).

When cocaine is applied to mucous membranes, systemic absorption occurs. Surveys have revealed that toxic reactions occur more often when cocaine is applied to the tracheobronchial tree than to other mucous membranes (43). The vasoconstrictive effect of cocaine does not retard its absorption through nasal mucous membranes (44), nor does fractional application allow use of a larger total dose, as detoxification occurs slowly. Peak plasma levels of cocaine occur 30–60 min after intranasal application, and the drug persists in plasma for 4–6 hr, in part due to slow absorption (45). Plasma cocaine levels after oral ingestion of cocaine are similar to those after intranasal application, perhaps explained by failure of the liver to metabolize the drug on hepatic first pass (46). This is in contradistinction to lidocaine, which when absorbed from the gastrointestinal tract is 70% metabolized on its first circulatory pass through the liver. This is important clinically; all the cocaine applied within the airway or swallowed will be absorbed and only slowly metabolized, whereas most of the lidocaine swallowed will be detoxified rapidly and does not add appreciably to the plasma lidocaine concentration. Cocaine is hydrolyzed slowly by plasma cholinesterase, and only a small proportion is metabolized in the liver or excreted unchanged (46). Therefore, cocaine must be used cautiously in patients with a plasma cholinesterase deficiency or atypical cholinesterase, and in patients taking cholinesterase inhibitors, such as echothiophate or neostigmine (47,48).

Hypertension, tachycardia, and cardiac arrhythmias are early signs and symptoms of sympathetic stimulation of a cocaine overdosage. Body temperature may rise due to interference with the temperature control center and to increased muscular activity and cutaneous vasoconstriction.

Because it is addicting, cocaine use is controlled by federal regulations and is only recommended for topical anesthesia. The drug has powerful cortical stimulating actions, causing excitement, euphoria, an increase in mental alertness, and elevated capacity for muscular effort. Illicit intranasal use of cocaine has caused severe complications and death from cerebral hemorrhage and ischemia attributed to cerebral vasospasm and rupture of a cerebral aneurysm secondary to a sudden rise in blood pressure (49,50).

Tetracaine

A derivative of *para*aminobenzoic acid, tetracaine is a potent and toxic local anesthetic with a longer duration of action than lidocaine or cocaine. It is used as a topical anesthetic in 0.5–1% concentrations, and 2% solution is available as a constituent in an aerosolized spray of Cetacaine (see Benzocaine, below). Absorption from the respiratory tract mucosa is rapid (17).

When the recommended dose has been exceeded, the first sign of toxicity can be sudden death without prodromal convulsions. The slow rate of hydrolysis by plasma cholinesterase may contribute to a high incidence of reactions. The comparative toxicities of tetracaine, cocaine, and lidocaine have been examined in rabbits after intravenous, intratracheal, intranasal, and intravesical application (51). The rapid rate of absorption of tetracaine is illustrated by the LD_{50} being equal to those after intravenous and intratracheal administration. Cocaine and lidocaine have similar toxicity when injected intravenously, but cocaine is two to three times more toxic than lidocaine when given by other routes. When applied to mucous membranes, toxicity from cocaine is midway between that resulting from most toxic tetracaine and least toxic lidocaine. An injected dose of tetracaine should not exceed 100 mg; therefore, the topically applied dose should be only about one-third that of the injected dose. Weisel and Tella (52) reported seven serious complications in 1000 bronchoscopies when the tetracaine dosage was limited to 40 mg (52). The systemic toxic effects of tetracaine are not easily reversed. Since its therapeutic margin of safety is so narrow, the drug is not recommended for tracheobronchial topical anesthesia.

Today, lidocaine and cocaine appear to be the choices for topical anesthesia, with lidocaine preferred for use in the respiratory tract and cocaine reserved for the nasal mucosa or ear, where vasoconstriction is desirable.

Benzocaine

The ethyl ester of *para*aminobenzoic acid, benzocaine is an ester-type local anesthetic agent, is water-insoluble, and is only useful topically. It is available in 10%, 15%, and 20% concentrations in prescription or nonprescription preparations for cutaneous use or use on mucous membranes. The onset of action is rapid, 15–30 sec, and the effective duration 5–10 min. Because of its short action, benzocaine alone has limited usefulness in endoscopic procedures. However, it can be combined with tetracaine to hasten the onset of anesthesia and prolong the duration of action. A mixture of 14% benzocaine, 2% butamben (butyl ester of *para*aminobenzoic acid), and 2% tetracaine, known as Cetacaine, is useful for oropharyngeal topical anesthesia. Americaine ointment, often used for lubricating endotracheal tubes, is a mixture of 20% benzocaine and 0.1% benzethonium chloride (53) (Fig. 2).

Overdosage of benzocaine can produce marked methhemoglobinemia (54,55). An intratracheal dose of 6 mg/kg produced in dogs up to 30% methhemoglobinemia after 6 hr. Neonates are especially susceptible because fetal hemoglobin is oxidized more readily than adult hemoglobin.

DELIVERY OF TOPICAL ANESTHETICS TO THE AIRWAY

Local anesthetics can be applied to mucous membranes with cotton-tipped applicators or pledgets or sprayed over the mucosa directly or via aerosol inhalation.

Nasal Passage

The passage of an endotracheal tube nasally is the most stimulating and painful part of awake nasotracheal intubation. The advancement of the fiberoptic bronchoscope through the nasal passage is reported as the most unpleasant portion of fiberoptic bronchoscopy (56–60). In addition, trauma to the nasal mucosa and bleeding during nasotracheal intubation is common. The use of vasoconstrictors or cocaine is commonly utilized to minimize the incidence of bleeding during nasal procedures.

The nasal mucosa may be anesthetized by the spraying of local anesthetic liquids, cotton tip applicators, pledgets or local anesthetic gel. If attempted without sedation, patient complaints are high with both lidocaine nasal spray and passing of anesthetic coated applicators through the nasal canal. Patients prefer lidocaine gel to lidocaine spray for nasopharyngeal anesthesia (27,56,60–62). If lidocaine gel is utilized, further spraying with 10% lidocaine on the nasal mucosa adds little to topical anesthesia and is not recommended (63). If topical anesthesia of the airway is applied after sedation is achieved, unpleasant recall is not a significant issue.

Cocaine is the only local anesthetic agent with vasoconstrictive properties, and because of this fact has been widely used in otolaryngology. The combination

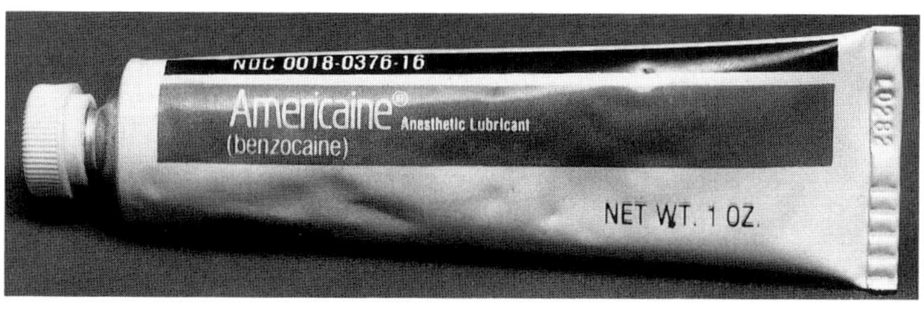

FIG. 2. Americaine ointment used to lubricate tracheal tube and for topical anesthesia of the oropharynx.

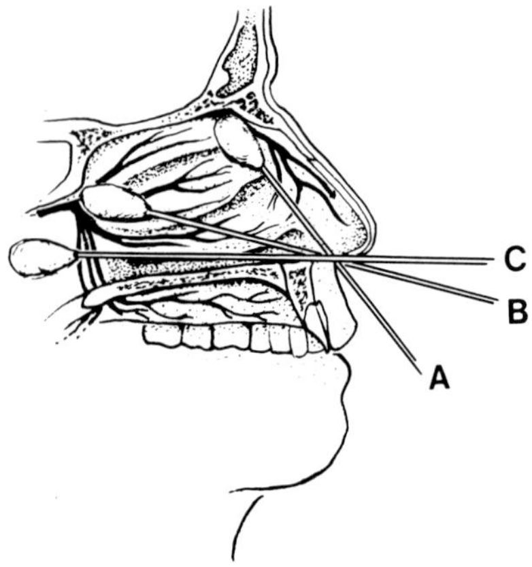

FIG. 3. Positions of cotton-tipped applicators soaked with topical anesthetic solution for producing analgesia of the nasal cavity. **A:** Blocks the branches of ethmoidal nerve. **B:** Blocks the sphenopalatine ganglion and branches of maxillary division of trigeminal nerve. **C:** Demonstrates the passageway for endotracheal tube and provides topical anesthesia for nasopharynx. Smooth, comfortable passage of four applicators tightly held together indicates that endotracheal tube, 7.5 mm internal diameter (ID), should pass with ease.

of neosynephrine and lidocaine is a suitable alternative to cocaine. Phenylnephrine provides rapid vasoconstriction (42), and retards the absorption of concurrently administered local anesthetic agents.

The nasal mucosa may be anesthetized with lidocaine gel, or two to three short sprays of 4–10% lidocaine, prior to the advancement of cotton-tipped applicators soaked with 4% lidocaine. The application of cotton-tipped applicators allows the entire nasotracheal passageway to be contacted and anesthetized. The applicators are also helpful in evaluating the patency of the nasal passage and the angle of endotracheal tube insertion.

To anesthetize the sphenopalatine ganglion and anterior ethmoid nerves, cotton-tipped applicators or pledgets soaked in 4–5% cocaine or a mixture of 3% lidocaine with 0.25% phenylephrine can be placed in the nose (Fig. 3). Allow 5 min for maximal effect; 1 or 2 ml are adequate for anesthetizing one side.

Oropharynx

Pretreatment with glycopyrrolate or atropine is a must to achieve good oropharyngeal topical anesthesia. Local anesthetics work better on dry mucous membrane that is not diluted and washed away by saliva. Increased saliva decreases contact time of local anesthetic with the mucosa and increases the amount swallowed.

A recent study demonstrated that pretreatment with 4 μg/kg of intravenous glycopyrrolate also enhanced the absorption of the lidocaine, and prolonged the analgesic action of topically applied lidocaine to the mucous membrane of the oral cavity (64). The subjects noted dryness of the mouth within 7 min (range 2–15 min) after injection of glycopyrrolate. The effect of topical lidocaine was dissipated in 40 min in patients who were pretreated with glycopyrrolate, compared to 20 min in a control group receiving saline injection.

Either a 4% solution or a 10% aerosol preparation of lidocaine sprayed into the oropharynx will abolish pain sensation and obtund gag and swallowing reflexes. Alternatively, local anesthetics may be applied with cotton swabs or pledgets to the anterior tonsillar pillars and base of the tongue. Lidocaine viscous solution, 2–4 ml gargled for 20–30 sec, will supplement the anesthesia of the oropharynx but is questionable for anesthetizing the hypopharynx, since the isthmus of the oropharynx is closed during gargle, preventing access of the fluid to the posterior pharyngeal wall (53). Local anesthetic jelly or ointment applied to the base of the tongue and anterior tonsillar pillars with a tongue blade will supplement oropharyngeal topical anesthesia.

Larynx and Trachea

Local anesthetics may be applied to the larynx and trachea by a direct spray through the fiberscope (the "spray as you go" technique), by percutaneous transcricothyroid injection, by aerosol inhalation, and by transoral spray using the laryngotracheal topical anesthetic (LTA) kit. Aerosol lidocaine prior to bronchoscopy will reduce the local anesthetic dose required for topical anesthesia of the airway during fiberoptic bronchoscopy (65).

The larynx, situated above the vocal cords, can be anesthetized by bilateral superior laryngeal nerve blocks.

Bronchi

A spray of local anesthetic through the fiberscope or by inhalation of nebulized local anesthetic is the preferred way of anesthetizing bronchial mucosa. The particles should range from 30–60 μ in diameter for best results.

Lidocaine sprayed or instilled to the lower airway can reach the alveoli where absorption is rapid and faster than from bronchi or bronchioles (30,66). Coughing during awake intubation or bronchoscopy limits the amount of lidocaine reaching the alveoli. Blood level of lidocaine is higher when patient is anesthetized (29).

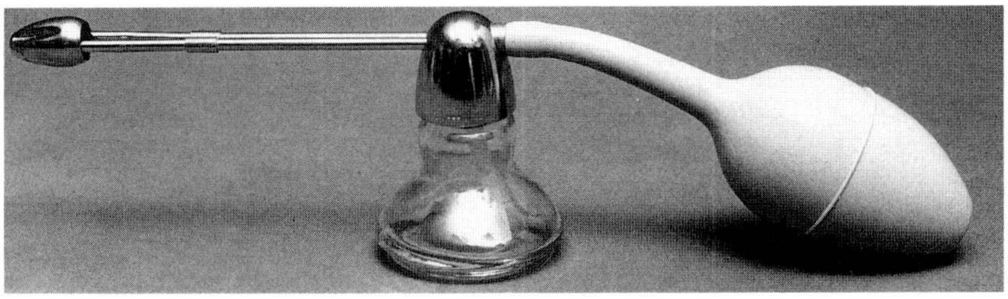

FIG. 4. DeVilbiss adjustable tip atomizer 15. (The DeVilbiss Co., Somerset, Pennsylvania 15501.)

TECHNIQUES OF APPLICATION

Spray

To deliver local anesthetics into the larynx and trachea, sprays and nebulizers with long delivery arms are needed, and a device to allow control of volume and anesthetic dose to be used is advisable (Fig. 4). A disposable prefilled syringe with a long plastic cannula that has multiple perforations at the tip (the LTA kit) is available for this purpose (Fig. 5). With the help of a laryngoscope, the cannula tip is advanced into the trachea under direct vision and the syringe contents quickly emptied to coat the tracheal walls.

The "spray as you go" method involves spraying topical anesthetic through the suction channel of an advancing fiberscope (67). The epiglottis and vocal cords are visualized through the fiberscope and sprayed directly. After 30–45 sec, the fiberscope is advanced into the trachea, and the anterior wall is sprayed. The fiberscope is further advanced toward the carina, and incremental doses of lidocaine are sprayed on the walls of the tracheobronchial tree.

The size of the fiberscope channel is important to this technique. A small suction channel (0.5–1.0 mm) enables the operator to use 0.2 ml of solution at a time, and produces a fine stream that reaches the targeted area. Most adult fiberscopes have larger suction channels (2–2.5 mm). The larger suction channel makes control of the injection stream of the small anesthetic volumes difficult, producing a less uniform spread of the anesthetic solution. This problem is overcome by passing a long angiographic or epidural catheter (internal diameter 0.5–1 mm), cut to the length of the fiberscope through the suction channel, through which the local anesthetic is sprayed (Fig. 6). The placing of a three-way stopcock at the hub of the epidural catheter will allow for suctioning and intermittent spraying without losing anesthetic solution during the suctioning. The three-way stopcock is closed to the syringe containing the anesthetic agent during suctioning and opened during spraying.

The "spray as you go" technique provides flexibility in selectively anesthetizing the respiratory passages. It is ideal for most awake tracheal intubations, especially in patients at risk of aspirating gastric contents. Since the topical anesthetic is applied to the vocal cords and trachea only *after* direct fiberoptic visualization, most of the lower airway is not anesthetized until the last few moments prior to intubation.

The "spray as you go" technique does not provide as good topical anesthesia as the transcricoid injection of lidocaine. In one comparative study the transcricoid technique required a lower dose of lidocaine, the cough rate was less during bronchoscopy, and the procedure was as acceptable to the patient (68) as the "spray as

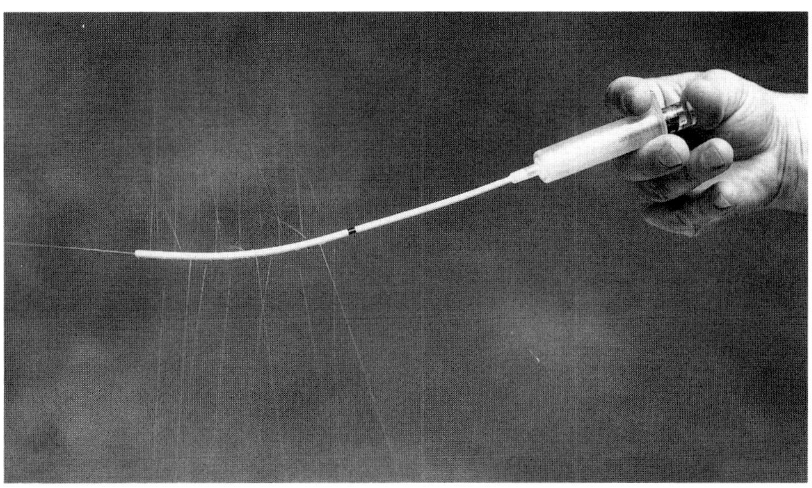

FIG. 5. Laryngotracheal topical anesthetic (LTA) spray kit. (Abbott Laboratories, North Chicago, Illinois.)

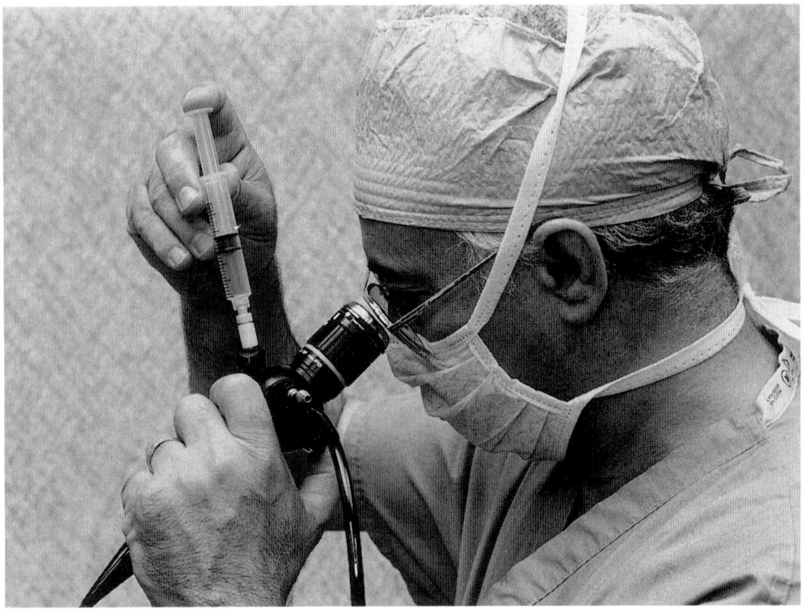

FIG. 6. Demonstrates injection of local anesthetic through epidural catheter, which can be passed through suction channel of the fiberscope.

you go'' technique. The cough induced by transcricoid injection is short lived, and is not associated with unpleasant sensation. The reduced rate of cough is a clear advantage of the cricothyroid injection method (68). In another study comparing transcricoid injection with bronchoscopic injection and nebulized lidocaine for bronchoscopy, both the patients and bonchoscopist preferred transcricoid injection (69).

The upper airway and the larynx usually is not well anesthetized by the ''spray as you go'' or nebulizer technique (69). However, transcricothyroid injection has more potential complications, but major complications are rare. Minimal mucosal bleeding at the needle entrance side is common. Occasionally blood from the puncture site trickles down the trachea, but does not produce any clinical problem in the patient with normal coagulation.(69)

Superior Laryngeal Nerve Block

These nerves can be blocked either topically or by infiltration. The internal branch of the superior laryngeal nerve, which supplies sensory innervation to the laryngeal mucosa, passes through the pyriform fossa and lies just beneath the mucosa. Cotton swabs soaked with local anesthetic placed firmly into the fossa with a curved forceps (Krause's forceps) will anesthetize this nerve. The contact should be maintained for 3–5 min to be effective. The superior laryngeal nerve block is confirmed by the development of hoarseness.

The external block of the internal branch of superior laryngeal nerve is performed by injecting 2–3 ml of 1% lidocaine bilaterally between the superior horn of the thyroid cartilage and the hyoid bone. Injection is done with a 23 or 25 gauge needle and after negative aspiration.

Translaryngeal Instillation

Percutaneous transcricothyroid membrane injection of a local anesthetic to provide topical anesthesia of the larynx and trachea was introduced in 1920 by Canuyt (70), advocated for bronchoscopy in 1948 (71), and described to facilitate tracheal intubation by Bonica in 1949 (72).

A needle is introduced into the larynx through the cricothyroid membrane (translaryngeal) or into the trachea through the space above or below the first tracheal ring (transtracheal) (Fig. 7). The landmarks are the thyroid and the cricoid cartilage and the cricothyroid space, triangular in shape, averaging 1–3 cm and usually easily identified. The vocal cords are located 1.5–2 cm superior to the cricoid ring behind the thyroid cartilage. The paired cricothyroid arteries communicate across the upper half of this membrane. The thyroid gland and isthmus lie inferiorly.

To begin this procedure, the supine patient's head is hyperextended, the thyroid notch palpated with the index finger, and the cricothyroid space felt immediately below, bounded inferiorly by the prominent cricoid ring. The skin is cleansed with alcohol and the patient instructed not to talk, swallow, or cough. A 20-gauge over-the-needle catheter connected to a syringe containing 3 ml of 4% lidocaine is inserted through the skin in the midline just above the cricoid ring and directed perpendicularly or slightly caudally into the trachea (Fig. 7). Loss of resistance and aspiration of air confirm placement in the airway (Fig. 8). The needle

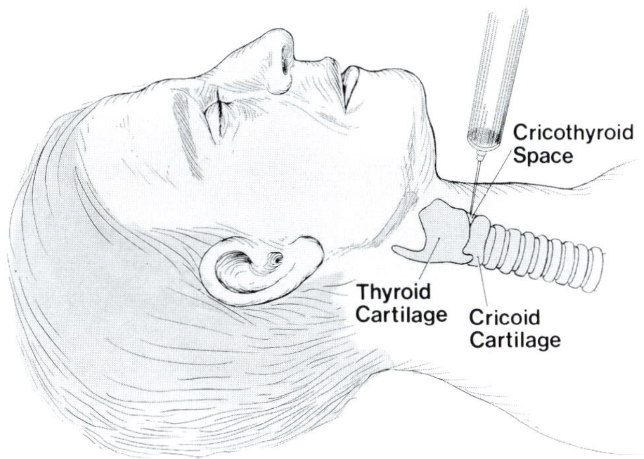

FIG. 7. Injection of lidocaine through cricothyroid membrane to produce topical anesthesia of the larynx and trachea.

is removed from within the catheter, the syringe is reattached to the catheter ensuring a tight seal, and aspiration is repeated to confirm correct placement of the catheter tip. With the catheter held by one hand, lidocaine is injected rapidly, the catheter removed, and an alcohol sponge firmly pressed over the injection site to prevent development of a subcutaneous hematoma and interstitial emphysema from air leak. The local anesthetic spreads from midtrachea to the oropharynx (73). Coughing induced by translaryngeal injection is brief, usually 4–8 sec, and immediately followed by return of regular respiration. A series of 200 patients underwent translaryngeal injections after receiving an average of 100 μg fentanyl and 10 mg of valium intravenously; 17% coughed severely, while 52% either did not cough or did so mildly (Table 1). The technique is simple, fast, easy to learn, and provides good topical

TABLE 1. *Severity of cough after translaryngeal injection of lidocaine graded by one observer*

None	Mild	Moderately severe	Severe
12 (6%)	92 (46%)	62 (31%)	34 (17%)

None, no coughs. Mild, one to five mild or single coughs. Moderately severe, strong single coughs or coughs with short periods of breath holding. Severe, severe fast coughs with prolonged periods of breath holding.

anesthesia in 92–95% of patients (73). It is especially effective in patients who resist oral application of topical anesthetics.

Potential complications include severe coughing—a major disadvantage of the technique, as blood pressure, heart rate, and intracranial pressure may increase. Pain, cellulitis, hematoma, transesophageal penetration, and subcutaneous emphysema at the site of injection have been reported. Intralaryngeal bleeding is rare if the injection is in the midline, but caution should be exercised in patients with a bleeding tendency (Fig. 9). The injection of the solution beneath the laryngeal or tracheal mucosa theoretically could produce airway obstruction. When the injection has been made during light thiopental anesthesia, severe laryngospasm has been reported (71,74).

Inability to palpate anatomic landmarks in obese patients with a short neck, enlarged thyroid, or severe flexion of the cervical spine constitute relative contraindications. Translaryngeal injection should be avoided when infection or malignant tumor is overlying the injection site.

Aerosol

Because of minimal respiratory tract stimulation, this approach is advantageous in patients with in-

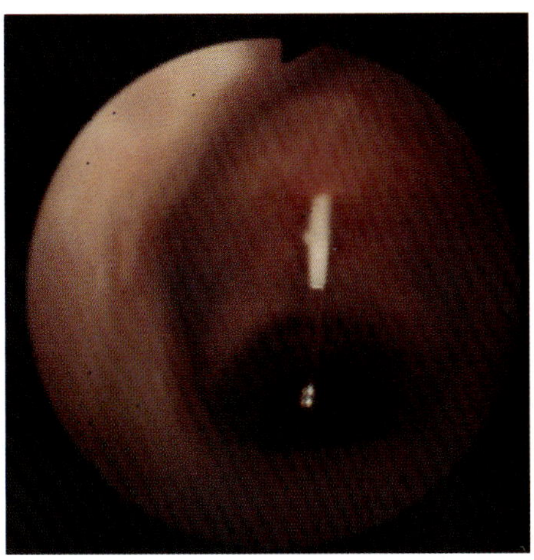

FIG. 8. Endoscopic view of 20-gauge catheter position inside the larynx.

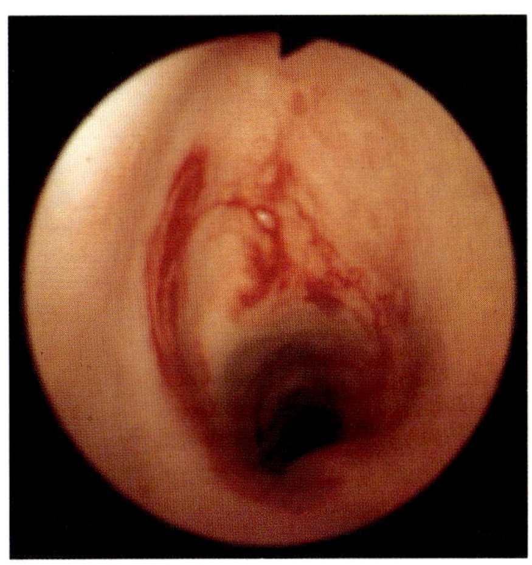

FIG. 9. Bleeding point after translaryngeal injection of lidocaine using 20-gauge catheter over the needle catheter.

creased intracranial pressure, an open eye injury, or severe coronary artery insufficiency (75–77). It is also an alternative when the landmarks are difficult to identify or are inaccessible.

A disposable breathing system with an attached nebulizer is used to deliver the aerosol (Fig. 10). The nebulizer is filled with 4–6 ml of 4% lidocaine to be nebulized by oxygen. The size of the particles delivered is important; those larger than 100 μ in diameter condense in the mouth and pharynx, while those 3 μ or less pass into the alveoli and are rapidly absorbed. Particle diameter must be between 10–30 μ to coat the mucosa of small bronchi, 30–60 μ for larger bronchi, and above 60 μ to affect mucosa of mainstem bronchi and trachea.

In preparation for aerosol inhalation, premedication to dry the mucosa should be given (glycopyrrolate, 0.2–0.3 mg, or atropine, 0.4–0.6 mg). In addition, fentanyl, 50–100 μg intravenously, is worthwhile to minimize irritation of the airway and coughing. The oxygen flow is gradually increased to 8–10 l/min and the patient instructed to breathe slowly and deeply through the mouth. For nasotracheal intubation, a mixture of 4 ml of 4% lidocaine and 1 ml of 1% neosynephrine is inhaled nasally through a face mask for 10–15 min to provide adequate topical anesthesia and shrink the nasal mucosa (76). Part of the solution is lost during nebulization and never reaches the patient. A loss of up to 50% or more occurs when nebulization is continuous during spontaneous breathing. About 20% is lost when using intermittent positive pressure ventilation (77,78). Peak plasma levels of lidocaine will be higher with intermittent positive pressure ventilation.

Advantages of aerosol inhalation include ease and simplicity of application and safety, as it is noninvasive, produces little discomfort, and is well accepted by patients. However, it consumes more time, possibly results in inadequate anesthesia of the larynx (76,79), and has limited application to small children and uncooperative adults. Nonetheless, both sedation and topical anesthesia of the airway obtund protective airway reflexes, so caution should be exercised in patients at risk of aspiration.

SYSTEMIC TOXIC REACTIONS

The most common toxic reaction to lidocaine as well as most other local anesthetic drugs involves the central nervous system (80) and is related to high plasma concentration (81).

While reactions may occur after use of any of the techniques of administration, they are most common after unintentional intravenous injection or because too large a volume or too concentrated a solution was topically applied to respiratory mucous membranes. The blood concentration of a local anesthetic is a function of the total dose given, of its rate of absorption and speed of distribution into tissues, and of metabolism and excretion. Tissue distribution is related in part to the protein binding and lipid solubility characteristics of a drug (82).

The blood concentrations achieved after use of lidocaine, the agent most commonly employed for topical anesthesia of the airway, has been the subject of many investigations (28,83–85). However, the conclusions of these studies are difficult to compare meaningfully because they involve many variables, each of which may affect rate of absorption and maximum blood concentrations measured. The variables are (a) dose of lidocaine used, (b) site and method of application, (c) whether the patient was awake or anesthetized, (d) whether the patient's breathing was spontaneous or controlled, (e) age, (f) body position during application of the drug, and (g) whether anticholinergic drugs were included in premedication.

Slower absorption from oropharynx and trachea may explain the 15–20 min required for lidocaine to reach maximal blood concentration. A more rapid ab-

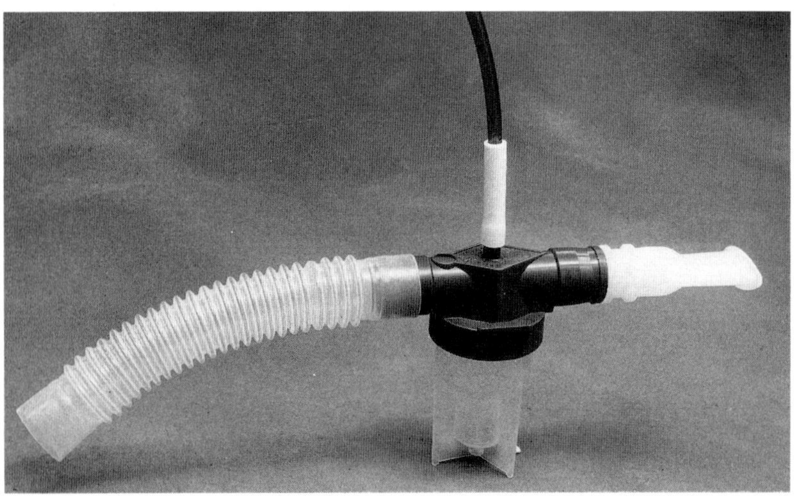

FIG. 10. An aerosol set for application of topical anesthesia to oropharynx, larynx, and trachea. Mouthpiece can be replaced by mask for producing anesthesia to nasal mucosa for nasotracheal intubation. (Seamless Hospital Products Co., Wallingford, Connecticut 06492.)

sorption from distal bronchi and alveoli produces maximal blood concentrations of lidocaine within 5 min. Nebulizers produce fine particles and promote rapid absorption because these particles travel into the small airways and alveoli (29). Korttila and associates (86) demonstrated that, after laryngotracheal spray, the peak level of lidocaine appeared in 15 min, while, after ultrasonic nebulization, that peak was attained in 5 min. When lidocaine is applied to the airway of a conscious patient, the drug is likely to be coughed into the pharynx and then swallowed; only a small portion of swallowed lidocaine reaches the systemic circulation (30,87). Telivuo (29) found that plasma concentrations of prilocaine given to conscious subjects were only 20–30% of those recorded in anesthetized patients. During spontaneous breathing in anesthetized patients, some of the drug sprayed into the trachea will be exhaled into the oropharynx, particularly if coughing occurs during spraying. Controlled ventilation causes a more peripheral spread of droplets within the respiratory tree, promoting greater absorption. Morrell (83) has shown that 10 mg lidocaine given by aerosol endotracheally produced a plasma concentration of approximately 0.1 μg/ml in spontaneous breathing patients and 0.15 μg/ml when ventilation was controlled.

The rate of lidocaine absorption from respiratory mucous membranes differs according to patient. Eyres and co-workers (88) sprayed 4 mg/kg of 4% lidocaine to the larynx and subglottic area and demonstrated a more rapid rise of local anesthetic to a similar peak plasma level (83) in younger children. In sitting patients, gravity aids the spread of drugs from the trachea toward the alveoli, resulting in faster absorption (32,67).

Use of lidocaine ointment or viscous solution for tracheal tube lubrication affects blood lidocaine concentration. Applying 2 ml of 5% lidocaine ointment to an endotracheal tube resulted in a mean plasma lidocaine level of 2.3 μg/ml at 20 min (89). Lidocaine blood concentrations in both conscious and anesthetized patients are unpredictable because of the many factors that influence the uptake, distribution, or metabolism of the drug (32,88,90–93).

Symptoms and Signs of Toxicity from Local Anesthetic

The initial symptoms of toxicity are those of central nervous system (CNS) stimulation characterized by apprehension, restlessness, hyperactivity, euphoria, and excitement; tinnitus, tingling of lips, bitter taste in mouth, vertigo, slurred speech, and tremors may also be noted. Medullary stimulation follows and is manifested by an elevation in pulse rate, blood pressure, and respiratory rate. With higher blood levels (8–12 mg/l), muscle twitching proceeding to convulsions and cardiorespiratory depression appear. The primary local anesthetic effect on the CNS is one of neurologic depression. The initial CNS hyperactivity characteristic of the early stages of toxicity is due to a depression of inhibitory neurons, which are most sensitive to local anesthetics. This leaves the excitatory neurons unopposed, ultimately allowing convulsions to develop (94). As local anesthetic levels rise further in the blood, the excitatory neurons are depressed, leading to cessation of respiration and vascular collapse. High blood levels of the drugs cause vasodilatation and diminish myocardial contractility, resulting in hypotension. Myocardial conductivity and contractility can be so reduced that severe bradycardia and cardiac arrest occur. If a sufficiently high blood level of local anesthetic develops in a relatively short time (20–25 mg/l), the excitatory phase may be absent, and respiratory and cardiovascular collapse occur precipitously. A toxic threshold can be considerably lower in sick, frail, and cachectic patients.

In men, convulsions appear at venous blood levels of 2–4 μg/ml of bupivacaine and etidocaine compared with more than 10 μg/ml of lidocaine (95). Seizures due to high plasma levels of lidocaine have been reported after intravenous as well as after topical application in both adults and children (22–24,96–100).

Benzocaine Induced Methemoglobinemia

Methemoglobinemia can result from exposure to benzocaine, which is the main ingredient of Cetacaine and Hurricaine aerosol sprays that are commonly used for topical anesthesia of the oropharynx. Patients develop bluish gray discoloration of the skin and mucous membrane. Most patients remain asymptomatic but begin to hyperventilate and become anxious. Cyanosis and neurological and cardiac dysfunction may develop when the methemoglobin level exceeds 30%. The diagnosis is confirmed by co-oximetry. Treatment is by intravenous injection of methylene blue (1–2 mg/kg). Recurrence of methemoglobinemia is a possibility and should be looked for.

Infants and elderly are at higher risk of developing methemoglobinemia (54,55).

Treatment of Systemic Reactions

Treatment of acute local anesthetic toxicity is supportive in nature, principally serving to prevent hypoxia and brain damage. With onset of early symptoms and signs, oxygen is administered by face mask and small incremental doses of thiopental (50 mg) or diazepam (5–10 mg) are injected intravenously to treat the excitement stage and prevent convulsions. If the reaction progresses to convulsions, vigorous treatment to suppress them and to prevent hypoxia, bodily injury, aspiration of vomitus, and respiratory arrest is necessary. Ventilation is assisted or controlled via bag and face mask, and thiopental or diazepam are continued as needed to abort the convulsions. However, sedatives and anticonvulsants must be used cautiously, as an excitatory phase can be followed by cardiovascular depression. When convulsions are severe and ventilation difficult to control by face mask, 1 mg/kg succinylcholine should be given intravenously to stop the muscle contractions. However, use of this drug should be limited to those skillful enough in airway management to ventilate the lungs effectively via a face mask and to readily intubate the trachea. The advantage of a muscle relaxant compared with high doses of anticonvulsant drugs is its lack of a cardiovascular depressant effect, which leads to vasodilatation and hypotension. But succinylcholine does not prevent brain cell hyperactivity, the factor that stimulates cerebral metabolism. With adequate pulmonary ventilation, high inspired oxygen concentrations, and an acceptable blood pressure, brain oxygenation and consequent cerebral function remain normal (101,102). If cardiovascular depression appears, vasopressors and positive inotropic agents may be necessary. Should hypotension develop, the rate of intravenous infusion of fluids should be increased and the patient's legs can be elevated as appropriate. Ephedrine 10–25 mg intravenously causes vasoconstriction and stimulates the myocardium. Bradycardia is of concern; atropine 0.4–0.6 mg intravenously may be beneficial. Should cardiac arrest develop, closed chest cardiac massage and full resuscitation are required and should be continued until cardiac rhythm is restored as the local anesthetic is metabolized and the blood level begins to decline.

Allergic Reactions

Hypersensitivity to local anesthetics is rare and is most likely seen with ester-type compounds. The allergen is *para*aminobenzoic acid, a metabolite of ester hydrolysis. Methylparaben, a preservative and antibacterial agent included in local anesthetic multidose vials, is chemically related to *para*aminobenzoic acid and may itself cause allergic reactions. Hypersensitivity to local anesthetics may manifest itself as an allergic dermatitis, asthmatic attack, or anaphylactic reaction.

Mild allergic manifestations are treated with antihistamines such as diphenhydramine hydrochloride 25–50 mg intravenously. Anaphylactic reactions are treated vigorously since there is a massive release of vasoactive substances that cause edema of the epiglottis, larynx, trachea, bronchi, and bronchioles. Vasodilatation causes peripheral blood pooling, impairing venous return and reducing cardiac output. Cardiac arrest can occur rapidly if treatment is not started immediately. Epinephrine 0.3–0.5 mg should be injected subcutaneously early, but if severe hypotension or cardiac arrest appears, it should be diluted and administered 0.1–0.2 mg intravenously. Other supportive treatment for hypotension, cardiac arrhythmias, laryngeal edema, or bronchospasm includes combinations of corticosteroids, antihistamines, and appropriate supportive measures.

Prevention of Toxic Reactions

1. A basic understanding of the pharmacokinetics and pharmacodynamics of topically applied and injectable local anesthetics should be appreciated.
2. Experience and knowledge of the different techniques used in applying topical anesthetics is required.
3. Diazepam or midazolam used as premedicants raise the convulsive threshold. Their use, however, does not justify exceeding the recommended doses of topical anesthetics.
4. Anticholinergics included with premedication decrease salivary secretions which interfere with the development of topical anesthesia by diluting the anesthetic, and with its contact on mucous membranes. Inadequate topical anesthesia necessitates use of additional anesthetic and increases the likelihood of overdosage.
5. Doses of local anesthetics should be reduced for patients with some illnesses. Debilitation, dehydration, electrolyte imbalance, congestive heart failure, and severe liver disease modify the absorption, distribution, metabolism, and excretion of topical anesthetics. The action of lidocaine is significantly prolonged in patients with heart failure or severe liver disease.
6. Administer the smallest volume and the lowest effective concentration of the local anesthetic.
7. Recommended doses are merely guidelines and do not constitute absolutely safe values. Reactions may occur after less than a recommended maximum dose has been given.
8. Fractional small doses of most anesthetic agents sprayed over a longer period of time result in a lower blood level than when an entire dose is applied at once.
9. Allow sufficient onset time for topical anesthesia to develop before applying additional doses. The time required for onset of action varies among agents and different concentrations of drugs.
10. The technique and site of application of local anesthetic are very important. Absorption is more rapid from the alveoli and small bronchi than from the trachea and pharynx.
11. Constant verbal contact with a patient and cardiovascular monitoring are essential for early detection and treatment of local anesthetic toxicity.

12. Drugs and equipment necessary to treat systemic reactions must be available, checked, and ready for immediate use before administration of any local anesthetic.

REFERENCES

1. Ovassapian A. Flexible bronchoscopic intubation of awake patients. *J Bronchology* 1994;1:240–245.
2. Langton JA, Murphy PJ, Barker P, Key A, Smith G. Measurement of the sentivity of upper airway reflexes. *Brit J of Anaesth* 1993;70:126–130.
3. Hinkle JE, Tantum KR. A technique for measuring the reactivity of glottis. *Anesthesiology* 1971;35:634–637.
4. Claeys DW, Lockhart CH, Hinkle JE. The effects of translaryngeal block and Innovar on glottic competence. *Anesthesiology* 1973;38:485–486.
5. Szereda-przestaszewska M, Widdicombe JG. Reflex effects of chemical irritation of the upper airways on the laryngeal lumen in cats. *Respiration Physiology* 1973;18:107–115.
6. Widdicombe JG. Sensory innervation of the lungs and airways. In: Cervero F, Morrison JFB, eds. *Progress in brain research,* vol. 67. Amsterdam: Elsevier Science Publishers B.V., 1986; 49–64.
7. Pontoppidan H, Beecher HK. Progressive loss of protective reflexes in the airway with the advance of age. *J Am Med Assoc* 1960;174:2209–2213.
8. Erskine RJ, Murphy PJ, Langton JA, Smith G. Effect of age on the sensitivity of upper airway reflexes. *Brit J of Anes* 1993; 70:574–575.
9. Groves ND, Rees JL, Rosen M. Effects of benzodiazepines on laryngeal reflexes. *Anaesthesia* 1987;42:808–814.
10. Murphy PJ, Lanston JA, Barker P, Smith G. Effect of oral diazepam on the sensitivity of upper airway reflexes. *Brit J of Anes* 1993:70;131–134.
11. Erskine RJ, Murphy PJ, Langton JA, Smith G. Upper airway reactivity in smokers and non-smokers. *Tenth World Congress of Anesthesiologists* 1992, The Hague, Holland. Abstract 197.
12. Mahajan RP, Murty GE, Singh P, Aitkenhead AR. Effect of topical anaesthesia on the motor performance of vocal cords as assessed by tussometry. *Anaesthesia* 1994;49:1028–1030.
13. Stuchartz G. Neural physiology and local anesthetic action. In: Cousins MJ, Bridenbough PO, eds. *Neural blockade in clinical anesthesia and management of pain,* 2nd ed. Philadelphia: JB Lippincott, 1988;25–45.
14. De Jong RH. Local anesthetics, St. Louis: Mosby-Year Book, 1994.
15. Adriani J, Zepernick R, Arens J, Authement E. The comparative potency and effectiveness of topical anesthetics in man. *Clin Pharmacol Ther* 1964;5:49–62.
16. Daos FG, Lopez L, Virtue RW. Local anesthetic toxicity modified by oxygen and by combination of agents. *Anesthesiology* 1962;23:755–761.
17. Perry LB. Topical anesthesia for bronchoscopy. *Chest* 1978; 73:691–693.
18. Adriani J, Campbell D. Fatalities following topical application of local anesthetics to mucous membranes. *JAMA* 1956;162: 1527–1530.
19. Boyes RN, Scott DB, Jebson PJ, Julian DG. Pharmacokinetics of lidocaine in man. *Clin Pharmacol Ther* 1971;12:105–116.
20. Le Lorier J, Larochelle P, Bolduc R, et al. Lidocaine plasma concentrations during and after endoscopic procedures. *Int J Clin Biopharm* 1979;17:53–55.
21. de Boer AG, Breimer DD, Mattie H, Pronk J, Gubbens-Stibbe JM. Rectal bioavailabililty of lidocaine in man: partial avoidance of "first-pass" metabolism. *Clin Pharmacol Ther* 1979; 26:701–709.
22. Panacek E, Beninger P, Albertson T. Lidocaine toxicity from intraurethral administration (letter). *Ann Emerg Med* 1984;13: 483–484.
23. Sundaram MBM. Seizures after intraurethral instillation of lidocaine. *Can Med Assoc J* 1987;137:219–220.
24. Wehner D, Hamilton GC. Seizures following topical application of local anesthetics to burn patients. *Ann Emerg Med* 1984; 13:456–458.
25. Wu FL, Razzaghi A, Souney PF. Seizure after lidocaine for bronchoscopy: case report and review of the use of lidocaine in airway anesthesia. *Pharmacotherapy* 1993;13:72–78.
26. Scavone JM, Greenblatt DJ, Fraser DG. The bioavailability of intranasal lignocaine. *Br J Clin Pharmacol* 1989;28:722–724.
27. Efthimiou J, Higenbottam R, Holt D, Cochrane GM. Plasma concentration of ignocaine during fiberoptic bronchoscopy. *Thorax* 1982;37:68–71.
28. Patterson JR, Blaschke TF, Hunt KK, Meffin PJ. Lidocaine blood concentrations during fiberoptic bronchoscopy. *Am Rev Resp Dis* 1975;112:53–57.
29. Telivuo L. An experimental study on the absorption of some local anaesthetics through the lower respiratory tract. *Acta Anaesth Scand (Suppl)* 1965;16:121–126.
30. Curran J, Hamilton C, Taylor T. Topical analgesia before tracheal intubation. *Anaesthesia* 1975;30:765–768.
31. Boster SR, Danzl DF, Madden RJ, Jarboe CH. Translaryngeal absorption of lidocaine. *Ann Emerg Med* 1982;11:461–465.
32. Chu SS, Rah KH, Brannan MD, Cohen JL. Plasma concentration of lidocaine after endotracheal spray. *Anesth Analg* 1975; 54:438–441.
33. Schuttler J. Pharmacokinetcs of drugs used for advanced cardiac life support. *Ann Fr Anesth Reanim* 1990;9:208–211.
34. Jebson P. Intramuscular lignocaine 2 percent and 10 percent. *Br Med J* 1971;3:566–567.
35. Scott DB, Jebson PJR, Braid DP, et al. Factors affecting plasma levels of lidocaine and prilocaine. *Br J Anaesth* 1972;44: 1040–1048.
36. Foldes FF, Molloy R, McNall PG, Koukal LR. Comparison of toxicity of intravenously given local anesthetic agents in man. *JAMA* 1960;72:1493–1498.
37. Covino BG, Vassallo HG. *Local anesthetics. Mechanisms of action and clinical use.* New York: Grune and Stratton, 1976.
38. Jones DA, McBurney A, Stanley PJ, et al. Plasma concentrations of lignocaine and its metabolites during fiberoptic bronchoscopy. *Br J Anaesth* 1982;54:853–856.
39. Schenck NL. Local anesthesia in otolaryngology. *Ann Otol* 1975;84:65–72.
40. Anderton JM, Nassar WY. Topical cocaine and general anesthesia: an investigation of the efficacy and side effects of cocaine on the nasal mucosa. *Anaesthesia* 1975;30:809–817.
41. Orr D, Jones I. Anesthesia for laryngoscopy: a comparison of the cardiovascular effects of cocaine and lignocaine. *Anaesthesia* 1968;23:194–202.
42. Gross JB, Hartigan ML, Schaffer DW. A suitable substitute for 4% cocaine before blind nasotracheal intubation: 3% lidocaine–0.25% phenylephrine nasal spray. *Anesth Analg* 1984; 63:915–918.
43. Feehan HF, Mancusi-Ungaro A. The use of cocaine as a topical anesthetic in nasal surgery—a survey report. *Plast Reconstr Surg* 1976;57:62–65.
44. Campbell D, Adriani J. Absorption of local anesthetics. *JAMA* 1958;168:873–877.
45. Van Dyke C, Barash PG, Jatlow P, et al. Cocaine: plasma concentrations after intranasal application in man. *Science* 1976; 191:859–861.
46. Wilkinson P, Van Dyke C, Jatlow P, et al. Intranasal and oral cocaine kinetics. *Clin Pharmacol Ther* 1980;27:386–394.
47. Jatlow P, Barash PG, Van Dyke C, et al. Cocaine and succinylcholine sensitivity: a new caution. *Anesth Analg* 1979;58: 235–237.
48. Verlander JM Jr, Johns ME. The clinical use of cocaine. *Otol Clin Am* 1981;14:521–531.
49. Lichtenfeld PJ, Rubin DB, Feldman RS. Subarachnoid hemorrhage precipitated by cocaine snorting. *Arch Neurol* 1984;41: 223–224.
50. Golbe LI, Merkin MD. Cerebral infarction in a user of freebase cocaine. *Neurology* 1986;36:1602–1603.
51. Astrom A, Persson NH. The toxicity of some local anesthetics after application on different mucous membranes and its relation to anesthetic action on the nasal mucosa of the rabbit. *J Pharmacol Exp Ther* 1961;132:87–90.

52. Weisel W, Tella RA. Reaction to tetracaine used as topical anesthetic in bronchoscopy. *JAMA* 1951;147:218–222.
53. Adriani J. *Labat's regional anesthesia*, 4th ed. St. Louis: Warren H. Green, 1985;650–690.
54. Severinghause JW, Xu-F-D, Spellman MJ. Benzocaine and methemoglobin: recommended actions. *Anesthesiology* 1991; 74:385–386.
55. Rodriguez LF, Smolik LM, Zbehlik AJ. Benzocaine-induced methemoglobinemia: report of a severe reaction and review of the literature. *Ann Pharmacother* 1994;28:643–649.
56. Webb AR, Woodhead MA, Dalton HR, Grigg JA, Millard FJC. Topical nasal anesthesia for fiberoptic bronchoscopy: patients' preference for lidocaine gel. *Thorax* 1989;44:674–675.
57. Gove RI, Wiggins J, Stablefort DE. A study of the use of ultrasonically nebulized lignocaine for local anesthesia during fiberoptic bronchoscopy. *Br J Dis Chest* 1985;79:49–59.
58. Johnson NMcI, Hodson ME, Clarke SW. Acceptability of fiberoptic bronchoscopy under local anaesthesia. *Practitioner* 1978;221:113–114.
59. Rees PJ, Hay JG, Webb AR. Premedication for fiberoptic bronchoscopy. *Thorax* 1983;38:624–627.
60. Webb AR, Doherty JF, Chester MR, et al. Sedation for fiberoptic bronchoscopy: comparison of alfentanil with papaveretum and diazepam. *Respir Med* 1989;83:213–217.
61. Sidu VS, Whitehead EM, Ainsworth QP, et al. A technique of awake fiberoptic intubation: experience in patients with cervical spine disease. *Anaesthesia* 1993;48:910–913.
62. Randell T, Yli-Hankala A, Valli H, Lidgren L. Topical anesthesia of the nasal mucosa for fiberoptic airway endoscopy. *Br J Anaesth* 1991;66:164–167.
63. Middleton RM, Shah A, Kirkpatrick MB. Topical nasal anesthesia for flexible bronchoscopy. *Chest* 1991;99:1093–1096.
64. Watanabe H, Lindgren L, Rosenberg, Randell T. Glycopyrronium prolongs topical anaesthesia of oral mucosa and enhances absorption of lignocaine. *Brit J of Anaesth* 1993;70:94–95.
65. Foster WM, Adam NH. Aerosolized lidocaine reduces dose of topical anesthetic for bronchoscopy. *Am Rev Respir Dis* 1992; 146:520–522.
66. Bromage PR, Robson JG. Concentration of lignocaine in the blood after intravenous, intramuscular, epidural and endotracheal administration. *Anaesthesia* 1961;16:461–478.
67. Fry WA. Techniques of topical anesthesia for bronchoscopy. *Chest* 1978;73:694–696.
68. Webb AR, Fernando SSD, Dalton HR, Arrowsmith JE, Woodhead MA, Cummin ARC. Local anaesthesia for fibreoptic bronchoscopy: transcricoid injection or the "spray as you go" technique? *Thorax* 1990;45:474–477.
69. Graham DR, Hay JG, Clague J, Nisar M, Earis JE. Comparison of three different methods used to achieve local anesthesia for fiberoptic bronchoscopy. *Chest* 1992;102:704–707.
70. Canuyt G. Les injections intratracheales par la voie intercricothyroidienne. *Soc De Med Et Chir Bordeaux,* 1920;249–259.
71. Harken DE, Salzberg AM. Transtracheal anesthesia for bronchoscopy. *N Engl J Med* 1948;239:383–385.
72. Bonica JJ. Transtracheal anesthesia for endotracheal intubation. *Anesthesiology* 1949;10:736–738.
73. Walts LF, Kassity KJ. Spread of local anesthesia after upper airway block. *Arch Otolaryngol* 1965;81:77–79.
74. Gold MI, Buechael DR. Translaryngeal anesthesia: a review. *Anesthesiology* 1959;20:181–185.
75. Abou-Madi M, Keszler H, Yacoub O. A method for prevention of cardiovascular reactions to laryngoscopy and intubation. *Can Anaesth Soc* 1975;22:316–329.
76. Bourke DL, Katz J, Tonneson A. Nebulized anesthesia for awake endotracheal intubation. *Anesthesiology* 1985;63: 690–692.
77. Venus B, Polassani V, Pham CG. Effects of aerosolized lidocaine on circulatory responses to laryngoscopy and tracheal intubation. *Crit Care Med* 1984;12:391–394.
78. Chinn WM, Zavala DC, Ambre J. Plasma levels of lidocaine following nebulized aerosol administration. *Chest* 1977;71: 346–348.
79. Faber LP. Flexible fiberoptic bronchoscopy. In: Berri G, ed. *Endoscopy*. New York: Appleton-Century-Crofts, 1976; 571–586.
80. Benowitz NL, Meister W. Clinical pharmacokinetics of lignocaine. *Clin Pharmacokinet* 1978;3:177–201.
81. Gianelly R, Von Der Groeben JO, Spivack AP, Harrison DC. Effect of lidocaine on ventricular arrhythmias in patients with coronary heart disease. *N Engl J Med* 1967;277:1215–1219.
82. Tucker GT, Mather LE. Pharmacology of local anesthetic agents. Pharmacokinetics of local anesthetic agents. *Br J Anaesth* 1975;47:213–224.
83. Morrell DF, Chappell WA, White IWC. Topical analgesia of the upper airway with lignocaine. *S Afr Med J* 1982;61:551–553.
84. Karvonen S, Jokinen K, Karvonen P, Hollmen A. Arterial and venous blood lidocaine concentrations after local anesthesia of the respiratory tract using an ultrasonic nebulizer. *Acta Anaesth Scand* 1976;20:156–159.
85. Boster SR, Danzl DF, Madden RJ, Jarboe CH. Translaryngeal absorption of lidocaine. *Ann Emerg Med* 1982;11:461–465.
86. Korttila K, Tarkkanen J, Tarkkanen L. Comparison of laryngotracheal and ultrasonic nebulizer administration of lidocaine in local anesthesia for bronchoscopy. *Acta Anaesth Scand* 1981; 25:161–165.
87. Scott DB, Littlewood DG, Covino BG, Drummond GB. Plasma lignocaine concentrations following endotracheal spraying with an aerosol. *Br J Anaesth* 1976;48:899–901.
88. Eyres RL, Bishop W, Oppenheim RC, Brown TCK. Plasma lignocaine concentrations following topical laryngeal application. *Anaesth Intens Care* 1983;11:23–26.
89. Sellers WFS, Dye A, Harvey J. Systemic absorption of lignocaine ointment from tracheal tubes. *Anaesthesia* 1985;40: 483–485.
90. Viegas O, Stoelting RK. Lidocaine in arterial blood after laryngotracheal administration. *Anesthesiology* 1975;43:491–493.
91. Smith RB. Uptake of lidocaine from the trachea. *Anesthesiology* 1976;44:269.
92. Pelton DA, Daly M, Cooper PD, Conn AW. Plasma lidocaine concentrations following topical aerosol application to the trachea and bronchi. *Can Anaesth Soc J* 1970;17:250–255.
93. Rosenberg PH, Heinonen J, Takasaki M. Lidocaine concentration in blood after topical anesthesia of the upper respiratory tract. *Acta Anaesth Scand* 1980;24:125–128.
94. Frank GB, Sanders HD. A proposed common mechanism of action for general and local anesthetics in the central nervous system. *Br J Pharmacol Chemother* 1963;21:1–9.
95. Covino BG. Clinical pharmacology of local anesthetic agents. In: Cousins MJ, Bridenbough PO, eds. *Neural blockade in clinical anesthesia and management of pain*, 2nd ed. Philadelphia: JB Lippincott, 1988;111–144.
96. Rothstein P, Dornbusch J, Shaywitz BA. Prolonged seizures associated with the use of viscous lidocaine. *J Pediatr* 1982: 101:461–463.
97. Giard MJ, Uden DL, Whitlock DJ, Watson DM. Seizures induced by oral viscous lidocaine (letter). *Clin Pharm* 1983;2: 110.
98. Mofenson HC, Caraccio TR, Miller H, Greensher J. Lidocaine toxicity from topical mucosal application. With a review of the clinical pharmacology of lidocaine. *Clin Pediatr* 1983;22: 190–192.
99. Fruncillo RJ, Gibbons W, Bowman SM. CNS toxicity after ingestion of topical lidocaine (letter). *N Engl J Med* 1982;306: 426–427.
100. Parish RC, Moore RT, Gotz VP. Seizures following oral lidocaine for esophageal anesthesia. *Drug intell Clin Pharm* 1985; 19:199–201.
101. Plum F, Posner JB, Troy B. Cerebral metabolic and circulatory responses to induced convulsions in animals. *Arch Neurol* 1968;18:1–13.
102. Moore DC, Bridenbaugh LD. Oxygen: the antidote for systemic toxic reactions from local anesthetic drugs. *JAMA* 1960; 174:842–847.

CHAPTER 5

Conscious Sedation

Andranik Ovassapian, M.D. and Tom C. Krejcie, M.D.

DEFINITION OF CONSCIOUS SEDATION

The term conscious sedation was introduced to differentiate light sedation from deep sedation. It is a state of mind obtained typically by the intravenous administration of a combination of anxiolytics, sedative/hypnotics, and/or analgesics that renders the patient relaxed yet allows the patient to communicate, maintain a patent airway, and ventilate adequately. Medications are administered intravenously in small incremental doses to allow time to observe maximum effects and avoid oversedation (1). The progression from conscious sedation to heavy or deep sedation increases the risk of loss of airway and protective reflexes. Anesthesiologists use conscious sedation frequently for awake tracheal intubation and procedures such as pulmonary artery catheter placement, diagnostic or therapeutic nerve blocks, and regional anesthetic techniques. Anesthesiologists perform the procedure and are also responsible for administering all medications and monitoring the patient. A trained individual should be present to assist in monitoring and admininstering medication.

REASONS FOR USING CONSCIOUS SEDATION

Manipulation of the airway in an awake patient without good topical anesthesia is stimulating, painful, and unpleasant. Patients have refused repeat awake tracheal intubation because of an unpleasant experience (2). Profound topical anesthesia will block the airway reflexes and unpleasant responses. However, an anxious and fearful patient may still complain of discomfort and be uncooperative. While anxiety is a normal and expected reaction that most adults can handle without pharmacologic intervention, patients appreciate being sedated and relaxed during procedures performed under local anesthesia (3–5). The goal of conscious sedation in performing tracheal intubation is to relieve anxiety while providing sedation, analgesia, and amnesia (1). Appropriate sedation is crucial in overcoming the patient's apprehension about perioperative pain and suffering (6).

The three common causes of "excitement" or "agitation" during procedures performed under local anesthesia are pain, anxiety, and unrecognized hypoxemia. Failure to recognize and distinguish between the causes will result in inappropriate therapeutic intervention and undesirable complications (7).

Pain should be treated by injecting additional local anesthetic drug. Rapid acting analgesics (e.g., fentanyl) are excellent choices to supplement the local anesthetic effect, minimizing pain and patient discomfort. Treatment of pain-induced agitation with anxiolytic and/or hypnotic drugs increases patient disorientation and communication difficulties, resulting in patients who are heavily sedated and have more drug-induced respiratory depression.

Management of anxiety induced agitation with potent analgesics (narcotics) is even more dangerous. In the absence of pain, the respiratory effect of narcotics will be profound, causing respiratory depression and hypoxemia (7). Treatment of hypoxemia includes supplemental oxygen therapy and, if possible, treatment of the cause of hypoxemia. The mandatory use of pulse oximetry can easily identify patients with hypoxemia and minimize the incidence of agitation caused by hypoxemia.

Minimizing the recall of unpleasant and painful stimuli is critical, thus inducing amnesia is a significant component of conscious sedation. Benzodiazepines and scopolamine are used to produce profound antegrade amnesia (lack of recall of events occurring after initiation of sedation) and mild retrograde amnesia (lack of recall of events occurring before sedation was begun).

PATIENT SELECTION

Not every patient is a candidate for an awake sedated tracheal intubation. Uncooperative, mentally impaired, or intoxicated patients often need deep sedation or general anesthesia to allow any kind of airway instrumentation. However, preoperative anxiety and fear expressed by a patient are not contraindications to an awake sedated intubation. These patients can benefit most from a well-conducted preoperative visit when the cause of the anxiety and fear should be explored and specific measures employed to minimize the fear (8). A detailed explanation of the technique and medications to be used to minimize the pain and anxiety will calm the patient. Anxious patients will often accept the physician's recommendation for an awake intubation if they are assured that after sedation the anxiety and fear will dissipate. Patients will also be assured if they know that the anesthesiologist will honor their request if they change their minds after sedation is induced and request to be asleep before intubation is attempted.

Appropriate premedication will supplement a good preoperative visit and further minimize fear and anxiety. Many anxious and fearful patients have managed awake intubation extremely well with the judicious use of sedation (9). Successful, atraumatic placement of an endotracheal tube in an awake sedated patient requires good topical anesthesia of the airway.

Various anxiolytic agents have been used as a premedicant. Diazepam (Valium™), 10 mg orally, or midazolam (Versed™), 2–4 mg intramuscular, provide good sedation and to a large extent amnesia. Intramuscular narcotics such as morphine (5–10 mg) and meperidine (Demerol™) (50–75 mg) should be prescribed as premedication only when specific indications such as pain or addiction to narcotics are present. Respiratory depression induced by narcotics, the possibility of nausea and vomiting, and the lack of amnesia are some of the reasons not to prescribe narcotics with each premedication order.

MONITORING STANDARDS

Maintaining verbal rapport with the patient is the most essential aspect of monitoring during conscious sedation. Talking, asking questions, and encouraging deep breaths are extremely helpful. When verbal contact with the patient is lost, either the patient is overly sedated or a major physiological disruption has taken place. These situations demand immediate attention.

Observation of the ventilatory pattern, chest wall movement, and patient color can all be helpful. However, clinical observation for recognition of the early signs of respiratory depression and hypoxemia has proven to be unreliable. It is on this basis that physiological monitoring is mandated by the American Society of Anesthesiologists (ASA) for patients subjected to Monitored Anesthesia Care (MAC) (10). Conscious sedation is often used as a part of MAC. Patient selection should be based on the underlying disease and the type of procedure being performed. Noninvasive monitoring of oxygenation by pulse oximetry, noninvasive blood pressure determination, and a continuous electrocardiogram is the minimum monitoring mandated by the ASA. The blood pressure and heart rate must be measured every 5 min; the ECG must be continuously displayed during the entire procedure. Most myocardial ischemic events can be detected by monitoring the V_5 precordial lead. Monitoring lead II simultaneously with lead V_5 increases the sensitivity of detecting myocardial ischemia.

Pulse oximetry can detect changes in oxygen saturation that are not apparent clinically. The clinical signs of adequacy of ventilation must continually be assessed during sedation. Accurate measurement of the exhaled CO_2 during conscious sedation is difficult. The capnometer, however, can be employed as a qualitative monitor of ventilatory rate and as an apnea monitor by sampling exhaled gas through a soft cannula near the nares (11–13).

Additional invasive monitoring may be necessary in high-risk patients. It should be emphasized that the use of monitoring devices should not distract the physician and/or assistant from basic clinical observation.

DRUGS USED FOR CONSCIOUS SEDATION

Basic Concepts of Pharmacokinetics and Pharmacodynamics

Pharmacokinetics (PK) is what the body does to a drug once it has been administered. It is based on determining the plasma/blood concentrations of a drug over time, that is, the drug concentration history. Pharmacodynamics (PD), on the other hand, is the effect a drug has on the body. It is based on the analysis of a measurable drug effect and relating this effect to drug concentration in the plasma/blood at any given time. Taken together, PK-PD analysis looks at the entire dose-response relationship, the relationship between an observed drug effect, and the dose of drug necessary to obtain that level of effect. A better understanding of the pharmacokinetics and pharmacodynamics of the various drugs used to provide conscious sedation provides a rational basis for the appropriate choice.

Historically, the pharmacokinetic description of drugs consisted of compartment volumes, intercompartmental and elimination clearances, and, most frequently, half-lives. These variables resulted from the mathematical description (modeling) of the plasma/blood concentration versus time profile of a drug. However, it has recently become obvious that none of these variables,taken alone or in simple combinations, can be used to predict the onset or offset of drug effect (response) (14). Although comparing half-lives is deeply entrenched in the literature and clinical thinking, comparing half-lives is not a rational method for selecting a drug (14). Therefore, two terms have been developed that are consistent with what can be clinically observed in terms of onset and offset of effect. The time to peak (maximum) effect (T_{max}) is the time it takes for the drug at the site of action (effect compartment), not in the plasma, to reach its maximum concentration. This time (T_{max}) can be significantly delayed from the time of maximum plasma concentration and is widely variable among drugs. Likewise, the decrement time (T_{dec}) is the amount of time required for the plasma drug concentration to decrease by a given percentage (i.e., a 50% decrease in plasma drug concentration, $T_{dec\ 50\%}$). The decrement time has far more clinical utility than an elimination half-life ($T_{1/2}$), which is the time required for the *amount* of drug in the body to decrease by 50%. The elimination half-life can be estimated from the plasma concentration decline only during the terminal elimination phase of the concentration history. During the terminal elimination phase, drug concentrations throughout all parts of the body are nearly equal to that of the plasma; therefore, the *change* in the *amount* of drug in the body can be estimated by changes in the plasma concentration of that drug. However, terminal elimination, and hence elimination half-life, typically occurs long after drug effect has dissipated, so it is of little clinical utility. The decrement time, on the other hand, can be calculated for any time period following drug administration and by definition is always shorter, usually much shorter, than the elimination half-life (15). Unfortunately, T_{max} and T_{dec} are not values commonly reported for most drugs. When available, however, this information is very useful.

A specific example of the decrement time as it applies to the effect compartment was first alluded to by Price in his classic study of the distribution of thiopental where he calculated prolongation of central nervous system drug concentrations following infusions of progressively longer durations (16). Shafer and Varvel, with more sophisticated pharmacokinetic simulations, applied this idea to commonly used opioids (17). Later, Hughes et al. described another application of the decrement time and coined the term context-sensitive half-time. The context-sensitive half-time, or the time required for the central compartment (plasma) drug concentration to fall by 50% (T_{dec} 50%), provides valuable insight into the actual time a patient may require to recover from the acute effects of a drug. This time varies not only among various drugs, but also depends on the context or drug administration scenario (the length of time the drug has been administered) (15). Basically, if a drug is administered as a bolus or a short duration infusion, the T_{dec}, and hence patient recovery, is quicker than it would be following a more prolonged infusion. These concepts and their application are nicely described in an editorial by Shafer and Stanski (18).

Although T_{dec} can be described with reasonable validity by analyzing either plasma or effect compartment concentrations, T_{max} can only be predicted using effect compartment concentration data in a mathematical simulation. Therefore, when reviewing this type of information, it is important to be aware of the concentrations being depicted. The most relevant data is that for the effect compartment, as it is this type of data that is truly predictive of drug effect and hence, the time course of patient response. Some of the pharmacokinetic literature include only plasma or central compartment drug concentrations and related variables. Predicting onset of drug effect using variables derived in this manner can be very misleading. Predictions or simulations of drug effect require that pharmacodynamic, not only pharmacokinetic, analysis be performed. This type of pharmacodynamic analysis entails some form of drug effect measurement (e.g., electroencephalogram) rather than just plasma drug concentration analysis. Once the pharmacodynamic analysis is completed, computer simulations are performed on the resultant data to derive the values for T_{max} and T_{dec}.

The basic idea to keep in mind when using sedative/hypnotics and/or analgesics to obtain a state of conscious sedation in a patient is to start low and go slow. This is the description of intravenous drug titration in which the maximum effect of one dose of the drug is ascertained before subsequent doses are administered (1). Although the *plasma* concentrations of the majority of the drugs used for this purpose reach their peak in the first minute after administration, the *effect* of that drug may not reach its peak for up to 5 min. Therefore, if multiple injections are made at too frequent an interval, the composite effect may not be seen until after the procedure has started, a time when the exaggerated effect of these drugs, including severe respiratory depression, is most likely to go unnoticed.

Anxiolytics and Hypnotics

Anxiolytic and sedative agents decrease patient anxiety and improve patient cooperation during procedures performed using local or topical anesthesia. Benzodiazepines are excellent agents and the most commonly used drugs for intravenous sedation. Benzodiazepines also increase the seizure threshold for local anesthetics (19), an additional advantage of bezodiazepines when local anesthetic agents are used. The three benzodiazepines used intravenously are diazepam (Valium™), midazolam (Versed™), and lorazepam (Ativan™).

Diazepam (Valium™)

Diazepam has been widely used for preoperative as well as conscious sedation. Intravenous doses of 5–10 mg diazepam produce antegrade amnesia for 30 min in 50–90% of patients, respectively (20). When given intravenously the onset of action is within 2–3 min, with peak effect (T_{max}) at 7–8 min. To avoid oversedation, diazepam should be given in incremental doses of 2.5 mg every 2–4 min because the individual dose response is widely variable (21).

The duration of effect is dose dependent. In low doses, rapid redistribution of diazepam is primarily responsible for termination of its clinical effect within 10–15 min. Diazepam is a long-acting sedative drug and patients should be warned that they may feel tired for a day or more after its administration.

An intravenous dose of 0.1 mg/kg of diazepam has little respiratory effect. A dose of 0.4 mg/kg depresses the ventilatory response to carbon dioxide and increases arterial carbon dioxide levels. Cardiovascular effects of diazepam are minimal in doses used for conscious sedation.

Diazepam, which is not water soluble, can cause pain during intravenous injection and may later result in phlebitis. Diazepam decreases muscle tone and, because of high lipid solubility, crosses the placenta and enters the fetal circulation. Diazepam administration has been linked with an increase in birth defects and should be avoided during the first trimester of pregnancy.

Midazolam (Versed™)

Presently, midazolam is the most widely used agent for conscious sedation (22). Midazolam provides effective amnesia and allows rapid recovery when used for conscious sedation.

Midazolam is a water soluble benzodiazepine with a rapid onset of action (23). It is three to four times more potent on a mg-per-mg basis than is diazepam in terms of sedation and amnesia (22). Midazolam, 5 mg intravenously (IV), produces sedation and anxiolysis within 1–2 min. Motor performance recovers in 34 min, and subjects are awake and walking within 73 min (22). Large doses of midazolam result in prolonged drowsiness and can induce respiratory depression. Cardiorespiratory arrest has been reported in the elderly during endoscopic procedures.

Plasma levels of midazolam and clinical end points have been correlated (23). At serum midazolam concentrations of 150–200 ng/ml, patients are sedated but are arousable and able to respond verbally. At concentrations of 100–150 ng/ml, patients are awake but appear drowsy. Amnesia is present at concentrations above 100 ng/ml, and sedation persists until concentrations decline to less than 75 ng/ml (23). Midazolam 0.1 mg/kg depresses ventilatory response to carbon dioxide as well as hypoxic ventilatory responses. The level of depression after midazolam 0.15 mg/kg is similar to that seen after diazepam 0.3 mg/kg in healthy subjects.

In adults less than 60 years old, administer 2 mg midazolam IV over the first 2 min, then wait at least another 2–3 min to administer additional drug if needed. In patients who are older than 60 years, the initial dose should be smaller (1–1.5mg IV over 2 min). Dose reduction is also indicated in debilitated patients while cautious use is advised in patients with preexisting respiratory dysfunction, such as patients with chronic obstructive pulmonary disease. Sedative responses may be exaggerated if the patient has received other CNS depressants such as opioids.

For tracheal intubation in conscious patients, the combination of midazolam 1–3 mg and fentanyl 50–150 μg provides effective sedation and analgesia. The combination of midazolam and opioids increases the incidence of apnea (24). In a clinical study in volunteers, Bailey et al. demonstrated that midazolam (0.05 mg/kg) alone produced no respiratory depression. Fentanyl (2 μg/kg) alone produced hypoxemia in 6 out of 12 subjects and a significant depression of the ventilatory response to CO_2, but did not cause apnea. The combination of midazolam and fentanyl increased the frequency of hypoxemia to 11 out of 12 subjects and produced apnea in 6 of the 12 subjects.

Midazolam can be given by infusion to provide a stable level of sedation during surgery and in intensive care unit patients. A satisfactory level of sedation should be achieved first by incremental titration of a loading dose using boluses or a rapid infusion. Loading doses of 0.01–0.07 mg/kg followed by a maintenance infusion rate of 0.04–0.10 mg/kg/hr have been used (19).

The receptor kinetics of diazepam and midazolam are identical despite different plasma pharmacokinetic profiles (22). Midazolam has a short elimination half-life (2–3 hr) and is metabolized in the liver by oxidation producing 1- and 4-hydroxy midazolam, which are inactive metabolites (25). Midazolam is highly protein bound (96%), mostly to albumin. The dissipation of clinical effect is primarily through the redistribution of the drug from active sites in the brain to inactive peripheral sites.

Lorazepam (Ativan™)

Lorazepam produces the most profound sedation and amnesia of the three benzodiazepines mentioned. However, its onset time of 5–20 min is very slow and, therefore, is not a suitable agent to produce fast-onset conscious sedation of short duration. Lorazepam is a good drug to use for sedation in patients with a high level of preoperative anxiety prior to long surgical procedures.

Benzodiazepines Antagonist (Flumazenil)

Flumazenil (Romazecon™) is a benzodiazepine antagonist that counteracts all CNS effects of benzodiazepines by a competitive antagonism at the CNS benzodiazepine receptors (26–28). Flumazenil counteracts the sedative, amnesic, muscle relaxant, and anticonvulsant effects of benzodiazepines. Flumazenil provides antagonist activity, whether given before, simultaneously with, or after the benzodiazepine (27).

Benzodiazepine withdrawal symptoms have been reported in benzodiazepine-dependent individuals. In addition, flumazenil may have weak, generalized central arousal activity (28). The clinical effects of bezodiazepines are dose related; low doses of midazolam cause anxiolysis, and higher doses cause hypnosis. Reversal of the benzodiazepine effect occurs in the opposite order of appearance (29). High doses of flumazenil are needed to reverse anxiolysis.

Flumazenil in doses of 0.2–0.4 mg has been used to reverse residual benzodiazepine sedation (30). Subjective awakening occurs in 1 min (31).

After IV injection, the peak level of flumazenil is reached in the plasma in 5 min and in the CNS (T_{max}) within 5–8 min. A lower protein binding (50%) contributes to its rapidity of action. Rapid distribution and a high liver extraction rate produce a relatively short duration of action. Flumazenil is metabolized in the liver to non-active metabolites.

The reported side effects, nausea and vomiting, occur in about 11% of anesthetized patients. Nausea is more common when flumazenil is given to patients after general anesthesia than after conscious sedation (32). Other transient side effects include tears, tremors, dizziness, and anxiety. An initial dose of 0.2 mg followed by incremental doses of 0.1 mg will minimize the side effects.

Flumazenil has basically no intrinsic toxicity. Doses of 100 mg IV have been well tolerated (27,28). Flumazenil reversal does not cause the hemodynamic changes that may be seen with naloxone (33,34).

Propofol (Diprivan™)

Propofol (*Diprivan*™) is a phenol derivative that has been used as an anesthetic (hypnotic) agent since 1989 (35). Propofol is prepared in a lipid emulsion for intravenous injection which causes an unpleasant burning sensation at the site of administration. This pain can be minimized by using a larger caliber, more proximal arm vein, or by preceding the injection of propofol with a small dose (10–20 mg) of 1% lidocaine.

Low-dose propofol infusions have also been used for sedation during various procedures, with superior recovery compared to midazolam or diazepam (35–39). The recommended dose of propofol when used as a continuous infusion for sedation is 25–75 μg/kg/min. However, a 40–60% dose reduction is required in the elderly, and the authors have noted very acceptable levels of sedation with as little as 1–2 mg/min. We have found that in average size adults, administration rate titration in mg/min, regardless of patient weight, is preferable as interindividual variability exceeds weight variability. Furthermore, by ignoring actual patient weight and concentrating on the actual drug administration rate, more finely tuned rate adjustments are possible with some of the commercially available infusion pumps. These pumps usually have a μg/kg/min rate setting as well as a patient weight setting. Because of the relatively large increments in the μg/kg/min settings, finer adjustments can be made by altering the body weight setting at any given infusion rate.

When amnesia and analgesia are needed, small doses of midazolam (2–3 mg) or fentanyl (50–100 μg) can be supplemented. Combining midazolam and propofol for sedation takes advantage of the rapid recovery from propofol, whereas the midazolam reduces intraoperative recall and anxiety.

Propofol suppresses airway reflexes, a desirable and beneficial feature for use during awake tracheal intubation. This is especially important considering that a reactive airway, due to poor topical anesthesia, is a major cause of failure in an awake intubation. Like any other hypnotic or narcotic agent, there is a wide variability in the responses of patients to propofol.

Propofol rapidly crosses the placenta and enters the fetal circulation. Neonatal elimination of propofol is slower than maternal and may contribute to slower recovery of the neonate when propofol is administered as an infusion during cesarean section (40,41).

The pharmacokinetic properties of propofol are unique, and contribute to its rapid recovery after IV injection. When an infusion of propofol is stopped, the concentration in the central compartment is much higher than that in the peripheral compartments. The decline of propofol concentration in the central compartment is due to metabolism and the continuing redistribution of the propofol from highly perfused to less perfused tissues. The decrease in the propofol level in plasma is fast, in part because of its higher metabolic clearance rate (15). Propofol is metabolized both by the liver and at extrahepatic sites (42).

Opioid Analgesics

Opioid analgesics are often administered in combination with sedative-hypnotic agents during conscious sedation to reduce the pain associated with procedures performed under local anesthesia. Opioids are also strong depressants of airway reflexes, a desirable feature when the airway is manipulated in an awake patient.

Selection of the type of opioid depends on its characteristics, duration of the procedure, and potential for side effects, especially histamine release.

Morphine

Morphine has been in clinical use for centuries and, along with meperidine, continues as the most prescribed analgesic after major surgical procedures. Because of its long duration of action, morphine is a less desirable agent for conscious sedation, especially during short procedures or for ambulatory patients.

For acute pain control or sedation, morphine in 1–2 mg doses is injected intravenously every 5–10 min until the desired level of analgesia is achieved.

Highly water soluble drugs like morphine are slow to penetrate the lipid membranes, including the blood brain barrier, and hence tend to have a slow onset of action. Morphine has a relatively long elimination half-life and slow redistribution to other tissues, accounting for its long duration of action.

Meperidine (Demerol™)

Meperidine, a more lipid soluble agent than morphine, is somewhat faster in onset of action. The side effects of meperidine, due to its anticholinergic properties, include tachycardia and delirium.

For conscious sedation or acute pain control, meperidine is injected in incremental doses of 10–20 mg until the desired level of sedation is achieved.

Fentanyl, Sufentanil, and Afentanil

These new short-acting synthetic opioids are highly lipid soluble, have faster onset, and shorter duration of action when compared to morphine (43).

Fentanyl is related to the phenyl piperidines and is 60 to 100 times more potent than morphine. Fentanyl is provided in solution at a concentration of 50 μg/ml. It may be stored at room temperature but must be protected from light. The onset of action is within 2 min of intravenous injection with its maximum respiratory depression effect (T_{max}) in 5–7 min. Fentanyl in doses of 1–2 μg/kg (0.5–2 ml in an average-size adult patient) combined with midazolam 15–40 μg/kg (1–3 ml in an average-size adult patient) is commonly used for conscious sedation for tracheal intubation under topical anesthesia. Airway reflexes are suppressed to some degree by 50–100 μg fentanyl, making instrumentation of the airway easier and less stressful during awake intubation. Patients who are habitual users of various addicting drugs, including alcohol, will need larger than customary doses of medications for sedation and analgesia.

Sufentanil is a derivative of fentanyl with a potency five to ten times greater than fentanyl (43). It is a fast-acting opioid with more rapid recovery than fentanyl. Sufentanil (50 μg/ml) should be diluted to a 5 μg/ml concentration to minimize the possibility of overdose and profound respiratory depression. Clinical experience with sufentanil for conscious sedation is much more limited than that with fentanyl. It does not have any special advantage over fentanyl (except for a somewhat shorter T_{max}) when used for conscious sedation. It is more likely to cause severe respiratory depression because of its extreme potency and ease in overdosing a patient during conscious sedation.

Alfentanil also is a synthetic derivative of fentanyl and is about ten times less potent than fentanyl. It has a rapid onset and much shorter duration of action compared to fentanyl. In doses of 10–20 μg/kg, combined with midazolam, alfentanil provides good sedation for awake tracheal intubation. The advantage of alfentanil as an opioid is its rapid and predictable onset. The T_{max} for alfentanil is 90 sec with a proportionally short recovery time.

Narcotics are strong respiratory depressants causing hypoxemia even with small intravenous doses. When used alone, opioid analgesics are not only poor sedatives, but also have a high incidence of undesirable side effects, such as respiratory depression, nausea, and pruritus (43). When sedation is the goal and the patient is free of pain, anxiolytics-hypnotics are recommended. The use of opioids in the absence of pain or painful procedure can produce more profound respiratory depression and may cause a dysphoric reaction.

The primary mechanism for termination of the synthetic opioids effect is redistribution from the central nervous system to other tissues following bolus dose administration.

Naloxone (Narcan™)

Naloxone is a pure μ-antagonist. It readily reverses all of the effects and side effects of the opioids including sedation and respiratory depression. Its use during or after conscious sedation should be judicious unlike its recommended usage in frank narcotic overdose. When used for undue sedation or respiratory depression a reverse titration technique is preferable. One ampule (0.4 mg, 1 ml) of Narcan™ is diluted in a 10 ml volume and 40 μg (1 ml of dilute solution) doses are injected intravenously at 2–4 min intervals until the patient has attained an acceptable level of consciousness. Large increases in the activity of the sympathetic nervous system, which are induced by the acute onset of pain from too rapid a reversal of the narcotic analgesics, have been reported. This has resulted in pulmonary edema even in young healthy patients (32,33).

GUIDELINES FOR SEDATION BY NON-ANESTHESIOLOGISTS

Increasingly, conscious sedation is provided to patients undergoing diagnostic and therapeutic procedures in dental offices, radiology suites, procedure rooms, and emergency departments. The use of sedatives and narcotics outside of operating rooms has been associated with major complications, including death (44,45).

A survey of members of the American Society for Gastrointestinal Endoscopy revealed a rate of 0.5% for sedation-related major cardiopulmonary complications (46). A recent report confirms the role of hypnotic doses of midazolam in decreasing oxygen saturation during gastrointestinal endoscopy (47). The presence of the gastroscope alone did not cause a decrease in oxygenation in patients subjected to gastroscopy without sedation and breathing room air. The group of patients who received sedation (an average of 4.5 mg of midazolam) for gastroscopy and without supplemental oxygen therapy, showed a decrease in oxygen saturation during the procedure. Nasal oxygen (2 l per min) prevented the decrease in oxygen saturation in the third group of patients who received sedation during gastrointestinal endoscopy (47).

Surveys and editorials have highlighted the danger of intravenous sedation and have emphasized the need for comprehensive guidelines and more intense monitoring during gastrointestinal endoscopy (44,47–52). Ventilatory arrests caused by oversedation during radiological studies in children have been reported (53,54). The danger of intravenous sedation in dental offices has also been acknowledged over the years, and guidelines aimed at minimizing major complications have been published. (55–58).

Iatrogenic injury is a major source of morbidity and mortality for patients (59–62). Practitioners not trained in the use of powerful hypnotics and analgesics for conscious sedation have contributed greatly to iatrogenic injury.

Inadequate knowledge of the pharmocology of drugs used for intravenous sedation, lack of experience in using these agents, inadequate monitoring during sedation, lack of readily available resuscitative equipment and experience in resuscitative techniques have all contributed to disastrous outcomes. Of 86 deaths associated with the intravenous use of midazolam reported to the Department of Health and Human Services, 78% were respiratory in nature and in 57% an opioid had also been administered (24). An anesthesiologist was in attendance in only three (3.5%) of the deaths.

For the above reasons, the Joint Commission on Accreditation of Healthcare Organizations (JCAHO) has established guidelines for the safe administration of conscious sedation (63). The intent of the guidelines is that regardless of where the conscious sedation is provided, the same degree of care, monitoring, and expertise needs to be applied. To achieve this goal, the JCAHO has mandated that the hospitals establish policies and procedural guidelines approved by the hospital administration and the medical staff. The guidelines should include a provision for privileging practitioners for administration of sedatives and narcotics. Anesthesiologists are expected to actively participate in formulating these guidelines and provide support to services that may need or seek such support. According to the JCAHO Accreditation Manual for Hospitals, the director of anesthesia is responsible for "the quality and appropriateness of anesthesia care provided by individuals in any department or service in the hospital."

A conscious sedation guideline for anesthesiologists

who participate in institutional policies governing the safe administration of sedation by non-anesthesiologists has been approved by the Executive Committee of the Department of Anesthesia of Harvard Medical School and has been published (64). This timely publication indicates that all basic care applied to a patient submitted to operation in the operating room should also be applied to patients undergoing diagnostic procedures performed outside the operating room. The objective of the guideline should clearly be stated, conscious sedation should be defined, the list of monitoring and other equipment should be compiled, and manpower needs should be addressed. The practitioner responsible for the treatment of the patient shall be appropriately trained. A minimum of two people (operator and monitor) should be present during procedures performed on a sedated patient. All physicians administering sedation should be trained in airway management and be able to use oropharyngeal and nasopharyngeal airways and apply positive pressure ventilation by bag and mask. The laryngeal mask airway, introduced recently in anesthesia practice, may play an important role in providing emergency airway support and ventilation (65).

Anesthesiologists should participate in the organization of a hospitalwide educational program to inform other practitioners of the guidelines for the use of sedatives and monitoring modalities.

Like administration of an anesthetic in the operating room, the details of the procedure and the sedatives and monitors used should be documented in the patient's chart. JCAHO demands the use of the ASA's physical status classification for each patient subjected to sedation for diagnostic and therapeutic procedures. A sample of a sedation monitoring record included with the article can be modified to meet the individual needs for various services (64).

Following sedation, postanesthesia care unit admission and discharge criteria guidelines should be followed strictly and applied both to inpatients and outpatients.

REFERENCES

1. Reed AP. Preparation of the patient for awake fiberoptic bronchoscopy. *Chest* 1992;101:244–253.
2. DeBoard JW, Ghia JN, Guilford WB. Caudal anesthesia in a patient with ankylosing spondylitis for hip surgery. *Anesthesiology* 1981;54:164–166.
3. Kvale PA. Is sedation necessary for flexible bronchoscopy? (Pro). *J Bronchology* 1994;1:246–249.
4. Colt HG. Is sedation necessary for flexible bronchoscopy? (Con). *J Bronchology* 1994;1:250–253.
5. Prakash UBS, Offord KP, Stubbs SE. Bronchoscopy in North America: the ACCP survey. *Chest* 1991;100:1668–1675.
6. Shevede K, Paoagopoulos G. A survey of 800 patients' knowledge, attitudes, and concerns regarding anesthesia. *Anesth Analg* 1991; 73:190–198.
7. Wansbrough SR, White PF. Sedation scales: measures of calmness or somnolence? *Anesth Analg* 1993;76:219–221.
8. Egbert LD, Battit GE, Turndorf H, Beecher HK. The value of the preoperative visit by an anesthetist. A study of doctor-patient rapport. *J Am Med Assoc* 1963;185:553–555.
9. Ovassapian A. Fiberoptic tracheal intubation. In: Ovassapian A, ed. Fiberoptic airway endoscopy in anesthesia and critical care. New York: Raven Press, 1990;57–79.
10. American Society of Anesthesiologists: Position on monitored care, Park Ridge, Ill. 1988.
11. Goldman JM. A simple, easy, and inexpensive method for monitoring ET_{CO2} through nasal cannulae (letter). *Anesthesiology* 1987;67:606.
12. Urmey WF. Accuracy of expired carbon dioxide partial pressure sampled from a nasal cannulae (letter). *Anesthesiology* 1988;68: 959–960.
13. Dunphy JA. Accuracy of expired carbon dioxide partial pressure sampled from a nasal cannulae (letter). *Anesthesiology* 1988;68: 960–961.
14. Youngs EJ, Shafer SL. Pharmacokinetic parameters relevant to recovery from opioids. *Anesthesiology* 1994;81:833–842.
15. Hughes MA, Glass PSA, Jacobs JR. Context-sensitive half-time in multicompartmental pharmacokinetic models for intravenous anesthetic drugs. *Anesthesiology* 1992;76:334–341.
16. Price HL. A dynamic concept of the distribution of thiopental in the human body. *Anesthesiology* 1960;21:40–45.
17. Shafer SL, Varvel JR. Pharmacokinetics, pharmacodynamics, and rational opioid selection. *Anesthesiology* 1991;74:53–63.
18. Shafer SL, Stanski DR. Improving the clinical utility of anesthetic drug pharmacokinetics. *Anesthesiology* 1992;76:327–330.
19. Philip BK. Supplemental medication for ambulatory procedures under regional anesthesia. *Anesth Analg* 1985;64:1117–1125.
20. Dundee JW, Pandit SK. Anterograde amnestic effects of pethidine, hyoscine and diazepam in adults. *Br J Pharmacol* 1972; 44:140–144.
21. Mandelli M, Tognoni G, and Garrattini S. Clinical pharmacokinetics of diazepam. *Clin Pharmacokinet* 1978;3:72–91.
22. Dixon J, Power SJ, Grundy EM, et al. Sedation for local anaesthesia: comparison of intravenous midazolam and diazepam. *Anaesthesia* 1984;39:372–376.
23. Kanto JH. Midazolam: the first water soluble benzodiazepine. Pharmacology, pharmacokinetics and efficacy in insomnia and anesthesia. *Pharmacotherapy* 1985;5:138–155.
24. Bailey PL, Pace NL, Ashburn MA, Moll JW, East KA, Stanley TH. Frequent hypoxemia and apnea after sedation with midazolam and fentanyl. *Anesthesiology* 1990;73:826–830.
25. Persson MP, Nilsson A, Hartvig P. Relation of sedation and amnesia to plasma concentrations of midazolam in surgical patients. *Clin Pharmacol Ther* 1988;43:324–329.
26. Klotz M, Kanto J. Pharmacokinetics and clinical use of flumazenil (RO 15–1788). *Clin Pharmacokinet* 1988;14:1–12.
27. Klotz M, Ziegler G, Ludwig L, Reimann IW. Pharmacodynamic interaction between midazolam and a specific benzodiazepine antagonist in humans. *J Clin Pharmacol* 1985;25:400–406.
28. Gross JB, Weller RS, Conrad P. Flumazenil antagonism of midazolam induced ventilatory depression. *Anesthesiology* 1991; 75: 179–185.
29. Amrein R, Hetzel W. Pharmacology of Dormicum (midazolam) and Anexate (flumazenil). *Acta Anaesthosiol Scand* 1990; 92(*Suppl*):6–15.
30. Brogden RN, Goa KL. Flumazenil. *Drugs* 1988;35:448–452.
31. White PF, Shafer A, Boyle WA III, Doze VA, Duncan S. Benzodiazepine antagonism does not provoke a stress response. *Anesthesiology* 1989;70:636–639.
32. Ricou B, Forster A, Bruckner A, et al. Clinical evaluation of a specific benzodiazepine antagonist. *Br J Anaesth* 1986;58: 1005–1011.
33. Prough DS, Raymond R, Bumgarner J, Shannon G. Acute pulmonary edema in healthy teenagers following conservative doses of intravenous naloxone. *Anesthesiology* 1984;60: 485–486.
34. Wride SR, Smith RE, Courtney PG. A fatal case of pulmonary edema in a healthy young male following naloxone administration. *Anaesth Intens Care* 1989;17:374–377.

35. Smith I, White PF, Nathanson M, Gouldson R. Propofol: An update on its clinical use. *Anesthesiology* 1994;81:1005–1043.
36. White PF, Negus JB. Sedative infusions during local and regional anestheesia: a comparison of midazolam and propofol. *J Clin Anesth* 1991;3:32–39.
37. Pratila MG, Fischer ME, Alagesan R, Alagesan R, Reinsel RÅ, Pratilas D. Propofol versus midazolam for monitored sedation: a comparison of intraoperative and recovery parameters. *J Clin Anesth* 1993;5:268–274.
38. Smith I, Monk TG, White PF, Ding Y. Propofol infusion during regional anesthesia: sedative, amnestic and anxiolytic properties. *Anesth Analg* 1994;79:313–319.
39. Randell T. Sedation for bronchofiberoscopy: comparison between propofol infusion and intravenous boluses of fentanyl and diazepam. *Acta Anesthesiol Scand* 1992;46:266–270.
40. Gin T, Yau G, Chan K, Gregory MA, Oh TE. Disposition of propofol infusion for Cesarean section. *Cand J Anaesthesia* 1991; 38:31–36.
41. Bacon RC, Razis PA. The effect of propofol sedation in pregnancy on neonatal condition. *Anaesthesia* 1994;49:1058–1060.
42. Shafer SL. Advances in propofol pharmacokinetics and pharmacodynamics. *J Clin Anesth* 1993;5(*Suppl*):S14–S21.
43. Mather LE. Clinical pharmacokinetics of fentanyl and its newer derivatives. *Clin Pharmacokinetics* 1983;8:422–446.
44. Arrowsmith JB, Gerstman BB, Fleischer DE, Benjamin SB. Results from the American Society for Gastrointestinal Endoscopy/ U.S. Food and Drug Administration collaborative study on complication rates and drug use during gastrointestinal endoscopy. *Gastrointest Endosc* 1991;37:421–427.
45. Daneshmend TK, Bell GD, Logan RF. Sedation for upper gastrointestinal endoscopy: results of a nationwide survey. *Gut* 1991;32:12–15.
46. Keeffe EB, O'Connor KW. 1989 American Society of Gastroenterology survey of endoscopic sedation and monitoring practices. *Gastrointest Endosc* 1990;36(3 *Suppl*):S13–S18.
47. Patterson KW, Noonan N, Keeling NW, Kirkham R, Hogan DF. Hypoxemia during outpatient gastrointestinal endoscopy: the effects of sedation and supplemental oxygen. *J Clin Anesth* 1995;7:136–140.
48. Fennerty MB, Earnest DL, Hudson PB, Sampliner RE. Physiologic changes during colonoscopy. *Gastrointest Endosc* 1990; 36:22–25.
49. Bell GD, McCloy RF, Charlton JE, et al. Recommendations for standards of sedation and patient monitoring during gastrointestinal endoscopy. *Gut* 1991;32:823–827.
50. Bell GD. Monitoring—the gastroenterologist's view. *Scand J Gastroenterol* 1990;179(*Suppl*):18–23.
51. Cousins MJ. Monitoring—the anaesthetist's view. *Scand J Gastroenterol* 1990(*Suppl*);179:12–17.
52. Nelson MD Jr. Guidelines for the monitoring and care of children during and after sedation for imaging studies. *Am J Roentgenol* 1993;160:581–582.
53. Fisher DM. Sedation of pediatric patients: an anesthesiologist's perspective. *Radiology* 1990;175:613–615.
54. Thompson JR, Schneider S, Ashwal S, Holden BS, Hinshaw DB, Hasso AN. The choice of sedation for computed tomography in children: a prospective evaluation. *Radiology* 1982;143: 475–479.
55. Campbell RL. Prevention of complications associated with intravenous sedation and general anesthesia. *J Oral Maillofac Surg* 1986;44:289–301.
56. Trieger N. Intravenous sedation in dentistry and oral surgery. *Int Anesthesiol Clin* 1989;27:83–91.
57. Litchfield NB. Complications of intravenous diazepam. An overall assessment of 16,000 cases and detailed studies of 6,000 cases. *Dent Anaesth Sedat* 1981;10:7–24.
58. Lowe T, Brook IM. Oxygen saturation during third molar removal with local anaesthetic alone and in combination with intravenous sedation. *Br Dent J* 1991;171:210–211.
59. Friedman M. Iatrogenic disease: addressing a growing epidemic. *Postgrad Med* 1982;71:128–129.
60. Brennan TA, Leape LL, Laird NM, et al. Incidence of adverse events and negligence in hospitalized patients. Results of the Harvard Medical Practice Study I. *N Engl J Med* 1991;324: 370–376.
61. Leape LL, Brennan TA, Laird N. The nature of adverse events in hospitalized patients. Results of the Harvard Medical Practice Study II. *N Engl J Med* 1991;324:377–384.
62. Bedell SE, Deitz DC, Leean D, Delbanco TL. Incidence and characteristics of preventable iatrogenic cardiac arrests. *J Am Med Assoc* 1991;265:2815–2820.
63. Joint Commission on Accreditation of Healthcare Organization (JCAHO): Accreditation Manual for Hospitals. Oakbrook Terrace, Illinois: JCAHO, 1991:269–280.
64. Holzman RS, Cullen DJ, Eichhorn JH, Philips JH. Guidelines for sedation by nonanesthesiologists during diagnostic and therapeutic procedures. *J Clin Anesth* 1994;4:265–276.
65. Calder I, Ordman AJ, Jackowski A, Croukard HA. The brain laryngeal mask airway. An alternative to emergency intubation. *Anaesthesia* 1990;45:137–139.

CHAPTER 6

Fiberoptic Tracheal Intubation in Adults

Andranik Ovassapian, M.D.

Since their introduction in the early 1900s, conventional tracheal intubation techniques have remained essentially unchanged, and limited to blind nasal and rigid laryngoscopic techniques. In 1967 a flexible fiberoptic choledochoscope was used to perform a difficult nasotracheal intubation in a patient with advanced rheumatoid arthritis (1). Five years later, a fiberoptic bronchoscope was used for nasotracheal intubation (2,3). The first series of fiberoptic intubations was reported by Stiles and her colleagues in 1972 (4).

Today the fiberscope's value in the management of the difficult tracheal intubation is well established (5–10). The fiberscope is an excellent and powerful airway management device in the hands of the skillful endoscopist. The use of the fiberscope need not be limited to patients for whom tracheal intubation proves, or may be considered, difficult. There are many circumstances in which the fiberscope provides a superior technique for tracheal intubation compared to conventional techniques (Table 1). In fact the rou-

TABLE 1. *Indications for fiberoptic intubation*

- Routine intubation (teaching and learning)
- Difficult intubation
  - Anticipated
    - History of previous difficult intubation
    - Physical evidence of difficult intubation
  - Unanticipated
    - Missed evidence of difficult intubation
    - Hidden causes
- Compromised airway
  - Upper airway pathology
  - Tracheal stenosis and compression
- Extension of neck not desirable
  - Unstable neck
  - Vertebral artery insufficiency
- High risk of dental damage
  - Poor, loose, or fragile teeth
  - Extensive dental restoration
- Awake intubation with topical anesthesia

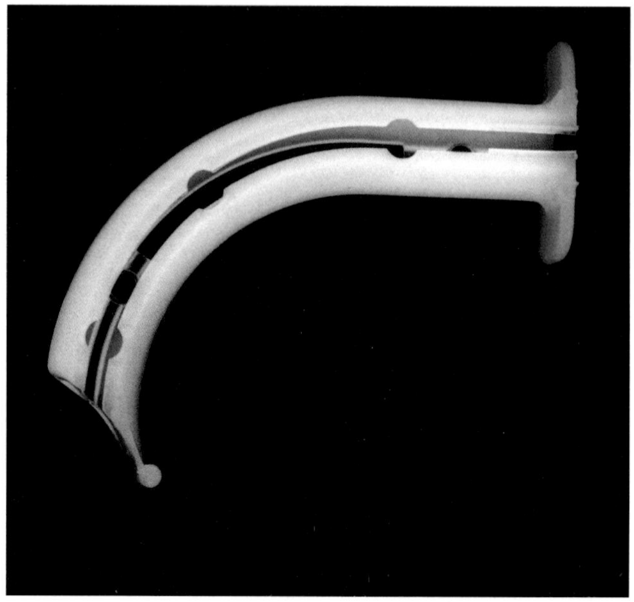

FIG. 1. Berman intubating/pharyngeal airway.

tine use of the fiberscope in tracheal intubation provides the first step in learning this fascinating, versatile airway skill (11).

Fiberoptic intubation is usually simple, fast, and easily accomplished when appropriate preparatory steps are taken. Many patients who might be denied a general anesthetic or subjected to tracheostomy because intubation by rigid laryngoscopy appeared difficult may be safely and easily intubated with the help of the fiberscope.

Several intubation techniques have been described, and various airway devices have been developed to facilitate fiberoptic tracheal intubation (12–18).

DEVICES TO AID FIBEROPTIC INTUBATION

Intubating Airways

These unique oral airways assist the endoscopist in keeping the fiberscope in the midline, aiding in exposure of laryngeal structures and maintaining an open oropharynx. The intubating airway also protects the fiberscope by preventing the patient from biting it.

Berman Intubating/Pharyngeal Airway

This airway is disposable and tubular along its entire length (Fig. 1). It was designed for blind orotracheal intubation (18). It has also been used and recommended for fiberoptic intubation. It has a longitudinal opening on its side which can be opened wide to disengage it from the endotracheal tube and then it can be removed from the patient's mouth. It is available in different sizes. Because of its length and tubular shape, the fiberscope cannot be maneuvered by bending its tip once it is placed through the airway. Therefore, if the distal end of the airway is not in line with the glottic opening, exposure of the cords can be accomplished only by partial withdrawal of the airway.

Ovassapian Fiberoptic Intubating Airway

This intubating airway provides an open space in the oropharynx and protects the fiberscope from being bitten by the patient. It provides a passage for the endotracheal tube and permits subsequent removal of the airway without disconnecting the endotracheal (ET) tube adapter (16) (Fig. 2).

The airway has a flat lingual surface, which minimizes rotation of the airway. The wide distal half of

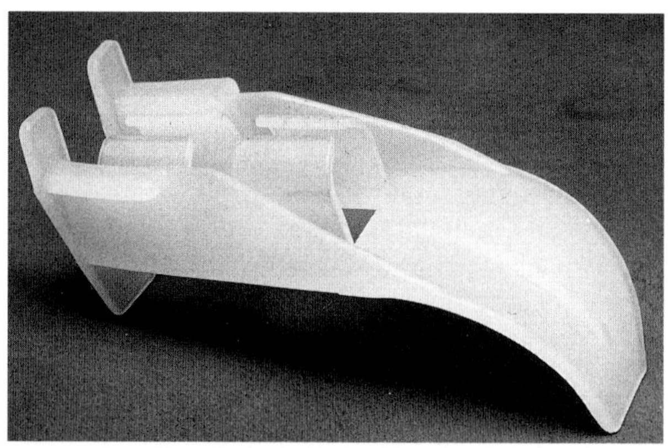

FIG. 2. Ovassapian fiberoptic intubating airway. (From ref. 34.)

the airway prevents the tongue and soft tissues of the anterior pharyngeal wall from falling back and obstructing the view of the glottis while maintaining an open space for maneuvering the tip of the fiberscope. The proximal half of the airway has a pair of guide walls that curve toward each other with a space between to allow passage of the fiberscope and endotracheal tube. The guide walls are flexible and permit removal of the airway from around the ET tube. This airway will accommodate an ET tube up to 9.0 mm inner diameter (ID).

Patil-Syracuse Endoscopic Airway

Designed for fiberoptic intubation, this airway has a small central groove on the lingual surface (13) (Fig. 3). A slit at the distal end of the airway allows the tip of the fiberscope to be manipulated in an anteroposterior direction but limits lateral manipulation. It is made of aluminum and is available in only one size.

Williams Airway Intubator

This airway was designed for blind orotracheal intubation, but its use in fiberoptic intubation has been described (15). The proximal half is cylindrical, while the distal half has an open lingual surface. It is made in two sizes (90 and 100 mm), which will admit up to a 8.5-mm ID ET tube (Fig. 4). The tip of the fiberscope cannot be maneuvered anteroposteriorly or laterally. If the distal end of the airway is not in line with the glottis, exposure of the vocal cords is difficult, requiring partial withdrawal of the airway. The adapter of the ET tube should be removed before intubation if the airway is to be removed following successful intubation.

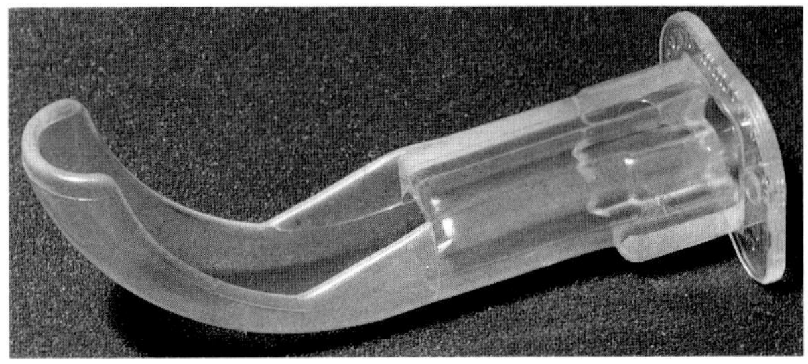

FIG. 4. Williams airway intubator.

Endoscopy Mask (Intubating Mask)

This device described by Mallios (12) in 1980 and by Patil and associates (13) in 1982 (Fig. 5), allows intubation with a fiberscope through a port/diaphragm in the mask. The diaphragm provides a seal, allowing positive pressure ventilation with a fiberscope in place.

Once the tip of the fiberscope is placed in the trachea, the ET tube is advanced over the fiberscope, through the diaphragm, and into the trachea. The intubating mask permits oral or nasal intubation. More recently, a new mask adapter for fiberoptic intubation of the anesthetized patient has been reported. The adapter consists of two parts: a rotating disk with an entrance port, and the adapter body which attaches to a Laerdal face mask (14).

An alternative to the endoscopy mask is to place an ET tube into a face mask, inflating the cuff to form a seal (19). A bronchoscopic swivel adapter is then placed between the tube and breathing circuit. This device allows for continuous anesthesia and positive pressure ventilation during fiberoptic intubation. The ET tube should be cut to the desired (shorter) length to allow adequate length for the fiberscope to enter the trachea (Fig. 6).

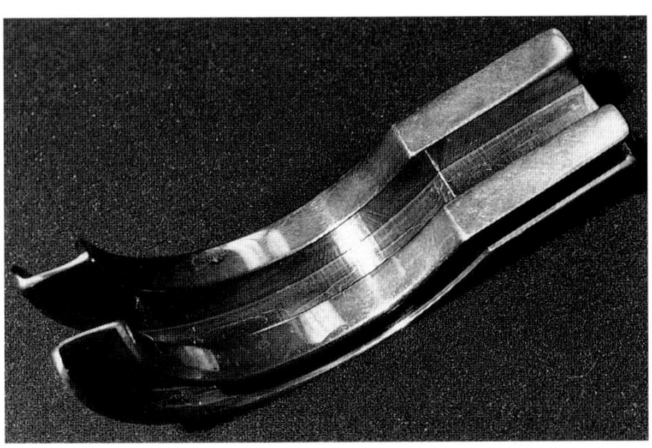

FIG. 3. Patil-Syracuse endoscopic airway.

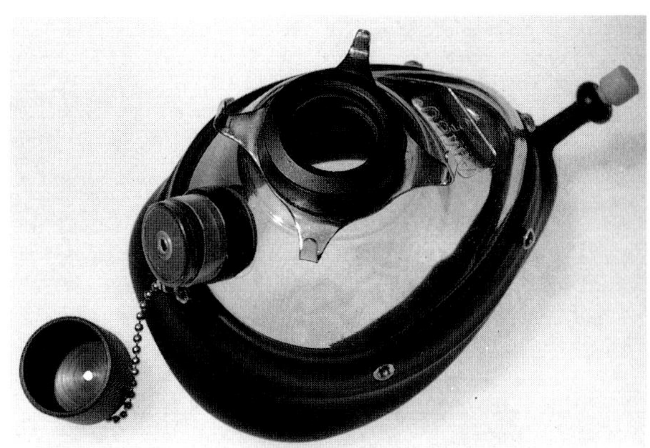

FIG. 5. Patil-Syracuse endoscopy mask.

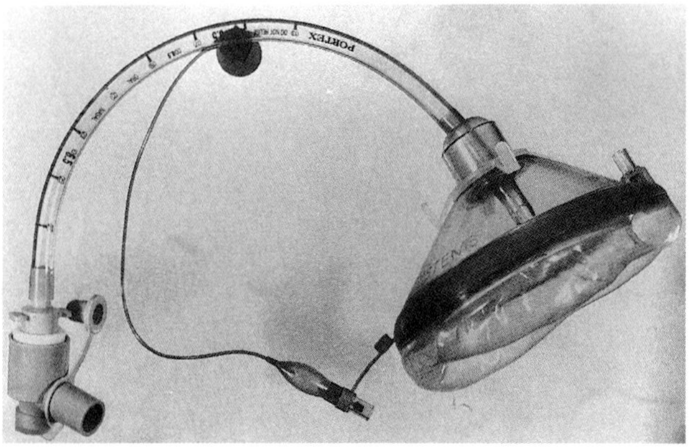

FIG. 6. Endotracheal tube with inflated cuff inside anesthesia mask (With permission, ref. 19.).

Malleable Tongue Retractor

This device is used to retract the tongue anteriorly to assist exposure of the glottis. It can be used for orotracheal or nasotracheal intubation (17).

PREPARATION FOR INTUBATION

Inspection of the Fiberscope

Prior to use, the fiberscope, light source, and ancillary equipment must be carefully checked and inspected to assure they are in proper working order. The light guide cable of the fiberscope is connected to the light source and the light intensity adjusted to an adequate level (Table 2).

The entire surface of the insertion cord is checked for defects. The angulation lever is manipulated to see that it functions smoothly. Then, holding the tip of the fiberscope a few millimeters away from some printing, the diopter ring is adjusted to insure a focused view and confirm that all lenses are clear.

TABLE 2. *Preparation and inspection of fiberscope*

Attach fiberoptic light guide cable to light source.
Adjust light intensity to adequate level of illumination.
Check insertion cord for abnormalities such as kinking, dents, wrinkles, or bite marks.
Check function of angulation lever.
Focus the fiberscope to your eyes.
Connect suction line and ensure proper functioning of suction.
Place the tip of the insertion cord and the endotracheal tube in warm water bath to prevent fogging of lens, soften endotracheal tube to ease passage, and minimize tissue trauma.
Lubricate insertion cord of fiberscope and the endotracheal tube.

The suction line is connected to the fiberscope, and water is suctioned to assure the channel is clear and working. In newer Olympus and Pentax model fiberscopes, suction is activated by a push button at the proximal end of the fiberscope handle. These newer fiberscopes also have a separate injection port located at the distal section of the handle which allows the installation of local anesthetics (Chapter 1).

The instillation of local anesthetics can be delivered through the working channel port of the fiberscope. The insertion cord of the fiberscope and the endotracheal tube are placed in warm water. This prevents fogging of the lens, and softens the ET tube, easing its passage through the intubating airway or nasal passage. The insertion cord of the fiberscope is lubricated with a water-soluble or local anesthetic lubricant before use.

The control section of the instrument is held by the left hand, and the angulation control lever is operated by the thumb. The angulation control lever is manipulated slowly and as little as necessary to guide the distal end of the insertion cord toward the target.

Control of the Fiberscope

The body of the fiberscope is held by the tips of the fingers so that the thumb position remains perpendicular to the angulation lever and controls movement of the fiberscope tip in a up/down direction, while the index finger controls the suction button. The tip of the fiberscope moves in the direction opposite to that of the angulation lever. An upward movement of the lever causes the tip to point downward, a downward movement causes the reverse. To move the tip of the fiberscope to the left or right, the fiberscope is rotated in the desired direction by the hand holding the body of the fiberscope.

The insertion cord should advance easily through the lumen of the ET tube. The hand that is not holding the scope should not grip the insertion cord tightly, as this will prevent the insertion cord to follow laterally directed movement of the fiberscope. The insertion cord should also be kept straight to avoid loop formation on its longitudinal axes. If a loop is formed, the tip of insertion cord will not follow the directional changes transferred by rotating the fiberscope body. The nonscope hand controls the advancement and withdrawal of the fiberscope.

Position of the Endoscopist

The endoscopist can be positioned either at the head of the table (head position), or at the side of the patient (side position). Advantages of the head position include: familiar orientation of airway anatomy by the anesthesiologist; easy access to equipment and drugs; no interference with surgical preparation or surgery. The main disadvantage of the head position is the position of physiologic monitoring devices which are often positioned to the side or back of the endoscopist and not easily viewed.

The main advantage of the side position is that it permits the endoscopist to face the patient and the monitoring devices. The disadvantages include: reversal of airway anatomy from the view familiar to the anesthesiologist; distance of the endoscopist from the anesthesia machine, airway equipment, and drugs; the position is unacceptable when surgery is in progress and may delay surgical preparation of the patient.

TABLE 3. *Indications for awake tracheal intubation*

Difficult or impossible mask ventilation
Acromegaly
Supraglottic mass
Morbid obesity
Compromised airway of various etiology
Difficult intubation
High risk for aspiration
Neurologic examination after intubation
Unstable cervical spine
Vertebrobasilar insufficiency
Self-positioning
Prone position
Lateral position
Outside the operating room
Ventilatory failure
Severely ill patients

Position of the Endotracheal Tube

Prior to performing fiberoptic intubation, the ET tube can be placed in either of two general positions. The tube can be partially inserted inside the intubating airway during orotracheal intubation or in the nostril in the case of nasotracheal intubation (tube-first technique). In the second general approach the ET tube is placed (loaded) over the fiberscope, which is then passed through the airway or the nostril (scope-first technique).

In the tube-first approach, the possibility of passing the tip of the fiberscope through the Murphy eye of the ET tube, rather than through its distal opening, should be kept in mind. If the fiberscope accidentally passes through the Murphy's eye, the ET tube may not advance over the fiberscope into the trachea. If the ET tube is advanced with force, removal of the fiberscope may not be possible, requiring removal of the tube and fiberscope together. Forceful removal of the fiberscope should be avoided. Forceful action may not only damage the fiberscope, but also cause a shearing of its plastic cover inside the trachea, leaving debris in the airway.

TRACHEAL INTUBATION OF THE CONSCIOUS PATIENT

The patient who has a history of failed intubation or upper airway pathology, or one expected to present a difficult airway, can benefit from awake fiberoptic intubation (Table 3). The application of good topical anesthesia and mild sedation makes fiberoptic intubation relatively easy in the awake patient. Maintaining spontaneous ventilation keeps the airway open, and the patient can swallow and clear secretions. Furthermore, having the patient phonate or breathe deeply can assist the endoscopist in locating the glottis when airway anatomy is distorted (9,20) (Table 4).

Patient Preparation

Preanesthetic preparation of the patient should include a detailed explanation of the procedure to optimize the patient's cooperation, appropriate preoperative medication to relax the patient, and administration of an antisialagogue drug to minimize secretions (21).

Conscious sedation is desirable for an awake intubation to minimize psychological trauma, provided that patient safety is not compromised. Depending on the patient's condition and the indication for awake intubation, an opiate, sedative hypnotic, or combination is used (22,23).

Strong depressants of the airway reflexes, opiates produce profound analgesia and facilitate oropharyngeal instrumentation while the patient is still capable of following verbal commands. However, narcotized patients are more susceptible to aspiration of gastric contents if regurgitation or vomiting occur.

Airway protective reflexes remain more active when a sedative such as diazepam or midazolam is used, but the patient may be less cooperative and react more

TABLE 4. *Tracheal intubation in conscious patient*

Advantages
Safest approach in patients with difficult airway
Maintains spontaneous ventilation
Keeps airway open
Time of intubation not limited
Patient can swallow the secretions
Deep breaths on command assist exposure of glottis
Allows postintubation neurologic examination
Disadvantages
Patient cooperation is needed
Possible patient discomfort
Gagging with poor topical anesthesia
Difficult in children and uncooperative patients

vigorously to instrumentation of the airway. A combination of fentanyl and diazepam (average dose, 1.5 μg/kg and 0.10 mg/kg, respectively), or fentanyl and midazolam (1.5 μg/kg and 30 μg/kg, respectively), has been used successfully for this purpose.

Drying agents are essential when intubation is carried out before induction of anesthesia. Excessive secretions interfere with the effectiveness of topical anesthesia, thereby leaving airway reflexes active, and are a major cause of patient discomfort and failure of the technique. In addition, instrumentation of the airway increases the flow of saliva. Increased secretions add to the difficulty of fiberoptic intubation (20–23).

The patient at a high risk for aspiration of gastric contents will benefit from premedication that increases gastric pH, reduces gastric volume, and enhances gastric emptying. Ranitidine HCL 150 mg orally, or Cimetidine 400 mg is given the night before surgery. The beta-2 blocking agent will increase the gastric pH and reduce gastric volume. Metoclopromide is a dopamine antagonist and has three different effects; it accelerates gastric emptying, increases the tone of the lower esophageal sphincter, and depresses the vomiting center in the medulla. Regurgitation and aspiration is more likely in anesthetized patients with a difficult airway, due to their attempts at breathing against an obstructed airway. The problem is further compounded by attempts at mask ventilation and the possibility of forcing air into the stomach. Both problems serve to open the gastroesophageal sphincter promoting regurgitation.

TABLE 5. *Steps of awake fiberoptic orotracheal intubation*

Titrate sedation.
Apply topical anesthesia.
Spray oropharynx with 4% or 10% lidocaine (4–6 sprays).
Inject 3 ml of 4% lidocaine through cricothyroid membrane.
or
Spray-as-you-go through fiberscope.
Apply lidocaine jelly to base of tongue.
Place intubating airway in patient's mouth.
Suction oropharynx gently through airway.
Place endotracheal tube in intubating airway about 5 cm.
Introduce fiberscope through the endotracheal tube, making sure to pass through distal lumen.
Identify the epiglottis and vocal cords. Advance fiberscope in trachea.
Pass endotracheal tube over fiberscope into trachea.
Confirm correct position of the endotracheal tube (3 cm above carina).
Attach breathing system. Reconfirm correct tube placement.
Tape the tube. Induce anesthesia.

Oral Approach

After lightly sedating the patient, topical anesthesia of the oropharynx is applied. Five or six sprays (50–60 mg) of 10% aerosolized lidocaine is applied to the palate, base of the tongue, and lateral pharyngeal walls. Translaryngeal injection of 3 ml of 4% lidocaine (120 mg) through the cricothyroid membrane provides topical anesthesia to the larynx and the trachea (Table 5). With experience, adequate topical anesthesia can be accomplished within 1 min.

To test its adequacy and supplement the topical anesthesia of the oropharynx, a local anesthetic jelly is spread on the base of the tongue using a tongue blade. In 94% of the cases, the topical anesthesia achieved is good to excellent for performing tracheal intubation (21). Additional topical anesthesia may be applied to the oropharynx if the patient reacts to the presence of the airway. Laryngeal topical anesthesia can be supplemented, if necessary, by spraying an additional 2 ml of 4% lidocaine (80 mg) through the fiberscope.

Establishing topical anesthesia prior to laryngoscopy will prevent coughing, swallowing, laryngeal spasm, and excessive salivation, all of which add to the difficulty of fiberoptic intubation. After gaining experience, topical anesthesia of the larynx and trachea may be achieved by spraying a local anesthetic through the working channel of the fiberscope rather than by injection through the cricothyroid membrane. Inhalation of local anesthetics through a nebulizer will also provide topical anesthesia of the upper airway and can be used in patients where severe coughing should be avoided (24). However, topical anesthesia of the airway using lidocaine has a duration of action of no more than 20 min and must be applied just before any attempt at intubation.

After obtaining adequate topical anesthesia, the head is placed in the normal intubating position. An intubating airway is placed in the mouth, the oropharynx is suctioned, and the lubricated ET tube is placed 4–5 cm inside the airway (tube-first approach). The fourth and fifth fingers of the right hand hold the ET tube to prevent premature advancement, while the index finger and thumb advance the fiberscope through it (Fig. 7). The endoscopist should look through the fiberscope to avoid passing the fiberscope through the Murphy eye of the ET tube.

As the fiberscope is advanced toward the oropharynx, the white pharyngeal surface of the airway, soft palate, and uvula will come into view (Fig. 8). With further advancement, the fiberscope enters into the oropharynx and its tip is deflected anteriorly to expose the epiglottis and vocal cords. In the presence of a large floppy epiglottis, the tip of the fiberscope should be manipulated under the tip of the epiglottis to visualize the vocal cords. By extending the head at the atlanto-

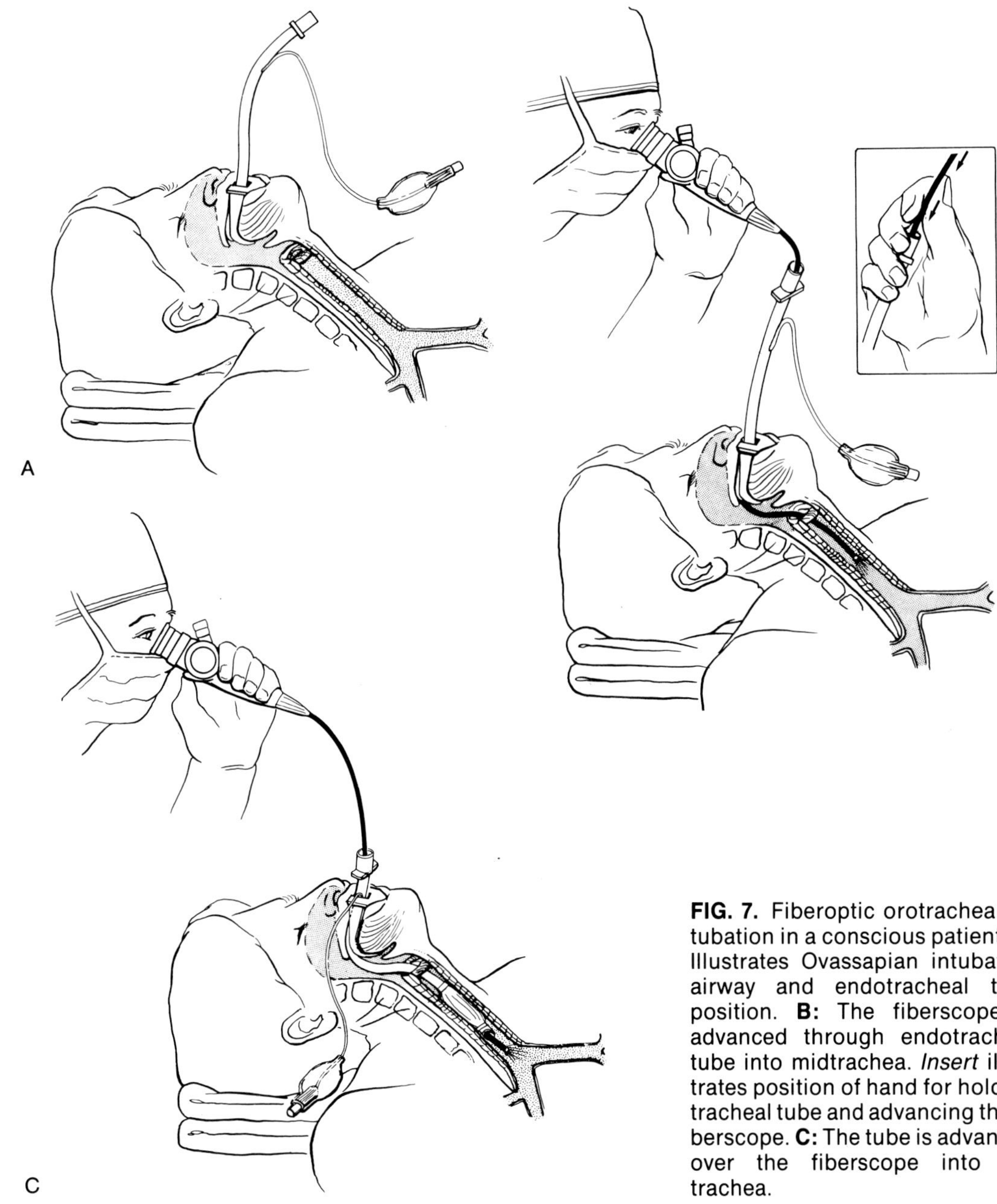

FIG. 7. Fiberoptic orotracheal intubation in a conscious patient. **A:** Illustrates Ovassapian intubating airway and endotracheal tube position. **B:** The fiberscope is advanced through endotracheal tube into midtrachea. *Insert* illustrates position of hand for holding tracheal tube and advancing the fiberscope. **C:** The tube is advanced over the fiberscope into the trachea.

occipital joint, keeping the mouth closed, the epiglottis will be kept away from the posterior pharyngeal wall. On occasions, a jaw thrust maneuver by an assistant or pulling the tongue forward may be required to facilitate glottic exposure.

After the vocal cords are exposed, they are maintained in the center of the field of view by fine manipulations of the control lever as the fiberscope is advanced. Without such maneuvering, the tip of the fiberscope often impinges on the anterior commissure or the anterior laryngeal wall. The flexing of the tip of the fiberscope posteriorly at this point will bring the laryngeal and tracheal lumen into view. The fiberscope is then advanced into the midtrachea, and the ET tube is advanced over the firmly held stationary fiberscope with a twisting motion into the trachea. The endoscopist should remove his eye from the fiberscope eyepiece and observe the endotracheal tube during this maneuver. It is important to ensure that the fiberscope is not pushed farther into the tracheobronchial tree during advancement of the ET tube. The tip of the ET tube is positioned 3–4 cm above the carina.

If an intubating airway is not used, the scope-first technique is applied. In this approach, the problem of the fiberscope being passed through the Murphy eye of the ET tube is avoided, but deviation of the fiberscope off of the midline is common.

In the obese patient and in most difficult airways, the

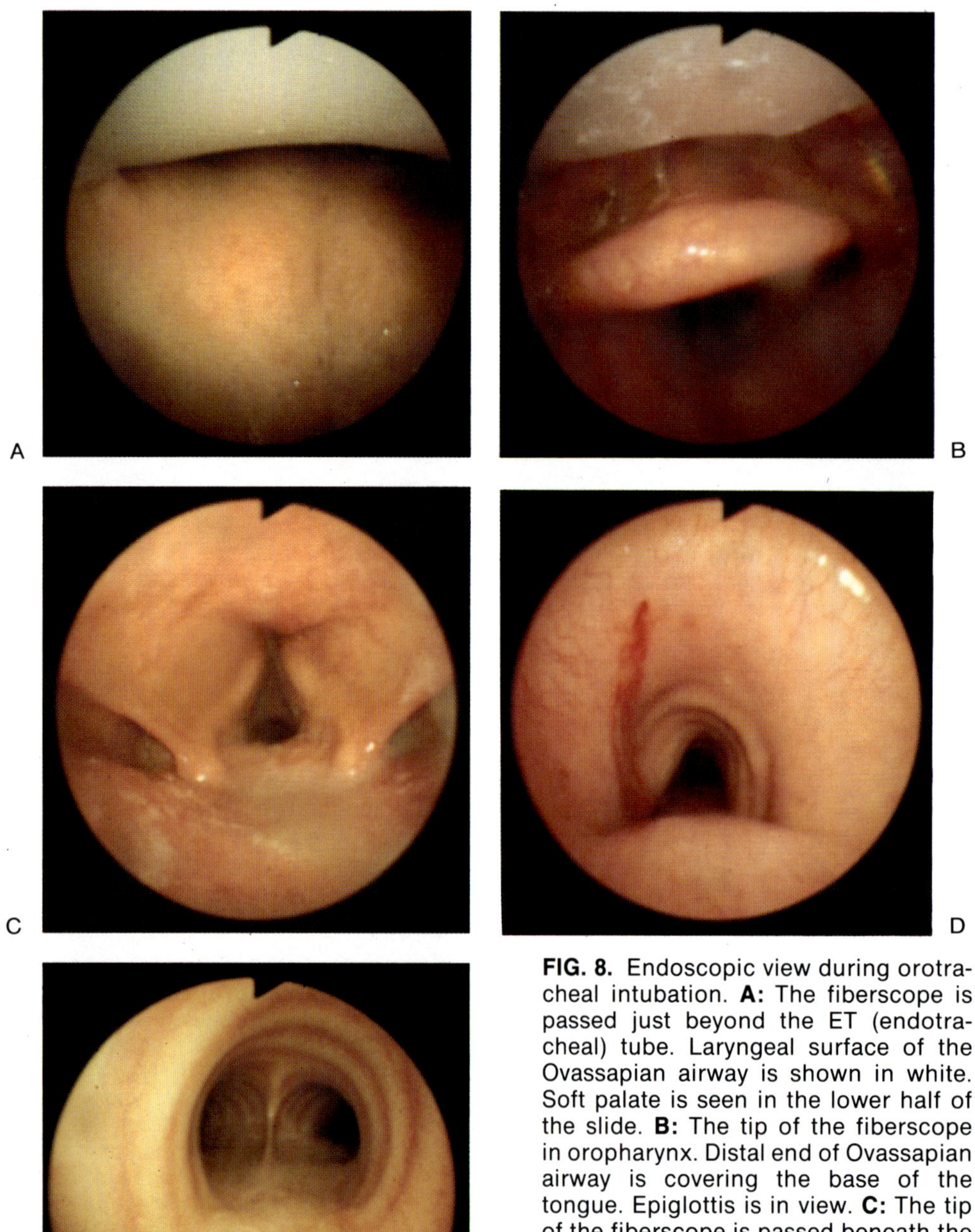

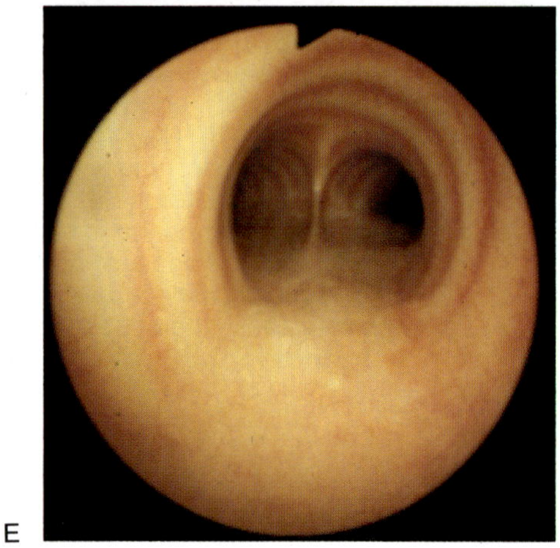

FIG. 8. Endoscopic view during orotracheal intubation. **A:** The fiberscope is passed just beyond the ET (endotracheal) tube. Laryngeal surface of the Ovassapian airway is shown in white. Soft palate is seen in the lower half of the slide. **B:** The tip of the fiberscope in oropharynx. Distal end of Ovassapian airway is covering the base of the tongue. Epiglottis is in view. **C:** The tip of the fiberscope is passed beneath the tip of the epiglottis. Glottis is in view. **D:** The tip of the fiberscope is passed just beyond the vocal cords. Anterior wall of larynx showing entry site of translaryngeal injection needle. **E:** The tip of the fiberscope in lower third of the trachea. Carina is in view.

use of the sitting position during application of topical anesthesia and intubation should be considered. The sitting position makes maintaining the sniffing position easier, and the local anesthetics gravitate toward the larynx and trachea (25).

The oral approach is usually slightly more difficult than the nasal approach because of the sharp curve leading from the oral cavity into the larynx (22,26,27) (Table 6). In 20–30% of patients, even though the fiberscope has entered the trachea, the ET tube impinges on laryngeal anatomy and cannot be advanced into the trachea (4,20,22). It is postulated that the tube catches on the arytenoids, interarytenoid muscle, epiglottis, or vocal cords, or that it lodges in the pyriform sinus (4). When this happens, the ET tube is pulled back over the fiberscope, rotated 90°counterclockwise to position the bevel of the tube posteriorly at the 6 o'clock position (22,28), and re-advanced during deep inspiration.

TABLE 6. *Advantages and disadvantages of orotracheal intubation*

Advantages	Disadvantages
Faster intubation	Mouth opening is required
Bacteremia unlikely	Cooperation of patient required
Larger diameter tube	Biting will occlude the tube
Less discomfort	Gagging is far greater than in nasal approach
	More difficult fiberoptic technique than nasal

In some patients, this maneuver may have to be repeated two to three times, particularly when a small-size fiberscope is used for placement of a large ET tube.

The larger the gap between the external diameter of the fiberscope and the ID of the ET tube, the more chance there is that the tube may not easily slide into the trachea (22,27). In two patients in our series, when repeated attempts at advancing an 8.5-mm ID tube over a small 4.0-mm fiberscope failed, the tube easily advanced when the small fiberscope was changed to a 6.0-mm fiberscope (22). Laryngospasm, due to poor topical anesthesia, may also prevent ET tube advancement. Additional topical anesthesia applied through the fiberscope will frequently remedy the problem.

Nasal Approach

Fiberoptic nasotracheal intubation is often easier than the oral approach because it is easier to a maintain midline position. In addition, the fiberscope is usually pointed straight at the glottis as it enters the oropharynx. Since there is no sharp turn to negotiate, the vocal cords are usually visible from a distance (Table 7) (7,9,20).

TABLE 7. *Advantages and disadvantages of nasotracheal intubation*

Advantages	Disadvantages
Easier fiberoptic technique	Takes more time to prepare
Mouth opening not required	Longer and smaller tube
Biting of fiberscope and tube not possible	Trauma and epistaxis common
Easier mouth care	Pressure necrosis of septum and nasal alai
Less laryngeal damage on short term	Bacteremia, sinusitis, otitis likely
Greater patient comfort	Submucosal tunneling
	Basilar skull fracture a possible contraindication

After selection of the most patent nostril, 4 or 5% cocaine is applied using cotton tip applicators to the nasal mucosa. This agent provides excellent topical anesthesia and shrinkage of mucosal tissue. The cotton tip swabs are gradually worked posteriorly along the floor of the nose until the applicator encounters the bony resistance of the posterior nasal pharynx. Spraying the nasal passages with 10% xylocaine prior to advancing the applicators may minimize the initial discomfort. However, most patients dislike the burning sensation and the taste of the lidocaine (29).

Laryngotracheal anesthesia is achieved by translaryngeal injection as described earlier, or by spraying through the fiberscope during the process of intubation. There is no need to apply topical anesthesia to the oropharynx, as the gag reflex is not stimulated by the nasal tracheal approach (20,22,30).

After sedation and application of topical anesthesia, an appropriate-size ET tube, softened in warm water, is lubricated generously, and gently inserted through the prepared nostril until the bend at the posterior nasopharynx is reached (tube-first technique). If it does not make the bend, it is pulled back, rotated 90° to the right or left, and reintroduced. If this maneuver is unsuccessful, the ET tube is pulled back, and the lubricated fiberscope is inserted into the tube and used as a guide to direct it into the oropharynx.

It is important to avoid passing the tube too far distally into the oropharynx as it may direct the fiberscope away from the midline and interfere with laryngeal exposure. The oropharynx is suctioned thoroughly through the ET tube, and the lubricated fiberscope is inserted through it into the oropharynx (Fig. 9). In 80–85% of patients, the epiglottis and vocal cords are seen with minimal or no manipulation of the fiberscope tip (20). In heavily sedated or edentulous patients, the tongue and pharyngeal tissue may block exposure of the larynx and vocal cords. Extension of the head, application of a jaw thrust, or pulling the tongue forward will help expose the vocal cords. The fiberscope is advanced into the midtrachea followed by the ET tube. In nasotracheal fiberoptic intubation, the problem of the ET tube meeting resistance and not entering the trachea is uncommon.

There are a number of advantages to the tube-first technique. It avoids the possibility of nasal secretions covering the lens of the fiberscope and obscuring the view. In addition, a tight nasal passage can be recognized when the fiberscope is being advanced. Once the fiberscope has passed through the ET tube into the trachea, advancing the tube over the fiberscope is easily accomplished. Disadvantages of the tube-first technique include a greater possibility of causing nasal bleeding and tears in the nasal mucosa secondary to the ET tube not making the bend into the oropharynx.

In performing the scope-first technique, the ET tube

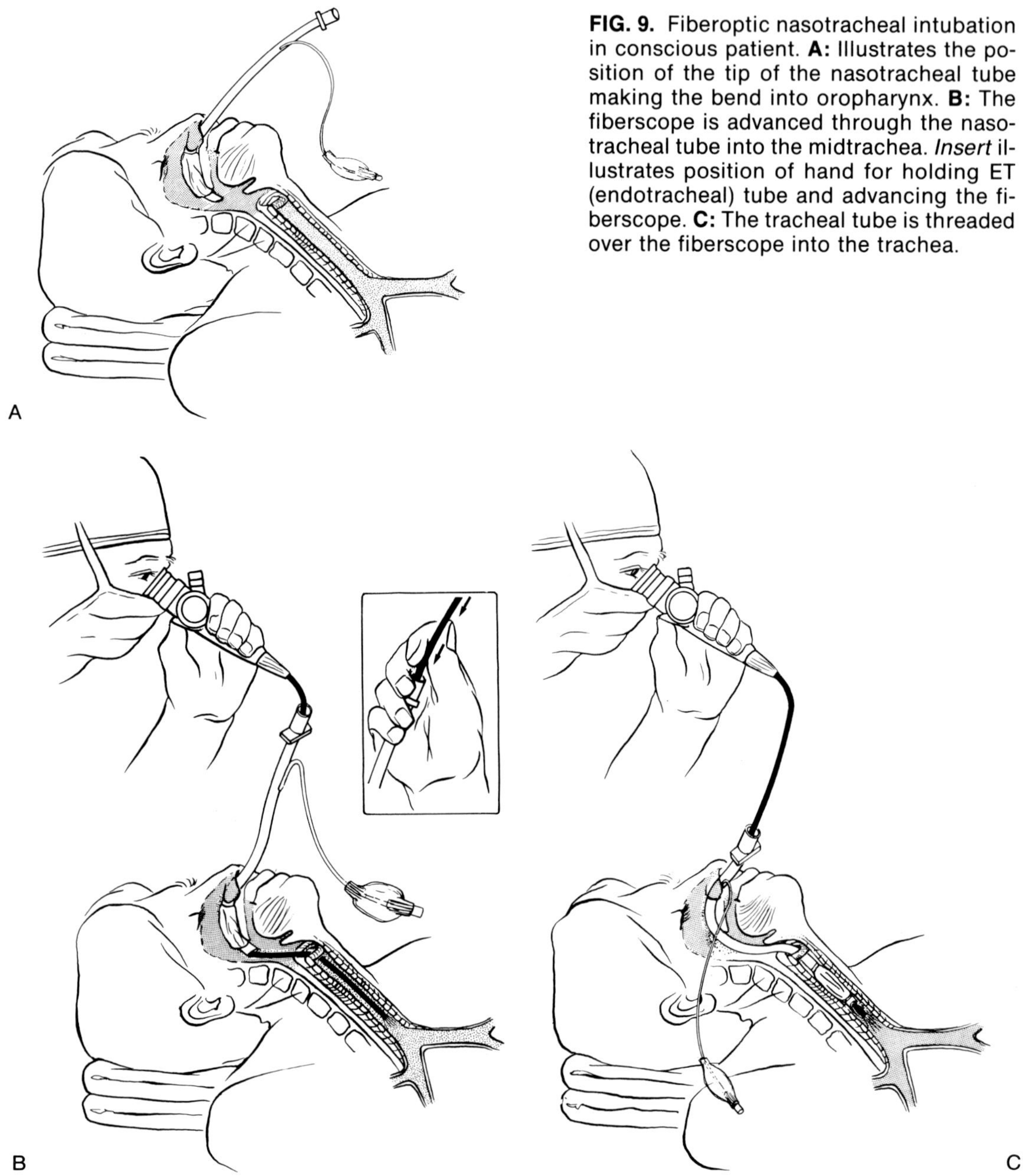

FIG. 9. Fiberoptic nasotracheal intubation in conscious patient. **A:** Illustrates the position of the tip of the nasotracheal tube making the bend into oropharynx. **B:** The fiberscope is advanced through the nasotracheal tube into the midtrachea. *Insert* illustrates position of hand for holding ET (endotracheal) tube and advancing the fiberscope. **C:** The tracheal tube is threaded over the fiberscope into the trachea.

is loaded over the insertion cord of the fiberscope. The fiberscope is then passed through the nostril and advanced through the glottis into the trachea. The ET tube is then advanced over the fiberscope into the trachea.

While the scope-first technique allows inspection of the nasal anatomy, it is difficult to judge the patency of nasal passages. After passage of the fiberscope into the trachea, the ET tube may not pass through the nose. If so, the procedure will have to be repeated using a smaller tube or trying the other nostril. Some endoscopists anesthetize both nostrils initially in the event that this may occur.

Anatomical Changes Affecting Nasal Intubation

Anterior septal deviation is common but does not interfere with intubation, since the problem usually involves cartilaginous, not bony, tissues. Nasal spurs may either be bony or cartilaginous and may compress the endotracheal tube, preventing passage. The movement of the tube over bony spurs can damage the ET tube cuff, or cause epistaxis.

The presence of large polyps will prevent nasal intubation. Small polyps usually respond well to topical vasoconstrictors and shrink. The presence of small polyps are not necessarily a contraindication to nasal intubation. Adenoidal tissue, quite common in children, is uncommon in adults. Osteophytes of the cervical spine can interfere with nasal intubation, deflecting the ET tube and fiberscope to the side, or anteriorly away from the glottic opening.

TRACHEAL INTUBATION UNDER GENERAL ANESTHESIA

Fiberoptic intubation under general anesthesia may be performed with the patient either breathing spontaneously or paralyzed with controlled ventilation.

Two major disadvantages of fiberoptic intubation under general anesthesia are the time limitation imposed by an apneic patient as well as the loss of tone of the tongue and pharyngeal tissues. This loss of tone serves to close the pharyngeal space, impairing visualization of the larynx (Table 8) (22).

To minimize apnea time and facilitate laryngeal exposure, an assistant is needed. The assistant is directed in four tasks: (a) to mount the ET tube on the lubricated fiberscope and have it ready to hand to the endoscopist as soon as the anesthesia mask is removed; (b) to apply a jaw thrust to maintain an open oropharynx; (c) to observe the apnea time; and (d) to monitor the patient. The endoscopy cart is placed at the head of the table on the left side of the patient, while the assistant stands on the patient's left side facing the endoscopist.

Oral Approach

After general anesthesia and muscle relaxation are established, the anesthesia mask is removed, the intubating airway is placed inside the mouth, and the oropharynx suctioned (Table 9). Ventilation by mask is resumed for 30–60 sec. The assistant at this time will have the fiberscope ready, with the endotracheal tube mounted on its insertion cord (Fig. 10). The anesthesia mask is removed; the endoscopist grasps the body of the fiberscope with his left hand, and the tip of the insertion cord with his right. The tip of the insertion cord is placed inside the intubating airway, and advanced into the oropharynx (scope-first technique).

TABLE 8. *Fiberoptic intubation under general anesthesia*

Advantages
Easy setup
Less preparatory time
Provides preoxygenation and denitrogenation
Easily applied for routine teaching
Disadvantages
Limitation of intubation time
Increase potential for hypoxemia
Immobile laryngeal structures

TABLE 9. *Steps of asleep fiberoptic intubation*

Establish general anesthesia and paralysis.
Place intubating airway into the mouth.
Suction the oropharynx.
Ventilate by mask, mild hyperventilation.
Assistant hands the fiberscope to the intubator.
Assistant exerts jaw thrust to help visualization of the glottis and monitors apnea time.
The fiberscope is passed through the airway, glottic opening, and into the trachea.
The endotracheal tube is threaded over the fiberscope through the airway and into the trachea.
Position of the tip of the tube is checked and fiberscope is removed.
For nasotracheal intubation, apply vasoconstriction to the nasal mucosa.
For spontaneously breathing patient apply topical anesthesia before advancing fiberscope into the trachea to minimize the risk of laryngospasm.

The assistant now applies a jaw thrust maneuver. This maneuver is vital, constituting the most important step in fiberoptic intubation under general anesthesia. If an intubating airway is not available, the assistant may pull the tongue forward away from the palate and posterior pharyngeal wall. This will move the epiglottis away from the posterior pharyngeal wall, thus assisting exposure of the vocal cords. The assistant may also use both hands to elevate the jaw while simultaneously opening the mouth by downward pressure on the chin (31). Forceful pulling of the tongue over the lower teeth may cause trauma and laceration of the tongue. Lung forceps or a mouth gag with tongue holder have been used to keep the tongue forward (32,33).

The intubating airway helps ensure that the fiberscope will remain in the midline position and thereby facilitates exposure of the vocal cords (34). After positioning the fiberscope in midtrachea, the endoscopist advances the ET tube with a rotating motion. If the advancing ET tube encounters resistance, it is pulled back, rotated 90° to the left or right, and then re-advanced. The assistant continues to apply a jaw thrust. The fiberscope is removed, and the breathing system is attached to the ET tube. In case of a prolonged intubation time, the position of the ET tube should be checked only after ventilation has been resumed.

Nasal Approach

General preparation, intubation technique, and assistant duties are similar to those for orotracheal intubation. Application of a vasoconstrictor to the nostril prior to intubation, before or after induction of anesthesia, is recommended to minimize bleeding.

The lubricated ET tube, mounted on the insertion cord of the fiberscope, is grasped by the anesthesiolo-

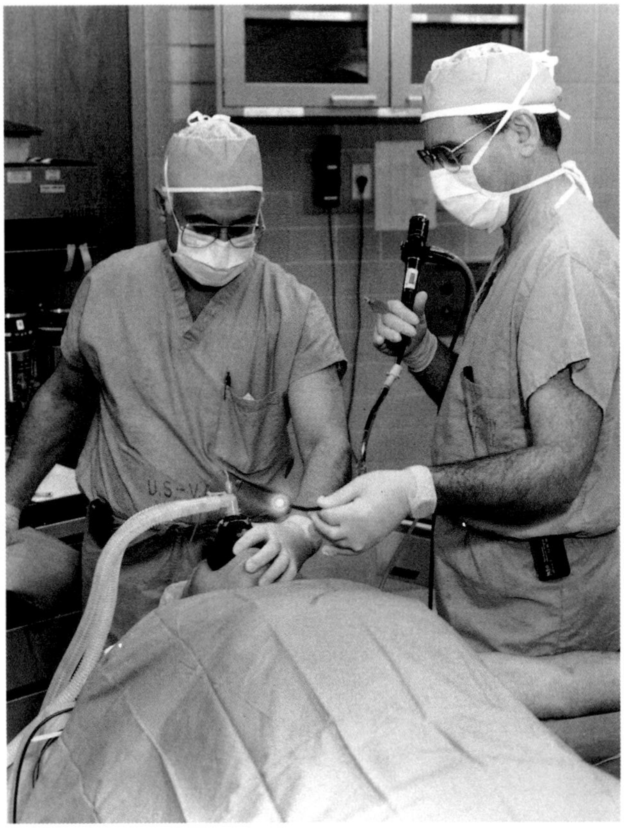

A

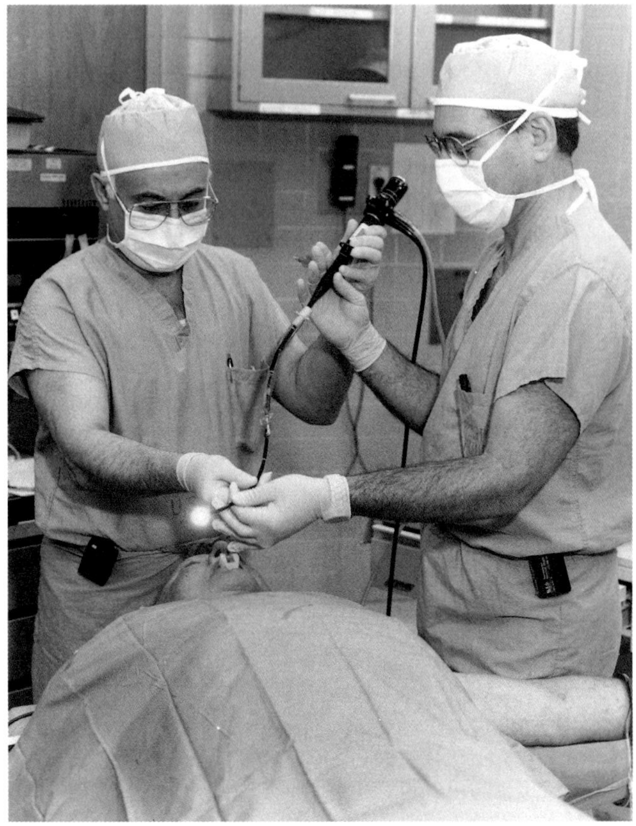

B

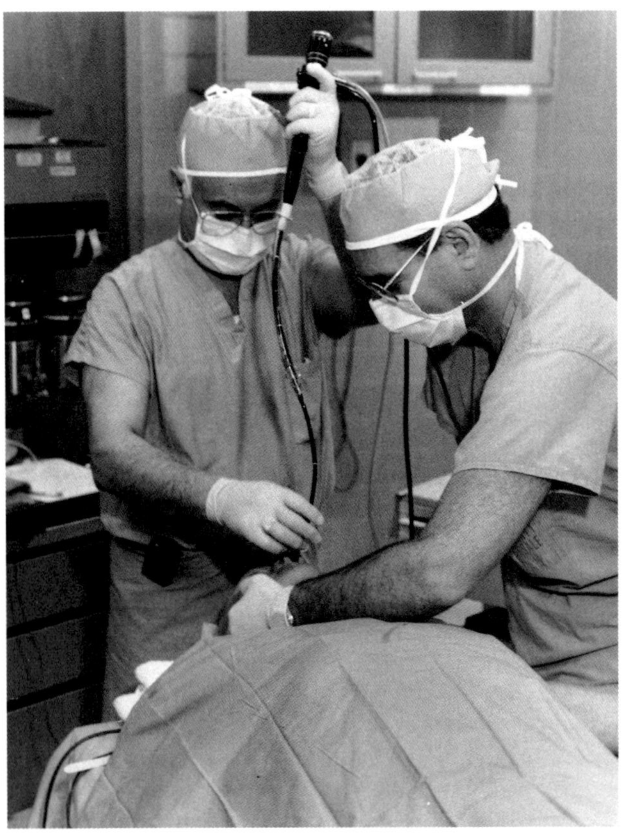

C

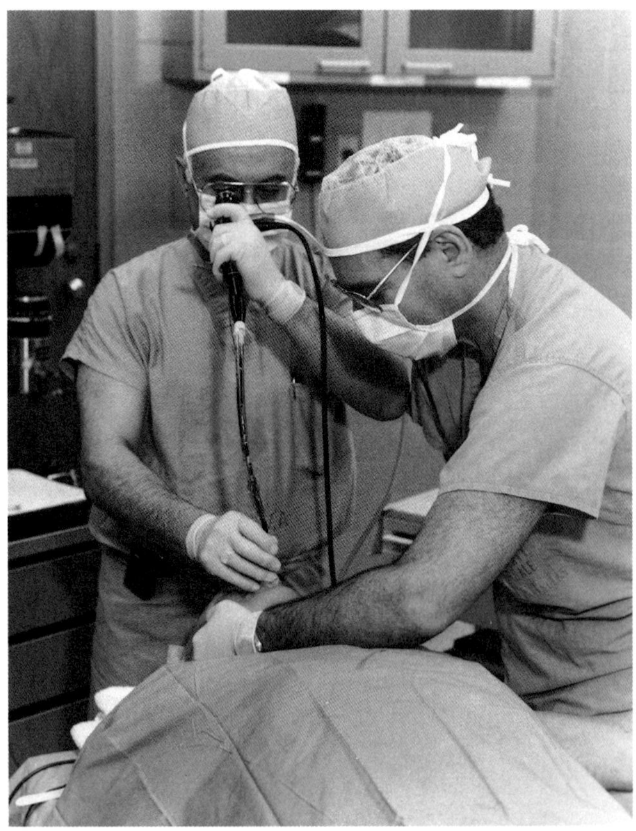

D

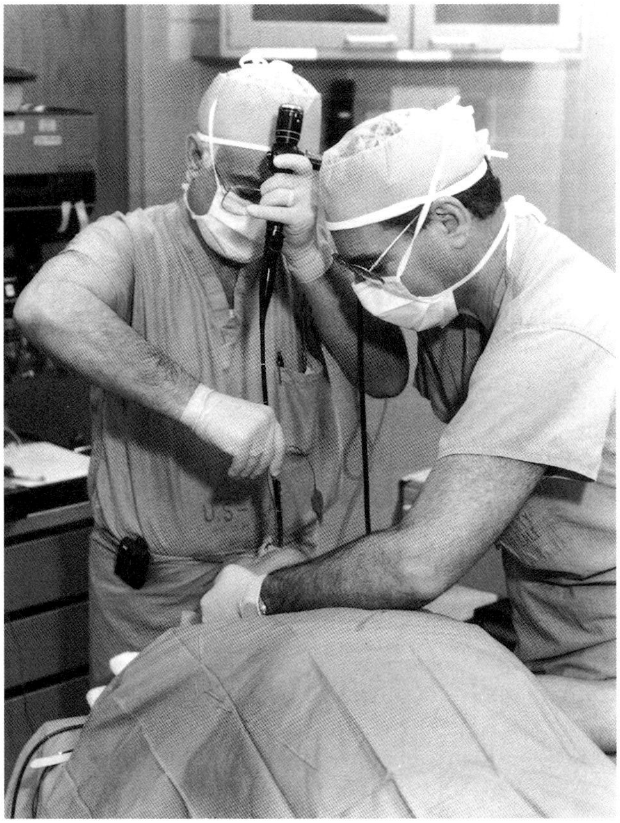

E

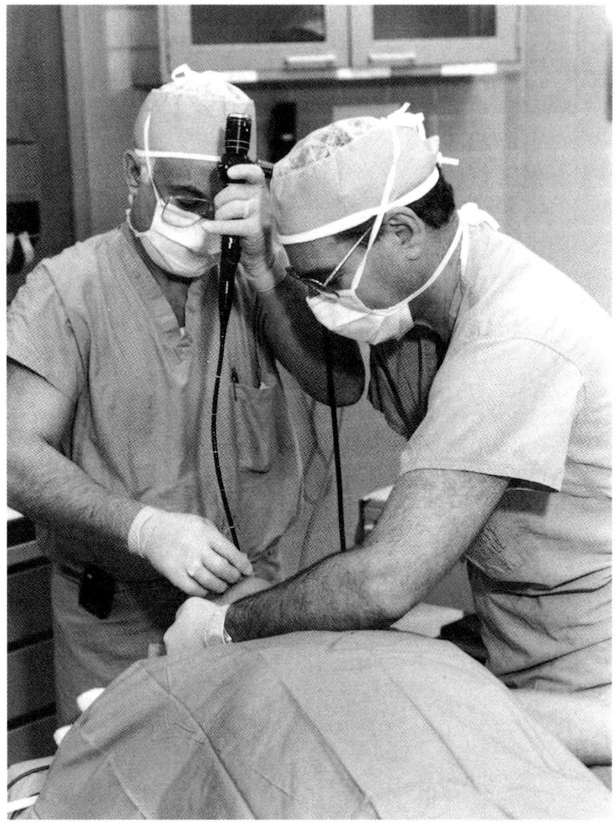

F

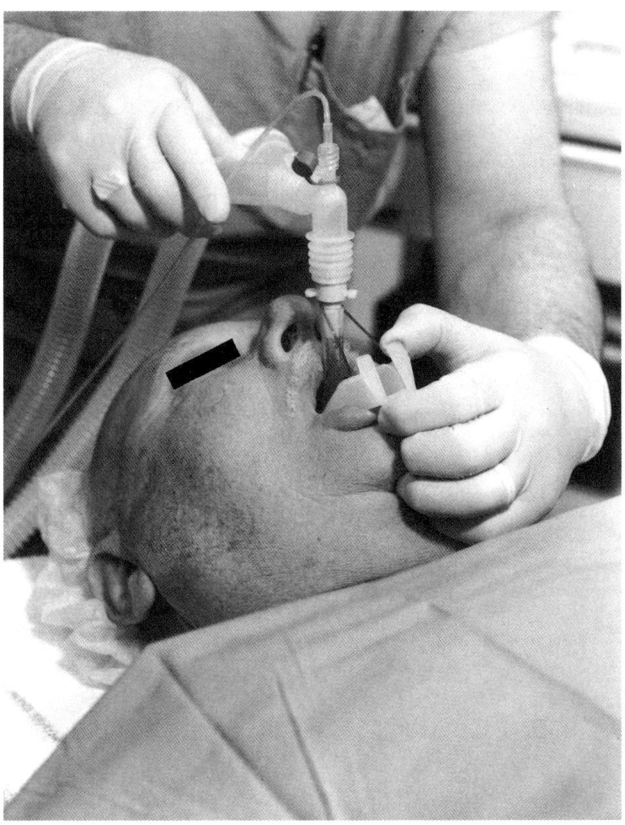

G

FIG. 10. Fiberoptic orotracheal intubation under general anesthesia. **A:** The assistant has the fiberscope ready for the operator. The patient is paralyzed, the intubating airway is in place, and the oropharynx has been suctioned. **B:** The operator receives the fiberscope from the assistant. **C:** The operator inserts the tip of the fiberscope inside the intubating airway. The assistant applies a jaw thrust as soon as the fiberscope has been passed to the operator. **D:** The operator looks through the fiberscope and advances the insertion cord through the airway and vocal cords into the trachea. **E:** The fiberscope has been passed into the trachea. The tube is rotated 45–90° during advancement. Note the position of the right hand. **F:** The tube has been placed in the trachea. **G:** The Ovassapian intubating airway is removed.

gist, as described earlier, as soon as the anesthesia mask is removed. The fiberscope tip is inserted into the selected nostril and advanced under direct vision toward the larynx and trachea. The assistant applies a jaw thrust maneuver to maintain an open oropharyngeal space. After midtracheal fiberscope placement, the endotracheal tube is threaded into the trachea.

Intubation Aided by Endoscopy Mask (Endoscopy Mask Technique)

To perform fiberoptic intubation by endoscopy mask technique, an assistant capable of administering anesthesia and maintaining mask ventilation is required (12,13). Anesthesia and ventilation are maintained with an endoscopy mask. An intubating airway is placed inside the mouth, the oropharynx is suctioned, and mask ventilation continued. The fiberscope, with the ET tube mounted on it (15-mm adapter removed), is advanced through the rubber diaphragm of the endoscopy mask port and into the intubating airway. The fiberscope is then passed through the vocal cords into the midtrachea (35,36).

The ET tube, in turn, is threaded over the fiberscope, through the endoscopy port and intubating airway, and into the trachea. After removing the fiberscope, the endoscopy mask is disengaged from the ET tube. The 15-mm ET tube adapter is replaced and connected to the anesthesia circuit. Caution should be exercised to avoid accidental injury to the face or eyes during placement of the ET tube adapter, which must be pushed securely into the ET tube. The use of an intubating airway is mandatory with this technique.

One of the shortcomings of the endoscopy mask is the danger of tearing its diaphragm and pushing it into the trachea (37,38). Diaphragm replacement is expensive, and segments remaining in the tracheobronchial tree may produce major problems. An alternative diaphragm made from a surgical glove is suggested to overcome these concerns with the manufacturer's diaphragm (39,40).

It is possible to use the endoscopy mask for nasotracheal intubation (35). However, the length of an uncut ET tube threaded over the fiberscope will prevent placement of the fiberscope tip in the midtrachea without advancing the ET tube through the diaphragm of the endoscopy port. When this occurs, the ET tube opens the system and positive pressure ventilation cannot be continued. Fiberscopes with insertion cords 60 cm in length, such as the Olympus LF-2, are long enough to reach midtrachea before the nasotracheal tube enters the endoscopy port.

Modified Endoscopy Mask Technique

To avoid the problems of instrument damage and fiberscope tip positioning described above, a modified endoscopy mask technique has been developed (22).

A lubricated ET tube is prepared with its 15-mm adapter loosely attached. A bronchoscopy swivel adapter is then mounted on the ET tube and its 15-mm side arm blocked with tape. The lubricated ET tube is passed through the diaphragm of the endoscopy mask port to about 10 cm (Fig. 11). Additional lubrication is then applied to the distal end of the ET tube.

General anesthesia and ventilation is maintained, using a regular anesthesia mask. After achieving an appropriate depth of anesthesia and complete relaxation, the regular anesthesia mask is removed. An oral intubating airway is placed, and the oropharynx suctioned. The endoscopy mask, with the inserted ET tube, is positioned over the face. Approximately 4 cm of the ET tube is inserted into the intubating airway. Anesthesia is continued with the endoscopy mask in place. The breathing system remains sealed.

The fiberscope is advanced through the swivel adapter and ET tube into the oropharynx and trachea. The ET tube is threaded over the fiberscope and into the trachea. The fiberscope, the 15-mm ET tube, and swivel adapter are removed together, leaving the ET tube in place. The endoscopy mask is then disengaged from the ET tube; the 15-mm ET tube adapter is firmly reattached, completing the procedure.

In nasotracheal intubation, the ET tube, with its loosely attached adapters, is mounted over the fiberscope prior to intubation. The breathing circuit will

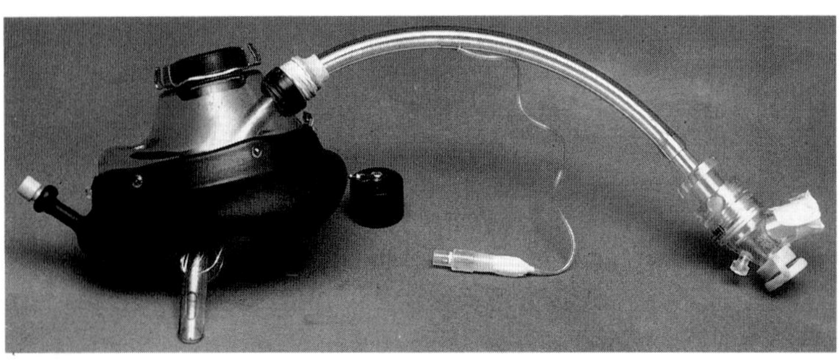

FIG. 11. Endoscopy mask mounted with endotracheal tube with loosely attached tracheal tube and bronchoscopy swivel adapters.

remain closed when the ET tube passes through the endoscopy port, due to the seal provided by the swivel adapter.

Intubation Using the Nasal Airway

In the anesthetized, spontaneously breathing patient, anesthesia may be maintained through a nasopharyngeal airway to allow time for unhurried tracheal intubation. Connected to the anesthesia breathing system, binasal airways are used for orotracheal intubation. An intubating airway is placed, and the fiberscope, mounted with an ET tube, is inserted through the airway to perform intubation (35).

In performing nasotracheal intubation, a nasopharyngeal airway, mounted with an ET tube adapter, is inserted in one nostril (41,42). The breathing circuit of the anesthesia machine is attached to the 15-mm adapter inserted in the nasal airway. The fiberscope, mounted with ET tube, is passed through the other nostril to perform tracheal intubation.

During either the oral or nasal approach, allow the patient to breath spontaneously to maintain the depth of anesthesia and allow time for an unhurried intubation. The fiberscope also allows the option of spraying a local anesthetic on the larynx to minimize laryngeal reaction and spasm. This may become necessary if the anesthetic depth proves inadequate for airway manipulation.

Intubation Using a Malleable Tongue Retractor

A malleable tongue retractor is useful in unassisted fiberoptic oral or nasotracheal intubation in the anesthetized patient (17). The last three digits of the left hand are used to hold the retractor, leaving the index finger and thumb free to advance the fiberscope (Fig. 12). The tongue retractor is placed in the mouth and, with gentle lifting pressure, the base of the tongue is pulled anteriorly to expose the epiglottis. The thumb and index finger of the left hand can now advance the fiberscope, while the right hand manipulates the fiberscope into the trachea. Alternatively, the retractor may be held by an assistant.

Rapid Sequence Induction and Intubation

The combination of a difficult intubation and full stomach in the patient scheduled for emergency surgery presents special problems. If the patient is uncooperative, intoxicated, or is a child, awake intubation to secure the airway prior to induction may not be a viable option. Under these conditions, general anesthesia using a rapid sequence induction technique is commonly employed. Compression of the cricoid cartilage to block passive gastric regurgitation into the oropharynx is part of this induction technique. Failure of tracheal intubation by rigid laryngoscopy during a rapid sequence induction leaves the patient's airway vulnerable to aspiration.

Fiberoptic intubation during rapid sequence induction, with cricoid pressure applied, is a technique that should be seriously considered. Advanced experience and confidence in the use of the fiberscope is necessary for success under these circumstances (43).

Mask ventilation, with cricoid pressure applied, is an acceptable practice when intubation fails. If mask ventilation is impossible, the possibility of airway obstruction due to the inappropriate application of cricoid pressure or the presence of hypertrophied lingual tonsils or other supraepiglottic masses should be considered.

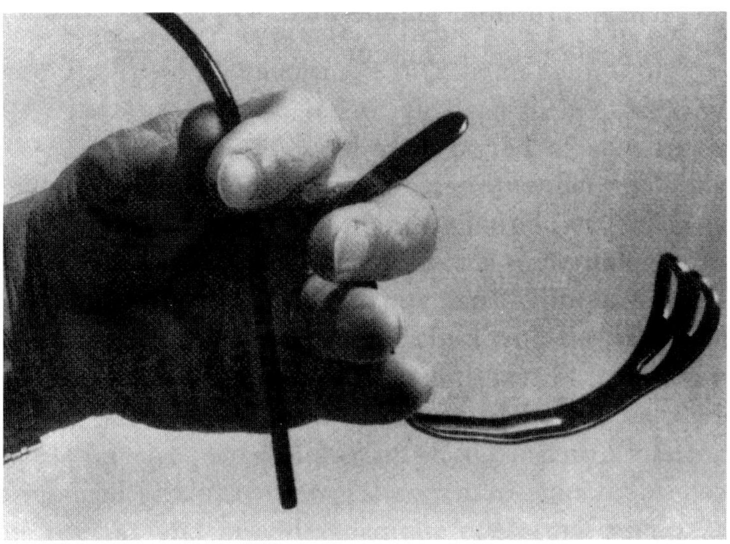

FIG. 12. Fiberoptic orotracheal intubation using malleable tongue retractor. Hand is positioned to advance fiberscope into the trachea while holding the retractor. The retractor will retract tongue forward, assisting in exposure of the epiglottis and cords. (From ref. 17.)

If mask ventilation proves difficult. Place the patient in five degrees of head down position and release the cricoid pressure. If mask ventilation is improved, proceed with intubation without cricoid pressure, or with adjustment of the degree of cricoid compression. It should be kept in mind that the risk of asphyxia under these conditions is much higher than the risk of regurgitation and aspiration.

The ability to perform rapid fiberoptic intubation in patients at high risk for aspiration may play an important role in diminishing major airway related catastrophes. Repeated unsuccessful attempts at blind nasal or rigid laryngoscopy traumatize the airway, frequently changing a manageable airway into an unmanageable one. A successful rapid fiberoptic intubation by an experienced endoscopist, before the airway is unduly traumatized, may prove a lifesaving measure.

A rapid sequence induction, incorporating fiberoptic intubation, may be used initially in a patient with a history of difficult intubation but known to be easily mask ventilated. One assistant should apply cricoid pressure, while another passes the fiberscope to the anesthesiologist and applies a jaw thrust maneuver (Fig. 13). Overly aggressive cricoid compression may block the endoscopist's view of the glottis (44). This problem is easily rectified by decreasing or releasing cricoid compression.

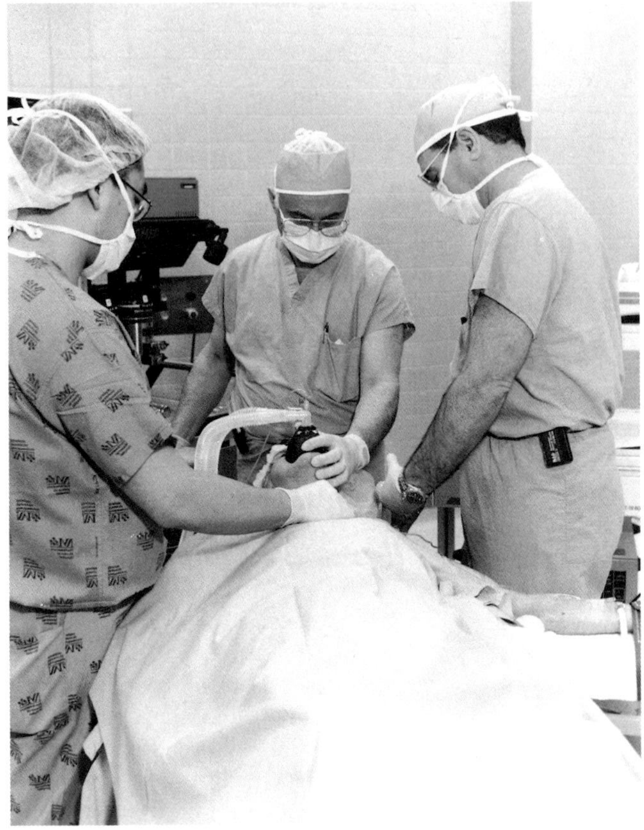

A

COMBINING FIBEROPTIC WITH OTHER INTUBATION TECHNIQUES

The fiberscope can be used in combination with other intubation techniques to secure an otherwise difficult airway. The fiberscope can be used in combination with a rigid laryngoscope, a laryngeal mask airway, or Combitube tube *in situ*. It can be used to correct a failed retrograde wire or "blind" nasal intubation attempt. The fiberscope may also be used as a light wand for tracheal intubation.

Fiberoptic Intubation Aided by Rigid Laryngoscopy

In patients with an oropharyngeal mass, upper airway edema, or posteriorly displaced epiglottis, the passage of a fiberscope beneath the epiglottis exposing the glottic opening may prove difficult. Combining rigid laryngoscopy with fiberoptic intubation is helpful under these circumstances (45–48).

The epiglottis is exposed using a rigid laryngoscope by a second anesthetist. The endoscopist, looking directly inside the mouth (not through the fiberscope), passes the tip of the fiberscope under the epiglottis (45). The tip of the fiberscope can also be further guided toward the glottis by the anesthetist performing

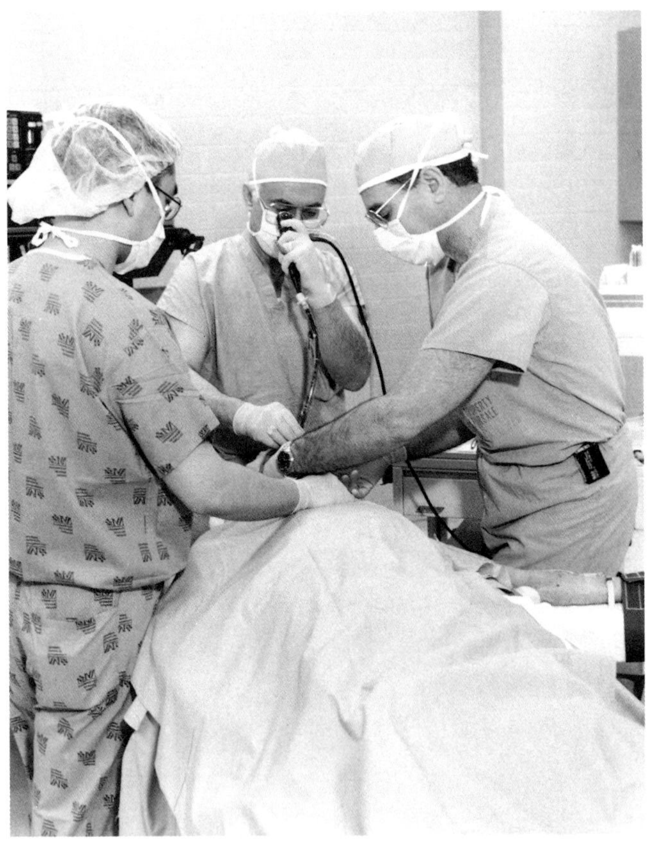

D

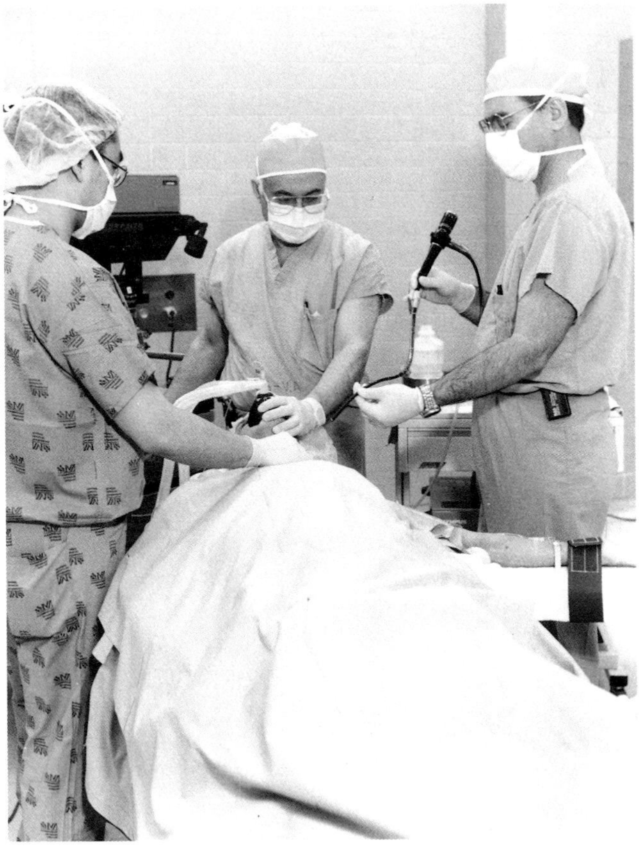

B

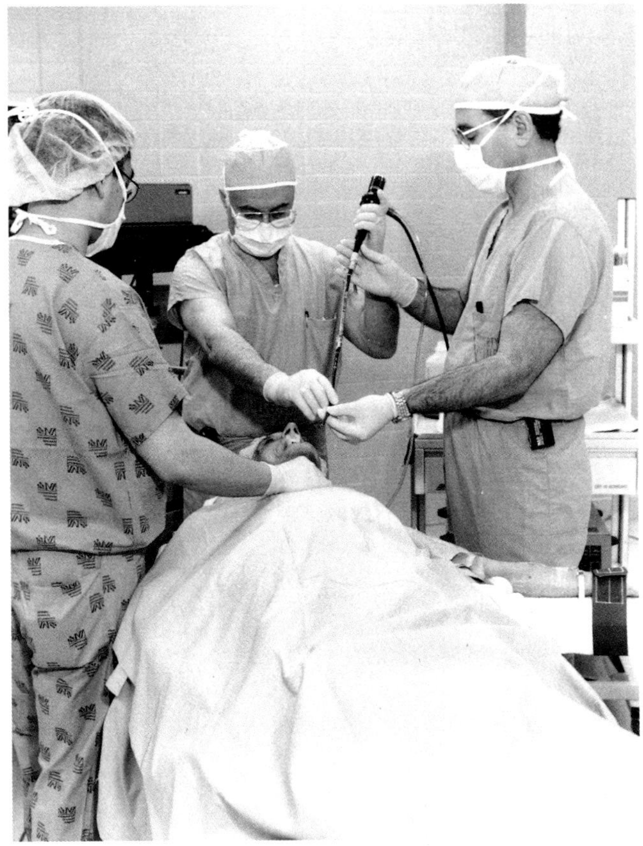

C

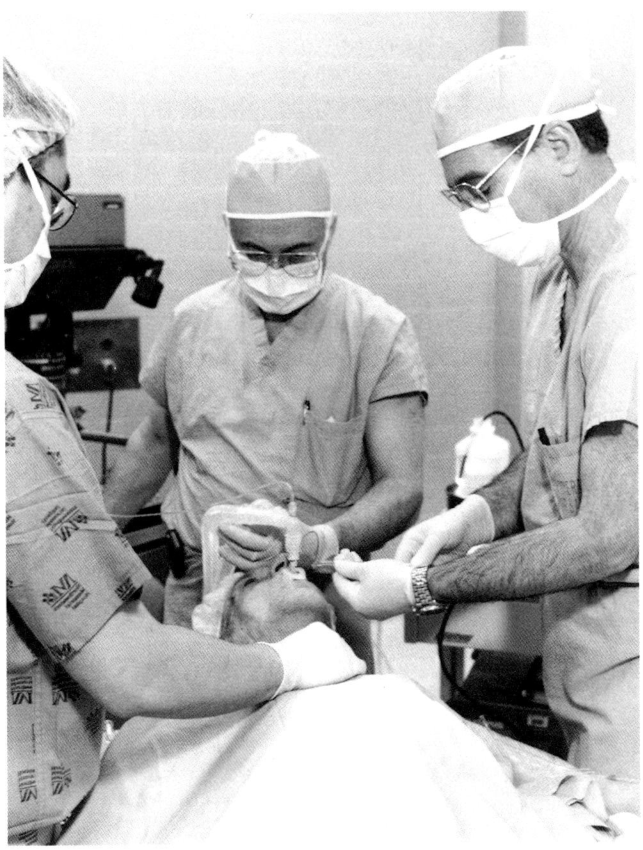

E

FIG. 13. Fiberoptically aided rapid sequence induction and intubation. **A:** First assistant on the right side of the operator applies cricoid pressure prior to induction of anesthesia. The second assistant on the left of the operator administers the induction agents. **B:** The second assistant has the fiberscope ready for the operator. **C:** The operator receives the fiberscope from the second assistant; jaw thrust is applied by the second assistant. **D:** The operator places the tip of the fiberscope through the intubating airway to perform intubation. **E:** Intubation is completed. The second assistant inflates the tracheal tube cuff; first assistant continues cricoid pressure until exhaled CO_2 is verified.

rigid laryngoscopy, while the endoscopist looks through the fiberscope eyepiece. This combined maneuver will allow easy exposure of the vocal cords and advancement of the fiberscope into the trachea.

The combined use of the rigid and fiberoptic laryngoscope is also useful in changing an existing endotracheal tube. Excessive pharyngeal soft tissue, edema of the airway, and copious secretions are common findings in difficult airway patients, interfering with fiberoptic visualization of the larynx. Rigid laryngoscopy helps in exposing the supraglottic area and allows for complete suctioning of secretions. In addition, a curved blade will lift the epiglottis, which may be embracing the ET tube, allowing passage of the fiberscope beneath the epiglottis. This is crucial in exposing the anterior commissure, permitting passage of the fiberscope alongside the existing tube into the trachea (Chapter 9).

Fiberoptic Intubation through a Laryngeal Mask

A number of case reports attest to the value of the laryngeal mask airway (LMA) in failed intubations and in restoring ventilation when it could not be achieved by a face mask. Tracheal intubation through the LMA has been successfully carried out in awake and anesthetized patients using blind or fiberoptic-aided techniques. Details of these intubation techniques are discussed in Chapter 12.

Fiberoptic Intubation with the Combitube In Place

The esophageal tracheal combitube (Combitube(R)) is recommended for rapidly establishing ventilation. The Combitube(R) will permit ventilation whether placed in the esophagus or trachea.

The Combitube(R) is not recommended for prolonged mechanical ventilation. Replacement of the Combitube(R) with an ET tube is necessary to avoid possible complications, and allow access for tracheal suctioning. The technique of fiberoptic intubation with the Combitube(R) in place is described in Chapter 13.

Fiberoptic and Blind Nasal Intubation

Two different techniques employing the fiberscope may be used to assist blind nasal intubation.

If the size of the nasal passage prevents passage of the fiberscope through the nasotracheal tube, the fiberscope may be introduced through the contralateral nostril. It can now be used to visualize the position of the tip of the tube, and assist in its passage through the vocal cord (49). Under fiberoptic observation, the nasotracheal tube and the patient's head are manipulated to direct the nasotracheal tube toward the larynx (Chapter 7).

In patients with a distorted and compromised airway, blind nasotracheal intubation, as well as fiberoptic exposure of the glottis, may fail. A combination of blind nasal and fiberoptic intubation techniques may prove successful (50).

The nasotracheal tube is advanced, gently and slowly, while listening to the breath sounds of the spontaneously breathing patient. The advancement of the tube is stopped when the breath sounds are loudest. In this position, the tip of the nasotracheal tube is a short distance from the glottic opening and the tube has passed beyond the distorted/obstructed airway.

The passage of a lubricated fiberscope through the nasotracheal tube brings the tip of the fiberscope close to the glottis, allowing easy identification of the epiglottis and glottic opening. The fiberscope is advanced into the trachea followed by the nasotracheal tube.

Fiberoptic and Retrograde Intubation

In the case of a failed retrograde intubation, a guide wire introduced through the cricothyroid membrane may be used to direct the fiberscope toward the glottis and trachea. Two different approaches are described below.

The ET tube that cannot be advanced over the guide wire into the larynx is left in place. The fiberscope is inserted into the ET tube and is advanced along the guide wire until it reaches the larynx. The fiberscope is then maneuvered and advanced into the trachea. The guide wire is removed, and the ET tube is threaded over the fiberscope into the trachea (51).

In the second approach, the guide wire is passed in a retrograde fashion through the suction channel of the fiberscope loaded with an ET tube (Fig. 14). The fiberscope is advanced over the guide wire into the trachea. The guide wire is removed, and the ET tube is threaded over the fiberscope into the trachea (52–54).

FIG. 14. Fiberoptic and retrograde intubation of the trachea. **A:** The guide wire is introduced into the trachea and mouth through the cricothyroid membrane. **B:** The guide wire is passed in a retrograde fashion through the suction channel of the fiberscope mounted with the endotracheal tube. **C:** The fiberscope is advanced over the wire into the larynx. **D:** The guide wire is cut at the entrance site in the anterior neck and is removed from above. The fiberscope is advanced into the midtrachea. **E:** The endotracheal tube is threaded over the fiberscope into the trachea. The fiberscope is removed, leaving the endotracheal tube in place.

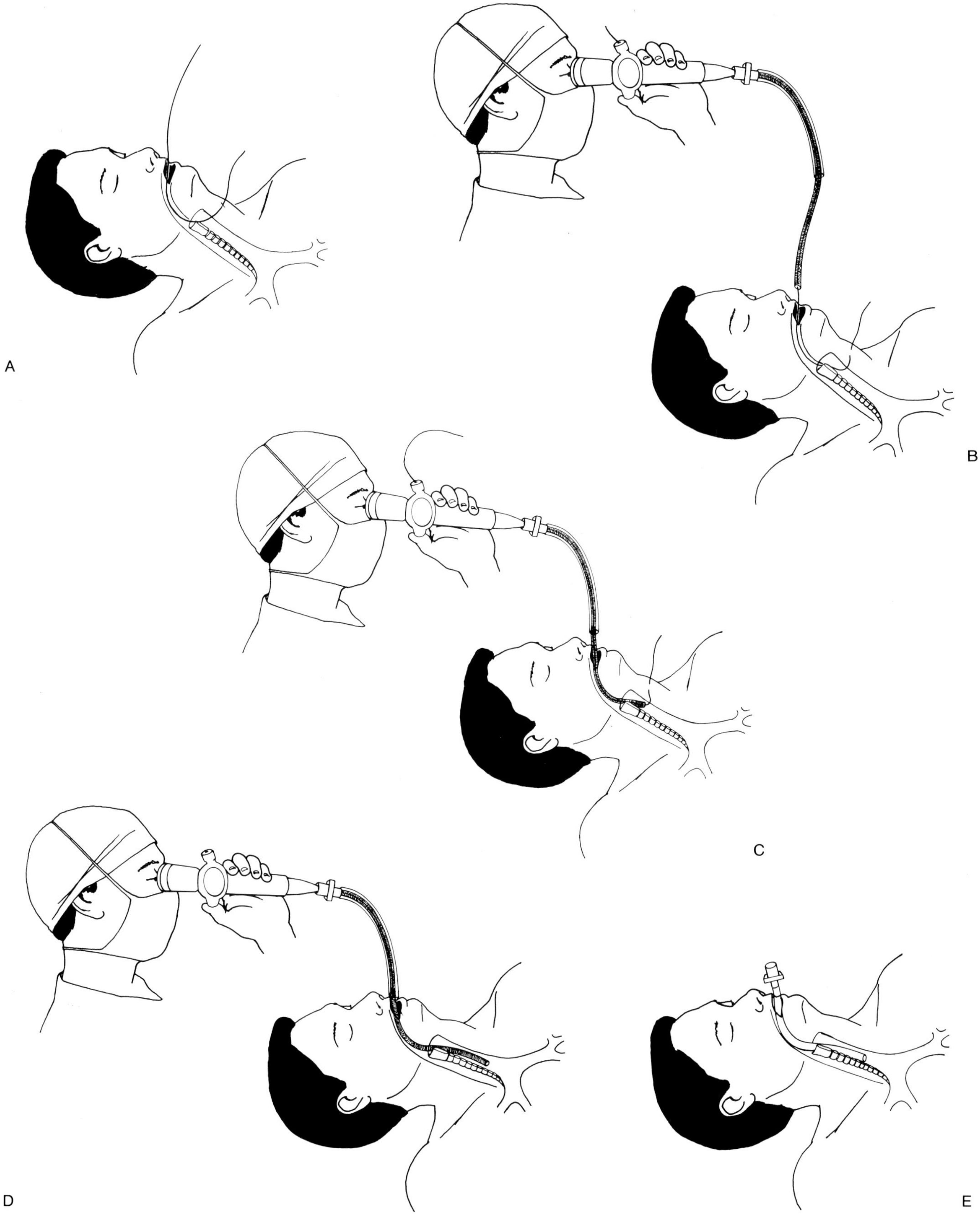
A
B
C
D
E

Gerrish and Weston (55) used the latter technique in a different circumstance. A fiberscope, loaded with an ET tube, was advanced into the trachea with great difficulty. The ET tube, however, would not advance into the trachea due to a tracheal stenosis secondary to a previous tracheostomy. Prior to removing the fiberscope, a guide wire was advanced through the suction channel into the trachea. The fiberscope was then removed. The fiberscope, reloaded with a smaller ET tube, was then rethreaded over the guide wire into the trachea, followed by the ET tube (Two-Stage Intubation, Chapter 7).

The Fiberscope as a Light Wand

The light wand is a stylet with a bright light on its tip. It is frequently used in blind tracheal intubations (Chapter 11). The light wand, loaded with an ET tube, is advanced blindly toward the trachea. Strong transillumination of the anterior neck confirms its tracheal entrance. The ET tube is then "railroaded" over the stylet into the trachea. If the light wand is not advanced sufficiently to reach the larynx, or it enters the esophagus, light is not transmitted through the anterior neck. When the light wand is off center, the light is detected lateral to the larynx in the anterior lateral neck.

The fiberscope has a strong light, allowing the instrument to be used as a light wand. This approach may prevent failure of a fiberoptic intubation when copious secretions or blood interfere with visualization of the airway anatomy. We have used the light wand technique on a few occasions, and it has been described by others (56,57).

The fiberscope, loaded with the ET tube, is passed through the intubating airway toward the larynx. While a jaw thrust maneuver is applied by an assistant, the fiberscope is advanced keeping its distal tip straight to facilitate passage beneath the epiglottis. When the fiberscope is judged to be immediately subglottic, the tip is deflected slightly downward (posteriorly) to facilitate entrance into the larynx. The position of the transilluminated light on the neck will dictate the maneuvers required to enter the trachea (Chapter 11).

CONFIRMING ENDOTRACHEAL TUBE POSITION

Unrecognized esophageal intubation has been responsible for many cases of anesthesia-related morbidity and mortality (58–61). Most of the commonly used methods of assessing tube position have been documented to fail under certain circumstances (62). A major advantage of fiberoptic intubation is that placement of the ET tube occurs under direct visual observation of the tracheal anatomy. Confirming ET tube position, and its relationship to the carina by fiberscope, after completion of intubation and tube taping assures that the ET tube is correctly placed.

The possibility of esophageal intubation does exist during fiberoptic intubation, and the practitioner should be alert to recognize and correct this misadventure immediately. In a patient with abnormal airway anatomy, in the presence of secretions, and in the uncooperative patient, it is possible that the fiberscope may be advanced into the esophagus instead of the trachea. The lumen of the esophagus is usually flat, with its anterior and posterior walls in direct contact. On occasion, however, the lumen of the esophagus is open and tubular, and may be mistaken for the trachea. When the tracheal rings are not satisfactorily identified, the fiberscope should be advanced further to expose the carina. The visualization of the tracheal bifurcation will confirm the tracheal position of the fiberscope and eliminate confusion as to its location.

It must also be kept in mind that placement of the fiberscope into the trachea does not guarantee tracheal placement of the ET tube. Upon threading of the ET tube, the fiberscope may be pulled out of the trachea and enter the esophagus. This is more likely to happen when a small-sized fiberscope is used for passage of a large ET tube (63). In addition, a correctly placed ET tube may inadvertently be withdrawn from the trachea while securing the tube.

The common methods of evaluating ET tube position should be applied for absolute certainty (64). Observation of symmetric bilateral movement of the upper chest wall, auscultation of the apical and midaxillary area, and auscultation of the epigastrium during ventilation should be performed after each intubation. The measurement of end-tidal CO_2 and exhaled tidal volume (while noting the characteristic feel of the reservoir bag and its refilling during exhalation) and condensation of water vapor in the ET tube lumen are all helpful in identifying correct tube placement.

Preoxygenation will delay the onset of cyanosis and cardiovascular signs indicative of hypoxemia, and therefore, delay recognition of an esophageal intubation (65,66). Esophageal intubation must be considered as a cause of hypoxemia, even when 5 to 10 min have elapsed after intubation. Clinical signs distinguishing esophageal and tracheal intubation may be misleading, especially once an operative procedure has begun, and other responsibilities of patient care are keeping the anesthesiologist busy.

The most reliable technique to confirm tracheal tube placement is measurement of end-tidal CO_2. Capnography provides a rapid and reliable way to confirm endotracheal placement of the tube (67–70). Face mask ventilation prior to tracheal intubation may inflate the stomach with exhaled air. The capnogram may show carbon dioxide in a few initial breaths. The CO_2 curves so produced are low, and disappear after five to six breaths (67,69,71).

It should be remembered that carbon dioxide elimination depends on cardiac output and pulmonary circulation (72). In a state of profound low blood pressure or cardiac arrest, the carbon dioxide curve may not be seen despite correct ET tube placement (72). In addition, carbon dioxide monitoring will not detect endobronchial intubation. The esophageal detector is another valuable device for confirmation of the correct endotracheal tube placement (73), however, a false positive result has been reported (74).

FIBEROPTIC INTUBATION IN TRAUMA AND EMERGENCY MEDICINE

Trauma to the head and neck may produce major acute or chronic anatomical changes. These changes may affect airway accessibility, making tracheal intubation or mask ventilation difficult.

The first paper describing the use of the fiberscope in airway management of the trauma patient was written by Mulder and colleagues in 1975. The paper described the successful use of the fiberscope in tracheal intubation of 14 trauma patients (6). Three patients had extensive soft tissue contracture of the head and neck secondary to thermal injury, six patients had complicated mandibular and facial fractures, and five patients had unstable cervical fractures or fracture dislocations.

Numerous papers have since been published describing fiberoptic intubation in trauma and emergency patients (75–80). The value of the fiberscope as a airway management tool in emergency room patients, and its limitations are presented in four related publications (76–79).

Schafermeyer reported a 76% success rate in 16 emergency intubations with fiberoptic techniques, compared to a 95% success rate with standard techniques (76). Failures were attributed to excessive secretions, bleeding, or operator inexperience. Delaney and Hessler reported a 13% failure rate in 60 intubation attempts, due to secretions, bleeding, agitation, airway obstruction, and status epilepticus (77). Their experience before using the fiberscope in emergency patients was limited to practice on mannequins under the guidance of an experienced anesthesiologist. Their learning curve indicated that after ten intubations, the time of their intubations plateaued at less than 4 min.

Mlinek reported a retrospective study of 35 emergency department intubation attempts over a 30-month period, with a success rate of 74% (78). Afilalo and colleagues report on 42 attempts at fiberoptic intubation over a 22-month period in emergency department patients (79). Most patients were intubated for respiratory failure, or airway protection. Three physicians performed the fiberoptic intubations, one of whom performed more than half. Their success rate was 72%. Failures were attributed to secretions, difficulty manipulating the fiberscope through the ET tube, prolonged intubation time in an unstable patient, and one case of retropharyngeal dissection by the ET tube.

Emergency physicians must master various intubation techniques since airway management holds utmost priority in management of the seriously ill or injured patient. While learning the technique of fiberoptic intubation is comparatively easy, true mastery only develops with extensive experience. The use of the fiberscope on a sporadic basis will not produce expertise in its full potential. The fiberscope should not be used for intubation alone, its value as a diagnostic and therapeutic tool in airway management is well established.

The familiarity of supportive emergency department staff with the technique is essential. The availability of good fiberscopes and equipment as well as organizing a fiberoptic cart for easy and fast accessibility are all critical for the liberal and successful use of this instrument. The routine use of the fiberscope in emergency departments will alleviate most of the shortcomings stated in the literature and dramatically improve the success rate of such intubations.

FIBEROPTIC INTUBATION IN OBSTETRICS

Failed intubation occurs in 1:300 anesthetics for cesarean section and accounts for 1:3 of all anesthetic-related maternal mortality (81,82). During pregnancy, several factors such as mucosal vascular engorgement, laryngeal edema, immobility of the floor of the mouth due to tongue engorgement, enlarged breasts, and obesity contribute to the difficult intubation.

Rapid sequence induction and intubation with application of cricoid pressure is routine in parturient patients subjected to general anesthesia. Application of cricoid pressure can contribute to failing to intubate (44,83,84).

The risk of regurgitation and aspiration of gastric contents is also high in pregnant patients, especially at term, and requires special attention. Furthermore, decreased functional residual capacity (FRC) due to weight gain and an enlarged uterus results in more rapid hemoglobin desaturation and hypoxemia during induction and intubation when no ventilation is attempted.

The high incidence of failed intubation, particularly in obese pregnant patients (85), the high risk of aspiration, and a decreased FRC all contribute to the risk of general anesthesia and airway-related complications. A general anesthetic plan should include pharmacologic preparation to minimize the sequela from aspiration, a careful approach, and a backup plan for management of a failed intubation, as well as the availability of two assistants during induction and intubation.

Familiarity with different intubation and ventilation techniques is a must to prevent or avoid airway disasters. The use of the fiberscope in the anticipated difficult or failed intubation in this group of patients can prove helpful. Unfortunately, to date, published data in this area remains very limited (86–88). Glassenberg, in a retrospective review of 1349 cesarean sections between 1980 to 1984, reports five (0.37%) failed intubations during cesarean section, four of these were successfully intubated with a blind nasal technique. In 1985, fiberoptic intubation was introduced in the obstetric unit. From 1985 to 1989, a total of 917 general anesthetics were administered for cesarean section; 127 suspected to present difficulty in intubation were intubated awake using a fiberoptic bronchoscope. There were two (0.2%) failures in the remaining 790 patients, both successfully intubated with using a fiberoptic bronchoscope. Despite using the fiberscope for 14% of the intubations after 1984, the improvement in the reported incidence of failed intubation (1:300 to 1:500) was not statistically significant. Half of the failed intubations occurred in parturient patients with normal appearing airways and were not anticipated. The two other reports involved single pregnant patients presenting with difficult intubation, both intubated awake and under somewhat rushed circumstances (87,88).

One should be aware of the effect of labor itself on the airway. Farcon and colleagues recently reported a case of changing Mallampati score during the course of labor in a healthy primigravida. On admission to hospital, the airway evaluation revealed Mallampati Class I–II. Repeat airway evaluation during labor revealed marked edema of the pharynx, changing the Mallampati Class to III–IV. The edema of oropharynx structures subsided within 12 hr postlabor with return of Mallampati Class to I–II (89).

PHYSIOLOGICAL RESPONSE TO FIBEROPTIC INTUBATION

Respiratory Effects

Stimulation of the upper airway without good topical or deep general anesthesia may induce laryngospasm. This nonspecific response to stimulation is seen whether rigid laryngoscopy, fiberscopic, or blind tracheal intubation is used. The afferent responses for laryngospasm are mediated by the glossopharyngeal nerve when the hypopharynx is stimulated, and by the vagus nerve when the laryngeal surfaces of the epiglottis, larynx, or bronchial tree are stimulated.

Bronchospasm can develop in susceptible patients, especially if intubated under light general anesthesia. The decrease in anatomical dead space is minimal and insignificant in patients with normal respiratory function. Airway resistance increases are greater with a small diameter ET tube (e.g., 6 mm ID) than with larger-sized tubes.

Cardiovascular Effects

Rigid laryngoscopy and tracheal intubation cause a sympathoadrenal response that increases arterial pressure, heart rate, and systemic vascular resistance. The release of norepinephrine from sympathetic nerve endings and epinephrine from the adrenal medulla is chiefly responsible for these changes. This response may place patients with coronary artery disease at an increased risk for myocardial ischemia during laryngoscopy and tracheal intubation (90).

Three factors contribute to the cardiovascular response: (a) apnea and the resultant increase in carbon dioxide levels; (b) compression of the tongue and stretching of the supraglottic tissues by the rigid laryngoscope; and (c) laryngotracheal stimulation by the ET tube.

Takeshima, in 1964, studied the effects of apnea time, rigid laryngoscopy, and rigid laryngoscopy followed by tracheal intubation on the magnitude of cardiovascular response (91).

Apnea by itself caused an increase in blood pressure of 20 mm Hg or more in 20% of the patients. Blood pressure began to increase 60– 90 sec after the onset of apnea. Two out of the ten patients studied showed increases in heart rate of 12–14 beats per min, 2–2.5 min after apnea began. The changes in blood pressure and heart rate noted after rigid laryngoscopy alone were similar to those seen with rigid laryngoscopy and intubation.

In another study, rigid laryngoscopy with or without intubation caused significant and similar increases in arterial pressure and circulating catecholamine concentrations. However, intubation resulted in significant increases in heart rate compared to rigid laryngoscopy alone (92).

Fiberoptic orotracheal intubation is achieved without significant tongue compression or stretching of the supraglottic tissues. Therefore, it seems logical that the overall cardiovascular response to fiberoptic intubation may be less compared to that of rigid laryngoscopy. However, Finfer et al. and Smith demonstrated that the pressor response to fiberoptic intubation under general anesthesia is similar or greater than that of rigid laryngoscopy and intubation (28,93). Vigorous pulling of the tongue may have contributed to the cardiovascular response. However, in a subsequent study, Smith and colleagues showed significant increases in heart rate and arterial pressure in both techniques of fiberoptic intubation (i.e., tongue traction versus through Berman airway) that were greater than changes noted in the Macintosh intubation group (94).

In a Finfer and associates study in 40 healthy adult patients, the time for fiberoptic intubation was significantly greater (mean 60 ± 22 sec) than for rigid laryngoscopic intubation (mean 36 ± 9 sec) (93). Schaefer and Marsch demonstrated that total intravenous anesthesia, with a continuous infusion of propofol and bolus doses of fentanyl, abolished the arterial pressure and heart rate responses to fiberoptic as well as Macintosh intubation (95).

Schaefer and colleagues also reported that the cardiovascular response to fiberoptic orotracheal intubation was similar under a balanced volatile technique using thiopental/enflurane, compared to total intravenous anesthesia with propofol (96). Fentanyl (6 μg/kg) suppresses the hypertensive and tachycardic response to fiberoptic and rigid laryngoscopic intubation (97).

The cardiovascular response to fiberoptic nasotracheal intubation in anesthetized patients was also investigated by Smith and colleagues (98). Sixty patients were randomly assigned in two groups. The first group was intubated with an Olympus LF-1 (4 mm) fiberscope, the second group by conventional Macintosh laryngoscopic and Magill forceps technique. The fiberoptic group showed less increase in systolic and diastolic pressures compared to the conventional group, but increases in heart rate were higher in the fiberoptic group. The magnitude of difference was clinically insignificant.

Controversial results have also been obtained on the hemodynamic response following awake fiberoptic intubation. Ovassapian and colleagues reported only a modest increase in arterial pressure (average 10 mm Hg) and heart rate (average 14 beats/min), during fiberoptic nasotracheal intubation, using topical anesthesia and intravenous sedation (99). Schrader and colleagues, in comparing awake oral fiberoptic with awake oral rigid intubation, found no differences in cardiovascular response in 75% of easy rigid intubations compared to the fiberoptic intubations. However, in 5 out of 20 rigid intubations that proved somewhat difficult, arterial pressure and heart rate increased significantly compared to the fiberoptic group (100).

Hawkyard and associates reported that awake fiberoptic nasotracheal intubation produced less arterial pressure and heart rate changes in comparison to rigid laryngoscopy (101). Randell and associates, supplementing diazepam sedation with alfentanyl 20 μg/kg, significantly dampened cardiovascular responses in awake fiberoptic nasotracheal intubations(102). Topical anesthesia of the trachea was sufficient to abolish the tracheal reaction to the fiberscope but failed to completely obtund the laryngeal reflexes. Alfentanyl totally abolished the protective reflexes of the larynx. Southerland and Sale found no significant increase in blood pressure and heart rate during fiberoptic awake orotracheal intubation (103). Their patients were also sedated with diazepam and fentanyl, and had good topical anesthesia.

More studies are needed to evaluate the cardiovascular responses to fiberoptic intubation in awake and anesthetized patients. The fiberoptic technique, intubation time, smoothness of intubation, size of the fiberscope, and size of ET tube used will contribute to the level of cardiovascular response. Deep placement of the fiberscope and touching the carina will further stimulate the cardiovascular system. Most studies do not comment on these particular issues, making data interpretation difficult.

CAUSES OF FAILURE OF FIBEROPTIC INTUBATION

The causes of difficulty in fiberoptic intubation differ from those of rigid laryngoscopy (20). A large floppy epiglottis or the presence of secretions or blood may contribute to a difficult fiberoptic intubation, but usually do not present special difficulty during tracheal intubation with a rigid laryngoscope. Conversely, a limited mouth opening, anterior larynx, or an unstable neck, which may contribute to difficult rigid laryngoscopy, often prove easy fiberoptic intubations. The causes of failure of fiberoptic intubation are summarized in Table 10.

Lack of Experience

Intense training in the technique(s) of fiberoptic intubation has not been available to most practicing anesthesiologists, nurse anesthetists, and critical care physicians. Self-instruction, without the guidance of an expert, is associated with such a high incidence of failure that many become disenchanted with the technique prematurely. The inexperienced operator lacks the

TABLE 10. *Causes of failure of fiberoptic intubation*

- Lack of experience
- Presence of secretions and blood
- Decreased space between the tip of the epiglottis and the posterior pharyngeal wall
  - Large, floppy epiglottis
  - Supraglottic cyst or mass
  - Inflammation or edema of the oropharynx
  - Severe flexion deformity of the cervical spine
- Distorted airway anatomy
- Inability to advance the endotracheal tube
- Inability to withdraw the endotracheal tube

technical dexterity in handling the fiberscope and knowledge of the special preparations critical to its successful use.

The Presence of Secretions and Blood

The objective lens at the tip of the fiberscope is easily covered with secretions and blood which interfere with the visualization of laryngeal structures (Fig. 15). The administration of an adequate dose of an antisialagogue and proper suctioning of secretions prior to intubation are important preliminary steps to intubation. In cases of unexpected difficult rigid laryngoscopy and tracheal intubation, fiberoptic intubation should be instituted as soon as possible prior to causing trauma and bleeding of the periglottic tissues.

The conscious patient can be asked to swallow or breathe deeply to clear secretions. Secretions can also be suctioned through the working channel of the fiberscope. If intubation attempts are unsuccessful, the fiberscope should be removed, its tip cleaned, and the oropharynx thoroughly suctioned before the next attempt at laryngoscopy. High-flow insufflation of oxygen through the suction channel helps to keep secretions away and improves exposure. However, one should be aware of the possibility of barotrauma to the lungs if the fiberscope is advanced through a narrowed airway during insufflation. Distension of the stomach can also occur during insufflation of oxygen if the fiberscope enters the esophagus. Fogging of the lens will also interfere with exposure of the laryngeal structures. Insertion of the fiberscope tip in warm water will prevent this problem.

Inadequate Topical Anesthesia

Instrumentation of the oropharynx will increase secretions and cause coughing, swallowing, and vomiting if topical anesthesia is inadequate. Swallowing or coughing will move the laryngeal structures out of the visual field. Laryngospasm is likely if poorly anesthetized vocal cords are touched with the fiberscope. Even if the fiberscope can be passed through the vocal cords, it may be impossible to pass the ET tube.

Decreased Space between the Tip of the Epiglottis and the Posterior Pharyngeal Wall

The gap between the tip of the epiglottis and posterior pharyngeal wall may be decreased for various reasons. This problem may make manipulation of the fiberscope under the epiglottis difficult.

In the presence of a large floppy epiglottis, application of a jaw thrust or pulling the tongue forward moves the epiglottis away from the posterior pharyngeal wall, correcting the problem (Fig. 16). If the problem is secondary to a supraglottic mass or inflammation and edema of the upper airway, the problem may not resolve with these maneuvers. In these circumstances, even if the fiberscope is advanced into the trachea, threading the ET tube over the fiberscope into the trachea may fail (Fig. 17). Anterior displacement of the base of the tongue with a rigid laryngoscope may be required to assist passage of the ET tube. In severe flexion deformity of the cervical spine, the entire larynx is pushed backward against the posterior pharyngeal wall, making fiberoptic intubation quite difficult.

Distorted Airway Anatomy

Distortion of the upper airway with deviation of the larynx due to prior surgery, mass, edema, or soft tissue

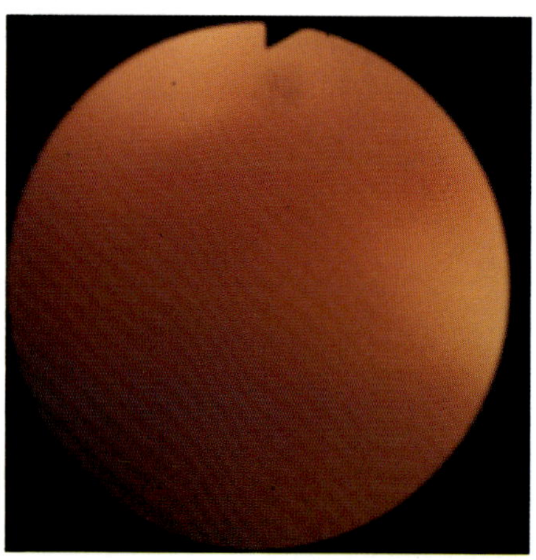

FIG. 15. Bloody secretions viewed through a fiberscope.

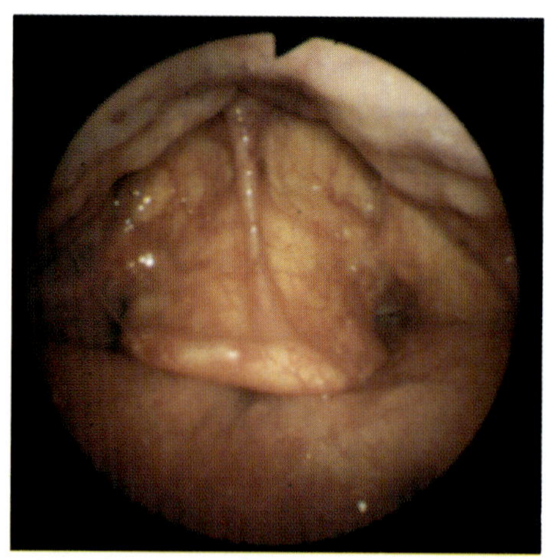

FIG. 16. Large, floppy epiglottis blocks the view of the glottis. A jaw thrust or pulling the tongue forward will move the tip of the epiglottis away from the posterior pharyngeal wall, making exposure of the glottis possible.

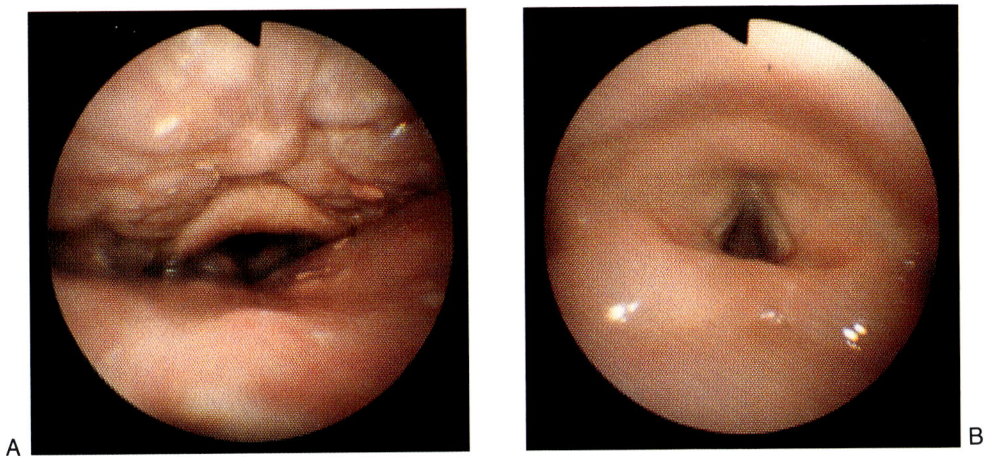

FIG. 17. **A:** A large, benign lymphoid mass at the base of the tongue compresses the epiglottis. The fiberscope was advanced into the trachea, but the endotracheal tube would not pass into the trachea. Rigid laryngoscopy was necessary to retract the tongue and assist passage of the tube into the trachea. **B:** Normal glottis.

contraction may contribute to difficulty with vocal cord exposure (Figs. 18 and 19). If attempting nasotracheal intubation, selecting the nostril on the side of the laryngeal deviation will assist in glottic exposure. In orotracheal intubation, the tip of the fiberscope should be directed toward the side to which the larynx is deviated. A deviated nasal septum may direct a nasotracheal tube away from the glottis. In severe cases, even though the fiberscope may enter the trachea, the ET tube may not follow.

Inability to Advance the Endotracheal Tube

Difficulty advancing the ET tube over the fiberscope into the trachea is a common occurrence during fiberoptic orotracheal intubation. The tip of the tube may easily catch on hypopharyngeal or laryngeal tissue. The arytenoids, interarytenoid muscle, vocal cords, and tip of the epiglottis are common sites of resistance.

Three contributing factors to this problem include: large differences in diameters between the fiberscope and the ET tube; the flexibility and design of the ET tube; and the technique selected, coupled with the expertise of the endoscopist.

Schwartz et al., under video observation, have demonstrated that the right arytenoid cartilage is the most common site for the ET tube to "hang-up" on when being threaded over the fiberscope (104). A 90° counterclockwise rotation of the tube turns the bevel of the tube to the 6 o'clock position, and the Murphy eye to the 12 o'clock position, permitting the ET tube to enter the trachea without resistance.

In the case of nasotracheal intubation, the obstruction encountered is usually the epiglottis. In this situation, the recommendation is to rotate the ET tube so as to place the tip of the tube at the 6 o'clock position before advancing (105). If the tip of the epiglottis is pushed up against the posterior pharyngeal wall, further advancement of the ET tube may only be possible by elevating the base of the tongue and epiglottis with a rigid laryngoscope blade.

The relationship between the size of the fiberscope and internal diameter of the ET tube is critical. The larger the gap between the fiberscope and ET tube, the greater the likelihood of difficulty in passing the tube. On rare occasions, despite all applied maneuvers, the ET tube will not enter the trachea until a larger-sized fiberscope or a smaller-sized ET tube is used. Failure to pass a 6.5-mm flexometallic tube over a 4-mm fiberscope has been reported secondary to decreased space between the epiglottis and the posterior pharyngeal wall (106).

If a large-size fiberscope (5 or 6 mm) is not available and an ET tube of 7.5 mm or larger is required, the gap between the tube and fiberscope can be minimized by placing a smaller-size ET tube into the ET tube being used (107). Fiberoptic intubation with a 4-mm fiberscope (Olympus LF-2 model) using a 7.0- and 8.0-mm ET tube for women and male patients, respectively, was associated with significant resistance to passage of the ET tube into the trachea in 90% of the cases. The placing of uncuffed 5.0-mm or 5.5-mm ID pediatric ET tubes, respectively, inside the larger adult tubes corrected the problem immediately. The tip of the pediatric tube protruded beyond the end of the larger tube, filling the space between the larger tube

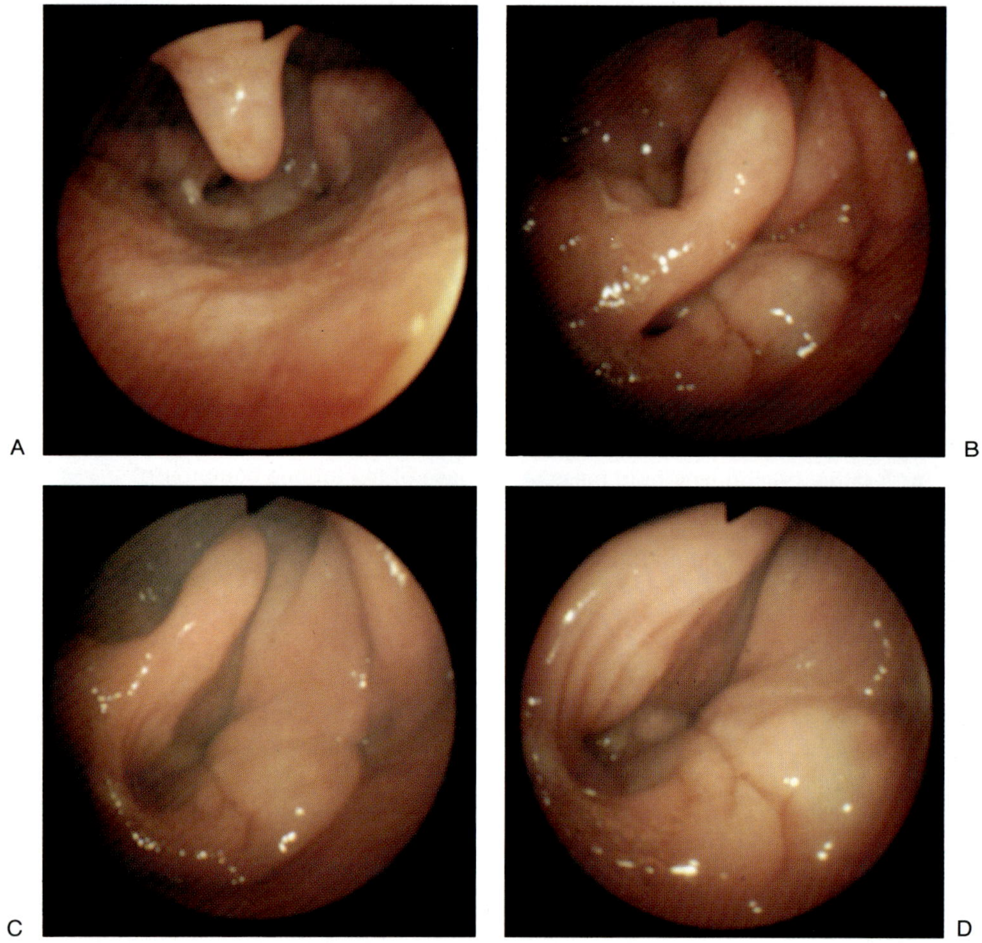

FIG. 18. Distorted laryngeal anatomy secondary to previous surgery. This patient had partial laryngectomy with rotation of the tip of the epiglottis to the left, sutured to the posterior pharyngeal wall. **A:** Advancement of the fiberscope through the oropharyngeal airway shows the tip of the uvula blocking the view of the larynx. **B:** Picture taken during exhalation. The opening of the glottis is blocked by the epiglottis. The tip of the epiglottis stretches from 12 o'clock to 7 o'clock. **C:** Picture taken during deep inspiration. The epiglottis is moved to open passage to the glottis. **D:** The tip of the fiberscope is beyond the tip of the epiglottis. Passage to the glottis in view, but not normal-looking. Intubation achieved within 2 min under topical anesthesia and light sedation.

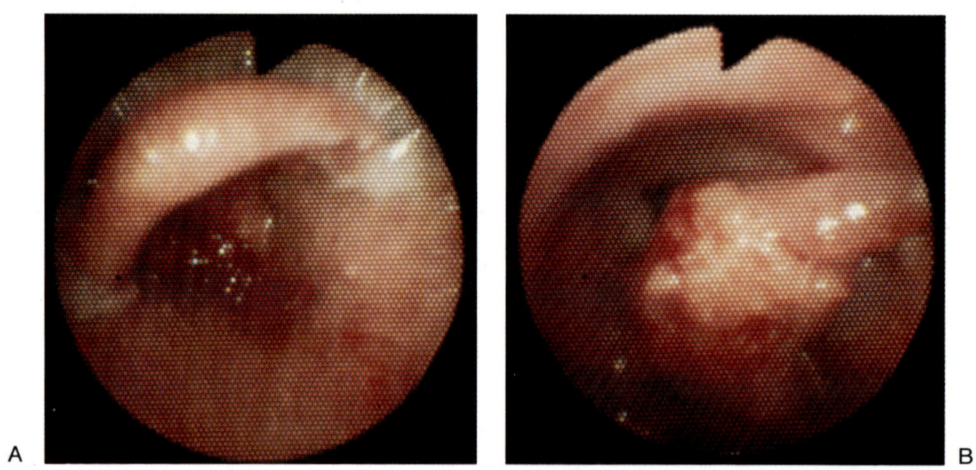

FIG. 19. Large squamous cell carcinoma of right aryepiglottic fold. **A:** Tip of the epiglottis in view. Lower portion of the tumor is also visible. **B:** The fiberscope is beyond the tip of the epiglottis. Tumor mass blocks the view of the glottis. The fiberscope was maneuvered to the upper left side over the mass and advanced toward the glottis.

and the fiberscope (Fig. 20). The placement of a second smaller tube through the intubating tube also prevents accidental passage of a small diameter fiberscope through the Murphy eye of the larger ET tube (107).

A manufacturing company (Rusch Incorporated, 2450 Meadowbrook Parkway, Duluth, Georgia) has introduced a special catheter "inner tube as an intubation aid" that fills the gap between the fiberscope and ET tube. The catheter tube is fitted inside the standard ET tube, and extends to a maximum of 3 cm beyond its tip. The inserted inner tube creates a tapered transition from the ET tube to the fiberscope, thus preventing impingement of the ET tube tip on arytenoid cartilage and hypopharyngeal or glottic structures.

Attention to technique is critical to successful use of the fiberscope. Fiberoptic orotracheal intubation conducted without use of an intubating airway tends to increase fiberscope deviation from the midline. If deviation occurs, the advancing ET tube has a greater tendency to catch the side of the epiglottis or other hypopharyngeal tissues.

The flexometallic (Anode) ET tubes have long been known to advance easily into the trachea (108). The flexometallic tubes are easier to pass, and less damaging to the tissues and fiberscope (109). In a prospective study, the ease of fiberoptic tracheal intubation was compared between regular ET tubes and flexometallic ET tubes (110). Nineteen out of 20 flexometallic intubations were successful on the first pass, compared to 7 out of 20 of the regular ET tubes. Of seven regular endotracheal tubes not placed in the trachea after three attempts, all were successfully intubated with flexometallic tubes of a comparable size. The authors attribute this success to the flexibility of the tube, which allows it to conform more easily to the fiberscope position (110).

In another randomized study, the influence of the ET tube tip on ease of advancement over the fiberscope was investigated. A new tracheal tube with a tapered tip and no bevel was designed and compared to a regular ET tube (111) (Fig. 21). Thirty patients were subjected to orotracheal and 30 to nasotracheal fiberoptic intubations. The patients were randomly assigned to receive either a regular or tapered tip tube. Intubations, without using an intubating airway or applying tongue traction, were then performed in these anesthetized, paralyzed patients. An assistant kept the lower jaw forward and open. In the orotracheal group 4 out of 15 regular ET tubes entered the trachea on the first attempt, compared to 14 out of 15 of the tapered tip tubes. In the nasotracheal group, 4 out of 14 standard ET tubes entered smoothly on the first attempt, compared to all 16 of the tapered tubes. The results indicate that removal of the gap between ET tube and fiberscope eliminates most of the difficulty encountered during fiberoptic intubations (111).

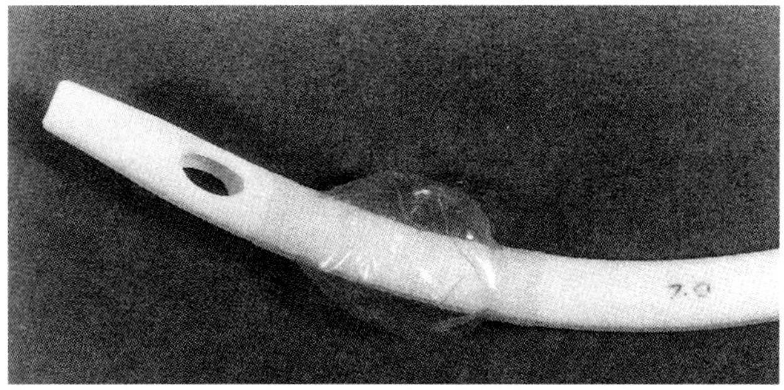

FIG. 21. Tapered-tip Moore endotracheal tube. (With permission, ref. 111.)

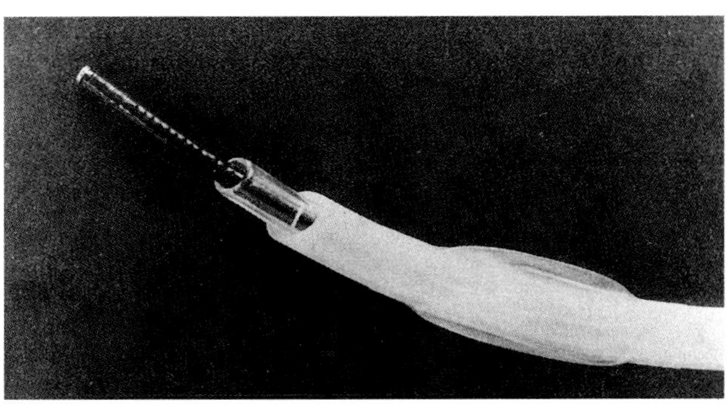

FIG. 20. Pediatric endotracheal tube inside larger ET tube to close the gap between the tube and fiberscope. (With permission, ref. 107.)

The avoidance of multiple attempts at ET tube advancement is important to avoid undue airway trauma. This is especially important in patients already judged to have difficult airways.

Inability to Remove the Fiberscope

If the fiberscope is passed through the Murphy eye of the ET tube, rather than through the distal lumen, withdrawal of the fiberscope may be prove difficult or damage the instrument (112,113) (Fig. 22). In this case, the fiberscope and ET tube should be withdrawn together as a unit. The intubation procedure may then be repeated.

To avoid this problem, pass the fiberscope through the ET tube under direct vision, identifying the distal lumen and the Murphy eye of the ET tube. If in doubt about the opening being viewed, follow the radio-opaque marker of the ET tube. The easily visible marker goes all the way down to the terminal opening. The loading of the ET tube over the fiberscope insertion cord prior to endoscopy also eliminates this error.

Poor lubrication of the fiberscope may make removal from the ET tube difficult. If the fiberscope's plastic cover is loose and force is applied, it may intussuscept over itself and occlude the ET tube lumen causing ob-

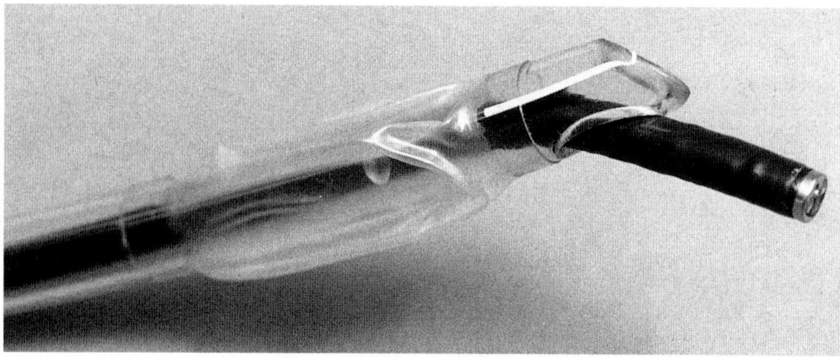

FIG. 22. Passage of the fiberscope through the Murphy eye of the endotracheal tube.

struction (114) (Fig. 23). Difficulty in removing the instrument from the ET tube may require removal of the tube and fiberscope together (114). On one occasion, the author was forced to remove a fiberscope and tube, due to the drying of water-soluble lubricant applied to the fiberscope, making movement of the fiberscope over the tube impossible.

SUCCESS RATE OF FIBEROPTIC INTUBATION

Relatively few large studies of fiberoptic intubation have been reported. Stiles et al. reported a 96% success rate in 100 fiberoptic intubations in a variety of patients (4). The fiberscope used did not have a suction channel, and the cause of failure in all four patients was attributed to the presence of copious secretions. Ovassapian et al. reported a 98.8% success rate in 413 awake nasotracheal intubations performed in patients with and without anatomic abnormalities (20). Eighteen of these patients had a history of difficult or failed intubation by conventional techniques.

Delaney and Hessler, after practicing fiberoptic intubation on a mannequin, used the fiberscope in 60 emergency room patients for nasotracheal intubation (77).

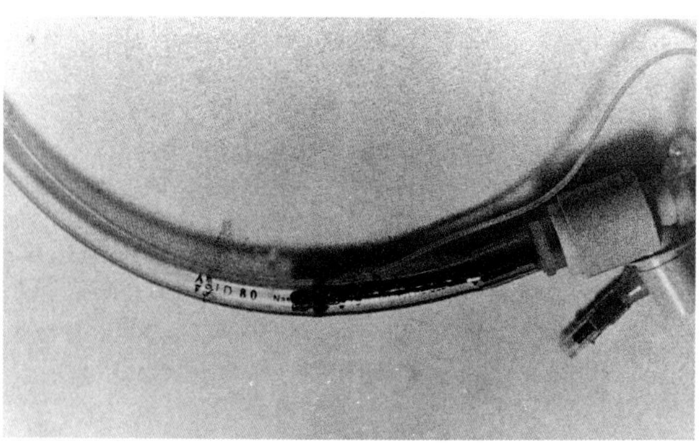

FIG. 23. Intussusception of the fiberscope inside the ET tube. (With permission, ref. 114.)

Despite their initial limited experience, they reported an 87% overall success rate. Their success rate on the last 37 patients in this series improved to 92%. This 92% success rate compares well with the other reports of blind nasal intubation conducted in the emergency room setting (115,116).

Northwestern Experience

The success rate at our institution was 98.6% in 1686 intubations performed under topical anesthesia with conscious sedation. In 345 intubations performed in anesthetized patients (Table 11), the success rate was 97.9%. Causes of intubation failure and the incidence of resistance to tracheal tube advancement is summarized in Tables 12–14.

The degree of difficulty in exposing the glottis was recorded in 1854 of 2031 intubations based on the following classification:

Not difficult—On initial introduction the fiberscope was properly aligned for good visualization of the cords, so little or no manipulation of the tip of the scope was needed.

Moderately difficult—Some manipulation of the fiberscope in all directions was necessary to locate the glottis.

Difficult—Extensive manipulation of the fiberscope in

TABLE 11. *Success rate of fiberoptic tracheal intubation*

Intubation type	Attempted (N)	Successful	Failed
Orotracheal			
Awake	974	958	16 (1.6%)
Anesthetized	335	328	7 (2.1%)
Nasotracheal			
Awake	712	704	8 (1.1%)
Anesthetized	10	9	1 (10%)
Total	2,031	1,999	32 (1.6%)

TABLE 12. *Causes of failure in 24 awake fiberoptic intubations*

Cause	N
Poor topical anesthesia	
Fiberscope in the trachea, but tube could not be advanced into the trachea	10
Gagging and vomiting—aborted the procedure	2
Severe cough and increase in blood pressure—aborted the procedure	1
Cords exposed, but fiberscope could not be advanced because of coughing and swallowing	1
Vocal cords not exposed	
Secretions and blood	5
Tumor and edema of the larynx	4
Tumor of the posterior pharyngeal wall	1
Total	24

TABLE 13. *Causes of failure in eight fiberoptic tracheal intubations in anesthetized patients*

Cause	N
Cords not exposed	
Secretions and/or tissues blocked the view	4
Poor light	1
Fiberscope placed in the trachea, but the tube could not be advanced	2
Cords exposed, but the fiberscope could not be advanced into the trachea	1
Total	8

TABLE 14. *Incidence of resistance to tracheal tube advancement during fiberoptic intubation*

Intubation type	Yes	No
Orotracheal		
Awake (*N*, 836)	245 (29.3%)	591 (70.7%)
Anesthetized (*N*, 291)	70 (24.1%)	221 (75.9%)
Nasotracheal		
Awake (*N*, 633)	38 (6.0%)	595 (94.0%)
Anesthetized (*N*, 9)	1 (11.0%)	8 (89.0%)
Total 1,769	354 (20.0%)	1,415 (80.0%)

all directions was necessary to identify the vocal cords, often with position changing.

Glottic exposure was considered easy in 65.4% of awake orotracheal and 79.8% of awake nasotracheal intubations. However, during general anesthesia, 82.4% of orotracheal intubations were easy. One should recall that all patients with a compromised airway, which adds considerably to the difficulty of laryngeal exposure, are in the awake group, while most anesthetized patients had normal airway anatomy (Table 15).

Exposure of the epiglottis and vocal cords was difficult in 101 intubations; there were various contributing factors (Table 16). Classification of their causes is somewhat arbitrary, since more than one cause is often present in an individual patient. Tumors or hematomas may contribute to intubation difficulty in different ways, depending on anatomic location. A supraglottic mass can block the view by pushing the epiglottis posteriorly, while a fungating mass arising in the vestibule may directly block the view of the cords.

If a cervical or oropharyngeal mass distorts the airway, use of the nostril on the opposite side of the mass usually provides easier and better fiberoptic exposure of the glottis. If airway deviation or distortion is caused by contraction of soft tissues of the oropharynx or neck, use of the nostril on the side of the contraction usually provides better exposure (20).

If translaryngeal injection fails to produce good topical anesthesia, supplemental local anesthetic can be sprayed through the working channel of the fiberscope. This approach was used in most patients with full stom-

TABLE 15. *Ease of laryngeal exposure in 1,854 intubations*

Intubation type	Each	Moderately difficult	Difficult
Orotracheal			
Awake (*N*, 899)	588 (65.4%)	251 (27.9%)	60 (6.7%)
Anesthetized (*N*, 312)	257 (82.4%)	42 (13.5%)	13 (4.1%)
Nasotracheal			
Awake (*N*,634)	506 (79.8%)	100 (15.8%)	28 (4.4%)
Anesthetized (*N*, 9)	7 (77.8%)	2 (22.2%)	0

TABLE 16. *Causes of difficult fiberoptic laryngeal exposure in 101 intubations*

Cause	N
Distorted airway anatomy (mass, hematoma, previous surgery, or radiation therapy)	34
Secretions/blood	26
Decreased space between the tip of the epiglottis and the posterior pharyngeal wall	25
Large, floppy epiglottis	8
Elevation of the floor of mouth and tongue due to edema and cellulitis	6
Supraglottic mass, causing dorsiflexion of the epiglottis	3
Obesity (obstructive sleep apnea)	4
Posterior displacement of the larynx due to severe flexion deformity of the cervical spine	4
Reactive airway (inadequate or no topical anesthesia)	10
Not recorded	6
Total	101

achs. Since the fiberscope and ET tube are held immediately above the vocal cords and topical anesthesia is achieved rapidly, the risk of aspiration with this method is negligible. It represents a safe alternative approach to the patient with a full stomach who is potentially a difficult intubation, or one with a limited mouth opening (117).

ADVANTAGES OF FIBEROPTIC INTUBATION

The primary advantage of fiberoptic intubation is its undoubted value in the management of a difficult tracheal intubation (Table 17). The fiberscope offers an excellent, effective, safe, often easy, and fast approach in patients who present difficult intubation problems with conventional techniques. Whenever movement of the head and neck is not possible or limited, and the opening of the mouth restricted, the fiberscope provides the best and most valuable approach for securing the airway.

Intubation of the trachea in the conscious sedated patient is well accepted, less stressful, and associated with lesser degrees of hypertension and tachycardia (99,100). The cardiovascular response to fiberoptic intubation under general anesthesia has not been shown to be more favorable compared with rigid laryngoscopy. Excellent visualization of the airway provides the opportunity to evaluate the airway prior to tube placement, differentiate the cause of airway compromise, and allow precise placement of the endotracheal tube, including for patients with tracheal compression (118). After completing intubation, the position of the tube is checked visually by reference to the carina, and thus avoids unrecognized esophageal and bronchial intubation.

TABLE 17. *Advantages of fiberoptic tracheal intubation*

Provides the best success in difficult intubation
Can be applied orally and nasally in all age groups
Provides evaluation of the airway prior to intubation
Avoids unrecognized esophageal and endobronchial intubation
Definitive check of tube position
Intubation can easily be performed with patient in sitting or lateral position
Only approach in patients with no access to anterior neck
Excellent patient acceptance of awake intubation
Less cardiovascular response during awake intubation
Ability to apply topical anesthesia, suction secretions, and insufflate oxygen during intubation
Excellent visualization of the airway
Less traumatic
Teaching attachment and video system

Fiberoptic intubation can easily be carried out with the patient in the supine, sitting, lateral, or prone position. The fiberscope provides the only hope for securing the airway and supplying general anesthesia in patients, where access to the anterior neck is not possible (119). Other advantages include less trauma and complete avoidance of tooth damage a common complication and the most common cause of malpractice suits against anesthesiologists (120–123).

Fiberoptic intubation is in fact the technique of choice in management of the difficult intubation and should be used initially, and not as a last resort, after repeated attempts using conventional techniques have failed. Fiberoptic tracheal intubation is critical to modern airway management. It should be mastered by all physicians involved in the care of patients who may present with a difficult airway or acute airway compromise.

DISADVANTAGES OF FIBEROPTIC INTUBATION

The two major disadvantages of the fiberscope are the cost of the instrument, and its size (Table 18). Fiberscopes are delicate instruments and require a separate light source for proper illumination during endoscopy; therefore, they occupy a larger space and need their own cart and setup. The cost and size of the fiberscope limit its practical availability in every anesthetizing location.

Cleaning, sterilization, and storage consume more time and resources. Its non-availability as a training tool leaves most anesthesiologists, and other physicians involved in airway management, lacking in the expertise and skills required for its effective use.

Other disadvantages include the ease with which relatively small amounts of secretions and blood can completely obscure the endoscopist's view, interfering with airway evaluation and tracheal intubation. Airway resistance is also increased as the fiberscope is advanced through the ET tube and the effective lumen allowing air exchange is compromised. The rigid bronchoscope provides a constant large lumen for air exchange. The small-size fiberscopes used in the neonate also lack a tip control mechanism and suction channel, limiting their value and maneuverability.

TABLE 18. *Disadvantages of fiberoptic tracheal intubation*

Expensive instrument
Delicate instrument
More difficult to clean and disinfect
Vision obscured easily by secretions and blood
Size of the instrument and light source

COMPLICATIONS

Some complications of tracheal intubation are solely related to the presence and effect of the endotracheal tube, while others are technique specific. Traumatic intubation using the rigid laryngoscope may cause laceration of oropharyngeal mucosa, damage to gums or teeth, and perforation of the pharynx and esophagus.

One case of laryngeal cyst attributed to fiberoptic nasotracheal intubation has been reported (124). A 16-year-old male with juvenile chronic arthritis was intubated under general anesthesia while breathing spontaneously. Topical anesthesia had been applied to the nose and larynx. Some firm manipulation was required to advance the ET tube over the fiberscope into the trachea. One month later the patient developed dysphagia and weight loss. A vocal cord mucosal cyst was then discovered. The cyst was removed, and his condition improved (124).

Additional complications include vocal cord paralysis due to high pressure of the ET tube cuff in the larynx. The cuff of the ET may be inflated below the vocal cords in the area of the thyroid cartilage, where it can damage the recurrent laryngeal nerve. Although precise placement of the tip of the ET tube is possible with the fiberscope, an error in measurement with the fiberscope may place the tube high in the larynx. This measurement error is not uncommon.

Complications in 2031 patients in our series of fiberoptic intubations were limited to laryngospasm in 51 patients, due to inadequate topical anesthesia; pain and/or hematoma at the translaryngeal injection site in 33 patients; gagging and/or vomiting in eight; and mild epistaxis in 70 of the 850 patients who had nasotracheal intubation (22). None of the patients with epistaxis required treatment by nasal packing.

In one patient who underwent awake orotracheal fiberoptic intubation, a small amount of gastric juice was noticed in the oropharynx before tracheal intubation; the fiberscope had entered the esophagus on the first attempt. There were no clinical or radiologic signs or symptoms of aspiration pneumonitis postoperatively. The fiberscope passed into the esophagus at least once during an intubation attempt on 49 occasions. While this is usually harmless, it may relax the cricopharyngeus muscle and facilitate regurgitation of gastric contents into the oropharynx if the esophagus contains gastric juice.

Respiratory depression and hypoxemia are relatively common with intravenous sedation. Since the oximeter was introduced into clinical practice, we routinely administer oxygen and use that monitor continuously during conscious sedation.

Information regarding recall in patients intubated awake was recorded in 808 orotracheal and 595 nasotracheal intubations. Among the 808 patients who had awake orotracheal intubation, 321 (39.7%) remembered the procedure, but only 41 (5.1%) recalled the procedure as somewhat unpleasant. In the 595 patients who had awake nasotracheal intubation, 292 (49.1%) remembered the procedure with 52 (8.7%) considering it unpleasant. Only nine (1.5%) of the awake nasotracheal group indicated that they would prefer not to go through the same procedure again (22). Most of the patients who had a vivid recollection of the intubation procedure and considered it unpleasant had received light or no sedation because of a severely compromised airway.

We did not find any lacerations resulting from tongue retraction, when used to open the pharyngeal space (125). Barotrauma of the lungs is possible if oxygen is insufflated through the suction channel of the fiberscope when it is advanced through a narrowed airway. The endoscopy mask diaphragm, covering the endoscopy port (as discussed earlier), can be pushed inside the oropharynx. This is a potential danger, and care should be exercised to avoid it (36).

Passage of the ET tube when threaded off of the fiberscope is a blind technique, and its tip may impinge on laryngeal structures. Error in measurement of ET tube tip distance from the carina may lead to high tube placement. If the cuff is inflated in the hypolarynx, the possibility of recurrent laryngeal nerve palsy may increase. Endobronchial intubation is also possible by mistaking upper and lower lobe bifurcation for the carina.

REFERENCES

1. Murphy P. A fiberoptic endoscope used for nasal intubation. *Anaesthesia* 1967;22:489–491.
2. Taylor PA, Towey RM. The broncho-fiberscope as an aid to endotracheal intubation. *Br J Anaesth* 1972;44:611–612.
3. Conyers AB, Wallace DH, Mulder DS. Use of the fiberoptic bronchoscope for nasotracheal intubation: a case report. *Can Anaesth Soc J* 1972;19:654–656.
4. Stiles CM, Stiles QR, Denson JS. A flexible fiberoptic laryngoscope. *JAMA* 1972;221:1246–1247.
5. Rucker RW, Silva WJ, Worcester CC. Fiberoptic bronchoscopic nasotracheal intubation in children. *Chest* 1979;76:56–58.
6. Mulder DS, Wallace DH, Woolhouse FM. The use of the fiberoptic bronchoscope to facilitate endotracheal intubation following head and neck trauma. *J Trauma* 1975;15:638–640.
7. Wang JF, Reves JG, Corssen G. Use of the fiberoptic laryngoscope for difficult tracheal intubation. *Alabama J Med Sci* 1976;13:247–251.
8. Messeter KH, Petersson KI. Endotracheal intubation with the fiberoptic bronchoscope. *Anaesthesia* 1980;35:294–298.
9. Edens ET, Sia RL. Flexible fiberoptic endoscopy in difficult intubations. *Ann Otol* 1981;90:307–309.
10. Ovassapian A, Doka JC, Romsa DE. Acromegaly—use of fiberoptic laryngoscope to avoid tracheostomy. *Anesthesiology* 1981;54:429–430.
11. Ovassapian A. *Fiberoptic airway endoscopy in anesthesia and critical care*. New York: Raven Press, 1990.

12. Mallios C. A modification of the Laerdal anesthesia mask for nasotracheal intubation with the fiberoptic laryngoscope. *Anaesthesia* 1980;35:599–600.
13. Patil V, Stehling LC, Zauder HL, Koch JP. Mechanical aids for fiberoptic endoscopy. *Anesthesiology* 1982;57:69–70.
14. Imai M, Kemmotsu Q. A new adapter for fiberoptic endotracheal intubation for anesthetized patients. *Anesthesiology* 1989;70:374.
15. Williams RT, Harrison RE. Prone tracheal intubation simplified using an airway intubator. *Can Anaesth Soc J* 1981;28:288–289.
16. Ovassapian A. A new fiberoptic intubating airway. *Anesth Analg* 1987(*Suppl*);66:S132.
17. Childress WF. New method for fiberoptic endotracheal intubation of anesthetized patients. *Anesthesiology* 1981;55:595–596.
18. Berman RA. A method for blind intubation of the trachea or esophagus. *Anesth Analg* 1977;56:866–867.
19. Higgins MS, Marco AP. An aid in oral fiberoptic intubation. *Anesthesiology* 1992;77:1236–1237.
20. Ovassapian A, Yelich SJ, Dykes MHM, Brunner EA. Fiberoptic nasotracheal intubation—incidence and causes of failure. *Anesth Analg* 1983;62:692–695.
21. Ovassapian A. Flexible bronchoscopic intubation of awake patients. *J of Bronchology* 1994;1:240–245.
22. Ovassapian A. Fiberoptic tracheal intubation. In: Ovassapian A, ed. *Fiberoptic airway endoscopy in anesthesia and critical care*. New York: Raven Press, 1990;57–79.
23. Reed AP, Han DG. The basics of awake intubation. In: Roberts JT, ed. *Clinical management of the airway*. Philadelphia: Saunders, 1994;147–157.
24. Southerland AD, Sale JP. Fiberoptic awake intubation—a method of topical anaesthesia and orotracheal intubation. *Can Anaesth Soc J* 1986;33:502–504.
25. Norton ML, Kyff J. Key medical considerations in the difficult airway: sleep apnea, obesity, and burns. In: Norton ML, Brown ACD, eds. *Atlas of the difficult airway*. St. Louis: Mosby Year Book, 1991;118–128.
26. Orringer MB. Endotracheal intubation and tracheostomy. Indications, techniques and complications. *Surg Clin North Am* 1980;60:1447–1464.
27. Witton TH. An introduction to the fiberoptic laryngoscope. *Can Anaesth Soc J* 1981;28:475–478.
28. Smith JE. Heart rate and arterial pressure changes during fiberoptic tracheal intubation under general anesthesia. *Anaesthesia* 1988;43:629–632.
29. Randell T, Yli-Hankala A, Valli H, Lindgren L. Topical anesthesia of the nasal mucosa for fiberoptic airway endoscopy. *Br J Anaesth* 1991;66:164–167.
30. Silberman HD, Wilf H, Tucker JA. Flexible fiberoptic nasopharyngolaryngoscope. *Ann Otol Rhinol Laryngol* 1976;85:640–645.
31. Lamb JD. Use of the fiberoptic laryngoscope. *Can Anaesth Soc J* 1982;29:181.
32. Lloyd EL. Fiberoptic laryngoscopy for difficult intubation. *Anaesthesia* 1980;35:719.
33. Pelimon A, Simunovic Z. Mouth gag and tongue holder for fiberoptic laryngoscopy. *Anaesthesia* 1985;40:386.
34. Ovassapian A, Dykes MHM. The role of fiberoptic endoscopy in airway management. *Semin Anesthesia* 1987;6:93–104.
35. Patil V, Stehling LC, Zauder HL. *Fiberoptic endoscopy in anesthesia*. Chicago: Year Book Medical Publishers, 1983.
36. Rogers SN, Benumof JL. New and easy techniques for fiberoptic endoscopy-aided tracheal intubation. *Anesthesiology* 1983;59:569–572.
37. Zorrow MH, Mitchell MM. Foreign body aspiration during fiberoptic assisted intubation. *Anesthesiology* 1986;64:303.
38. Williams L, Teague PD, Nagia AH. Foreign body from a Patil Syracuse mask. *Anesth Analg* 1991;73:359–360.
39. Davis K. Alterations to the Patil-Syracuse mask for fiberoptic intubation. *Anesth Analg* 1992;74:472–473.
40. Thomas JG. An alternative diaphragm for Patil-Syracuse mask. *Anesth Analg* 1992;74:473.
41. Wangler MA, Weaver JM. A method to facilitate fiberoptic laryngoscopy. *Anesthesiology* 1984;61:111.
42. Lu GP, Frost EAM, Goldiner PL. Another approach to the problem airway. *Anesthesiology* 1986;65:101–102.
43. Ovassapian A, Krejcie TC, Joshi CW. Fiberoptic vs rigid laryngoscopy for rapid sequence intubation of the trachea. *Anesth Analg* 1992(*Suppl*);74:S229.
44. Georgescu A, Miller JN, Lecklinter ML. The Sellick maneuver causing complete airway obstruction. *Anesth Analg* 1992;74:457–459.
45. Ovassapian A. The difficult intubation. In: Ovassapian A, ed. *Fiberoptic airway endoscopy in anesthesia and critical care*. New York: Raven Press, 1990;135–148.
46. Johnson C, Hunter J, Ho E, Bruff C. Fiberoptic intubation facilitated by a rigid laryngoscope. *Anesth Analg* 1991;72:713.
47. Couture P, Perreault C, Girard D. Fiberoptic bronchoscopic intubation after induction of general anesthesia: another approach. *Canad J Anaesth* 1992;39:99.
48. Russell SH, Hirch NP. Simultaneous use of two laryngoscopes. *Anaesthesia* 1993;48:918.
49. Alfery DD, Ward CF, Harwood IR, Mannino FL. Airway management for a neonate with congenital fusion of the jaws. *Anesthesiology* 1979;51:340–342.
50. Ovassapian A, Mesnick PS. The art of fiberoptic intubation. Anesthesiology clinics of North America 1995;13:391–409.
51. Tobias R. Increased success with retrograde guide for endotracheal intubation. *Anesth Analg* 1983;62:366–367.
52. Lechman MJ, Donahoo JS, McVaugh M III. Endotracheal intubation using percutaneous retrograde guide wire insertion followed by antegrade fiberoptic bronchoscopy. *Crit Care Med* 1986;14:589–590.
53. Carlson CR, Perkins HM, Veltkamp S. Saving a difficult intubation. *Anesthesiology* 1986;64:537–538.
54. Gupta B, McDonald JS, Brooks JHJ, Mendenhall J. Oral fiberoptic intubation over a retrograde guidewire. *Anesth Analg* 1989;68:517–519.
55. Gerrish SP, Weston GA. The use of a biopsy brush wire as a bronchoscope guide. *Anaesthesia* 1986;41:444.
56. Skinner AC. Glottic illumination by fiberscope. *Anaesthesia* 1983;38:1100–1101.
57. Whitlock JE, Calder I. Transillumination in fiberoptic intubation. *Anaesthesia* 1987;42:570.
58. Utting JE, Gray TC, Shelley FC. Human misadvanture in anaesthesia. *Can Anaesth Soc J* 1979;26:472–478.
59. Keenan RL, Boyan CP. Cardiac arrest due to anesthesia: a study of incidence and causes. *JAMA* 1985;253:2373–2377.
60. Caplan RA, Posner KL, Ward RJ, Cheney FW. Adverse respiratory events in anesthesia: A closed claims analysis. *Anesthesiology* 1990;72:828–833.
61. Cheney FW, Posner KL, Caplan RA. Adverse respiratory events infrequently leaking to malpractice suits. A closed claims analysis. *Anesthesiology* 1991;75:932–939.
62. Birmingham PK, Cheney FW, Ward RJ. Esophageal intubation: a review of detection techniques. *Anesth Analg* 1986;65:886–891.
63. Moorthy SS, Dierdorf SF. An unusual difficulty in fiberoptic intubation. *Anesthesiology* 1985;63:229.
64. Howells TH, Riethmuller RJ. Signs of endotracheal intubation. *Anaesthesia* 1980;35:984–986.
65. Pollard BJ, Junius F. Accidental intubation of the oesophagus. *Anaesth Intens Care* 1980;8:183–186.
66. Warden JC. Accidental intubation of the oesophagus and preoxygenation. *Anaesth and Intens Care* 1980;8:377.
67. Guggenberger J, Lenz G, Federle R. Early detection of inadvertent oesophageal intubation: pulse oximetry vs. capnography. *Acta Anaesth Scand* 1989;33:112–115.
68. Ionescu T. Signs of endotracheal intubation. *Anaesthesia* 1981;36:422.
69. Linko K, Paloheimo M, Tammisto T. Capnography for detection of accidental oesophageal intubation. *Acta Anaesth Scand* 1983;27:199–202.
70. Murray IP, Modell JH, Early detection of endotracheal tube accidents by monitoring carbon dioxide concentration in respiratory gas. *Anesthesiology* 1983;59:344–346.
71. Sum Ping St. Esophageal intubation. *Anesth Analg* 1987;66:483.

72. Burton GW. Measurement of inspired and expired oxygen and carbon dioxide. *Br J Anaesth* 1969;41:723–729.
73. Wee MYK. The esophageal detector device. Assessment of a new method of to distinguish esophageal from tracheal intubation. *Anaesthesia* 1988;43:27–29.
74. Calder I, Smith M, Newton M. The esophageal detector device. *Anaesthesia* 1989;44:705.
75. Davies JR. The fiberoptic laryngoscope in the treatment of cut throat injuries. *Br J Anaesth* 1978;50:511–513.
76. Schafermeyer RW. Fiberoptic laryngoscopy in the emergency department. *Am J Emer Med* 1984;2:160–163.
77. Delaney KA, Hessler R. Emergency flexible fiberoptic nasotracheal intubation: a report of 60 cases. *Ann Emerg Med* 1988; 17:919–926.
78. Mlinek EJ, Clinton JE, Plummer D, Ruiz E. Fiberoptic intubation in the emergency department. *Ann Emerg Med* 1990;19: 359–362.
79. Afilalo M, Guttman A, Stern E, Lloyd J, Colacone A, Tselios C, Dankoff J. Fiberoptic intubation in the emergency department: A case series. *J Emerg Med* 1993;11:387–391.
80. Bullingham A, Hampson–Evans D, Palazzo M. An impaled neck. Management of difficult airway access. *Anaesthesia* 1994;49:866–869.
81. Lyons G. Failed intubation. Six years experience in teaching maternity unit. *Anaesthesia* 1985;40:759–762.
82. Reports on confidential inquiries into maternal death in England and Wales 1982–1984. London: HMSO, 1985.
83. Shorten GD, Alfille PH, Gliklich RE. Airway obstruction following application of cricoid pressure. *J. Clin Anesth* 1991;3: 403–405.
84. Wright WJ, Chammey AR, Howells TH. The determination of effective cricoid pressure. *Anaesthesia* 1983;38:461–466.
85. Hood DD, Dewan DM. Anesthetic and obstetric outcome in morbidly obese parturients. *Anesthesiology* 1993;79: 1210–1218.
86. Glassenberg R, Vaisrub N, Albright G. The incidence of failed intubation in obstetrics. Is there an irreducible minimum? *Anesthesiology* 1990;73:A1061.
87. Burns AM, Dorje P, Lawes EG, Nielsen MS. Anesthetic management of cesarean section for a mother with pre-eclampsia, the Klippel–Feil syndrome congenital hydrocephalus. *Br J Anaesth* 1988;61:350–354.
88. Fayek SS, Isaac PA, Shah J. Awake fiberoptic intubation in a 38 week pregnant patient with submandibular abscess. *Inter J Obst Anesthesia* 1994;3:103–105.
89. Farcon EL, Kim HM, Manx GF. Changing Mallampati score during labor. *Can J Anaesth* 1994;41:50–51.
90. Kleinman B, Henkin RE, Glisson SN, El–Etr AA, Bakhos M, Sullivan H, Montoya A, Pifarre R. Qualitative evaluation of coronary flow during anesthetic induction using thallium—201 perfusion scans. *Anesthesiology* 1986;64:157–164.
91. Takeshima K, Noda J, Higakik M. Cardiovascular response to rapid anaesthesia induction and endotracheal intubation. *Anesth Analg* 1964;43:201–208.
92. Shribman AJ, Smith G, Achola KJ. Cardiovascular and catecholamine responses to laryngoscopy with and without tracheal intubation. *Br J Anaesth* 1987;59:295–299.
93. Finfer SR, Mackenzie JM Saddler, Watkins TG. Cardiovascular responses to tracheal intubation: A comparison of direct laryngoscopy and fibreoptic intubation. *Anaesth Intens Care* 1989;17:44–48.
94. Smith JE, Mackenzie AA, Scott-Knight, VCE. Comparison of two methods of fibrescope-guided tracheal intubation. *Br J Anaesth* 1991;66:546–550.
95. Schaefer HG, Marsch SCU. Comparison of orthodox with fibreoptic orotracheal intubation under total IV anaesthesia. *Br J Anaesth* 1991;66:608–610.
96. Schaefer HG, Marsch SCU, Strebel SP, Drewe J. Cardiovascular effects of fibreoptic oral intubation. *Anaesthesia* 1992;47: 1034–1036.
97. Smith JE, King MJ, Yanny HF, Pottinger KA, Pomirska MB. Effect of fentanyl on the circulatory responses to orotracheal fibreoptic intubation. *Anaesthesia* 1992;47:20–23.
98. Smith JE, Mackenzie AA, Sanghera SS, Scott-Knight VCE. Cardiovascular effects of fibrescope-guided nasotracheal intubation. *Anaesthesia* 1989;44:907–910.
99. Ovassapian A, Yelich SJ, Dykes MHM, Brunner EA. Blood pressure and heart rate changes during awake fiberoptic nasotracheal intubation. *Anesth Analg* 1983;62:951–954.
100. Schrader S, Ovassapian A, Dykes MHM, Avram M. Cardiovascular changes during awake rigid and fiberoptic laryngoscopy. *Anesthesiology* 1987;67:A28.
101. Hawkyard S, Morrison A, Doyle L, Croton R, Wake P. Fiberoptic intubation: attenuating the hypertensive response to laryngoscopy and intubation. *Br J Anaesth* 1989;63:624P.
102. Randell T, Valli H, Lindgren L. Effects of alfentanil on the responses to awake fiberoptic nasotracheal. *Acta Anaesthesiologica Scandinavica* 1990;34:59–62.
103. Southerland AD, Sale JP. Fiberoptic awake intubation: a method of topical anesthesia and orotracheal intubation. *Can Anaesth Soc J* 1988;33:502–504.
104. Schwartz D, Johnson C, Roberts J. A maneuver to facilitate fiberoptic intubation. *Anesthesiology:* 1989;470–471.
105. Katsnelson T, Frost EAM, Farcon E, Goldiner PL. When the endotracheal tube will not pass over the flexible fiberoptic bronchoscope. *Anesthesiology* 76:152–152, 1992.
106. Telford RJ, Searle JF, Boaden RW, Baier F. Use of a guide wire and ureteral dilator as an aid to awake fiberoptic intubation. *Anaesthesia* 49:691–693,1994.
107. Marsh NJ. Easier fiberoptic intubation. *Anesthesiology* 1992; 76:860–861.
108. Hodkgin JE, Rosenow EC, Stubbs SE. Diagnostic and therapeutic techniques in thoracic medicine. Oral introduction of the flexible bronchoscope. *Chest* 1975;68:88–90.
109. Calder I. When the endotracheal tube will not pass over the flexible fiberoptic bronchoscope. *Anesthesiology* 1992;77:398.
110. Brull SJ, Wiklund R, Ferris C et al. Facilitation of fiberoptic orotracheal intubation with a flexible tracheal tube. *Anesth Analg* 1994;78:746–748.
111. Jones HE, Pearce AC, Moore P. Fiberoptic intubation. Influence of tracheal tube tip design. *Anaesthesia* 1993;48:672–674.
112. Ovassapian A. Failure to withdraw flexible laryngoscope after nasotracheal intubation. *Anesthesiology* 1985;63:124–125.
113. Nichols KP, Zornow MH. A potential complication of fiberoptic intubation. *Anesthesiology* 1989;70:562–563.
114. Siegel M, Coleprate P. Complication of fiberoptic bronchoscope. *Anesthesiology* 1984;61:214–215.
115. Damzle DF, Thomas DM. Nasotracheal intubation in the emergency department. *Crit Care Med* 1980;8:677–682.
116. Iserson KV. Blind nasotracheal intubation. *Ann Emerg Med* 1981;10:468–471.
117. Ovassapian A, Krejcie TC, Yelich SJ, Dykes MHM. Awake fiberoptic intubation of the patient at high risk of aspiration. *Br J Anaesth* 1989;62:13–16.
118. Prakash UBS, Abel MD, Hubmayr RD. Mediastinal mass and tracheal obstruction during general anesthesia. *Mayo Clin Proc* 1988;63:1004–1011.
119. Ovassapian A, Land P, Schafer MF, et al. Anesthetic management for surgical correction of severe flexion deformity of the cervical spine. *Anesthesiology* 1983;58:370–372.
120. Wright RB, Manfield FFV. Damage to teeth during the administration of general anesthesia. *Anesth Analg* 1974;53:405–408.
121. Burton JF, Baker AB. Dental damage during anaesthesia and surgery. *Anaesth Intens Care* 1987;15:262–268.
122. Solazzi RW, Ward RJ. The spectrum of medical liability cases. *Intern Anesth Clin* 1984;22:43–59.
123. Holzer JF. Current concepts in risk management. *Intern Anesth Clin* 1984;22:91–116.
124. Smith BL. Laryngeal cyst following fiberoptic intubation. *Anaesthesia* 1986;41:430–431.
125. El-Ganzouri, El-Baz N, Ford E, et al. Training residents in fiberoptic intubation in the operating room. *Anesthesiology* 1988;69:A805.

CHAPTER 7

Pediatric Fiberoptic Intubation

Melissa Wheeler, M.D. and Andranik Ovassapian, M.D.

The child with a difficult airway is a challenge for any anesthesiologist. Traditional approaches to this problem have relied on "tricks" using a rigid laryngoscope, such as laryngeal pressure, retromolar approach, and the use of intubating stylets or "blind" techniques. Repeated unsuccessful attempts with a rigid laryngoscope may lead to airway trauma and subsequent edema, turning a difficult airway into an impossible airway and a life-threatening problem. Children are particularly at risk for airway edema and obstruction because of the relatively small size of the airway structures. An alternative to this scenario is early and preemptive use of the techniques of fiberoptic laryngoscopy and intubation. Currently available fiberscopes may be utilized with endotracheal (ET) tubes as small as 2.5-mm inner diameter (ID) and therefore virtually no child is "too small" for fiberoptic management of the airway (Table 2, Chapter 1).

EQUIPMENT

The Fiberscope

The Olympus LF-P can be used for ET tubes as small as 2.5-mm ID, with the 15-mm adapter removed (Fig. 1). It has no working channel, therefore suctioning, insufflation of 0_2, and "spray-as-you-go" application of topical anesthesia are not possible. However, prelaryngoscopic application of topical anesthesia and suctioning as well as provision of 0_2 by nasal cannula, endoscopic mask, or "blow by" can circumvent the lack of a working channel.

The Olympus LF-2 (4-mm outer diameter) and the Pentax FI-P10 (3.6-mm OD) models have a working channel and are suitable for ET tubes size 4.5-mm ID and greater. For some brands of ET tubes, a 4.0-mm ID ET tube will fit over the Pentax F1-P10.

Other ultrathin fiberscopes are manufactured but do not have tips that can be directed. These scopes can be used to check the position of an ET tube but are unsuitable for use in intubation.

Ancillary Equipment

Ancillary equipment to facilitate pediatric fiberoptic tracheal intubation is more limited than that for adult intubation. At present, intubation airways designed to facilitate orotracheal intubation are only available for adult-sized patients. A modification of the Guedel-type oropharyngeal airway has been described for use in

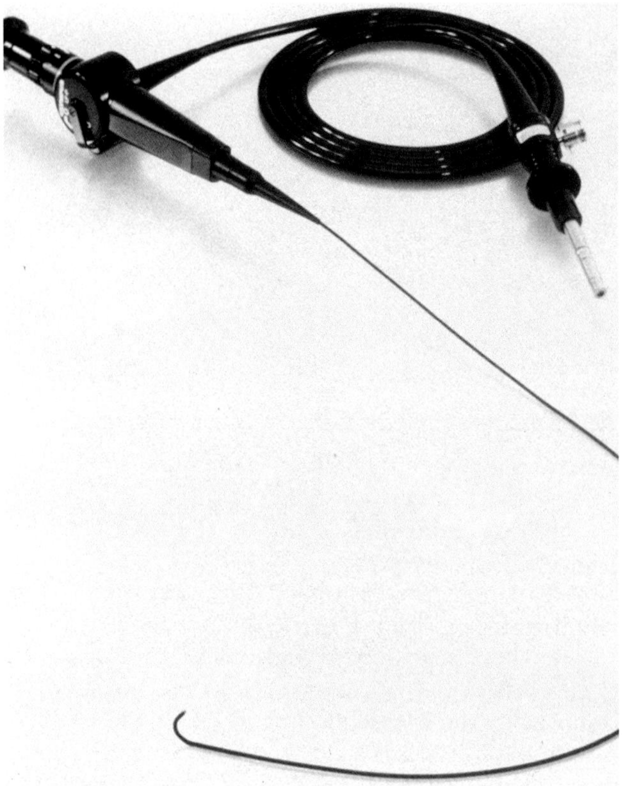

FIG. 1. Olympus LF-P intubation fiberscope.

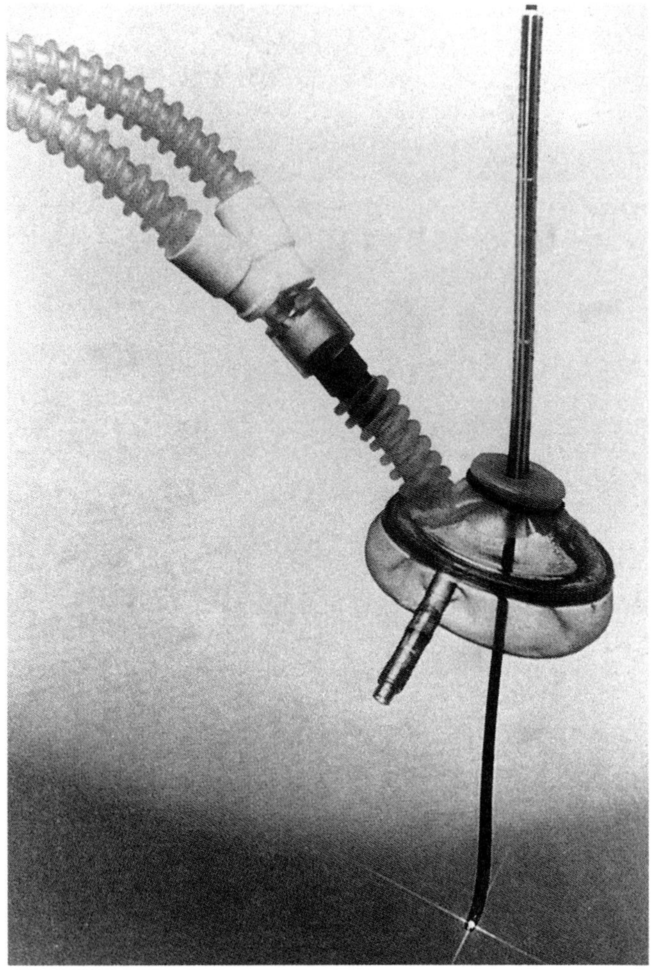

FIG. 2. Modified pediatric face mask for fiberoptic intubation. (With permission, ref. 2.)

children. A strip is cut from the convex surface of the oropharyngeal airway (1). It is suggested that the modified oropharyngeal airway should be slightly smaller than that used to assist ventilation so as to allow adequate visualization of the glottis. This modified oropharyngeal airway is *not* an effective bite block, however, and serves only to assist in maintaining a midline position.

Ventilating face masks for pediatric fiberoptic intubation are available commercially, such as the Patil-Syracuse mask, or can be made by modifying standard pediatric face masks (Fig. 2) (2).

INDICATIONS

All applications of the techniques of fiberoptic endoscopy described for adults may be utilized in children. These include securing and evaluating the airway, changing the ET tube, checking the tube position and patency, tracheobronchial toilet, and nasogastric tube placement.

The techniques for these applications are similar but not identical to those for adults. In particular, the techniques of fiberoptic intubation deserve special consideration. A summary of 17 reports of the use of a fiberscope to assist in difficult pediatric intubation is presented in Table 1 (3–19). Anesthesiologists who report the use of a fiberscope for intubation of children with difficult airway remark on the superiority of this technique to other airway management options (4,6,14,18). These clinicians comment on the ease of endotracheal tube placement, the decreased trauma, and the ability to visually confirm correct endotracheal tube placement (4,6,14,18).

EVALUATION AND PREDICTION OF THE DIFFICULT PEDIATRIC AIRWAY

Although not specifically designed for children, the American Society of Anesthesiologists (ASA) practice guidelines for the difficult airway provide a sound approach for evaluation and prediction of the difficult airway for any patient. This approach relies primarily on an airway history and physical examination and secondarily on diagnostic tests (20).

TABLE 1. *Fiberoptic intubation for pediatric airway management: case reports*

Author	Ref.	Patient age	Precipitating disease	Indication for intubation	Complications
Alfery, et al. '79	3	Newborn[a]	Fusion of the jaws	Examination of the jaw	none
Rucker, et al. '79	4	22 children: 18 months–16 years	Trauma, asthma, seizures, Reye's syndrome, croup, pneumonia, epiglottitis, encephalitis	Ventilatory failure or impending ventilatory failure	none
Berthelsen, et al. '85	5	6 months[b]	History of difficult intubation	Intraocular surgery	none
Kleeman, et al. '87	6	3 children: 3–30 months	Ankylosis of TMJ (cong.), Pierre Robin syndrome	Plastic surgery	none
Gouverneur '87	7	2 weeks[a]	Klippel-Feil syndrome	Ventriculoperitoneal shunt	none
Howardy-Hansen and Berthelsen '88	8	3 days[c]	Pierre Robin syndrome	Esophageal atresia repair	none
Baines, et al. '89	9	6 years	Swollen tongue	Airway obstruction	none
Wilder and Belani '90	10	12 years	Hurler's syndrome	Incarcerated umbilical hernia	pulmonary edema
Tassony, et al. '90	11	4 children: 4–9 years	Noma (gangrenous stomatitis)	Various surgical procedures	20 intubations; 1 epistaxis
Audenaert, et al. '91	12	20 children: 1 day–17 years[d]	Amyoplasia, cerebral palsy, congenital anomalies, arthrogryposis with Klippel-Feil, Hurler's, Hallerman-Streiff, Pierre Robin and Schwartz-Jampel syndromes, C_1-C_2 subluxation, Still's disease	Various surgical procedures	2 O_2 desaturations
Montgomery, et al. '91	13	13 years	Goldenhar's syndrome	Harrington rod instrumentation	none
Monrigal, et al. '91	14	10 infants: 9 days–6 months	4 with history of difficult intubation, 6 with "facial abnormalities"	Various surgical procedures	none
Scheller and Schulman '91	15	1 month[c]	Pierre Robin syndrome	Pyloromyotomy	none
Finer and Muzyka '92	16	23 neonates: 31.5–60 weeks postconceptual age	Goldenhar's, Pierre Robin, and Larsen's syndromes, micrognathia, stridor, failed intubation, hydrocephalus	Respiratory failure, various surgical procedures	transient desaturation
Suriani, et al. '92	17	29 months[c]	Pierre Robin syndrome	Cleft palate repair	none
Asada, et al. '94	18	8 years	Farber's syndrome	Excision of airway granulomas	none
Roth, et al. '94	19	20 infants: 1–24 months	Healthy children (prospective study)	Various surgical procedures	2 had barky cough at 24 h

[a] Intubation under fiberoptic observation
[b] Three-stage technique
[c] Two-state technique
[d] Retrograde-assisted technique
(Tables 1 and 2 with permission: Benumof, Jonathan L.,ed. *Airway Management-Principles and Practice*. Philadelphia; Moseby Yearbook, Inc., 1995:304–305.)

Airway History

Children often have different reasons for airway difficulty than do adults, and the importance of the airway history is based upon the recognized association between the difficult airway and congenital, acquired, and traumatic disease states. Congenital anomalies are common and those historically associated with the potential difficult airway should be recognized. Examination of previous anesthetic records, if available, is crucial and may provide useful airway management information.

A primary feature of many syndromes associated with difficult airway management is micrognathia (e.g., Pierre Robin syndrome, Treacher Collins's syndrome, Nager's syndrome, Goldenhar's syndrome). Micrognathia results in a decreased potential displacement space for the tongue and therefore increases the likelihood that the glottis will be difficult to visualize during laryngoscopy. Those patients with syndrome-associated micrognathia are usually easily recognized and often have a history of airway-related problems, such as obstructive apnea, snoring, "noisy" breathing, or a history of difficult intubation or difficult mask ventilation. Even in a patient who appears to be "normal," a history of any of these problems should alert the practitioner to the possibility of difficult airway management.

A less obvious deformity, such as a short neck (associated with Larsen's and Down's syndromes) or the Klippel-Feil syndrome (synostosis of the cervical vertebrae), will limit the ability to align oral, pharyngeal, and laryngeal axes and will therefore result in difficult intubation.

Other congenital anomalies associated with difficult airway management are reviewed in refs. 21 and 22.

Airway Physical Examination

Many evaluation schemes involving complex calculations of measured patient parameters, either directly or by X ray, have been developed. None, however, are universally applicable, practical, sensitive, specific, and predictive, and no system for evaluation of the pediatric airway has been devised and rigorously tested. The tools used to make an educated guess about a possibly difficult airway must be extrapolated from studies of adults and what is known about the syndrome-related, difficult pediatric airway.

Physical examination should evaluate the chin for any degree of micrognathia, the neck for shortening or limited mobility, the mouth opening, and the temporal mandibular joint mobility. If the patient is able to cooperate, the Mallampoti classification may be utilized (23). Estimations of submandibular space are, by definition, variable by age, and one that is normal is difficult to describe. To a great degree all examination criteria are subjective, and although increasing pediatric experience will increase the ability to pick up more subtle clues of abnormal or potentially difficult airways, no test and no person is immune to missing the occasional difficult airway.

PREPARATION FOR FIBEROPTIC INTUBATION IN CHILDREN

Equipment Preparation

Preparation of the fiberscope is essentially the same as for adults. However, special care must be taken to avoid excessive bending or direct blows to the small-sized pediatric insertion cords, as they are very delicate and easily broken. Special plastic sheaths are provided to protect the fiberscopes when they are not in use, including after the intubation is complete. The plastic sheath is sterilized along with the fiberscopes. If you are using the LF-P which has no working channel, have suction catheters prepared with tape over the thumb control port so that these may be utilized with one-handed operation if necessary.

For intubations performed under spontaneous ventilation, supplemental oxygen should be provided. Options include pediatric nasal cannula or oxygen "blow by" from the circuit for the sedated patient. For the anesthetized patient the circuit can be attached to an oral or nasal airway, or an endoscopic or laryngeal mask airway, with an endoscopic swivel adapter attached. The last two techniques can be used in the anesthetized and paralyzed patient with controlled ventilation. Insufflation of oxygen through the suction channel of the fiberscope has been suggested to provide oxygen and clear secretions from the airway. Possible problems include insufflation of oxygen into the stomach and barotrauma to the lung if exhalation is blocked by the fiberscope or airway pathology and the oxygen flow rate is high.

Patient Preparation and Anesthetic Options

The age and maturity of the child with a potentially difficult airway affects his ability to cooperate with traditional conscious sedation techniques used for securing the difficult airway in an adult. The anesthetic technique must be tailored to the airway problem and the maturity of the child.

For very young infants, intubation under topical anesthesia may be the safest approach to secure the airway. Alternatively, infants and children through preschool age may be heavily sedated with ketamine to preserve spontaneous ventilation. Ketamine is a potent hypnotic as well as analgesic agent which produces a "dissociative" anesthesia. In most circumstances, ketamine preserves adequate spontaneous ventilation while providing anesthesia to prevent reaction to airway manipulation. It may be used alone or in conjunction with midazolam. Another attractive feature of ketamine is that it has many routes for administration. If an intravenous (IV) line is difficult or impossible to obtain, a small intramuscular, intranasal, oral, or rectal dose can be effectively used for heavy sedation. An IV line can then be secured and further sedation, if necessary, may be given intravenously.

Ketamine has not been widely used in adult anesthesia because of its high incidence of psychomimetic emergence reactions (24). However, these reactions are less common in children, particularly if ketamine is combined with midazolam (25,26). Also, ketamine can produce increased upper airway secretions that might interfere with fiberoptic airway management, but a preoperative antisialagogue in conjunction with preendoscopy suctioning of the airway will alleviate this problem. There are anecdotal reports of "hyperreactive" airway reflexes when ketamine is used. However, adequate ketamine or ketamine-midazolam doses combined with good suctioning and skilled endoscopy techniques are the best defense against airway reactivity. In fact, ketamine is a commonly described anesthetic agent for the fiberoptic airway management of young children with difficult airways, and no problems with increased airway reactivity have been noted (3,5,8).

Older children and adolescents may cooperate with a technique of midazolam and fentanyl sedation if the methodology and reasons for proceeding with this technique are carefully and thoughtfully presented to them and their parents. The addition of small doses of droperidol can add a "neuroleptic" dimension to the anesthetic, which may increase patient acceptance. This drug also decreases the incidence of nausea and vomiting, which can occur in the extremely anxious child.

For the child who is extremely anxious and in whom a mask airway is not expected to be difficult, a gentle halothane induction may be the best alternative. With adequate depth of anesthesia and supplemented with topical anesthesia, intubation can then be attempted on the spontaneously breathing patient. Alternatively, controlled ventilation may be gradually assumed to assure the child's airway can be managed by mask. If mask ventilation is easily performed, a short-acting muscle relaxant can be given and fiberoptic intubation begun. This approach obviates any risk of laryngospasm or of sudden patient movement, which can occur with sedation or light anesthesia with spontaneous ventilation. However, time for fiberoptic intubation will be decreased because of the patient's apnea.

Propofol infusion, titrated to provide a more profound degree of sedation but maintain spontaneous ventilation, is another anesthetic option. However, the technique is tricky, and advanced experience is required because of the risk of oversedation and apnea. But propofol has the advantage of quick awakening after the infusion is discontinued, unlike titrated doses of ketamine. Propofol is useful in those patients for whom conscious sedation is not an option.

All fiberoptic techniques will be more successful if a preoperative antisialagogue is administered either intramuscularly or intravenously before proceeding with the fiberoptic intubation.

Topical Anesthesia: Special Considerations

For tracheal intubation of the patient who is sedated, or is under light general anesthesia with spontaneous ventilation, topical anesthesia of the airway will improve patient acceptance, prevent laryngospasm, and increase the success rate of intubation. All techniques used in adults may be used in children with a few caveats. Keep in mind the smaller size of the patient and the subsequent restrictions on the volumes and amount of local anesthetic that can be used. Cetacainec™ spray and Americainec™ ointment, because of their ingredient benzocaine, may cause methemoglobinemia in infants and it is best to avoid them in this age group (27). Translaryngeal injection is technically difficult in infants less than 6 months of age and should therefore be avoided in these children.

TABLE 2. *Lidocaine nebulizer—suggested doses*

Patient weight (kgs)	cc of 4% lidocaine	cc of .9 normal saline
10–14.9	.5	.5
15–19.9	1.0	1.0
20–24.9	1.5	.5
25–29.9	2.0	—
30–34.9	2.5	—
35–39.9	3.0	—
40–44.9	3.5	—
45 and up	4.0	—

Nebulized lidocaine is ideal for young children. Children seem to get a better anesthetic effect from this technique than do adults. Also, many children have used nebulizers in the treatment of asthma or bronchospastic disease and therefore readily accept the lidocaine nebulizer. Suggested volumes based on weight are given in Table 2.

PEDIATRIC FIBEROPTIC INTUBATION TECHNIQUES

Single-Stage Intubation

Oral Approach

The single-stage intubation or routine technique is the traditional adult technique (tube over the fiberscope). This is the method of choice if a small directable-tip fiberscope is available.

The patient should be positioned to assure the greatest possibility of success. The arms are tucked and a strap is placed over the legs. For infants, a papoose-style technique is useful. This technique keeps arms restrained but maintains a free excursion of the chest and abdomen. Head position should be neutral or extended rather than sniffing to assure a better angle for visualization of the larynx.

To begin fiberoptic intubation, the assistant should provide a jaw thrust. This brings the tongue up off the posterior pharynx and provides an unobstructed view

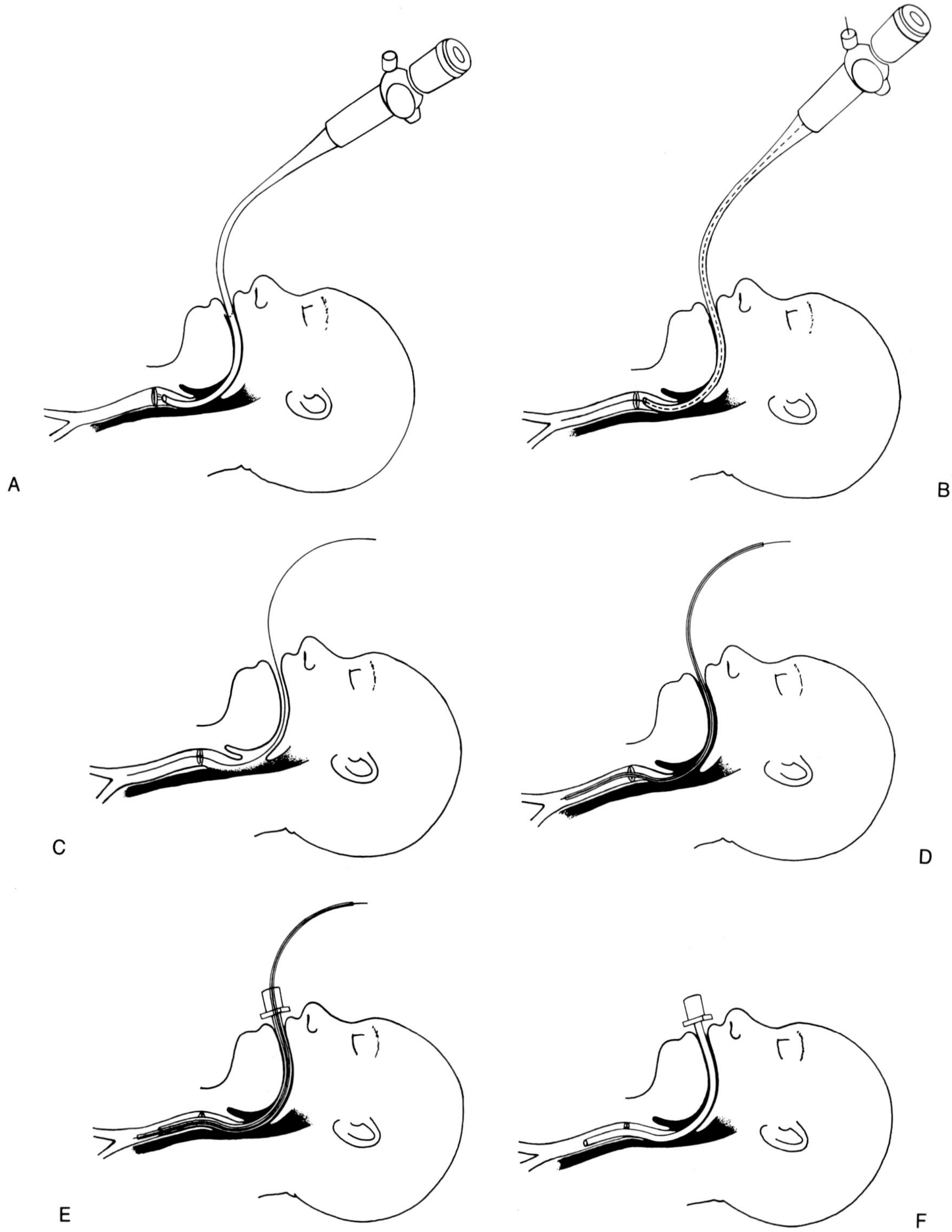

FIG. 3. Two-stage fiberoptic tracheal intubation using guide wire and catheter described by Stiles (29). **A:** The fiberscope is introduced through the mouth, and the tip is positioned at the level of the vocal cords. **B:** The guide wire is inserted into the suction channel and is advanced into the trachea under visual observation. **C:** The fiberscope is removed, leaving the guide wire inside the trachea. **D:** The catheter is advanced over the guide wire into the trachea. **E:** The endotracheal tube is threaded over the guide wire and catheter into the trachea. **F:** The catheter and guide wire are removed, leaving the endotracheal tube in place.

of the larynx. The mouth should then be suctioned. It is important to place the fiberscope into the mouth in a midline position. This is especially critical in small infants and neonates because it is easy to confuse the anatomy if the initial central position is not assured. A good method is to look directly at the fiberscope (not through the fiberscope) while it is being placed into the mouth, and then rest the right hand on the patient's face while holding the insertion cord of the fiberscope in the midline position. The fiberscope is advanced using the fingers of the right hand, while directing the fiberscope tip with the thumb of the left hand. When needed, the body of the fiberscope may be rotated to change the orientation of the tip of the fiberscope. It is extremely important to keep the insertion cord taut so that all motion of the left hand (both rotation and lever manipulation) will be directly translated to the tip of the fiberscope.

If the view through the fiberscope is a "pink mass," pull back the fiberscope so that recognizable structures will come into view. The most common mistake, particularly if one is used to adult airways, is to advance the fiberscope too deeply, thus entering the esophagus. Occasionally, a "pink mass" is seen because a jaw thrust is not adequate to free the pharyngeal space. In this circumstance, the tongue must be pulled forward with a gauze or gauze-wrapped towel clamp.

Keep in mind that several anatomic differences between adults and children will affect the fiberoptic technique. The airway distances are much shorter in neonates, infants, and young children compared to those of adults. Therefore, these structures will come into view very quickly. Thus, strict midline placement and advancing the fiberscope only when recognizable landmarks come into view are very important. Remember also that neonates and infants have a larynx which is more cephalad, vocal cords which are angled more anteriorly, and an epiglottis which is more angular, long, and stiff than those of adults (28). These differences make it critical that the larynx be approached with the fiberscope in the midline position, not from the sides of the mouth. If the approach is not midline, the insertion cord may not pass easily through the glottis.

Also, recall that the cricoid cartilage is the narrowest portion of the airway in children, as opposed to the glottic opening in adults. For this reason, uncuffed endotracheal tubes are used in children. This presents a problem unique to intubating children: an inability to effectively ventilate or protect the airway after ET tube placement because the inserted tube is too small. One solution is to use a tube changer to switch to an ET tube a half-size larger. The fiberscope can then be used to help confirm the correct placement of the new ET tube.

Alternatively, the fiberscope can be loaded with the new ET tube and the tip directed to the larynx. An assistant can then withdraw the old tube as the fiberscope is directed through the glottis. The new ET tube is then advanced into the trachea and the fiberscope removed as usual.

Also, the opposite problem can occur, i.e., the ET tube which you are attempting to insert is too large for the child's glottis. If the ET tube will not pass easily into the glottis, first try turning the tube 90° counterclockwise, then 180° in the opposite direction. If these maneuvers are not successful, the tube may be too large. At this juncture, there are several options.

If the airway was easily visualized and a smaller-size ET tube will fit over the fiberscope, it is usually best to redo the intubation with the appropriate-size ET tube. If the approach to the airway was difficult, a guide wire can be passed through the working channel under direct vision. The fiberscope is removed, the appropriate-size tube is loaded onto the fiberscope, and then the fiberscope is threaded over the wire to assist in directing the scope to the larynx. The new tube is then placed as usual. (*See* Two-Stage Intubation Technique).

If the fiberscope does not have a working channel, the tube can be "wedged" gently in the larynx to serve as a guide for a wire or a ventilating stylet. The larger tube can then be removed and the appropriate-size tube is threaded over the guide into the trachea. (*See* Three-Stage Intubation Technique).

Nasal Approach

The single-stage or routine technique of fiberoptic intubation may be performed nasally rather than orally but be aware of the possibility of sheared adenoid tissue, particularly in children between 2 and 6 years of age, when adenoid tissue can be very hypertrophied. Potential advantages of the nasal approach are that it avoids the possibility of a sedated child biting on the fiberscope and it may help to maintain a midline position. However, the oral approach with good jaw thrust is easily performed and avoids the potential problems of shearing adenoid tissue and of creating a nasal bleed. If a nasal approach is necessary, neosynephrine or oxymetazoline (Afrine™) drops may be used to vasoconstrict the nasal passages. This may ease placement and decrease the possibility of bleeding. Also, an oral airway may be used to keep the tongue away from the hypopharynx and thus assist visualization of the larynx.

Two-Stage Intubation

The two-stage intubation technique can be used in infants and small children when the fiberscope avail-

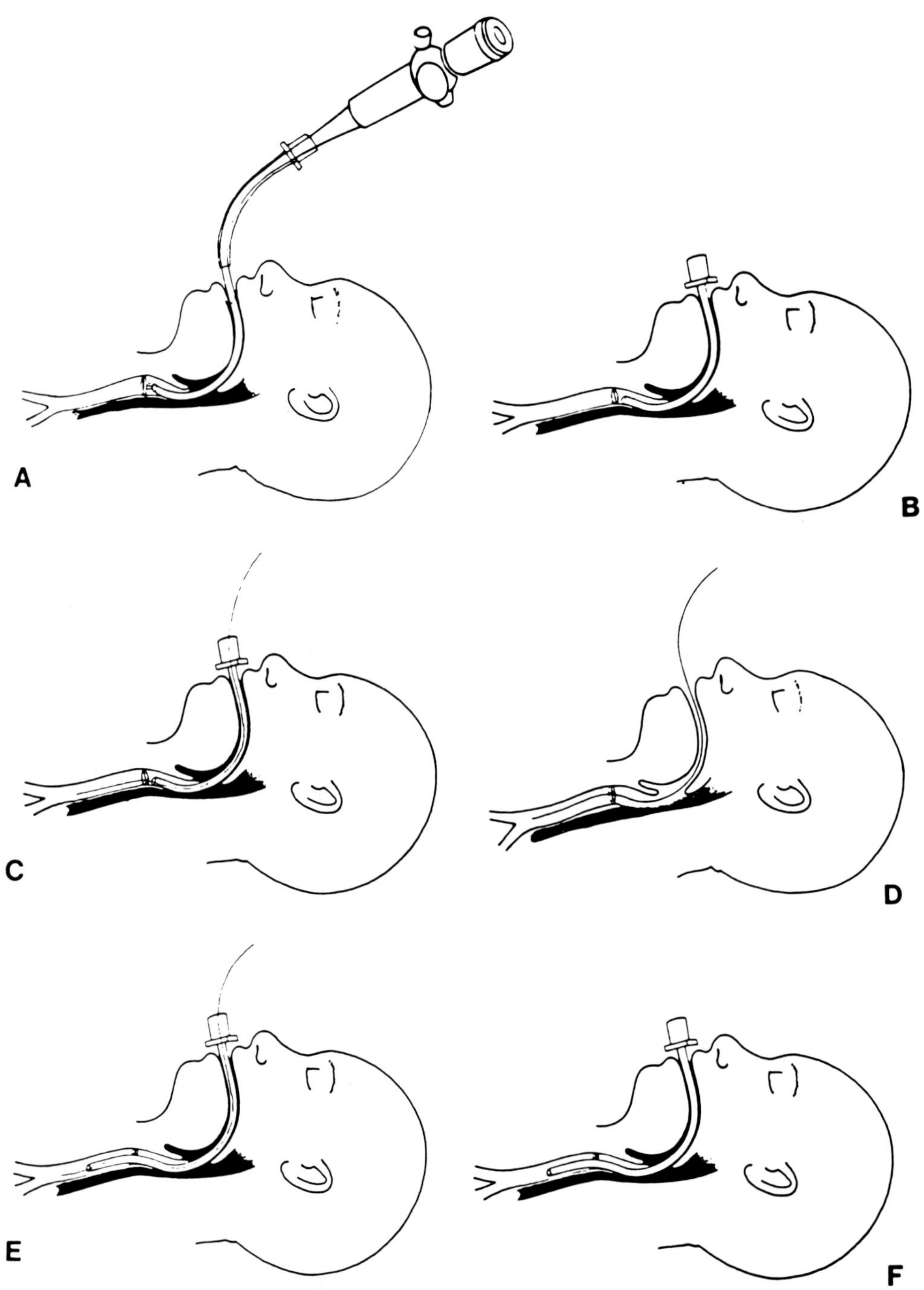

FIG. 4. Three-stage tracheal intubation technique. **A:** The fiberscope loaded with the endotracheal tube is introduced through the mouth, and the tip is positioned at the level of the vocal cords. **B:** The endotracheal tube is advanced over the fiberscope into the mouth, and the tip of the tube is positioned on top of the vocal cords. The fiberscope is removed, leaving the endotracheal tube in place (stage one). **C:** The guide wire or a catheter is advanced into the trachea through the endotracheal tube. **D:** The larger endotracheal tube is removed, leaving the guide wire inside the trachea (stage two). **E:** An appropriate-size endotracheal tube is advanced over the guide wire into the trachea (stage three). **F:** The guide wire is removed leaving the endotrachael tube in place.

able is too large to pass through the appropriate-size ET tube. The technique as described by Stiles is cumbersome, however, and a single-stage technique is preferred when possible. The original technique requires a fiberscope with a working channel, a standard cardiac catheter, and a guide wire with the proximal connector removed (29).

Stage one is as follows. The cardiac catheter and guide wire are passed through the working channel of the fiberscope to within 1 inch of its distal portion. The fiberscope is placed in the mouth and positioned at the top of the vocal cords. The guide wire is advanced under direct observation through the glottis into the trachea. The fiberscope is removed, leaving the guide wire in place. The patient is ventilated by mask while an assistant passes the cardiac catheter over the guide wire (Fig. 3).

Stage two involves threading the ET tube over the guide wire and catheter into the trachea. The catheter/guide wire combination is then removed leaving the ET tube in place.

This technique has been utilized for the intubation of three infants with the Pierre Robin syndrome (8,15,17). However, these authors found that threading of the cardiac catheter over the guide wire, which Stiles described as necessary to stiffen the wire and facilitate tube placement, was an unnecessary step. The endotracheal tube was easily passed directly over the guide wire into the trachea in all cases.

Modification of this technique when the fiberscope has no working channel has also been described (30). The authors used a number 8 French red rubber catheter attached by waterproof tape to the insertion cord of the fiberscope. The larynx was visualized in the usual fashion and then a cardiac catheter/guide wire was threaded through the rubber catheter into the trachea. With the guide wire in position, the fiberscope was then withdrawn, and an ET tube was passed into the trachea over the guide wire. A disadvantage of these techniques is that visual confirmation of endotracheal tube placement and position is not possible.

Three-Stage Intubation

A three-stage fiberoptic intubation technique for infants was described in 1985 (5). This approach is another alternative which can be used when the fiberscope is both too large and lacks a working channel. For this technique, an ET tube that is larger than the larynx of the infant is advanced over the fiberscope and positioned on top of the vocal cords (stage one). The fiberscope is then removed and a tube changer or catheter is advanced into the trachea through the ET tube (stage two). The larger tube is then removed and the appropriate-size ET tube is threaded over the tube changer into the trachea (stage three) (Fig. 4). This technique was used successfully in a 6-month-old whose operation had been previously canceled because of failure to intubate (5).

Intubation under Fiberoptic Observation

This technique is another alternative to nasotracheal intubation when the fiberscope is too large to pass through the appropriate-size ET tube. For this technique, the fiberscope is introduced through one nares while the ET tube is passed through the second nares. The tube is manipulated into the glottis while the glottis and the tip of the tube are observed through the fiberscope (Fig. 5) (3). Alternatively, a small ureteral catheter may be more easily manipulated into the glottic entry than the tube. This catheter may then be used as a stylet to pass the ET tube into the trachea (7). Spontaneous ventilation is preserved and supplemental O_2 is administered via the ET tube during manipulations (3,7). These techniques were used successfully in two neonates, one with congenital fusion of the jaws and a second with Dandy-Walker syndrome associated with Klippel-Feil, micrognathia, hypoplasia of the soft palate, and anteversion of the uvula (3,7).

A disadvantage of these techniques is that a minimum of two people, and ideally a third person, is needed to perform the manipulations. One person performs the fiberoptic laryngoscopy to expose the larynx and ET tube, a second person holds and manipulates the head of the patient, and the third person manipulates the tube or catheter into the larynx. Use of a

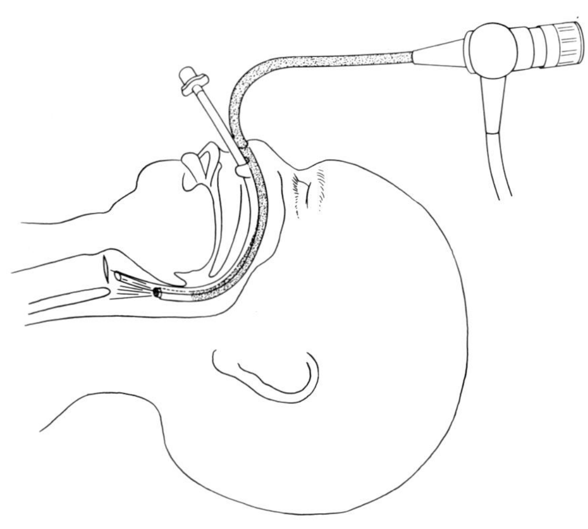

FIG. 5. Tracheal intubation under fiberoptic observation. The fiberscope is introduced through the contralateral nostril to expose the larynx and the tip of the nasotracheal tube. Manipulation of the nasotracheal tube to pass through the vocal cords is performed under visual observation.

video fiberscope will facilitate this technique, as both clinicians can use the screen for exposure and manipulation of the tube. Additionally, these techniques are time consuming. One group of authors reports that "after 40 minutes . . . the trachea was successfully intubated" (3). The other group does not state a specific time but refers to multiple attempts at direct tube placement before finally resorting to placement of the ureteral catheter.

Retrograde-Assisted Fiberoptic Tracheal Intubation

This technique has also been advocated for use in children with difficult airways (12). The authors believe this pairing of methods offers several advantages over isolated conventional retrograde or fiberoptic intubation. With regard to retrograde intubation, difficulties with the blind passage of the endotracheal tube over a wire, which can occur because of pediatric airway anatomy, are overcome by the use of the fiberscope to stiffen the wire and allow visualization of the glottis. With regard to standard fiberoptic intubation, the guide wire improves the likelihood of finding the glottis quickly, even in the presence of secretions (Chapter 6).

The technique as described by the authors requires some specialized equipment including a ventilating bronchoscopic mask, a long guide wire, and a grabbing forceps or hook. It also requires a fiberscope with a working channel, which may not be readily available in the ultrathin sizes needed for infants and neonates. The technique poses the potential risk of guide wire damage to airway structures. The authors' suggestions for safe and successful use of this technique include obtaining a 2 MAC level of anesthesia before cricothyroid puncture and withdrawal of the guide wire in a caudal direction to help maintain scope position in the airway. Although the authors only described the use of translaryngeal lidocaine in one case, its use prior to passage of the wire seems reasonable to blunt airway reflexes (12).

Fiberoptic Intubation through Laryngeal Mask Airway

A two-stage fiberoptic intubation through laryngeal mask (LMA) has been described (31). The technique involves the use of LMA, fiberscope with a suction channel and a guide wire. The technique permits the use of an adult fiberoptic bronchoscope for infants and children and allows ventilation during intubation (Chapter 12).

COMPLICATIONS OF PEDIATRIC FIBEROPTIC INTUBATION: A REVIEW OF CASE REPORTS

In a review of 17 articles reporting 134 pediatric fiberoptic intubations performed in 114 patients, a total of six complications were specifically noted (Table 1). A few authors referred in a nonspecific way to "transient desaturation," or the need to stop the procedure to give 0_2 before successfully completing intubation (11,16). None of these authors used supplemental 0_2 during the procedure. In 2 of 20 patients who required fiberoptic intubation for a variety of illnesses, saturations of 86% and 89% were noted (12). However, no supplemental oxygen was being used in these patients, and saturations rapidly returned to normal with administration of supplemental oxygen. In a study performed at our institution, of 20 patients intubated by fiberscope, 2 patients were noted to have a barky cough reported by the parents at 24 hr. These coughs resolved without consequence (19). It should be noted that in a control group of 20 children intubated with rigid laryngoscope, 2 also had a barky cough at 24 hr posttreatment and these children also resolved their cough without consequence (19). In a report of 20 intubations performed in four children with gangrenous stomatitis who had multiple procedures, one episode of epistaxis was reported (11).

In a 12-year-old child with Hurler's syndrome who had successful fiberoptic intubation, postobstructive pulmonary edema after transient laryngospasm was reported (10). Hurler's syndrome is a mucopolysaccharidase deficiency which results in deposition of mucopolysaccharides in tissues causing facial and airway deformities. These deformities make airway management extremely difficult. Fiberoptic intubation under conscious sedation has been suggested for safe airway management (32).

Postobstructive pulmonary edema has been described in normal children because of acute airway obstruction associated with forceful respiratory attempts (33). The technique of intubation does not contribute to the development of this complication. The authors felt that in this case inadequate topical anesthesia during prolonged intubation attempts contributed to laryngospasm and suggested that superior laryngeal nerve block, translaryngeal injection of local anesthetic, or spraying of the larynx through the bronchoscope may have prevented laryngeal spasm (10).

Complications reported during pediatric fiberoptic intubation are few and mostly preventable. The administration of supplemental 0_2 during intubation is mandatory and could have prevented the cases of desaturation. The one instance of epistaxis occurred in a child in whom nasal vasoconstriction was not applied (11). The barky cough which occurred in our study was not unique to the fiberoptic intubation, but occurred with equal frequency in rigid intubation (19).

LEARNING AND DEVELOPING SKILLS IN PEDIATRIC FIBEROPTIC INTUBATION

As emphasized for the adult application of the fiberscope, maneuvering and handling of the instrument is best learned on a model before applying the fiberscope to patients. Those familiar with the use of fiberscopes in adults quickly acquire dexterity with the smaller pediatric scopes.

As is advised for treatment of adult patients, first-time use of the pediatric fiberscope should not be on the difficult pediatric airway. Practice on normal pediatric airways is mandatory and safe. Our study revealed no difference in complications between rigid and fiberoptic tracheal intubation. Time to complete intubation was longer in the fiberoptic group (13.6 + 0.95 versus 22.8 + 1.75), but well within an acceptable and reasonable time frame.

The key to success is an understanding of the pediatric patient, especially the anatomic and physiologic characteristics that differ from those of adults, so that fiberscopic and anesthetic techniques can be tailored to this special patient population.

REFERENCES

1. Wilton NCT. Aids for fiberoptically guided intubation in children. *Anesthesiology* 1991;75:549–550.
2. Frei FJ, Ummenhofer W. A special mask for teaching fiber-optic intubation in pediatric patients. *Anesth Analg* 1993;76:450–461.
3. Alfery DD, Ward CF, Harwood IR, Mannino FL. Airway management for a neonate with congenital fusion of the jaws. *Anesthesiology* 1979;51:340–342.
4. Rucker RW, Silva WJ, Worcester CC. Fiberoptic bronchoscopic nasotracheal intubation in children. *Chest* 1979;76:56–58.
5. Berthelsen P, Prytz S, Jacobsen E. Two-stage fiberoptic nasotracheal intubation in infants: a new approach to difficult pediatric intubation. *Anesthesiology* 1985;63:457–458.
6. Kleeman PP, Jantzen JPAH, Bonfils P. The ultra-thin bronchoscope in management of the difficult paediatric airway. *Can J Anaesth* 1987;34:606–608.
7. Gouverneur JM, Veyckenans F, Licky M, Verellen G, Gribomont BF. Using an ureteral catheter as a guide in difficult neonatal fiberoptic intubation. *Anesthesiology* 1987;66:436–437.
8. Howardy-Hansen P, Berthelsen P. Fibreoptic nasotracheal intubation of a neonate with Pierre Robin syndrome. *Anaesthesia* 1988;43:121–122.
9. Baines DB, Goodrick MA, Beckenham EJ, Overton JH. Fibreoptically guided endotracheal intubation in a child. *Anaesth Intensive Care* 1989;17:354–356.
10. Wilder RT, Kumar GB. Fiberoptic intubation complicated by pulmonary edema in a 12-year-old with Hurler syndrome. *Anesthesiology* 1990;72:205–207.
11. Tassony E, Lehmann C, Gunning K, Coquoz E, Montandon D. Fiberoptically guided intubation in children with gangrenous stomatitis (noma). *Anesthesiology* 1990;73:348–349.
12. Audanaert SM, Montgomery CL, Stone B, Akins RE, Lock RL. Retrograde-assisted fiberoptic tracheal intubation in children with difficult airways. *Anesth Analg* 1991;73:660–664.
13. Montgomery G, Dueringer J, Johnson C. Nasal endotracheal tube change with intubating stylette after fiberoptic intubation. *Anesth Analg* 1991;72:713–718.
14. Monrigal JP, Granry JC, LeRolle T, Rod B, Cavellat M. Difficult intubation in newborns and infants using an ultra-thin fiberoptic bronchoscope. *Anesthesiology* 1991;72:A1044.
15. Scheller JG, Schulman SR. Fiber-optic bronchoscopic guidance for intubating a neonate with Pierre-Robin sequence. *J Clin Anesth* 1991;3:45–47.
16. Finer NN, Muzka D. Flexible endoscopic intubation of the neonate. *Pediatr Pulmonol* 1992;12:48–51.
17. Suriani RJ, Kayne RD. Fiberoptic bronchoscopic guidance for intubating a child with Pierre-Robin syndrome. *J Clin Anesth* 1992;4:258–259.
18. Asada A, Tatekawa S, Takekazu T, Masanori H, Masato H, Kazutoshi I, Mitsugu F. *Anesthesiology* 1994;80:206–209.
19. Roth AG, Wheeler M, Stevenson GW, Hall SC. Comparison of a rigid laryngoscope with the ultrathin fibreoptic laryngoscope for tracheal intubation in infants. *Can J Anaesth* 1994;41:1069–1073.
20. Practice guidelines for management of the difficult airway. A report by the American Society of Anesthesiologists Task Force on management of the difficult airway. *Anesthesiology* 1993;79:413–414.
21. Jones AEP, Pelton DA. An index of syndromes and their anaesthetic implications. *Can Anaesth Soc J* 1976;23:207–226.
22. Katz J, Steward DJ. *Anesthesia and uncommon pediatric diseases,* 2nd ed. Philadelphia, W. B. Saunders Company, 1993.
23. Mallampoti SR, Galt SP, Gugino LD, Desai JP, Waraksa B, Freiberger D, Lui PL. A clinical sign to predict difficult tracheal intubation: a prospective study. *Can Anaesth Soc J* 1985;32:429–434.
24. White PE. Ketamine update: its clinical uses in anesthesia. *Seminars Anesth* 1988;7:113–126.
25. Hollister GR, Burn JMB. Side effects of ketamine in pediatric anesthesia. *Anesth Analg* 1974;53:264–267.
26. Cartwright PD, Pingel SM. Midazolam and diazepam in ketamine anesthesia. *Anaesthesia* 1984;39:439–442.
27. Hughes JR. Infantile methemoglobinemia due to benzocaine suppository. *J Pediatr* 1965;66:797.
28. Eckenhoff JE. Some anatomic considerations of the infant larynx influencing endotracheal anesthesia. *Anesthesiology* 1951;12:401–410.
29. Stiles CM. A flexible fiberoptic bronchoscope for endotracheal intubation in infants. *Anesth Analg* 1974;53:1017–1019.
30. Ford RWJ. Adaptation of the fiberoptic laryngoscope for tracheal intubation with small diameter tubs. *Can Anaesth Soc J* 1981;28:479–480.
31. Hasan MA, Black AE. A new technique for fiberoptic intubation in children. *Anaesthesia* 1994;49:1031–1033.
32. Sjogren P, Pedersen T, Steinmetz H. Mucopolysaccharidoses and anaesthetic risks. *Acta Anaesthesiol Scand* 1987;31:214–218.
33. Ondjhane K, Bowen AD, Oh KS, Young CW. Pulmonary edema complicating upper airway obstruction in infants and children. *Can Assoc Radiol J* 1992;43:278–282.

CHAPTER 8

Fiberoptic-Aided Bronchial Intubation

Andranik Ovassapian, M.D.

Surgical procedures related to the chest and mediastinal structures, are increasingly being performed under thoracoscopic technique (1,2). The deflation of the operative lung is an absolute necessity for such procedures performed under general anesthesia. Unlike open thoracotomy, where the surgeon has the option of manually compressing the lung, this option is not available with thoracoscopic approach, making separation of the lung an absolute necessity. The anesthesiologist must therefore be versatile in providing safe one-lung anesthesia in all patients subjected to thoracoscopy, to avoid complications (2), unnecessary case delays, or cancellation of the procedure.

Introduction and improvement of disposable double-lumen endobronchial tubes (DLTs), combined with fiberoptic-aided bronchial intubation techniques (3) and improved techniques of oxygenation and monitoring of oxygenation during anesthesia, have made one-lung anesthesia (OLA) a safe procedure.

The purpose of this chapter is to emphasize the role and importance of the fiberoptic bronchoscope in the placement of endobronchial tubes and blockers. For more detailed coverage of thoracic anesthesia, readers are referred to several excellent published textbooks (4–7).

INDICATIONS FOR SEPARATION OF THE LUNGS

Endobronchial tube placement is indicated in the anesthetic management of intrathoracic operations (4–7) and for a variety of purposes in critically ill patients, where separation of the lungs and selective lung ventilation are desired (Table 1) (8–10). The most common indication for OLA is to facilitate dissection and surgical exposure during intrathoracic operations. Thoracoscopic procedures performed under general anesthesia almost always require this technique.

Various types of endobronchial tubes and blockers have been developed for separation of the lungs (11–16). The Robertshaw double-lumen endobronchial tubes are the most commonly used endobronchial tubes for this purpose (12). This chapter will cover the various indications and fiberoptic techniques used in the placement of the Robertshaw double-lumen tube, Univent® tube, and Fogarty catheter endobronchial blockers used to achieve lung separation.

TABLE 1. *Indications for separation of the lungs*

Surgical
- Absolute indications
  - To prevent contamination of nonoperative lung from secretions and blood
  - To provide adequate ventilation in the presence of a large bronchopleural fistula
  - To allow open rupture of giant lung cyst and pneumothorax
  - Thoracoscopic procedures
- Relative indications
  - To improve surgical exposure
    - Pulmonary resections
    - Esophageal surgery
    - Thoracic aortic aneurysm repair
    - Other intrathoracic procedures

Nonsurgical
- Bronchopulmonary lavage
  - Pulmonary alveolar proteinosis
- Differential lung ventilation
  - Unilateral pulmonary insufficiency
    - Severe atelectasis
    - Pulmonary contusion
  - Management of pulmonary hemorrhage

EQUIPMENT

Bronchial Catheters

Bronchial catheters used to achieve lung separation can be broken down into four general categories listed below.

1. *Double-Lumen Endobronchial Tubes.* These tubes are the most popular and commonly used tubes to establish separation of the lungs. The double-lumen tubes provide independent access to either lung, allowing for two- or one-lung ventilation. The DLTs consist of two tubes joined together and separated at their proximal ends (Fig. 1). These tracheal tubes have a distal bronchial curvature that facilitates bronchial intubation. A bronchial cuff is located at the distal end of the bronchial tube. The tracheal cuff is located proximal to the opening of the tracheal lumen and seals the trachea when inflated. The tubes are designed for right or left bronchial intubation.

Tubes designed for intubation of the right main stem bronchus have a window in the lateral aspect of the bronchial cuff (ventilation slot), permitting ventilation of the right upper lobe, which takes off closer to the carina than its left-sided counterpart. When properly positioned, with the bronchial and tracheal cuffs inflated, the DLTs provide a separate airway for each lung.

In 1949, Carlens (17) designed a DLT for intubation of the left bronchus. A small carinate hook, located at the takeoff of the bronchial tube, is meant to prevent undue deep placement of the endobronchial tube and lend stability to the tube. Unfortunately, the hook also increases the difficulty of passing the tube through the vocal cords. It may also produce trauma to the respiratory tract and contribute to malpositioning of the tube (18).

In 1959, Bryce-Smith (19) and White (20) independently designed a similar DLT for right bronchial intubation. In 1962, Robertshaw (21) introduced a DLT without a carinate hook, designed for either right or left bronchial intubation. The Robertshaw tube has a larger lumen, and provides lower resistance to gas flow than the equivalent-sized Carlens or White tube (22,23).

Introduced in 1978, the disposable Robertshaw DLT (Broncho-Cath®, NCC Division, Mallinkrodt, Inc., Glen Falls, New York 12801) is made of clear polyvinyl chloride (PVC). The advantages of PVC tubes include a softer and more flexible structure, thin-walled tracheal and bronchial cuffs, a more gentle distal curve, and a greater inside-to-outside diameter. When positioned in the trachea, the PVC tubes also allow observation of the humidity of the exhaled air (24). The bronchial cuff is blue, making for easy identification during fiberoptic bronchoscopy. The Broncho-Cath® Robertshaw right- and left-sided DLT is available in five sizes: 28, 35, 37, 39, and 41 French (Fr). The 28 Fr left-sided DLT is for use in children (Table 2). The outer diameter, inner lumen diameter, and tracheal cuff of the right-sided tube are similar to those of the left-sided tube. The ventilation slot of the right-sided tube is 11 mm long and 5 mm wide. The inflation volume to 25 cm H_2O pressure, requires 5 ml for the left bronchial cuff and 16 ml for the tracheal cuff.

At least three companies are manufacturing disposable polyvinyl left- and right-sided DLTs. The designs of the left-sided tubes are similar and have similar volume/pressure characteristics. However, the Sheridan design (Sheridan Catheter Corp., Route 40, Argyle, New York) requires a higher mean bronchial cuff pressure (27 ± 17 cm H_2O) to seal the bronchus than the Broncho-Cath® (17.6 ± 8.5 cm H_2O) or Rusch (14.1 ± 8.6 cm H_2O) tubes (Rusch Inc., 2450 Meadowbrook Parkway, Duluth, Georgia). The potential for trauma to the bronchus may be higher with high intracuff pressures during prolonged one-lung ventilation (25).

The designs of the right-sided DLT differ significantly between manufacturers, to accommodate the short right main stem bronchus and provide ventilation to the upper lobe bronchus (Figs. 2,3). The design of the right-sided bronchial cuff of the Broncho-Cath® DLT is unique. The cuff lies at an oblique angle in relationship to the axis of the bronchial portion of the tube. The portion of the bronchial cuff seen with the flexible bronchoscope at the carina represents the upper margin of the medial (distal) portion of the bronchial cuff, and lies 8–10 mm below the upper border

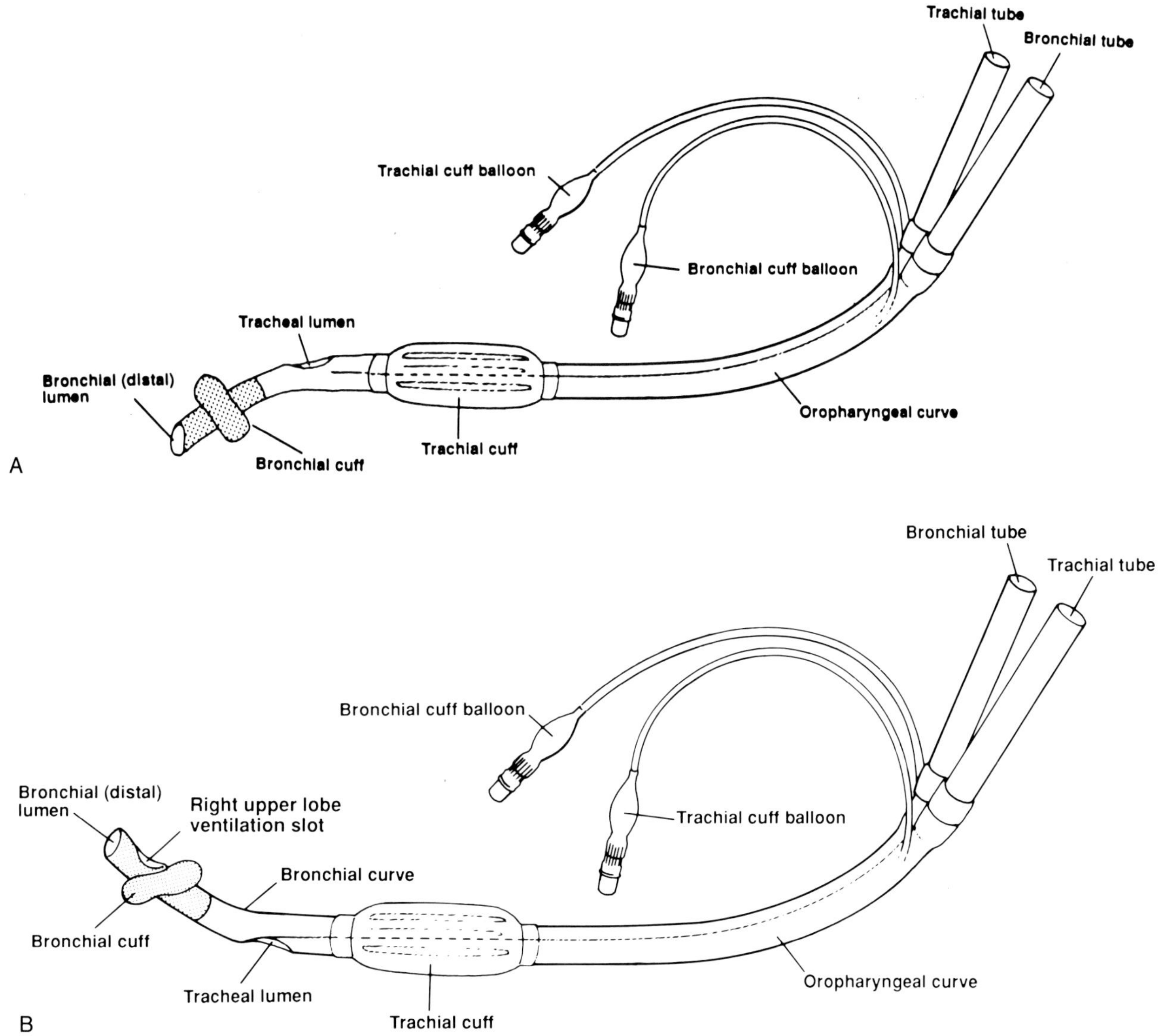

FIG. 1. A: Drawing of a left-sided double-lumen Robertshaw-type endobronchial tube. **B:** Drawing of a right-sided double-lumen Robertshaw-type endobronchial tube (Broncho-Cath design).

TABLE 2. *Characteristics of left-sided BronchoCath endobronchial tubes*

Outer diameter French size (Fr)	Distance from bronchial tip to: Separation of two lumens (cm)	Upper border of tracheal cuff (cm)	Distal opening of tracheal lumen (cm)	Approximate equivalent inner lumen diameter[a]: Bronchial (mm)	Tracheal (mm)	Cuff length: Bronchial (cm)	Tracheal (cm)
28	33	10.6	5.6	4.5	4.5	1.2	4.5
35	33	12.9	6.7	6.0	6.0	1.4	4.5
37	33	13.0	6.7	6.5	6.5	1.4	4.5
39	33	13.5	7.1	7.0	7.0	1.4	4.5
41	33	13.8	7.1	7.4	7.4	1.4	4.7

[a] The lumen is D-shaped rather than circular. Equivalent size will not be helpful for selection of fiberscope size.

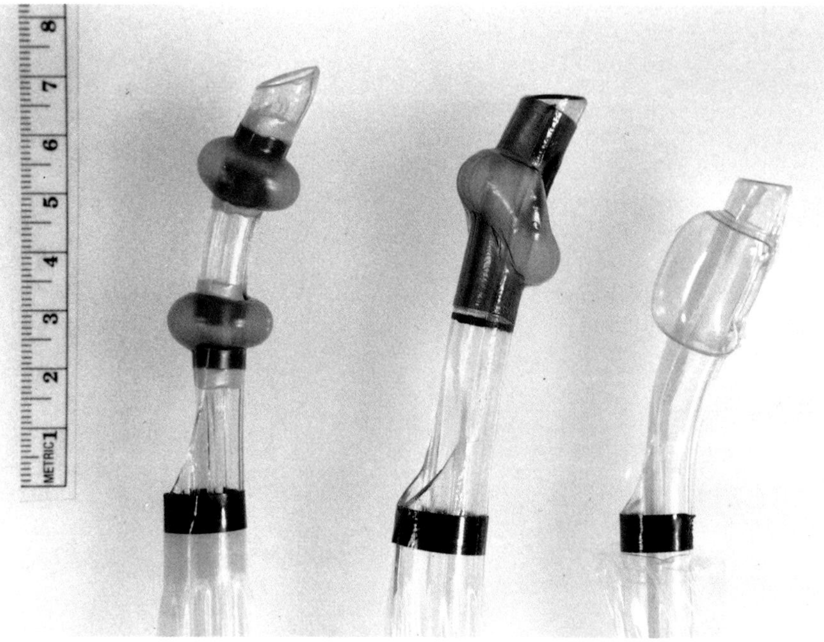

FIG. 2. Photographic demonstration of the distal portion of the bronchial cuff of three different right-sided double-lumen endobronchial tubes. **A:** Sheridan; **B:** Mallinkrodt (Broncho-Cath); **C:** Rusch. The more recent design of Rusch right-sided DLT has incomplete circular cuff at the lower half of the bronchial cuff (not shown).

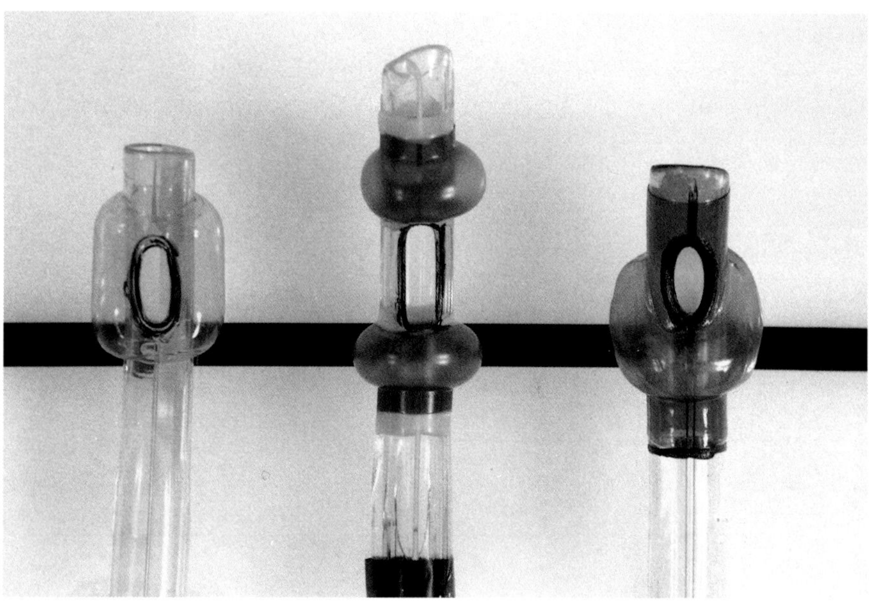

FIG. 3. Demonstrates the size and shape of the bronchial cuff window (upper lobe ventilation slot) of the three different types of right-sided DLT endobronchial tubes. **A:** Rusch; **B:** Sheridan; **C:** Mallinkrodt. A larger size ventilation slot does not provide wider margin of safety. The diameter of the right upper lobe bronchus is about 10 mm and the length of the bronchus intermedius limits the depth of insertion of the bronchial tube.

of the lateral (proximal) portion of the right bronchial cuff (Fig. 4). It is the lateral (proximal) aspect of the bronchial cuff that contacts the lateral wall of the main stem bronchus or the trachea, and therefore has the potential of occluding the orifice of the right upper lobe bronchus.

The bronchial cuff design of the Rusch endobronchial tube is circular at its proximal end, above the ventilation slot, forming an incomplete circle at its distal portion located around the ventilation slot. The Sheridan design incorporates two small circular cuffs, at the proximal and distal end of the ventilation slot. The comparative benefits of the various cuff designs have not been explored in any significant detail. The author has used the Broncho-Cath® right-sided tube exclusively, and has had very good success with it.

2. *The Univent® Tube*. The combination of an endotracheal tube and blocker was first introduced in 1953 (11). The concept never received much popularity until the introduction of the Univent® tube (Fugi Systems Co., Ltd., Tokyo, Japan) in 1981 by Inoue et al. (13,26).

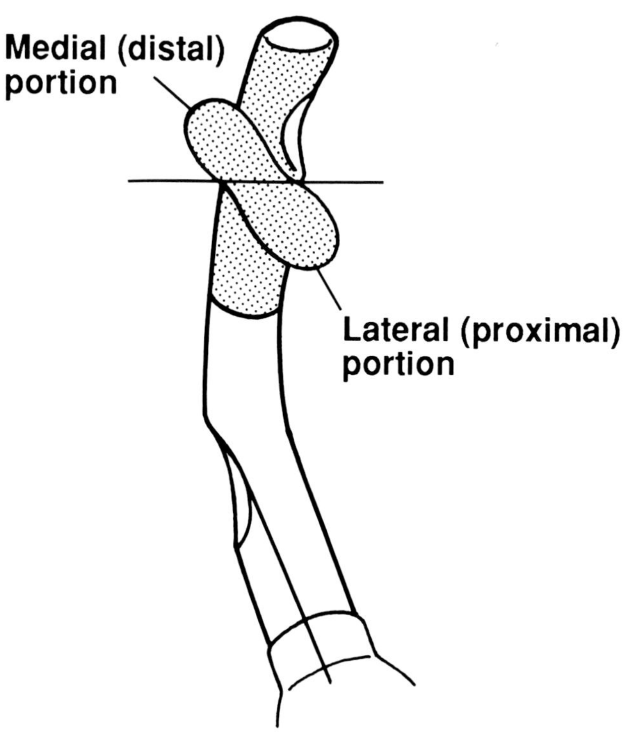

FIG. 4. Schematic presentation of the tip of the Broncho-Cath (Mallinkrodt) right-sided Robertshaw-type DLT. The line divides the bronchial cuff into medial (distal) and lateral (proximal) portions. The lateral (proximal) portion of the cuff will block the right upper lobe bronchus if the tube is advanced too far down into the main stem bronchus. The most proximal placement possible is when the upper border of the medial (distal) portion of the bronchial cuff lies at the level of the carina. The length of the bronchial cuff from the upper border of the lateral (proximal) portion to the lower border of the medial (distal) portion is about 18 mm. The length of the lateral (proximal) portion of the cuff to the beginning of the ventilation slot is about 10 mm in a 39 Fr DLT.

The Univent® tube is a new form of endobronchial blocker. The silicone tube is available in 0.5-mm inner diameter (ID) increments from 6.00- to 9.00-mm ID sizes (Table 3). The external diameter of the Univent® tube, compared to a regular endotracheal tube, is larger for comparable ID-sized tubes. The increased diameter is due to the increased space required by the endobronchial blocker and the thicker wall of the Univent® tube.

The Univent® tube's movable blocker consists of a stiff catheter housed in a secondary channel (conduit), positioned in the anterior wall of a regular-shaped endotracheal tube (Fig. 5). The 3-mm blocker is hollow, with a lumen of 1 to 1.5 mm, which allows for suctioning of secretions and oxygen delivery. The blocker is fully retractable into the main tube, and can be extended to 12 cm beyond the tip of the main tube.

The blocker's shaft has seven circular marks at its proximal end. A double circle marks the point where the blocker is fully retracted inside the tube's conduit. The next two single circular marks are spaced 3 cm apart, and are followed by four other circular marks 1 cm apart. The tip of the blocker is slightly bent to allow for easier insertion into the targeted main stem bronchus. The blocker can be fixed in the desired position with a cap and a band stopper.

The tip of the blocker is hard and can cause tracheobronchial injury if repeated attempts are made during blind placement (27). Dislodgment of the mold cap at the tip of the blocker has been reported (28). The blocker's blue-colored cuff requires a larger volume of air to provide a seal, compared to the bronchial cuffs of a DLT. The manufacturer recommends 6–7 ml of air to provide an appropriate seal.

TABLE 3. *Physical characteristics of the Univent® tubes*

	Outer diameter*		
Inner diameter[a] (mm)	Lateral (mm)	Anterior-posterior (mm)	Measured[b] circumference (mm)
6.0	10.0	11.0	34
6.5	10.5	11.5	
7.0	11.0	12.0	
7.5	11.5	12.5	36
8.0	12.0	13.5	39
8.5	12.5	14.0	
9.0	13.0	14.0	42

[a] Information provided by company
[b] From Slinger P. Con: The Univent® tube is not the best method of providing one-lung ventilation. *J Cardioth Vascul Anesth* 1983;7:108–112.

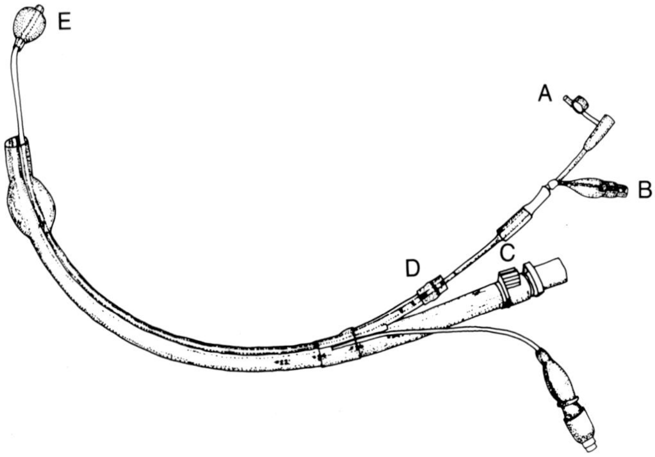

FIG. 5. Drawing of a Univent® tube with bronchial blocker advanced beyond the tip of the main tube. **A:** Bronchial blocker plug for capping the lumen of the blocker when one-lung ventilation is not applied. This cap should not be engaged (bronchial blocker lumen open) during one-lung ventilation. **B:** Bronchial blocker cuff pilot valve. **C:** Hand stopper secures the bronchial blocker shaft and prevents its movement when blocker is positioned and the shaft of it is pushed inside the stopper. **D:** Movable cap on the shaft of the bronchial blocker to seal off the leak between the blocker shaft and its conduit. **E:** Bronchial blocker cuff.

The blocker cuff exhibits high-pressure characteristics when it is fully inflated during one-lung ventilation (29). The use of continuous suction through the bronchial blocker lumen, allows for complete collapse of the operative lung, with reduction of the required cuff air volume to 3–5 ml for inflation of the blocker cuff (29).

3. *Bronchial Blockers.* Several types of bronchial blockers have been introduced since 1934 (11). Fogarty embolectomy catheters, available in varying sizes, are suitable as bronchial blockers in pediatric and adult patients (13–16). Bronchial blockers are introduced into the bronchus of the operative lung, while the nonoperative lung is ventilated through a tracheal or contralateral endobronchial tube. Using this technique, the suctioning of bronchial secretions or ventilation of the operative lung are not possible without losing the separation of the lungs.

4. *Single-Lumen Endobronchial Tubes with One or Two Cuffs.* These tubes were the first to be used for OLV. Single-cuffed tubes have only a bronchial cuff, while double-cuffed tubes in this category have a bronchial and a tracheal cuff. Typically the tubes are positioned in the bronchus of the nonoperative lung. Inflation or suctioning of the operative lung cannot be performed during lung separation (11). The single-lumen endobronchial tube is mainly of historic interest and rarely used today (12).

Fiberscopes

In 1973, Davis (30) suggested that the fiberscope might prove helpful in the positioning of endobronchial tubes. In 1974, Prithvi Raj et al. (31) used a fiberoptic laryngoscope to guide a left-sided Robertshaw DLT into the left main stem bronchus. Small-diameter fiberscopes have been used for tracheal, bronchial intubation and positioning of DLTs (32–36). They have also been used to verify the position of DLTs placed "blindly" (37,38) and to identify and correct malpositioned DLTs (3,33,39).

Fiberscopes with a 4.8-mm-diameter insertion cord will pass easily through the tracheal lumen of a 39 Fr or larger DLT, and through the bronchial lumen of a 41 Fr DLT tube, although tightly. The fiberscope should be well lubricated to ease passage and to avoid damage to the insertion cord's plastic covering. Fiberscopes of 4 mm or less in diameter will pass through the tracheal and bronchial lumens of 35 to 41 Fr DLTs. Fiberscopes with a 60-cm insertion cord allow evaluation of the main stem bronchi, while the tip of the DLT remains in the trachea. The new generation of small fiberscopes provides a wide field of view, combined with adequate suction capability, greatly facilitating their use.

SELECTION OF THE DOUBLE-LUMEN TUBE

The preferred approach is to intubate the bronchus of the nonoperative lung, leaving the main bronchus of the operative lung free (7,40). This procedure allows for unimpeded bronchial surgery, and eliminates the possibility of the DLT being inadvertently sutured in place (Table 4) (41).

About one-half of the thoracic procedures will be on the left hemithorax, necessitating the use of a right-sided DLT. Anatomical variations of the right bronchial tree may interfere with the proper placement of a right-sided DLT (Fig. 6).

TABLE 4. *Intubating the nonoperative bronchus*

Logic
Pneumonectomy and bronchoplasty possible without interruption
Compression blockade of the tracheal lumen inconsequential
Eliminates the possibility of suturing or clamping of the endobronchial tube
Endobronchial mass or lesions are avoided
Problems
Approximately half of the time the right bronchus needs to be intubated.
Positioning of right-side tube is more difficult

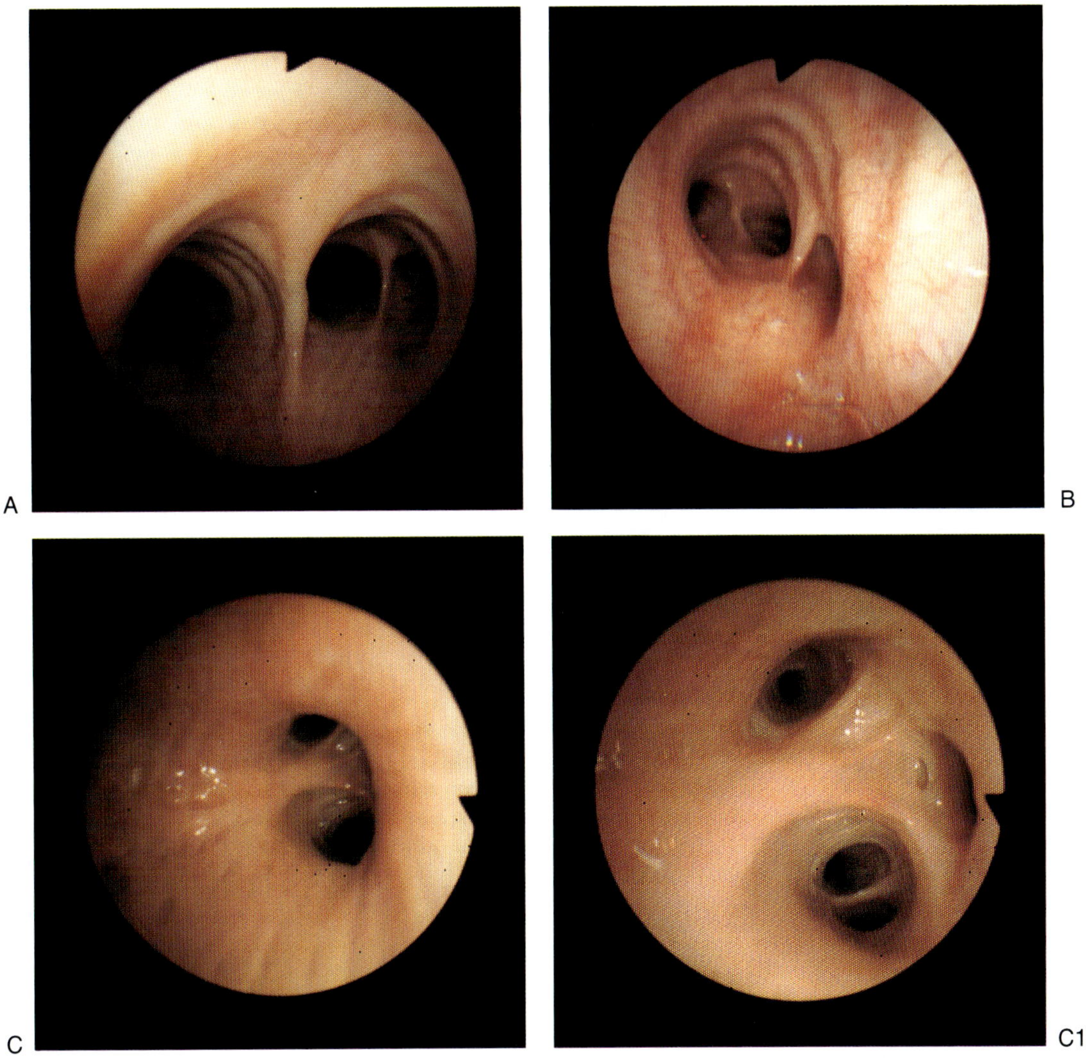

FIG. 6. Some anatomical variations of right bronchial tree encountered during bronchial intubations. **A.** High take off of right upper lobe bronchus. Placement of presently available right-sided double-lumen tubes will not be possible in this patient. **B.** Trifurcation of the trachea. Right upper lobe bronchus takes off from the lower trachea (far right opening). **C.** Low take off of right upper lobe bronchus. Shows the upper lobe bronchus opening at 3 o'clock just below to the bronchus of the middle lobe. The lower lobe bronchus not in view. The length of the right main stem bronchus was about 4 cm. A right-sided double-lumen tube was used in this patient without positioning the bronchial cuff window against the right upper lobe bronchus opening. All three, upper, middle, and lower lobes bronchi openings remained distal to the tip of the bronchial tube. **C1.** Fiberscope is advanced inside the upper lobe bronchus to visualize the three segments of the right upper lobe.

Under most circumstances, however, the left main stem bronchus is intubated with a left-sided DLT, due to its relative ease of placement and high margin of safety (42,43). In some cases, anatomical variations make left tube placement impossible (Fig. 7) (44,45). In addition, in some patients isolated ventilation of the dependent left lung is inadequate, compromising the safety of left-sided OLV (Table 5) (46).

The malposition of left-sided DLTs have been reported to be as high as right-sided DLTs (46,47). The frequency of intubating the wrong bronchus by blind technique is greater with left-sided than right-sided DLTs (47–50). If the left main stem bronchus takeoff is more acute than usual, the distal opening of the left DLT bronchial lumen is frequently forced against the medial wall of the main stem bronchus (Fig. 8). The resultant effect produces various degrees of obstruction and otherwise interferes with pulmonary gas flow. Partial bronchial obstruction may cause air entrapment, poor gas exchange, and hypoxemia. The distal

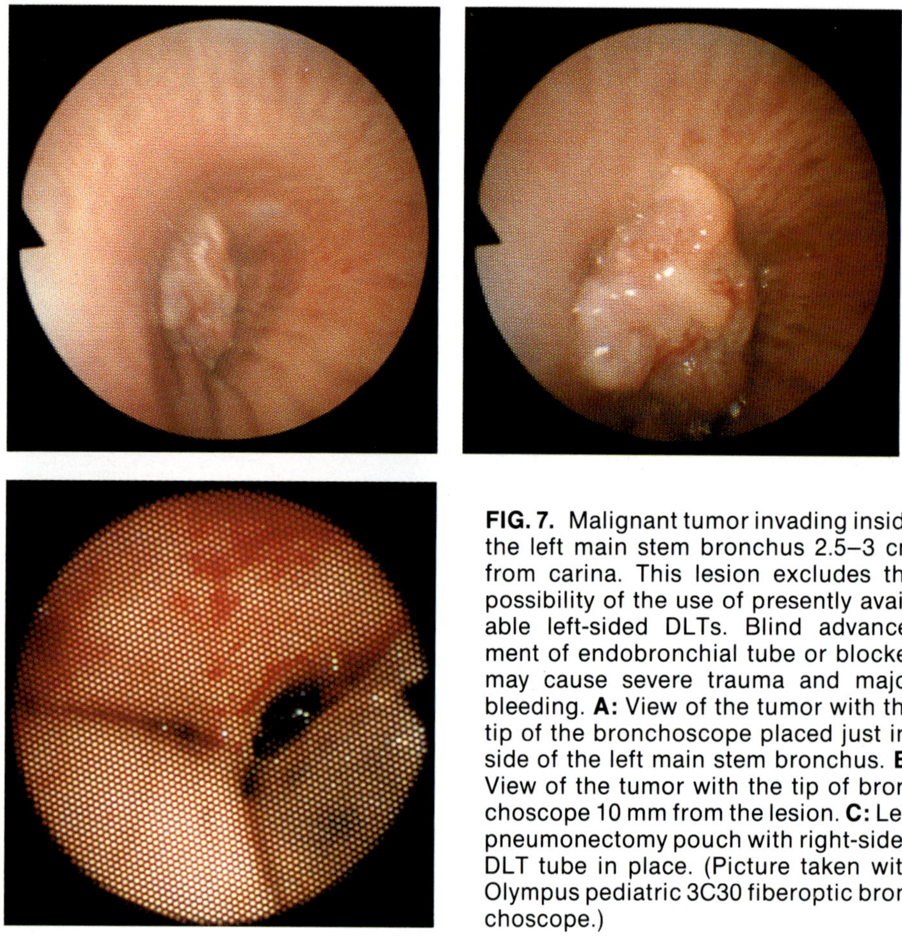

FIG. 7. Malignant tumor invading inside the left main stem bronchus 2.5–3 cm from carina. This lesion excludes the possibility of the use of presently available left-sided DLTs. Blind advancement of endobronchial tube or blocker may cause severe trauma and major bleeding. **A:** View of the tumor with the tip of the bronchoscope placed just inside of the left main stem bronchus. **B:** View of the tumor with the tip of bronchoscope 10 mm from the lesion. **C:** Left pneumonectomy pouch with right-sided DLT tube in place. (Picture taken with Olympus pediatric 3C30 fiberoptic bronchoscope.)

DLT tracheal lumen opening may also be pushed against tracheal wall, causing a partial or complete airway obstruction.

A prominent aortic arch and aneurysm of the arch of aorta that pushes the trachea to the right often interferes with left bronchial intubation, especially when blind technique is applied. An aneurysm of the thoracic descending aorta compressing the left main stem bronchus, may interfere with left-sided bronchial intubation as well (51,52).

Some practitioners recommend that the bronchus of the operative lung be routinely intubated, since most of the problems encountered with DLTs relate to bronchial intubation (53). In addition, such problems as upper lobe atelectasis of the operative lung would be easily recognized when the chest wall is opened. In general, difficulties with ventilation of the operative lung will prove of less consequence. The logic and shortcomings of intubating the operative lung is summarized in Table 6.

TABLE 5. *Intubating the left bronchus routinely*

- Logic
  - It is easy to position
  - It has high margin of safety
- Problems
  - Poor ventilation of the left lung is common despite good separation of lungs
  - Anatomical variation or pathological changes may interfere with bronchial intubation
  - Approximately half of the time left side will be the operative lung with the disadvantages stated in Table 6

Intubating the operative side bronchus leaves the DLT tracheal lumen vulnerable to being pushed against the tracheal wall. Thus exposing the airway to possible occlusion or a ball valve action, resulting in poor ventilation and hyperinflation of the dependent lung (46,54) (Fig. 9).

The largest DLT that can be easily passed should be selected for intubation. This is usually 39–41 Fr for average to large adult males, and 35–37 Fr for adult women. Proper tube size selection decreases air volume required to inflate the bronchial cuff, and minimizes airway resistance during OLV. In children and infants either a single-lumen tracheal tube or combination of a Fogarty catheter and a tracheal tube, can be used to separate the lungs.

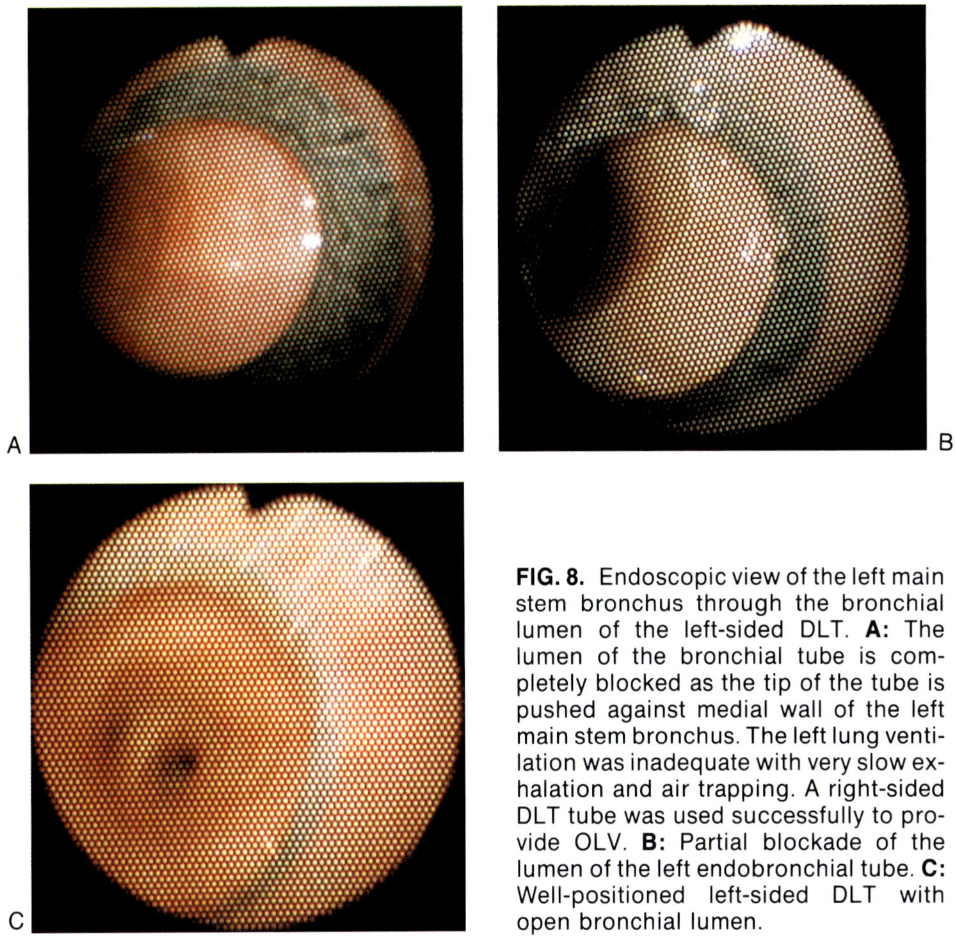

FIG. 8. Endoscopic view of the left main stem bronchus through the bronchial lumen of the left-sided DLT. **A:** The lumen of the bronchial tube is completely blocked as the tip of the tube is pushed against medial wall of the left main stem bronchus. The left lung ventilation was inadequate with very slow exhalation and air trapping. A right-sided DLT tube was used successfully to provide OLV. **B:** Partial blockade of the lumen of the left endobronchial tube. **C:** Well-positioned left-sided DLT with open bronchial lumen.

Chest X-rays should carefully be studied in patients who are candidates for one-lung anesthesia. A distorted trachea may interfere with blind intended bronchial intubation and with ventilation of the lung through the tracheal lumen. A sharp takeoff of the left main stem bronchus may interfere with ventilation of the left lung even though separation is achieved.

The ideal approach is to intubate the bronchus of the nonoperative lung, leaving the operative bronchus free (3,7,40). This eliminates the possibility of the tracheal tube being clamped or sutured in place (41). Thus in the ideal circumstance, one-half of the patients subjected to thoracotomy will require right-sided endobronchial tube placement.

TABLE 6. *Intubating the operative lung bronchus*

Logic
Ventilation difficulties due to malpositioned endobronchial tube are less consequential.
Atelectasis of the upper lobe is easily recognized.
Problems
Suturing, clamping, or cutting the endobronchial tube or damaging the bronchial cuff is possible.
For pneumonectomy, the endobronchial tube should be pulled out.
Difficult for surgeon to perform bronchoplasty.
Tracheal lumen vulnerable to being pushed against tracheal wall causing air trapping and poor ventilation.

The developed techniques of fiberoptic bronchoscopic positioning of the right-sided DLT (3) have largely resolved the technical difficulties of blind placement and its associated high incidence of failure (48–50). The continued discouragement of right-sided DLT placement and the routine use of a left-sided DLT for all intrathoracic procedures is no longer a valid recommendation. The fiberoptic bronchoscope is a tool that all clinicians using or intending to use DLTs must be thoroughly familiar with.

TRACHEAL PLACEMENT OF DOUBLE-LUMEN TUBES

The following items are required for fiberscopic DLT placements:

A DLT with connectors.
Rigid laryngoscope with a Macintosh blade.

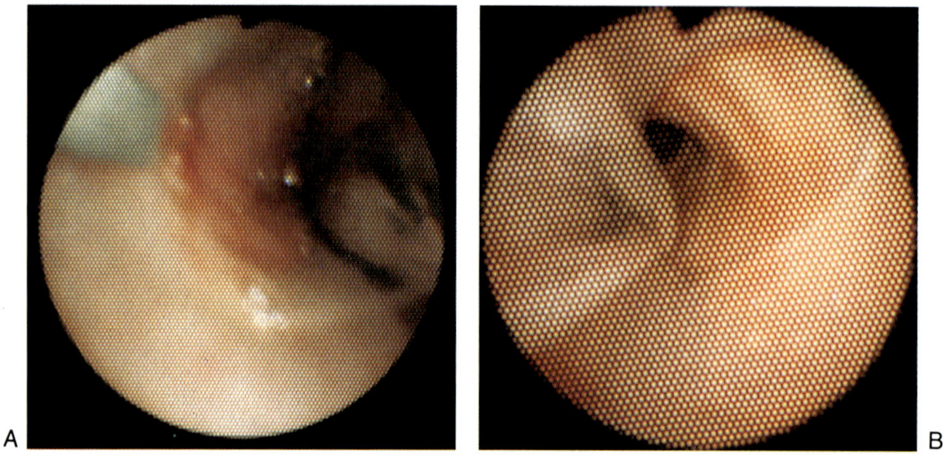

FIG. 9. Endoscopic view of the distal opening of the tracheal lumen of a right-sided DLT. **A:** Tracheal lumen is unobstructed with good view of the trachea and right main stem opening. **B:** Tracheal lumen is partially blocked by the tracheal wall.

Two swivel adapters with a bronchoscopy port (if the DLT connector lacks an endoscopy port) (Fig. 10).
A fiberscope with insertion cord of 4 mm or less.
A bottle of warm sterile water.
A large Kelly clamp.
One 10-ml and 5-ml syringe, clear lubricating jelly, and 1 in adhesive tape.

The tracheal and bronchial cuffs are tested for leaks. The tube is checked to ensure that both lumens are patent and the interluminal septum is intact. The stylet of the bronchial lumen is left in place to assist tracheal intubation using a rigid laryngoscope.

After the patient has been anesthetized and paralyzed, the larynx is exposed by rigid laryngoscopy and the Robertshaw DLT inserted into the trachea with the tip of the bronchial tube facing anteriorly. To achieve this position, the left-side tube is rotated 90° clockwise, conversely the right-side tube is rotated 90° counterclockwise. Once the tip of the bronchial tube passes through the glottic opening, the stylet is removed and the tubes are rotated 90° back to their original position. The bronchial tube should now be pointing toward its respective main stem bronchus (Figs. 11 and 12).

In the case of a DLT with a carinate hook, once the tip of the bronchial tube passes the glottis, the stylet is removed, and the tube is rotated 180° in the opposite direction (left-side DLT counterclockwise, right-side DLT clockwise) to bring the carinate hook anteriorly prior to its passage through the glottis. This prevents the carinate hook catching on the glottic "chink." After passing the carinate hook through the glottis, the DLT is rotated 90° in the appropriate direction to place the tube in its normal anatomic tracheal position (Figs. 13 and 14). The tracheal cuff is then inflated, and the patient mechanically ventilated.

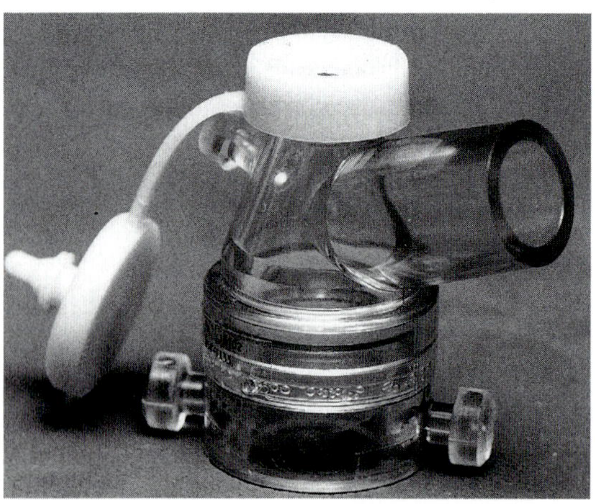

FIG. 10. Swivel bronchoscopic adapter.

ENDOBRONCHIAL PLACEMENT AND POSITIONING OF DOUBLE-LUMEN TUBES

Fiberoptic bronchoscopy provides an easy, safe, and accurate means of positioning the DLT. It is particularly helpful, when severe lung disease limits the use of auscultation in checking DLT placement, or when the patient is already prepped and draped and the chest cannot be reached for auscultation. It has also proved of invaluable help when abnormalities of the left main stem bronchus are present (46,47). If technical problems are encountered after patient positioning or during surgery, the fiberscope can be used for evaluation of DLT position and correction of any tube malposition.

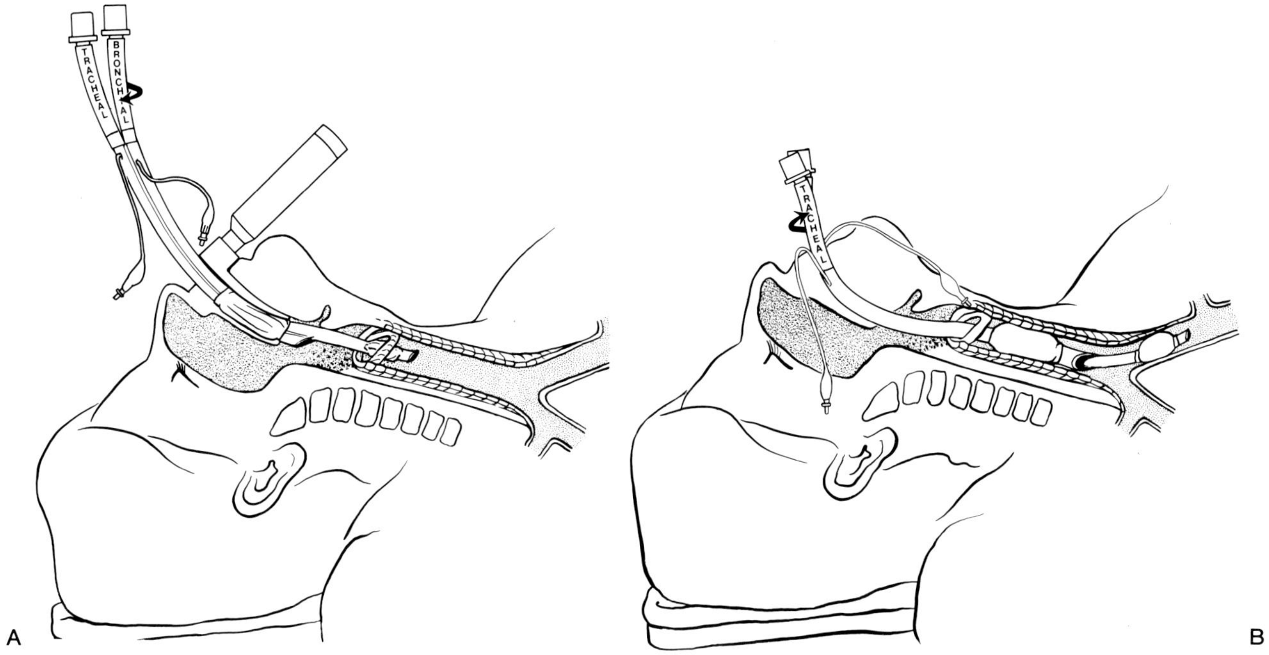

FIG. 11. Tracheal placement and bronchial position of the left-sided Robertshaw-type DLT. **A:** The tube is held 90° rotated to the right to bring the tip of the bronchial tube to the 12 o'clock position. After the tip has passed the vocal cords, the tube is rotated 90° to the left so that the bronchial lumen is pointed toward the left main bronchus. **B:** Proper position of endobronchial tube.

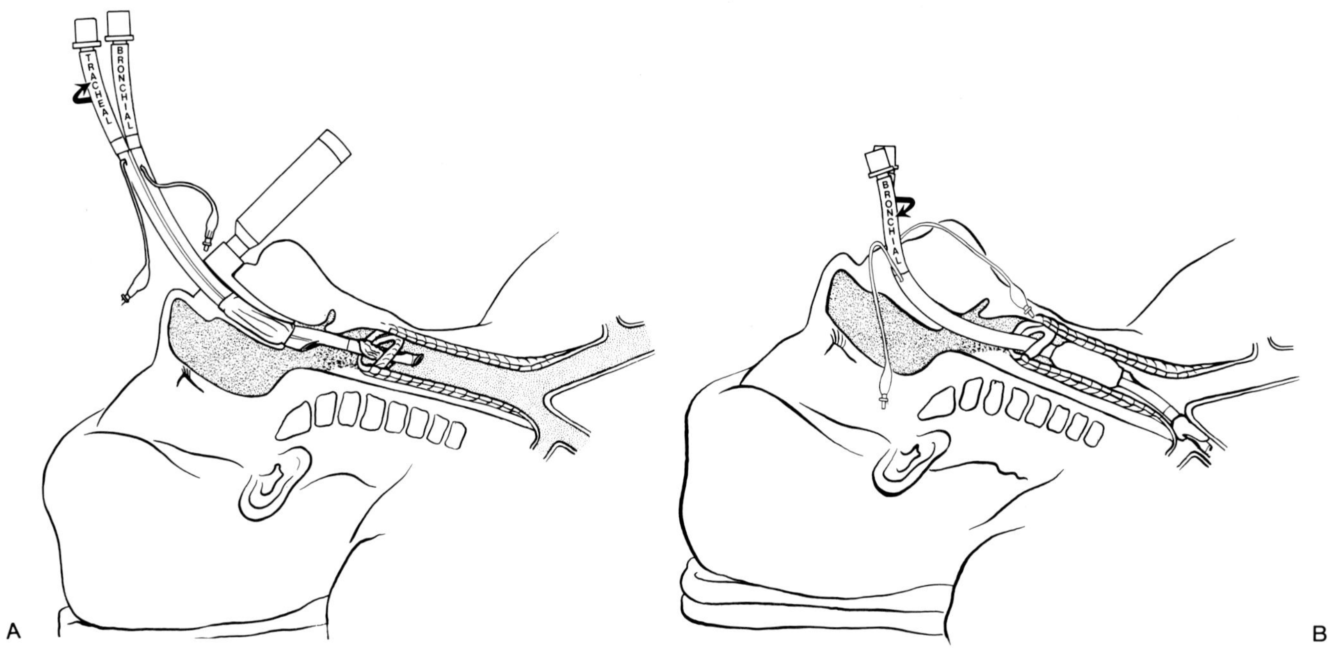

FIG. 12. Tracheal placement and bronchial position of the right-sided Robertshaw-type DLT. **A:** The tube is held 90° rotated to the left to bring the tip of the bronchial tube to the 12 o'clock position. After the tip has passed the vocal cords, the tube is rotated 90° to the right so that the bronchial lumen is pointed toward the right main bronchus. **B:** Proper position of endobronchial tube.

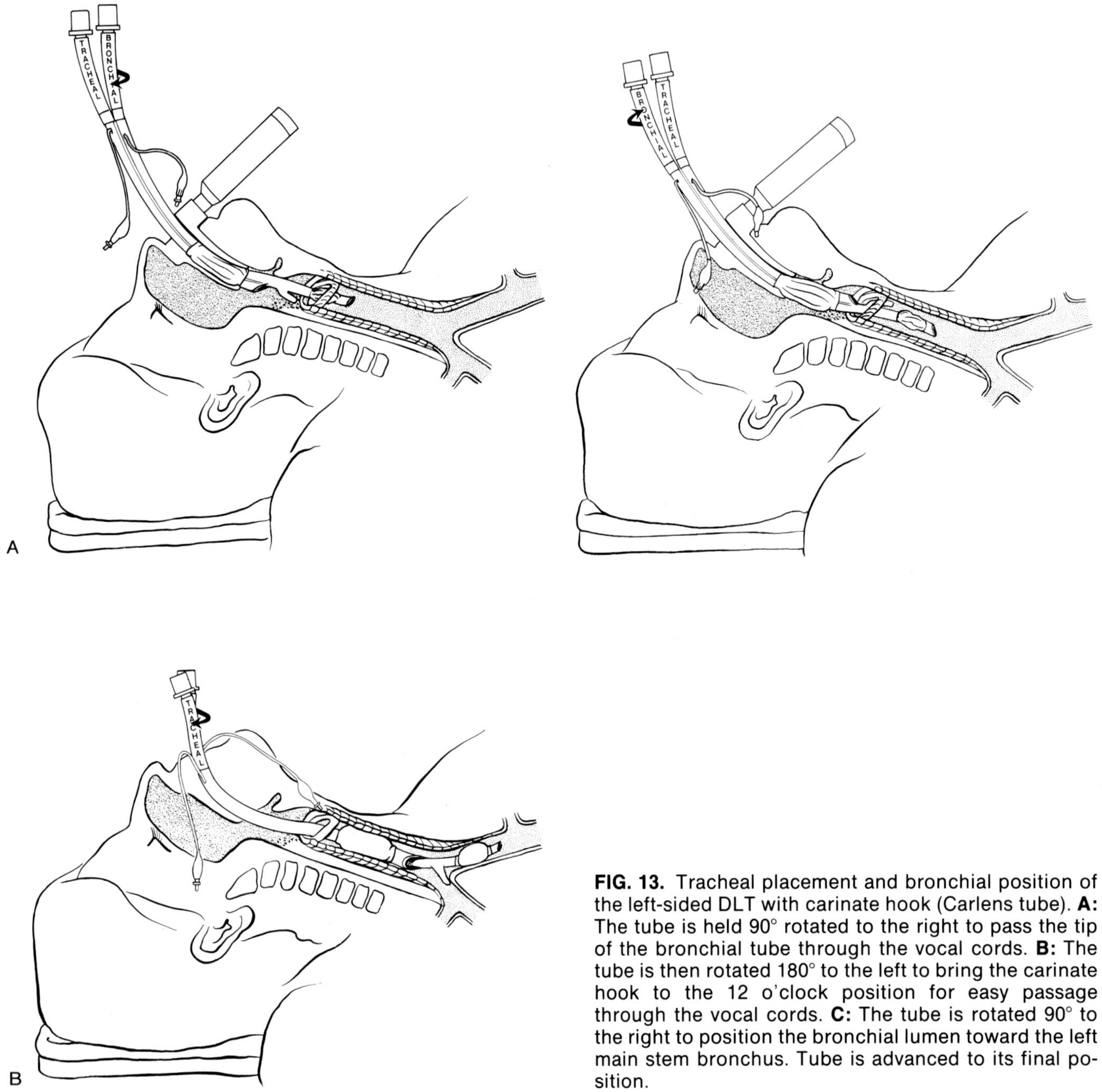

FIG. 13. Tracheal placement and bronchial position of the left-sided DLT with carinate hook (Carlens tube). **A:** The tube is held 90° rotated to the right to pass the tip of the bronchial tube through the vocal cords. **B:** The tube is then rotated 180° to the left to bring the carinate hook to the 12 o'clock position for easy passage through the vocal cords. **C:** The tube is rotated 90° to the right to position the bronchial lumen toward the left main stem bronchus. Tube is advanced to its final position.

Left-Sided Double-Lumen Tube

After the left-sided DLT is positioned in the trachea, it is connected to the anesthesia machine breathing circuit, and mechanical ventilation is initiated. The fiberscope is inserted through the bronchoscopy adapter of the tube's bronchial lumen, then into the left main stem bronchus. The length, patency, and integrity of the bronchus are evaluated, and the tip of the fiberscope positioned 10 mm above the level of the orifice of the left upper lobe bronchus (Fig. 15). The DLT tracheal cuff is deflated, the fiberscope is held stationary, and the tube advanced over the fiberscope into the left bronchus. The tip of the tube is advanced until it just passes the tip of the fiberscope.

The tracheal cuff is inflated to secure the tube, and the fiberscope is advanced beyond the bronchial lumen to visualize the orifice of the upper lobe bronchus and ensure that the tube does not impinge on it. The fiberscope is then passed down the tracheal lumen of the DLT to visualize the carina and the opening of the right main stem bronchus. If the bronchial cuff is noted to

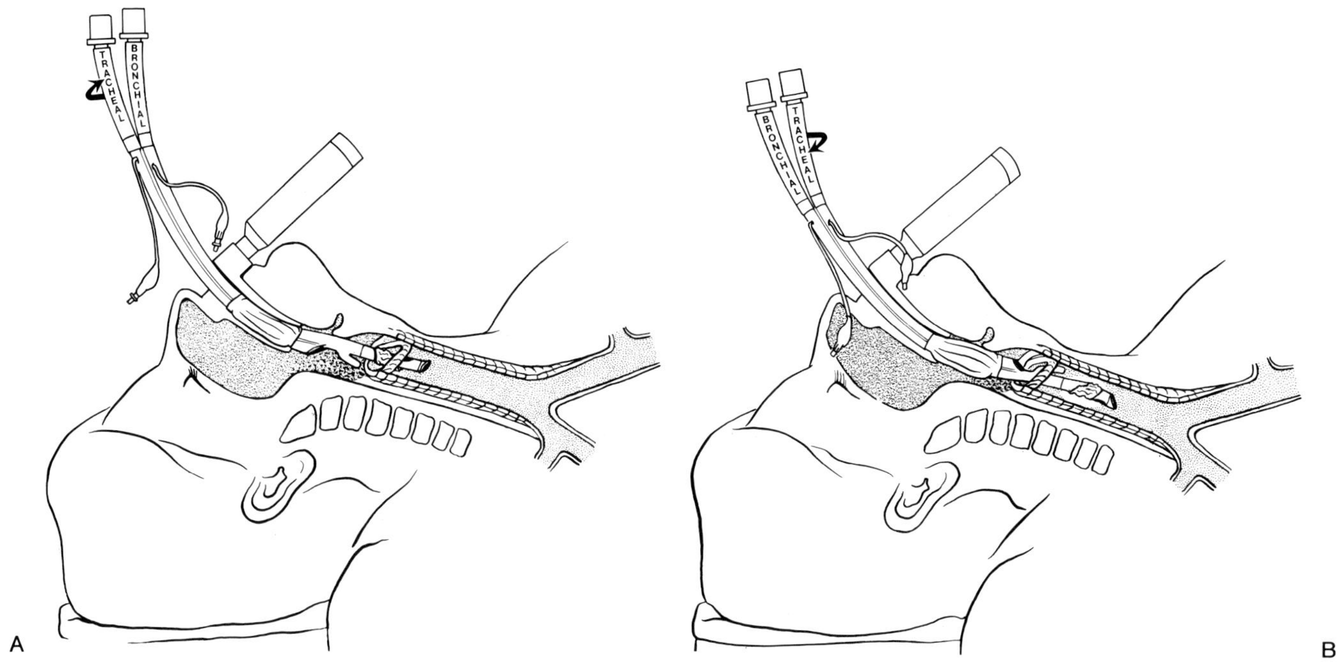

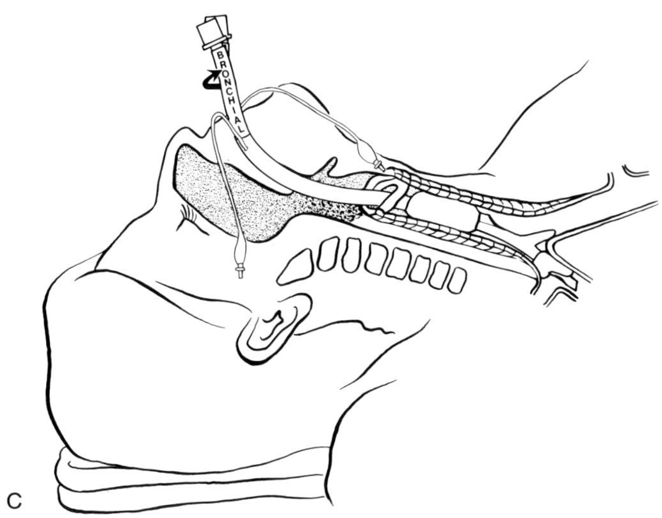

FIG. 14. Tracheal placement and bronchial position of the right-sided DLT with carinate hook (White tube). **A:** The tube is held 90° rotated to the left to pass the tip of the bronchial tube through the vocal cords. **B:** The tube is then rotated 180° to the right to bring the carinate hook to the 12 o'clock position for easy passage through the vocal cords. **C:** The tube is rotated 90° left to position the bronchial lumen toward the right main stem bronchus.

be herniating over the carina, the tracheal cuff is deflated and the tube is advanced until the proximal edge of the bronchial cuff lies 3–5 mm inside the bronchus. If the proximal edge of the bronchial cuff is not visible at the carina, the tube is withdrawn 2–4 mm. The fiberscope is maintained in this position, and the bronchial cuff is inflated by the minimal leak technique under direct fiberscope observation.

The tracheal lumen connector limb is clamped, and its suction port opened to the air. The patient is now being ventilated solely through the bronchial lumen. The anesthesiologist listens for air leak at the open tracheal lumen connector, and the bronchial cuff is inflated until an airtight seal is obtained.

Due to the limited volume capacity of bronchial cuffs, relatively small changes in cuff volume will produce large increases in intracuff pressure. The use of a cuff pressure controller has been shown to be more sensitive in accurately maintaining cuff pressure at the minimal leak level, even when nitrous oxide is being used (55).

The resting bronchial cuff volumes of disposable DLTs vary widely amoung the different tube sizes and brands. The inflation of the bronchial cuff above the resting volume sharply increases the intracuff pressure. If the bronchial cuff of a properly placed DLT requires more than its resting volume to create a seal, it is likely to be the wrong size for that patient (56). If

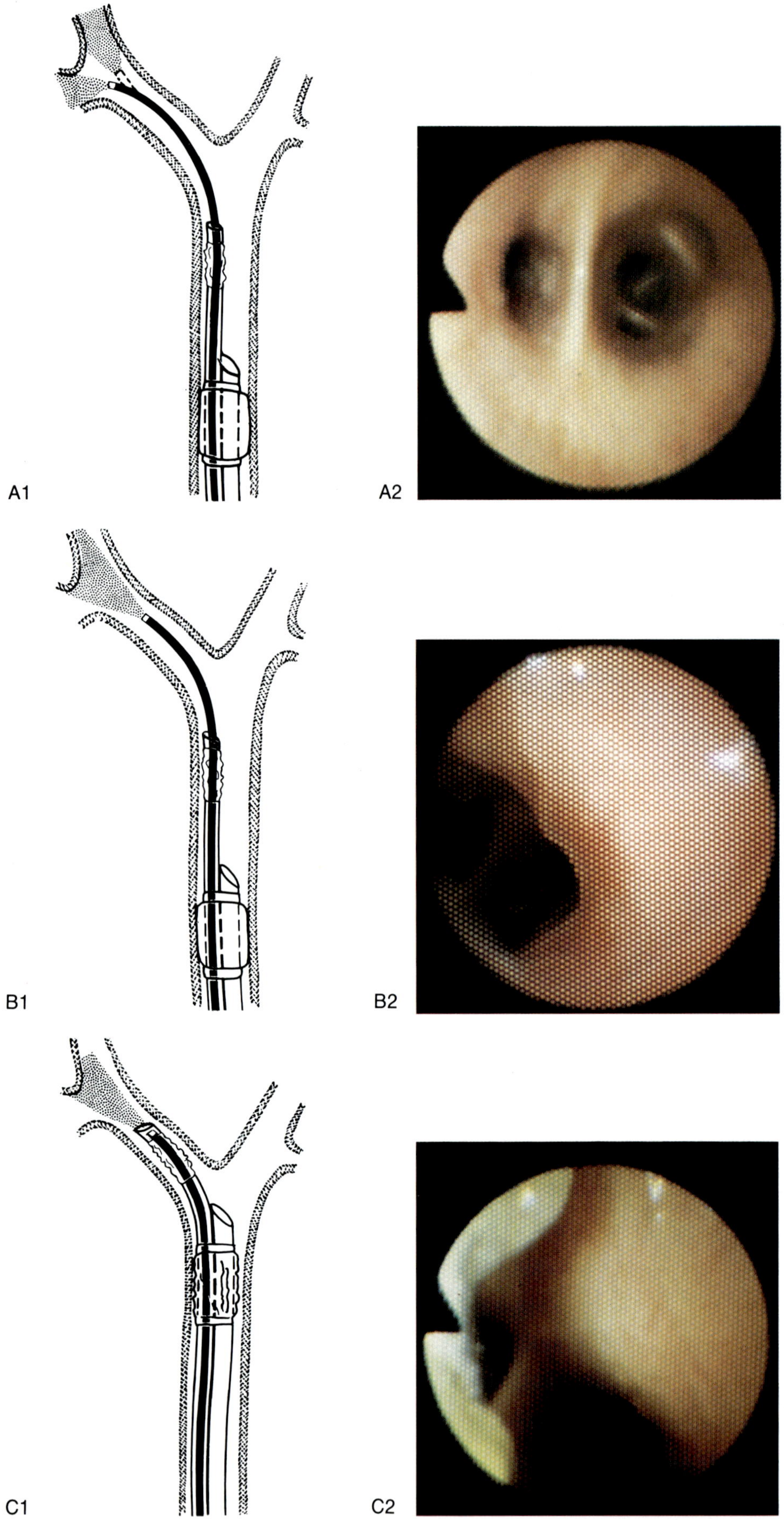
A1
A2
B1
B2
C1
C2

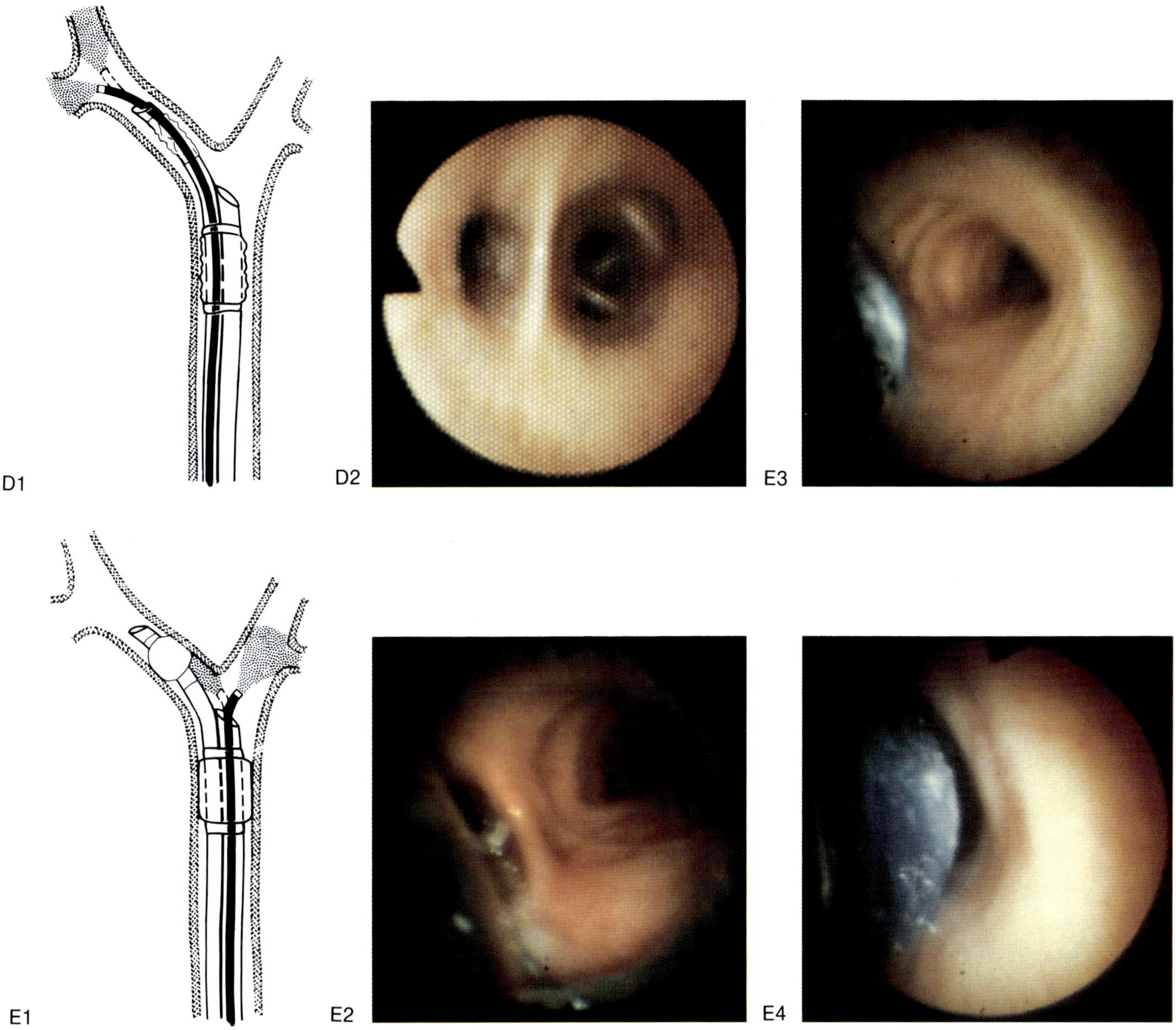

FIG. 15. Schematic demonstration of fiberoptic placement and positioning of the left-sided DLT with corresponding endoscopic pictures. **A1:** The fiberscope is passed through the bronchial lumen into the left main stem bronchus. The patency, length, and anatomy of the left main stem bronchus and the position of the upper and lower lobe bronchi are evaluated. **A2:** Endoscopic view of the left upper and lower lobe bronchi orifices. **B1:** The fiberscope is withdrawn slightly, and its tip is positioned 10 mm above the origin of the left upper lobe bronchus. **B2:** Endoscopic view of the left upper and lower lobe bronchi orifices with the tip of the fiberscope positioned 15 mm above the origin of the left upper lobe bronchus. **C1:** The tracheal cuff is deflated, and the tube is advanced over the fiberscope into the left main stem bronchus until it comes into view beyond the tip of the fiberscope. **C2:** Endoscopic view of the tip of the bronchial lumen visible distal to the tip of the fiberscope above the left upper lobe bronchial orifice. **D1:** The fiberscope is advanced beyond the bronchial lumen to visualize the left upper lobe bronchus once again. **D2:** Left upper and lower lobe bronchi orifices. **E1:** The fiberscope is passed through the tracheal lumen to check the position of the bronchial cuff and the opening of the right main stem bronchus. **E2:** Endoscopic view of the open right main stem bronchus and the bronchial tube positioned in the left main stem bronchus. This represents proper positioning of the endobronchial tube. **E3:** Endoscopic view of the bronchial tube blue cuff herniates out of the left main stem bronchus. **E4:** Inflating the bronchial cuff with 2 ml of air partially blocks the right main stem bronchus (unsatisfactory position) (with permission, ref. 3).

the endobronchial tube is fit tightly inside its respective main stem bronchus, a cuff volume less than resting volume will be needed to maintain it as a low-pressure cuff.

The clamp is now removed from the tracheal lumen, and the tracheal cuff is deflated and reinflated using the minimal leak technique. The bronchial cuff should remain inflated during patient positioning, remaining so until surgery is completed and lung separation is no longer required.

If the distance between the carina and orifice of the left upper lobe bronchus is short, repeated observations through both tube lumens may be necessary to ensure proper position is maintained and to avoid blockage of the left upper lobe bronchus. When a left-sided DLT is correctly placed, the opening of the tracheal lumen should lie 2–3 cm above the carina. The tip of the bronchial lumen should not occlude the left upper lobe bronchus, and the bronchial cuff should be confined to the inside of the left main stem bronchus.

A second approach may be used for positioning the left-side DLT. After inspection of the left bronchus, the fiberscope is pulled back and rotated 90° to the left so as to position its tip at the distal opening of the left bronchial lumen (Fig. 16). The tracheal cuff is deflated, and the fiberscope and tube advanced together into the left bronchus until the left upper lobe orifice is visualized. The tip of the bronchial tube is positioned 5–10 mm above the takeoff of the left upper lobe bronchus (Fig. 17). The rest of the procedure remains unchanged from that already described. The first approach technique is preferred for placement of the left-sided endobronchial tube because of high incidence of the left-sided tube entering into the right main stem bronchus when not guided over the fiberscope.

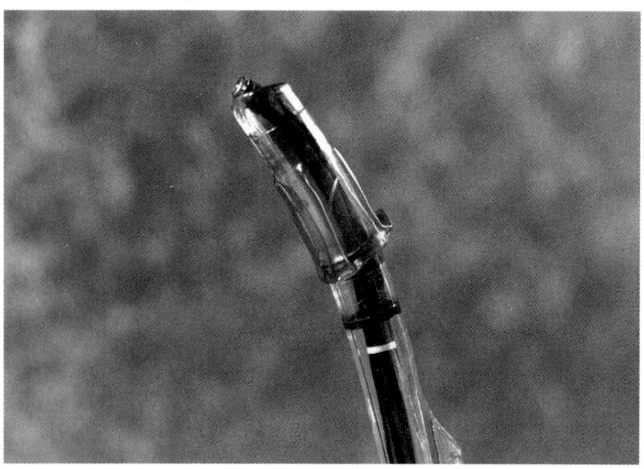

FIG. 16. Demonstrates the position of the tip of fiberscope at the distal opening of the bronchial lumen of a left-sided DLT.

Right-Sided Double-Lumen Tube

The ability to evaluate the anatomy of the right bronchial tree is vital for rapid and accurate placement of the right-sided double-lumen tube. Aberrant anomalies (e.g., the tracheal bronchus that arises from the right tracheal wall above the carina) may be easily missed (57,58). The practice of blind placement of the endobronchial tube, and use of the fiberscope solely to check the position of the endobronchial cuff, results in unnecessary confusion, repeated intubation attempts, and airway trauma (59).

Proper positioning of the right-sided DLT is technically more difficult due to the short and variable length of the right main stem bronchus. In addition, any anatomic compression of the tracheobronchial tree by aortic aneurysm, tumor, or other obstruction can make placement of a right-sided tube particularly difficult (60,61).

After tracheal intubation the fiberscope is passed through the bronchial lumen of the DLT and into the right main stem bronchus. The length, patency, and integrity of the bronchus is evaluated. The fiberscope is then withdrawn into the lumen of the bronchial tube. The tip of the fiberscope is rotated 90° clockwise and positioned at the proximal end of the side window in the bronchial cuff (Fig. 18). The position of the tip of the fiberscope is such that the operator can see the lateral and lower window borders and the tracheal wall, but not the upper border of the window. The distal opening of the tube allows viewing of the lower trachea and main stem bronchus.

While viewing through the window opening of the tube, the tube and fiberscope are advanced into the right main stem bronchus. The tube is then further advanced until the opening of the right upper lobe orifice appears through the bronchial cuff window. The tube is again advanced until the distal edge of the window passes 1–2 mm beyond the distal border of the right upper lobe bronchial orifice (Fig. 19).

The fiberscope is then advanced until it reaches the midpoint of the bronchial tube window, allowing visualization of the right upper lobe bronchial lumen. The fiberscope is then rotated back to its neutral position and advanced toward the distal end of the tube, allowing for visualization of the right middle and lower lobe bronchial openings. Finally, the fiberscope is inserted into the tracheal lumen to inspect the position of the bronchial cuff.

In a second approach to right-sided endobronchial intubation, the fiberscope is advanced through the bronchial lumen of the DLT and into the right main stem bronchus. The fiberscope is then rotated 90° clockwise and the tip deflected upward at 90°. The fiberscope is advanced in this position, until the orifice of the right upper lobe is visualized. At this point, the

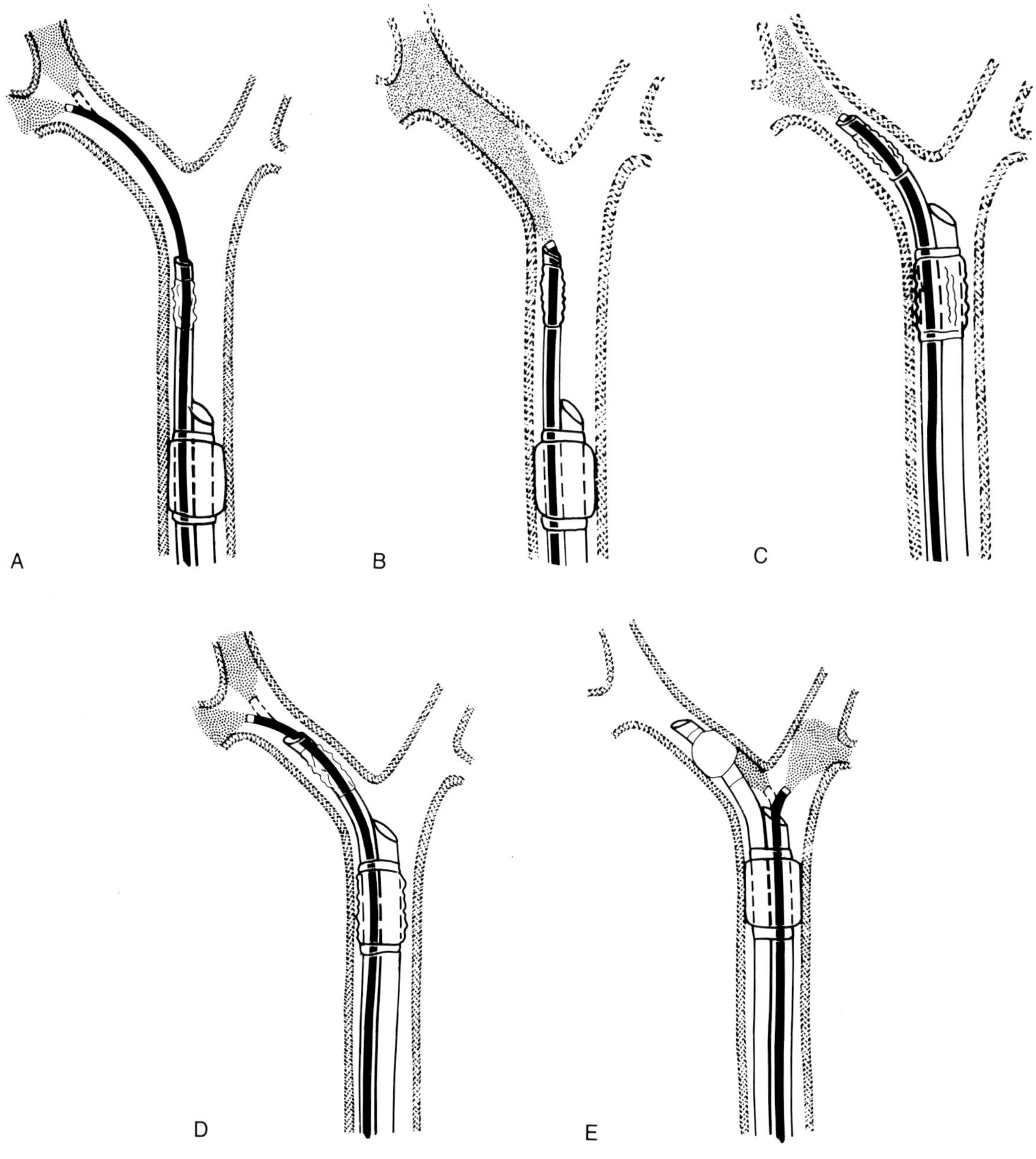

FIG. 17. Schematic demonstration of alternate approach to fiberoptic placement and positioning of the left-sided DLT. **A:** The fiberscope is passed through the bronchial lumen into the left main stem bronchus. The patency, length, and anatomy of the left main stem bronchus and the position of the orifice of the left upper lobe bronchus are evaluated. **B:** The fiberscope is pulled back and its tip is positioned at the level of the distal opening of the bronchial lumen (Fig. 16). The fiberscope is 90° rotated to the left with the tip angled anteriorly toward the lateral wall of the trachea. **C:** The tracheal cuff is deflated; the tube and fiberscope are advanced together inside the left main stem bronchus until the orifice of the left upper lobe comes into view. At this point the tip of the fiberscope is 10–15 mm above the left upper lobe orifice. The tube is advanced further to position the distal end of the tube about 5 mm above the orifice of left upper lobe bronchus. **D:** The fiberscope is passed beyond the tip of the tube to visualize left upper lobe bronchus once again. **E:** The fiberscope is passed through the tracheal lumen to check the position of the bronchial cuff and the opening of the right main stem bronchus.

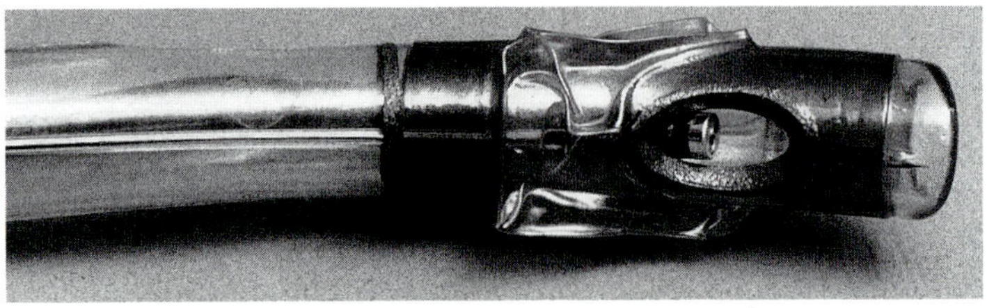

FIG. 18. Demonstrates the position of the tip of the fiberscope at the proximal border of the right-sided DLT cuff window.

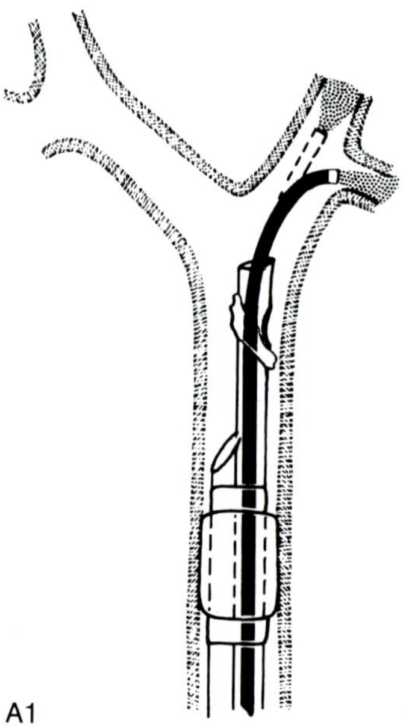

A1

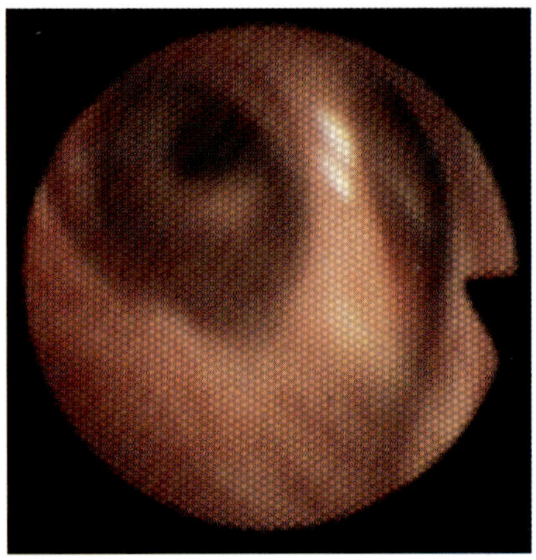

A2

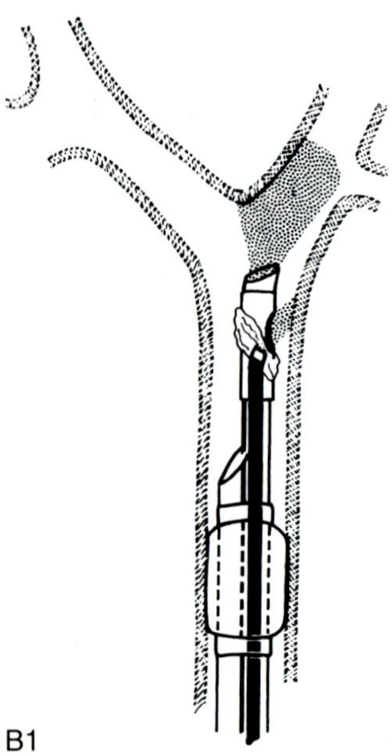

B1

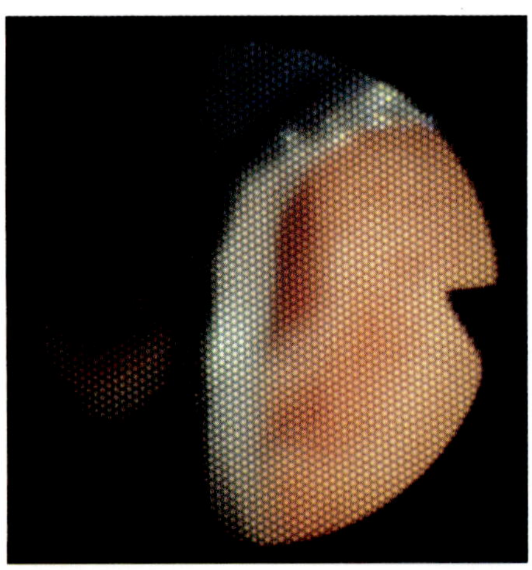

B2

FIG. 19. Schematic demonstration of fiberoptic placement and positioning of the right-sided DLT with corresponding endoscopic pictures. **A1:** The fiberscope is passed through the bronchial lumen into the right main stem bronchus. The patency, length, and anatomy of the right main stem bronchus and the position of the orifice of the right upper lobe bronchus are evaluated. **A2:** Right upper lobe bronchus orifice and bronchus intermedius. **B1:** The fiberscope is then withdrawn inside the bronchial lumen until its tip is placed at the proximal border of the bronchial cuff slot (Fig. 18). **B2:** The tip of the fiberscope at the proximal border of the bronchial cuff slot showing the window of the bronchial tube (right upper lobe ventilation slot) and the tracheal wall.

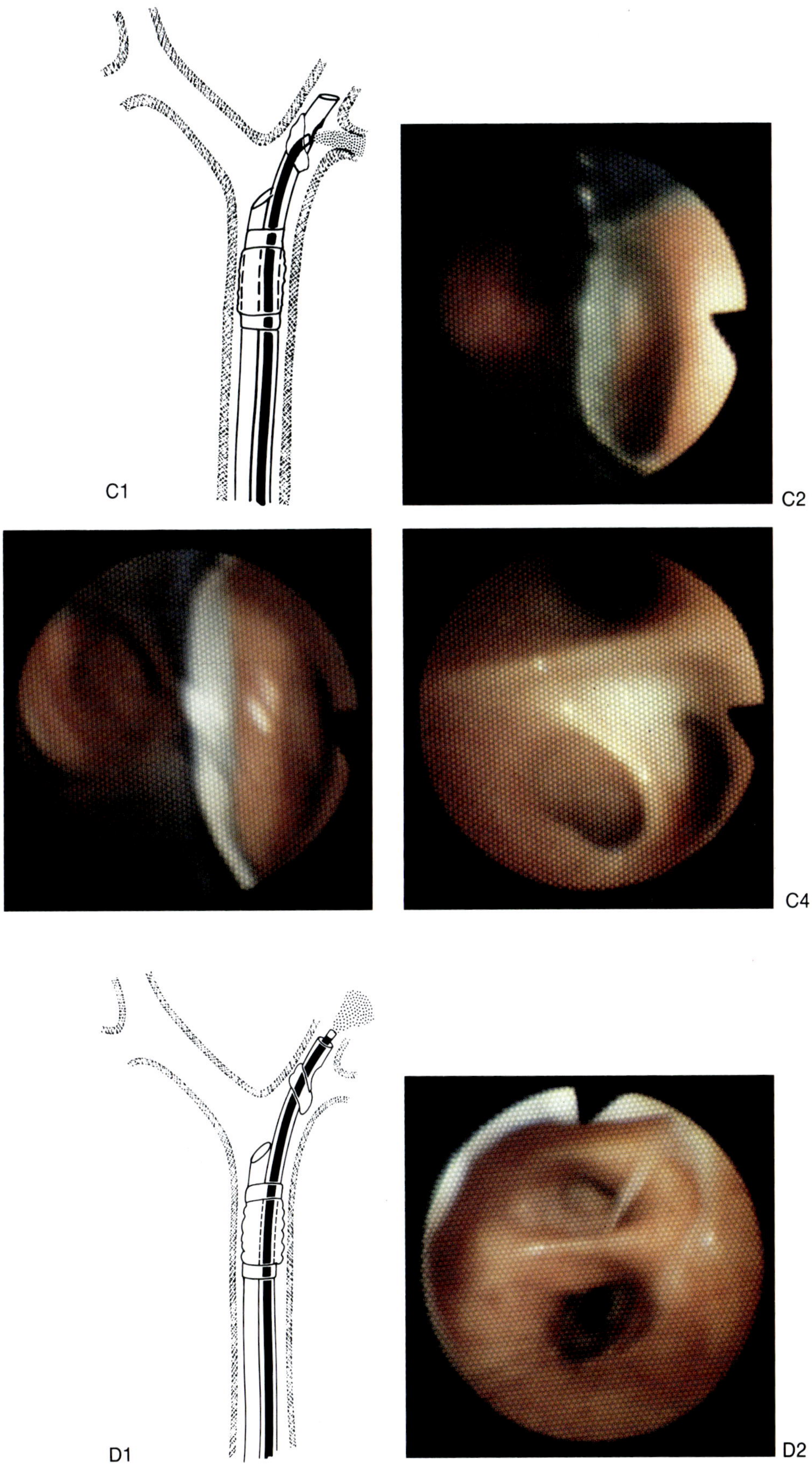

FIG. 19. *Continued.* **C1:** The tracheal cuff is deflated, and the tube and the fiberscope are then advanced together inside the right main stem bronchus until the orifice of the right upper lobe comes just into view through the window of the bronchial cuff. **C2:** Endoscopic view of the partial opening of the right upper lobe bronchus comes into view. **C3:** The bronchial cuff window in perfect position against right upper lobe bronchus orifice. The distal border of the bronchus orifice is at the level of the distal border of the bronchial cuff window. **C4:** The fiberscope is advanced through the bronchial cuff window (ventilation slot) to bring into view the three segments of the right upper lobe. The view confirms correct positioning of the tube. **D1:** The fiberscope is then passed beyond the distal opening of the bronchial tube to visualize the right middle and lower lobe bronchial orifices. **D2:** Endoscopic view of the right middle and lower lobe bronchial orifices.

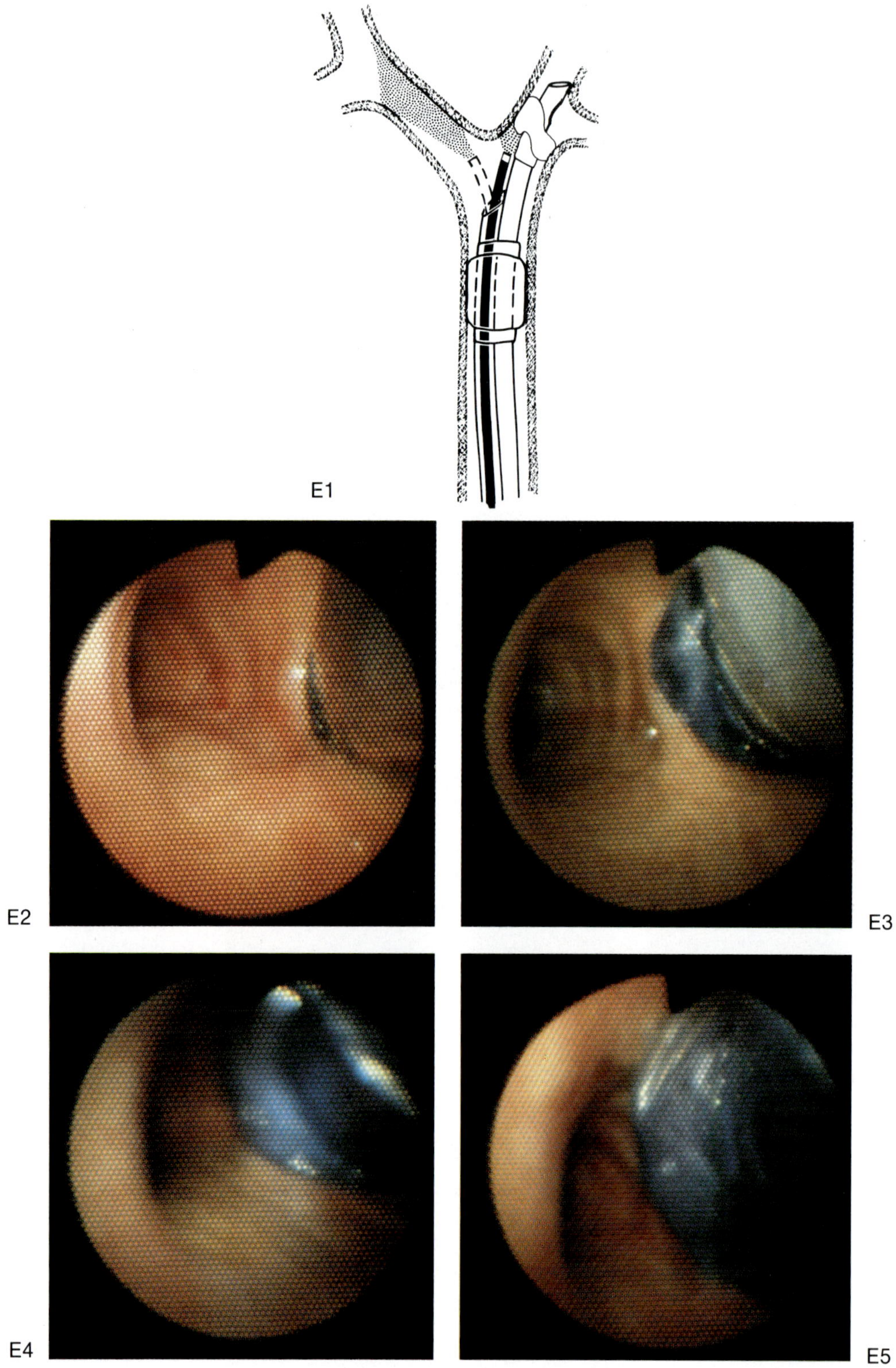

FIG. 19. *Continued.* **E1:** The fiberscope is passed through the tracheal lumen to check the position of the bronchial cuff and the opening of the left main stem bronchus. **E2:** Endoscopic view of the left main stem bronchus opening and the endobronchial tube inside the right main stem bronchus. The bronchial cuff is not visible. This is a satisfactory position of the right-sided endobronchial tube. **E3:** Same as E2 except that the upper edge of the blue bronchial cuff is visible at the level of the carina. This is an acceptable position, but it is more prone to dislodgment. **E4:** The bronchial tube blue cuff herniates out of the right main stem bronchus. **E5:** Inflating bronchial cuff with 2.5 ml of air partially blocks the left main stem bronchus (unsatisfactory position). (From ref. 3.)

fiberscope is held stationary, and its tip is returned to the neutral position.

The tracheal cuff is deflated, and the tube is advanced over the stationary fiberscope into the right bronchus. When the distal end of the bronchial tube comes into view, it is passed beyond the tip of the fiberscope (Fig. 20). In this position, the window of the bronchial cuff lies opposite the orifice of the right upper lobe bronchus. The fiberscope is then withdrawn inside the bronchial lumen to visualize the orifice of the right upper lobe through the window of the bronchial cuff.

The fiberscope is now inserted into the tracheal lumen to inspect the position of the bronchial cuff as previously described. The fiberscope is maintained in this position, and the bronchial cuff can be inflated by the minimal leak technique under visual observation.

The oblique design of the Broncho-Cath® right-

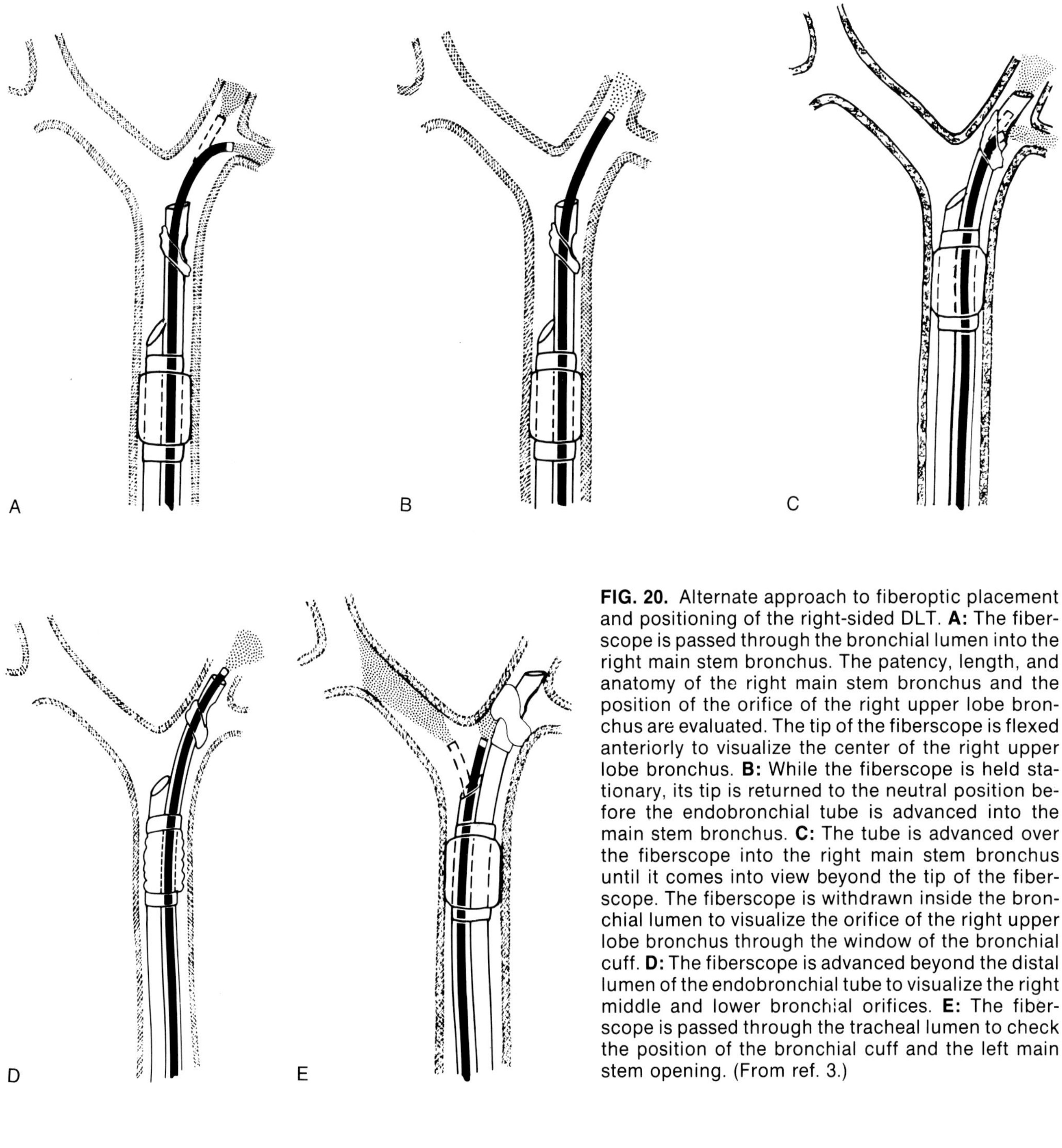

FIG. 20. Alternate approach to fiberoptic placement and positioning of the right-sided DLT. **A:** The fiberscope is passed through the bronchial lumen into the right main stem bronchus. The patency, length, and anatomy of the right main stem bronchus and the position of the orifice of the right upper lobe bronchus are evaluated. The tip of the fiberscope is flexed anteriorly to visualize the center of the right upper lobe bronchus. **B:** While the fiberscope is held stationary, its tip is returned to the neutral position before the endobronchial tube is advanced into the main stem bronchus. **C:** The tube is advanced over the fiberscope into the right main stem bronchus until it comes into view beyond the tip of the fiberscope. The fiberscope is withdrawn inside the bronchial lumen to visualize the orifice of the right upper lobe bronchus through the window of the bronchial cuff. **D:** The fiberscope is advanced beyond the distal lumen of the endobronchial tube to visualize the right middle and lower bronchial orifices. **E:** The fiberscope is passed through the tracheal lumen to check the position of the bronchial cuff and the left main stem opening. (From ref. 3.)

sided DLT bronchial cuff (Fig. 4) allows placement of this tube when the right main stem bronchus is as short as 10 mm. The upper border of the medial (distal) portion of the right-sided DLT bronchial cuff is often positioned at the level of the carinate ridge. With high airway pressures during OLV and during positioning, it is therefore more likely to be displaced.

In patients with permanent tracheostomy requiring intrathoracic surgical intervention, a DLT may be placed through the tracheostomy stoma (62). A left-side DLT has been placed through tracheostomy stoma on three occasions at our institution (Fig. 21). Although passage of the tube through the stoma is easier than through the mouth, the bronchial placement and positioning require careful attention to detail. Under these circumstances, the tracheal cuff usually lies at or partially outside the tracheal stoma (62). The use of a shorter version of a left-sided DLT, Broncho-Trach (Sheridan Catheter Corp., Argyle, New York) in patients with tracheostomies has been reported (63).

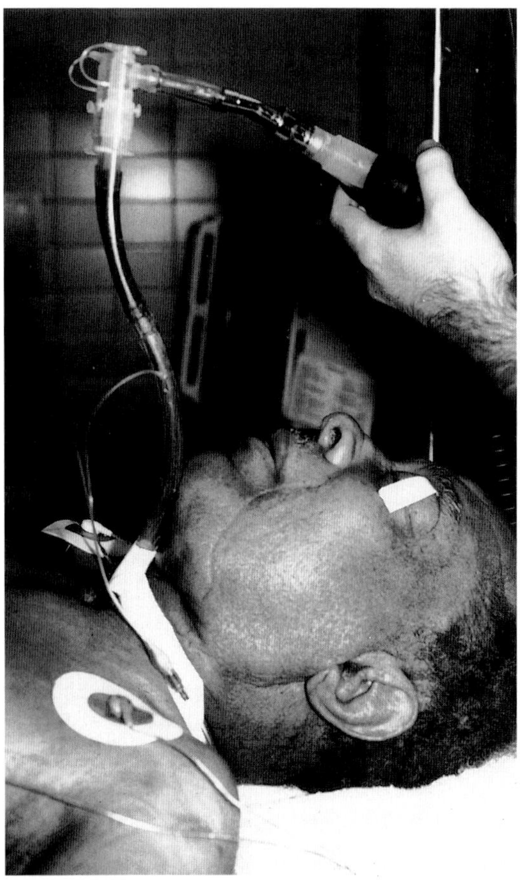

FIG. 21. Left-sided Robertshaw DLT placed through tracheostomy stoma. Patient had total laryngectomy for squamous cell carcinoma of the larynx 5 years prior to this admission.

Verifying the Functional Status of Double-Lumen Tubes

Double-lumen tube separation of the lungs does not guarantee proper ventilation of each respective lung. Unobstructed ventilation of the nonoperative lung is critical to successful OLV. The following applied steps are used to assure the correct placement and functioning of the DLT.

1. The mechanical ventilator is set at a tidal volume of 10 ml/kg at a rate of eight breaths/min. The lungs are auscultated bilaterally, and chest wall movement observed. The exhaled tidal volume is noted and recorded, along with peak and plateau airway pressures. The expiratory flow pattern and the appearance of humidity in both tube lumens is observed.
2. The tracheal lumen connector tube should be clamped and the suction port opened to the air. Breath sounds, with good associated chest-wall movement, should be present only on the bronchial side. There should be no air leak through the tracheal lumen. The exhaled tidal volume should show a decrease of not more than 10–15%, and peak airway pressure should not increase by more than 50%, compared with two-lung ventilation. The expiratory flow pattern should remain unchanged.
3. The clamp should then be placed on the bronchial lumen connector tube and the suction port opened to air. Breath sounds should be present only on the tracheal side. Tidal volume, peak airway pressure, and expiratory flow pattern should change little from one lung to the other (Table 7).
4. The lumens of the PVC tubes should "fog" with water vapor with equal intensity during exhalation. A slow, incomplete appearance and clearance of the water vapor "fog," may indicate poor airflow through that lumen.

After completion of these procedures, two-lung ventilation should be resumed. Tincture of benzoin should be applied to the tube and patient's face prior to securing the DLT with adhesive tape applied around the neck.

Immediately before lateral positioning, the tube should be disconnected from the anesthesia circuit and held in place with one hand while the other hand supports the back of the head. This serves to minimize movement of the neck. Cervical flexion may cause up to 2.5 cm of distal movement, leading to upper lobe obstruction. Cervical extension may lead to accidental extubation of the bronchus (64). After the patient is in the lateral position, all of the above procedures are repeated.

Placement of a DLT is considered unsatisfactory if the wrong bronchus is intubated, if separation of the lungs is incomplete, if the tidal volume decreases by

TABLE 7. *Tidal volumes and peak airway pressures during one-lung ventilation*

	Supine		Lateral	
	TV	PAP	TV	PAP
Left-sided tube (*N* = 16)				
Two-lung ventilation	756 ± 67	24 ± 4	760 ± 64	24 ± 4
Left-lung ventilation	700 ± 84	36 ± 4	708 ± 67	36 ± 4
Right-lung ventilation	714 ± 75	35 ± 4	715 ± 70	36 ± 4
Right-sided tube (*n* = 16)				
Two-lung ventilation	785 ± 75	23 ± 3	787 ± 84	23 ± 3
Left-lung ventilation	722 ± 67	35 ± 4	733 ± 65	34 ± 3
Right-lung ventilation	711 ± 72	34 ± 4	735 ± 63	34 ± 4

Abbreviations: TV, tidal volume of 10 to 12 ml/kg. PAP, peak airway pressure (cm H_2O). All values are means ± SD.

more than 15%, if the peak airway pressure increases by more than 50%, or if the expiratory flow rate of either lung slows markedly upon changing to OLV.

If there is any question regarding positioning or obstruction, the fiberscope should be passed through the DLT tracheal lumen to check the positions of the bronchial cuff and the tracheal lumen opening in relationship to the tracheal wall. If these positions appear satisfactory, the fiberscope is passed through the bronchial lumen to ensure the tip of the bronchial tube is not pressing against the bronchial wall or blocking the orifice to the upper lobe bronchus. In right-sided tubes, the position of the window in the bronchial cuff relative to the orifice of the right upper lobe bronchus should be reconfirmed.

In the presence of advanced lung disease, or of lung tissue loss, a more exaggerated change of tidal volume and airway pressure is expected when switching from two-lung ventilation to one-lung ventilation (Table 8). This may or may not be accompanied by changes in the exhaled airflow pattern.

In restrictive lung pathology (e.g., empyema, acute atelectasis of one lobe, or main stem bronchus obstruction), the pattern of airflow does not change relative to two-lung ventilation when each lung is ventilated individually. However, tidal volume may drastically decrease, with concomitant substantial increases in airway pressure (Table 8, Cases 1, 2, and 3) (Fig. 22).

Case 4 illustrates the findings in a patient who had prior left upper lobectomy, well compensated by the remaining lower lobe. Upon changing from bilateral to left-lung ventilation, modest changes in volume and pressure were noted. The patient was now to undergo a right thoracotomy. Two attempts at OLV resulted in a decrease in oxygen saturation levels to 90% in 5 min.

Case 5 illustrates findings where the tracheal lumen of a right-sided DLT impinged against the wall of the trachea. In severe cases of this nature, ventilation is impaired, airway pressure rises, tidal volume decreases, and airflow slows. In this case, lateral positioning of the patient improved the situation sufficiently to allow for successful OLV.

The patient in Case 6 suffered restrictive lung disease secondary to asbestosis. Compared to patients with normal lung compliance, at any given tidal volume, peak airway pressures remained significantly elevated in this patient. Airflow, however, remained normal.

Patients with bronchospasm will show similar increases in airway pressure associated with decreased tidal volumes and a poor airflow pattern. In patients with reactive airways, this condition is sometimes encountered after bronchial intubation under light anesthesia.

In cases where auscultation of the lungs proves limited or unreliable, the modalities described will provide the information necessary to confirm proper tube placement. End-tidal CO_2 and pressure/volume loop monitoring of each lung have been suggested for assessing proper placement of a DLT(65). The shape, height, and rhythm of the end-tidal CO_2 waveforms, as well as the flow/volume loops from each lung, are compared (66,67). The presence of partial airway obstruction or decreased ventilation is easily detected.

SUCCESS AND FAILURE RATE OF DOUBLE-LUMEN TUBE PLACEMENT

In a retrospective review of 214 DLT placements, the incidence of difficult intubation, failed tracheal intubation, and improper tube placement was 50% with the red rubber Carlens tubes, 22.5% with the red rubber Robertshaw tubes, and 4% with the PVC Robertshaw tubes (24). One-lung ventilation was abandoned in 9.6% of patients in the red rubber Robertshaw group, and in 2% of patients in the PVC group. In three patients (one in each group), a single-lumen tube was substituted for the DLT, due to failure to intubate the trachea (24).

In a prospective study using both left- and right-sided tubes, initial placement of the tube was unsatisfactory

TABLE 8. *Tidal volumes, peak and plateau airway pressures during one-lung ventilation in six patients with various kinds of pulmonary pathology*

	TV						PAP/PP					
	Supine			Lateral			Supine			Lateral		
Case #	BO	LO	RO	BO	LO	RO	BO	LO	RO	BO	LO	RO
1	725	450	675	700	500	650	36/30	65/65	38/32	36/30	68/68	40/32
2	870	830	820	860	600	820	20/10	30/20	28/22	28/22	52/40	30/22
3	720	720	250	750	750	250	30/20	30/20	50/50	32/24	32/24	50/50
4	750	725	750	750	650	700	26/18	42/32	34/24	26/20	42/30	34/28
5	800	300	700	750	450	675	30/24	70/50	46/40	32/24	56/40	46/40
6	750	750	750	750	650	700	34/28	50/50	44/38	34/30	58/56	42/38

Abbreviations: TV, tidal volume of 10 to 12 ml/kg; PAP, peak airway pressure (cm H_2O); PP, plateau pressure (cm H_2O); BO, bilateral ventilation; LO, left-lung ventilation; RO; right-lung ventilation

Case 1. Male, 98 kg, with left-side emphysema managed with right-sided DL tube. Left-lung ventilation with the same ventilator tidal volume setup generated high pressures with a much smaller tidal volume. The flow of air was the same, and the picture did not change when the patient was placed in the right lateral decubitus position.

Case 2. Male, 87 kg, with acute atelectasis of the left upper lobe caused by a left endobronchial tube. When the patient was turned to the right lateral decubitus position, separation of lungs was rechecked. Left-lung ventilation showed decreased tidal volume and increased airway pressure, with no change in the exhaled airflow pattern. No adjustments were made until the chest was opened. Left upper lung, as was suspected, was collapsed by the endobronchial tube, which had been advanced too far. The tube was withdrawn and repositioned with an immediate change of tidal volume and airway pressure to their original values.

Case 3. Male, 60 kg, with tumor sitting on right main stem bronchus and carina (Fig. 14). Opening of right main stem could not be visualized. Left-sided DLT was placed for thoracotomy and drainage. Right-lung ventilation generated high pressures and tidal volume of 250 ml. Peak airway and plateau pressures are equal.

Case 4. Male, 90 kg, who had a left upper lobectomy in the past, now scheduled for a right thoracotomy for a coin lesion with a left-sided DLT. Tidal volume shows little change from two-lung ventilation to one-lung ventilation. However, PAP generated by left-lung ventilation is higher and that of the right lung is lower than expected when compared to PAP during two-lung ventilation. This reflects low capacity of the left lung which contributes to higher PAP during two-lung ventilation. Tidal volume and airway pressure changes are more dramatic with acute loss of lung volume (acute atelectasis) as in Case 2 which had time to compensate for loss of the left upper lobe.

Case 5. Male, 75 kg, for left thoracotomy. Right-sided DLT was easily placed, but the tracheal lumen was pushed against the tracheal wall. This resulted in poor exhalation airflow, small tidal volumes, and very high peak and plateau pressures. On turning the patient to the right lateral decubitus position, the situation was improved enough to conduct one-lung ventilation by readjusting the tidal volume.

Case 6. Male, 84 kg, for left thoracotomy. The patient had stiff lungs due to asbestosis. All recorded airway pressures were high compared with a similar-size patient (Case 2) with normal lung compliance. PP and PAP were elevated further on OLV. Exhaled airflow showed no change.

in 27% of patients. In 12% of the patients, OLV was abandoned, either because correct placement could not be achieved or because of persistent hypoxemia (68).

In a retrospective review of 78 patients, Black and Harrison (50) reported problems in 11.5% of red rubber Robertshaw tube placements. In a prospective study of 59 cases, however, they reported problems in 37.2% of their patient sample. In 8.5% of these cases, the use of the DLT had to be discontinued. Clinical observation and evaluation of blindly positioned DLTs did not identify marginally positioned tubes, nor did they iden-

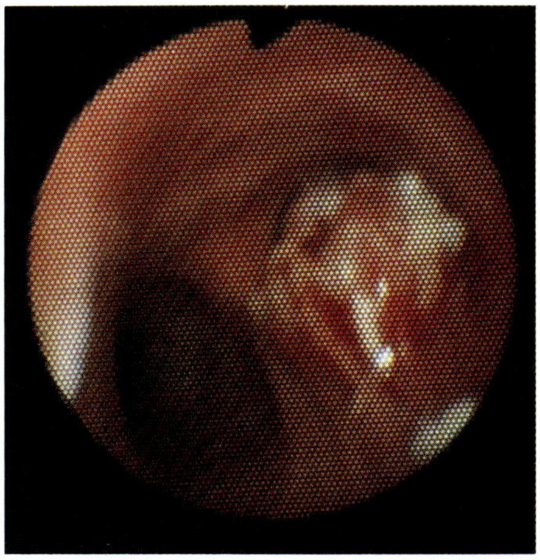

FIG. 22. Infiltration of tumor has almost completely blocked the right main stem bronchus, an accidental finding in a patient scheduled for a right thoracotomy. Four weeks prior to surgery, fiberoptic bronchoscopy was reported normal. The planned operation was canceled. Considering that blind advancement of left-sided DLT has a 20% chance to enter into the right main stem bronchus, that approach would have been dangerous in this case.

tify air trapping (50) and atelectasis of the left upper lobe (69–71).

The bronchoscopic evaluation of blindly placed DLTs shows a large number of marginally placed endobronchial tubes. Common findings show the bronchial cuff resting above the carina (3,39,54), the bronchial tube advanced too far into the main stem bronchus (3,54), and concentric constriction of the endobronchial lumen due to overinflation of the bronchial cuff (38,39,54).

A summary of 46 right-sided and 110 left-sided Robertshaw disposable DLT placements at VA Lakeside Medical Center is presented in Tables 9 and 10 (46,72). All right-sided tubes were positioned with the aid of a fiberscope. Left-sided tubes were either positioned with the aid of a fiberscope or the tube position was confirmed by fiberscope after blind placement. Airway complications or tube malfunction during surgery was evaluated and corrected whenever possible with the aid of a fiberscope.

Rigid laryngoscopic intubation of the trachea with a right-sided DLT was successful in 43 patients. In two patients with prior histories of difficult intubation, awake fiberoptic tracheal intubations with a 39 Fr DLT were performed.

In one patient, due to a failed rigid laryngoscopy, asleep fiberoptic intubation with a single-lumen tube was performed for a flexible bronchoscopy prior to thoracotomy. After the completion of the bronchoscopy, the endotracheal tube was changed to a 39 Fr DLT, using a fiberoptic bronchoscope.

TABLE 9. *Results of 43 right endobronchial intubations*

Leak around bronchial cuff	
Tube partially pulled out	7
Nasogastric tube in right main stem	1
Tracheal lumen against tracheal wall	3
OLV	
Used as needed	41
Not used (1 not suitable, 1 not needed)	2
Abandoned	0
Duration of one-lung ventilation (min), mean (SD)	97 (53)
Lowest P_aO_2 during one-lung ventilation (FIO_2 1.00)	
63–80 mm Hg (2 on FIO_2 = 0.5)	4
81–100 mm Hg	8
>100 mm Hg	29

FIO_2, fraction of inspired oxygen; OLV, one-lung ventilation.

TABLE 10. *Results of 110 left endobronchial intubations*

Satisfactory placement	100
Unsatisfactory	10
Incomplete separation	1
Tip of tube against bronchial wall; effect of positioning	
Not changed	2
Improved	3
Worsened	4
One-lung ventilation	
Not used (no need)	12
Used as needed	98
Abandoned (poor ventilation)	3
PaO_2 during one-lung ventilation	
<60	7
60–80	35
80–100	22
<100	28
Not recorded	6

Lowest PaO_2 recorded was 54 mm Hg, which improved when oxygen concentration was changed from 50% to 100%.

In 43 patients, separation of the lungs using a right-sided DLT was successful. In three patients, a short right main stem bronchus precluded the use of a right-sided DLT (72). A left-sided DLT was used in two of these patients, and a Univent tube with endobronchial blocker in the third. In 41 patients, OLV (ranging from 30 to 230 min) was tolerated well (Table 9). The lowest PaO_2 values obtained during OLV ranged between 61 and 80 mm Hg in four patients. Two of these patients had an FIO_2 of 0.5.

In seven (16%) of the patients, a leak around the bronchial cuff or decreased ventilation of the lung indicated displacement of the tube during the operative procedure (Table 9). Bronchoscopic examination confirmed cephalad displacement of the tube, with the bronchial cuff herniating partially into the trachea. In each case, the tracheal and the bronchial cuffs were deflated and the tube was advanced into the desired position.

In one patient, a nasogastric tube passed to deflate the stomach inadvertently entered the right main stem bronchus, causing a large leak at the bronchial cuff seal (Fig. 23). The leak stopped after the nasogastric tube was removed. In three patients the tracheal lumen was partially blocked by compression against the tracheal wall, one while in the supine position, and two upon lateral decubitus positioning. Postoperative chest roentgenogram showed good expansion of the right lung in all patients.

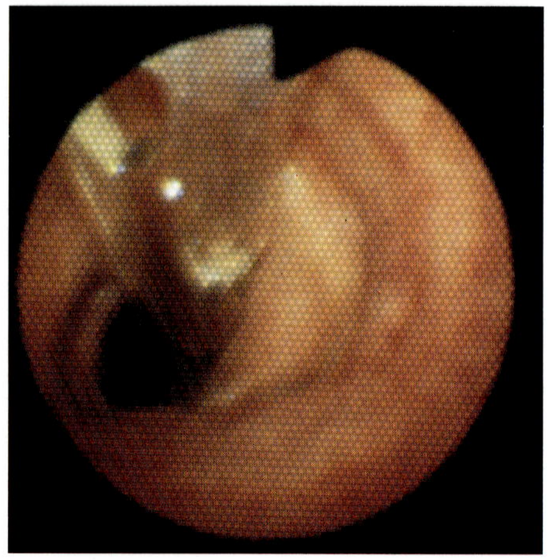

FIG. 23. Nasogastric tube in right bronchus intermedius. Right lower lobe opening is in view. The *black arrow* is at the right side of the nasogastric (NG) tube. The hole in the NG tube is clearly shown at the 11 o'clock position.

Separation of the lungs was achieved in all but one of 110 left-sided DLT intubations. The cause of this one failure could not be identified. All other improperly placed or dislodged tubes, were successfully corrected with the help of the fiberscope.

In nine patients, ventilation of the left lung in the supine position was unsatisfactory, secondary to the tip of the tube lying against the medial wall of the main stem bronchus. Turning the patients laterally improved ventilation in three patients, led to no improvement in two, and worsened the situation in four. One-lung ventilation was discontinued in 3 patients (Table 10). One-lung ventilation was not necessary in another 12 patients. The duration of OLV in the remaining 95 patients was 20–180 min (average, 75 min).

The most common problem encountered with the left-sided DLT, is its tip lodging against the medial bronchial wall, due to the anatomic configuration of the left main stem bronchus. This positioning produces increases in the peak and plateau airway pressures, and lowers the tidal volume. Turning the patient laterally, may change the position of the tip of the bronchial tube, improving or worsening the problem in some cases (Table 11). If ventilation remains poor in the left dependent lung after lateral positioning, OLV cannot be utilized. If the left lung is the operative lung, then poor left lung ventilation is not a significant problem, since that lung is collapsed during surgery.

Auscultation as a check of tube placement is unreliable, so bronchoscopic assessment of tube position

TABLE 11. *Tip of the bronchial tube of a left-sided Robertshaw DL tube lying against the medial bronchial wall (effect of positioning)*

		TV						PAP/PP					
		Supine			Lateral			Supine			Lateral		
Case	Wt (kg)	BO	LO	RO	BO	LO	RO	BO	LO	RO	BO	LO	RO
1	71	750	550	700	725	700	650	30/20	70/40	42/22	35/20	52/30	42/30
2	60	725	300	700	700	300	700	26/12	60/30	40/20	32/18	70/40	42/22
3	77	800	700	750	775	650	775	20/14	32/30	28/20	22/16	44/40	24/20

Abbreviations: TV, tidal volume of 10 to 12 ml/kg; PAP, peak airway pressure (cm H_2O); PP, plateau pressure (cm H_2O); BO, bilateral ventilation; LO, left-lung ventilation; RO, right-lung ventilation.

Case 1. Left lateral decubitus position improved the situation; left-lung tidal volume increased and airway pressure decreased after positioning.

Case 2. Left lateral decubitus position did not improve the situation; left-lung tidal volume remained the same, with somewhat higher airway pressure.

Case 3. Left lateral decubitus position worsened the situation; left-lung tidal volume decreased and airway pressure increased substantially.

TABLE 12. *Advantages of fiberoptic positioning of DLTs*

Anatomical anomalies and pathological conditions are recognized prior to intubation
Endoscopic evaluation of the right main stem bronchus assists in selecting the appropriate endobronchial tube
Correct placement is readily achieved
Technical problems are easily identified
A malpositioned tube is easily corrected
Repeated attempts at blind placement are avoided
Intubation of the wrong bronchus is minimized
Trauma to the bronchial tree is minimized

should be performed in every patient. Fiberoptic bronchoscopy revealed malpositioning of 38–78% of left-sided, and up to 83% of right-sided DLTs (39,44,47,73). Intubation of the wrong bronchus using a blind approach has been reported between 14% to 30%, with left-sided DLTs (47–50,73,74).

In the case of abnormal bronchial anatomy, the failure to examine the tracheobronchial tree prior to insertion of an endobronchial tube and blocker not only delays the successful separation of the lungs, but may contribute to airway trauma, secondary to repeated blind attempts at positioning (59). Routine use of fiberoptic bronchoscope for evaluation of the tracheobronchial tree and positioning of endobronchial tubes and blocker will avoid a substantial number of stated complications (Table 12).

THE DIFFICULT INTUBATION

Problems with tracheal intubation are not infrequent when using DLTs, due to the tubes' large size and bulk (24,50). The fiberscope provides a useful tool under such circumstances. Awake fiberoptic endobronchial intubation is indicated in known or anticipated cases of difficult intubation (46,72,75). The technique requires good topical anesthesia, adequate conscious sedation, and assistance in maintaining soft tissue support. The intubating airway is not applicable to DLT use.

In the case of a failed rigid laryngoscopic intubation on an anesthetized and paralyzed patient, fiberoptic intubation can be utilized. The tongue is first held and pulled out of the mouth by an assistant. This maneuver helps to maintain a relatively unobstructed channel allowing for easier identification of the glottis and passage of the fiberscope into the trachea (46).

The fiberscope is inserted through the bronchial lumen of the DLT, and advanced into the oropharynx, through the vocal cords, and into the trachea. The DLT is then unloaded off of the fiberscope into the trachea.

The large size of a DLT, combined with its curved tip, makes passing a DLT slightly more difficult than a single-lumen endotracheal tube. To assist in its passage, the tube is rotated to bring the tip of the bronchial lumen to the 6 o'clock position to negotiate the tip of the epiglottis. After passing the epiglottis, the tip is rotated to the 12 o'clock position to facilitate passage into the trachea (46).

If this maneuver proves unsuccessful, an assistant is asked to hold the body of the fiberscope so that the operator can use the nondominant hand to pull the patient's jaw and tongue forward while using the dominant hand to manipulate the tube into the trachea. The operator can also use a rigid laryngoscope to lift the base of the tongue and epiglottis to assist passage of the DLT over the fiberscope into the trachea.

The tracheal cuff of a DLT is prone to damage during tracheal intubation, as it lies against the upper teeth. It is essential to check the tracheal cuff after each unsuccessful intubation attempt. The placing of a plastic guard on the upper incisors will minimize the problem.

DIAGNOSTIC BRONCHOSCOPY PRIOR TO THORACOTOMY

The performance of fiberoptic bronchoscopy by the surgeon immediately prior to a thoracotomy procedure is a common medical practice. Fiberoptic bronchoscopes of 5 mm or larger are often preferred by surgeons for this procedure, and an airway of a larger internal diameter than provided by the double-lumen tube is required.

In the past we routinely used a single-lumen endotracheal tube for the bronchoscopy procedure, which would be replaced with a DLT prior to pàtient positioning for thoracotomy. The introduction of the laryngeal mask airway has changed our prior practice. We now routinely utilize the laryngeal mask airway for bronchoscopy, replacing it with the required DLT after completion of the procedure (Chapter 12). The laryngeal mask airway allows examination of the larynx and upper trachea. If the laryngeal mask is not available, or is unsuitable in a particular patient, an 8.5- to 9-mm single-lumen tube is placed in the trachea, which allows adequate lumen size for the procedure.

If tracheal intubation with a single-lumen tube proves difficult, its replacement with a DLT will usually prove to be a more difficult challenge. In such cases the fiberscope may be used to change the tube. The fiberscope passed through the bronchial lumen of the DLT is advanced next to the orotracheal tube and into the trachea. An assistant deflates the cuff of the endotracheal tube and extubates the patient. The DLT is then advanced over the fiberscope into the trachea, as previously described above (72).

POSITIONING OF THE UNIVENT® ENDOBRONCHIAL BLOCKER

Prior to tracheal intubation, the tracheal and blocker cuffs are tested for leaks. The blocker cuff and shaft is generously lubricated and moved back and forth inside the tube conduit, ensuring free movement of the blocker. The blocker is fully retracted into the main body of the endotracheal tube, and the trachea intubated.

After tracheal intubation, the endobronchial blocker is advanced through its conduit and directed into the intended bronchus. To facilitate passage of the blocker into the bronchus, the Univent® tube is turned 90° toward the operative side (tube rotation method). The 90° rotation of the main tube is necessary to control the direction of the blocker tip. The blocker tip cannot be manipulated by movement of the blocker's proximal shaft.

Blind positioning of the blocker is not recommended. The blocker may enter the wrong bronchus under these circumstances (76). Repeated attempts at blind placement may also cause tracheal and bronchial injuries (27). In addition, the ability to judge the proper depth of blocker insertion by auscultation alone is difficult, leading to repeated and time-consuming auscultation of the lungs.

Fiberscopic placement of the blocker can be achieved by two different methods. In one approach the tip of the Univent® tube is positioned 3–5 mm above the carina. A bronchoscopy adapter is placed on the main 15 mm tube adapter, and the fiberscope advanced through the tracheal tube lumen to expose the carina. An assistant advances the blocker toward the intended bronchus. If necessary, fiberoptic manipulation is applied to direct the blocker toward the intended bronchus. The fiberscope is used to guide the depth of bronchial blocker insertion, depending on whether collapse of the entire lung or only the lower lobe is desired.

If entering the left bronchus, the bronchial cuff is positioned just above the left upper lobe takeoff to block the entire lung (Fig. 24). To block the entire right lung, the balloon is positioned just opposite the right upper lobe bronchus to give it more stability and less chance for dislodgment. To block only the lower lobes of the right and left lungs, the balloon is positioned just beyond the opening of the respective upper lobe bronchus.

The bronchial cuff is inflated with 4–7 ml of air under fiberoptic observation, and the blocker fixed in place with the cap and band stopper. The cap stopper will also prevent air leakage around the blocker shaft. After verifying isolation of the lung, the balloon is deflated leaving the blocker in place.

In the second approach the fiberscope is passed through the Univent® tube into the desired main stem bronchus. The tube is then advanced over the fiberscope and positioned at the entrance of the main stem bronchus. The blocker is now advanced beyond the tip of the tube into the bronchus. While the blocker is held in position, the tracheal cuff is deflated and the tube pulled back to the desired position in the trachea.

The bronchial blocker is fixed in place. Its cuff is inflated to check the correct position of the blocker and then deflated. The fiberscope is now removed and the tube taped in place. In either technique, if difficulties are experienced in advancing the blocker, deflating the tracheal cuff and rotating the patient's head toward the operative (intended) side, may facilitate advancement of the blocker into the bronchus (77).

When commencing one-lung ventilation, the main tube is disconnected from the anesthesia machine. The surgeon is asked to compress the lung for rapid deflation, and the blocker cuff is then inflated. This approach helps promote a rapid deflation of the operative lung.

The advantages of the Univent® tube for intrathoracic operations include its easier tracheal placement compared to DLTs, the successful positioning of the blocker may be easier compared to proper placement of DLTs, long-term intubation is possible without tube changing, and fiberoptic bronchoscopy before or after surgery is possible through the main tube (26,78).

The Univent® tube, like all bronchial blockers, does not allow for simultaneous bilateral pulmonary ventilation and lung separation. This fact characterizes its chief disadvantage. In some patients, pulmonary isolation is necessary from the initiation of anesthesia to prevent contamination of the dependent lung. Some patients are unable to tolerate one-lung ventilation. The possibility of maintaining adequate ventilation by high-frequency jet ventilation through the Univent® blocker lumen has been suggested. However, there are no published reports regarding the feasibility, ease of use, and drawbacks or possible complications of this technique.

In regard to this issue, the value of the DLT in the management of acute pulmonary hemorrhage should be emphasized. The main risk for these patients lies in the danger of asphyxiation. The prompt and expeditious isolation of the lungs is of critical import in such cases. Although the Univent® tube is used successfully in some cases of pulmonary hemorrhage (79,80), there are several problems associated with the use of bronchial blockers under these circumstances (81).

If the side of hemorrhage is not known, correct placement of a bronchial blocker is likely to be delayed. Furthermore, blockers leave no access to the involved lung, which would allow for monitoring of bleeding, diagnostic evaluation, etc. The left-sided DLT is an ideal instrument under these circumstances.

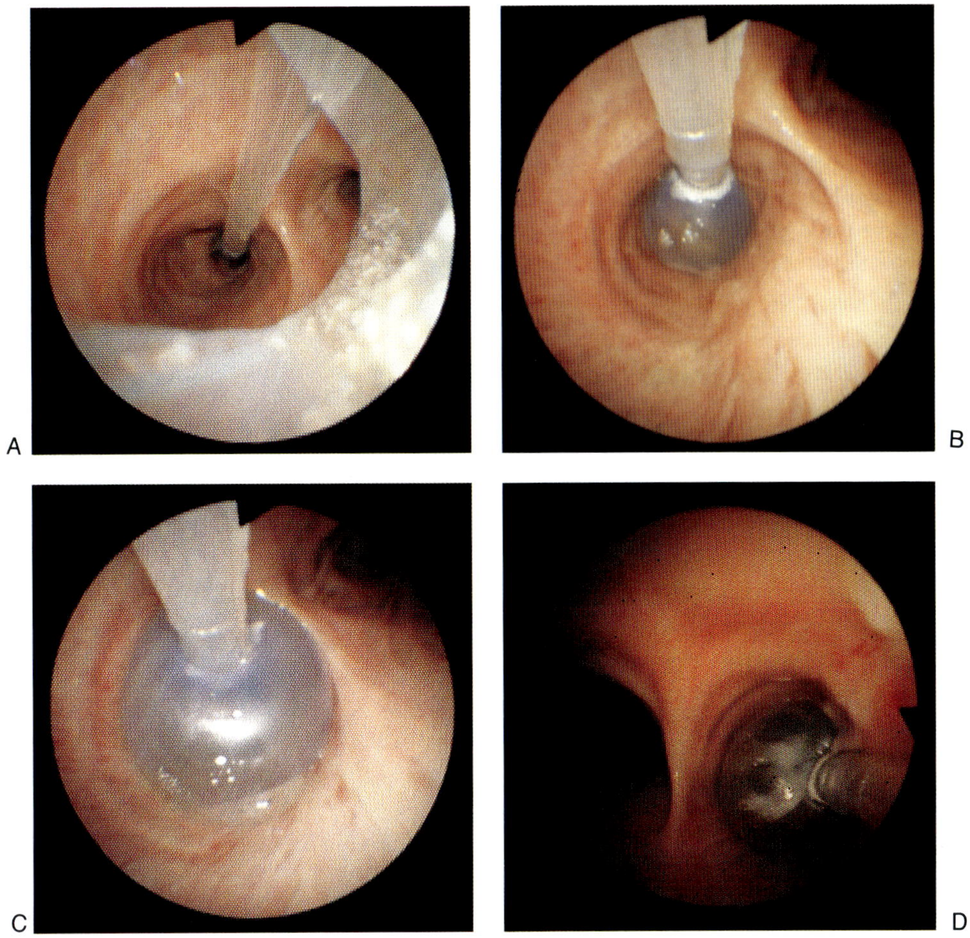

FIG. 24. Endoscopic view of positioning the Univent tube blocker and its balloon position in left and right main stem bronchi. **A:** Shows the tip of the Univent main tube about 3 cm above the carina and the blocker inside the left main stem bronchus. **B:** Shows the balloon in its most distal position possible while achieving separation of the entire left lung. The balloon is positioned at the level of left upper lobe bronchus takeoff. **C:** The balloon of the blocker at the most proximal position possible to provide separation of the left lung avoiding herniation over the carina blocking the right main stem bronchus. **D:** Shows the position of the balloon in right main stem blocking the entire right lung.

A blindly placed DLT allows for unobstructed bilateral lung isolation, without impairing the clinician's ability to locate the general site of hemorrhage. Should the left-sided DLT inadvertently enter the right main stem bronchus, with blockage of the right upper lobe, oxygenation may still remain adequate. The DLT is also the only intubating device that permits adequate access to the nonventilated lung, for techniques such as pulmonary lavage, while protecting the ventilating lung.

Because of its relative ease of intubation, the Univent® endotracheal tube may prove useful in patients with upper airway abnormalities. It should be kept in mind that the smallest available Univent® tube (6.0-mm ID) corresponds to an 8.5-mm ID endotracheal tube (Table 3). The measured external circumference of a 6.0-mm ID Univent tube is 33 Fr, not much smaller than the standard 35 Fr DLT (81). The high takeoff of the right upper lobe bronchus excludes the use of Univent® tube or other endobronchial blockers for right side thoracotomy (Fig. 6A).

If the Univent® tube is left in place for postoperative ventilatory support, precautions should be taken to avoid accidental injury to the patient (82). In one postoperative patient, the retracted bronchial blocker inadvertently moved beyond the tip of the main tube. A technician correcting an air leakage around the tracheal cuff, inadvertently inflated the bronchial cuff, which obstructed the main tube lumen causing severe patient distress. Fortunately, the problem was immediately recognized by the anesthesiologist, who deflated the bronchial cuff before any harm to the patient ensued (82).

When the patient is left intubated with a Univent® tube, precautions should be taken to avoid similar accidents. The bronchial blocker should be retracted fully inside the conduit, and the shaft of the blocker should be taped to the main tube to prevent advancement of the blocker into the trachea. In addition, the bronchial blocker cap and pilot balloon should be taped to prevent accidental opening of the cap, which will cause a leak in the system or accidental inflation of the blocker balloon. It is vital to provide in-service training to all medical and paramedical personnel managing patients with a Univent® tube.

The Success and Failure Rate of the Univent Tube

The number of clinical research papers on the Univent tube is limited. In one report of 50 cases, blind placement of the Univent tube was satisfactory in 90% of the patients studied (83). The fiberoptic bronchoscope was used for successful placement in five cases. In one instance, satisfactory deflation of the lung could not be achieved; in another patient, hypoxemia and hypercarbia developed from partial blockade of the Univent® tube by secretions. On two occasions, the blocker was dislodged after patient positioning in the lateral decubitus position. The blocker was then repositioned with the aid of a bronchofiberscope (83).

In another series involving eight patients, blind placement was unsuccessful on seven occasions. The fiberoptic bronchoscope was used for successful positioning in four of these patients. A satisfactory seal could not be achieved in three patients, and the Univent® tube was replaced with a double-lumen tube (27).

Case reports describing the sucessful use of the Univent® tube in aortic aneurysm repair, lung transplantation, bronchopulmonary fistula repair, and management of hemoptysis have been published (78,80,84). The Univent® tube is claimed to be less traumatic than DLT placement, and therefore a better choice for patients on anticoagulants (85). The Univent® tube, like the DLT, can be placed through a tracheostomy stoma to provide isolation of the lungs.

FIBEROPTIC-AIDED PLACEMENT OF A FOGARTY CATHETER BRONCHIAL BLOCKER

The Fogarty embolectomy catheter has been utilized as a bronchial blocker in children and adults requiring one-lung anesthesia (13–15). The catheters are available in various sizes (inflated balloon diameter, 5–14 mm).

After the establishment of general anesthesia and muscle relaxation, a Fogarty catheter with the tip angled toward the intended bronchus is placed in the distal trachea under rigid laryngoscopy. This is followed by tracheal placement of a single-lumen endotracheal tube. Mechanical ventilation is initiated. To visualize the Fogarty catheter, a fiberscope is inserted through the tracheal tube bronchoscopy adapter and advanced beyond the distal end of the endotracheal tube. The tracheal cuff is deflated, and the Fogarty catheter is manipulated so its angled tip is directed toward the intended bronchus (Fig. 25).

The tip of the fiberscope can be used to help direct the catheter into the bronchus. In blockade of the left-lung, the balloon of the Fogarty catheter is positioned immediately above the orifice of the left upper lobe bronchus to provide better stability (Fig. 25). In blockade of the right lung, the tip of the catheter is placed just beyond the right upper lobe orifice, and the balloon inflated to occlude the main stem bronchus (Fig. 26).

Fogarty catheters can also be guided into a lobar bronchus to produce atelectasis of either upper or lower lobe. This technique allows only one selected lobe to be blocked in a patient who may not tolerate collapse of an entire lung.

The Fogarty catheter can be used to block the operative lung when the position of a DLT is not satisfactory or the DLT becomes nonfunctional due to leak of the bronchial cuff. In such cases, the Fogarty catheter is passed through the DLT lumen, providing ventilation to the operative lung. The bronchial tube is pulled back to allow adequate space in the main stem bronchus to position the Fogarty catheter balloon at or above the origin of the respective upper lobe bronchus. It is preferable to leave the tip of the DLT bronchial tube inside the bronchus, as this will prevent dislodgment of the Fogarty catheter.

If the nonoperative pulmonary bronchus is intubated, the Fogarty catheter is passed through the DLT tracheal lumen into the operative lung bronchus and positioned as described above. The DLT bronchial cuff is then deflated and the DLT pulled back to allow proper ventilation of the nonoperative lung. A small-sized Foley catheter has been used under these circumstances (86).

→

FIG. 25. Fiberoptic positioning of Fogarty catheter as a bronchial blocker in the left side main stem bronchus. **A:** Fogarty catheter in the lower trachea. **B:** The endotracheal tube in place with cuff inflated. The Fogarty catheter is seen beyond the tip of the endotracheal tube. **C:** The fiberscope is advanced through the endotracheal tube and visualizes the Fogarty catheter. The tracheal cuff is deflated and the Fogarty catheter is advanced into the left main stem bronchus. **D:** The Fogarty catheter cuff is inflated to block the main stem bronchus. **E:** The fiberscope is removed, leaving the Fogarty catheter in place. **F:** Endoscopic view of Fogarty catheter balloon positioned in left main stem.

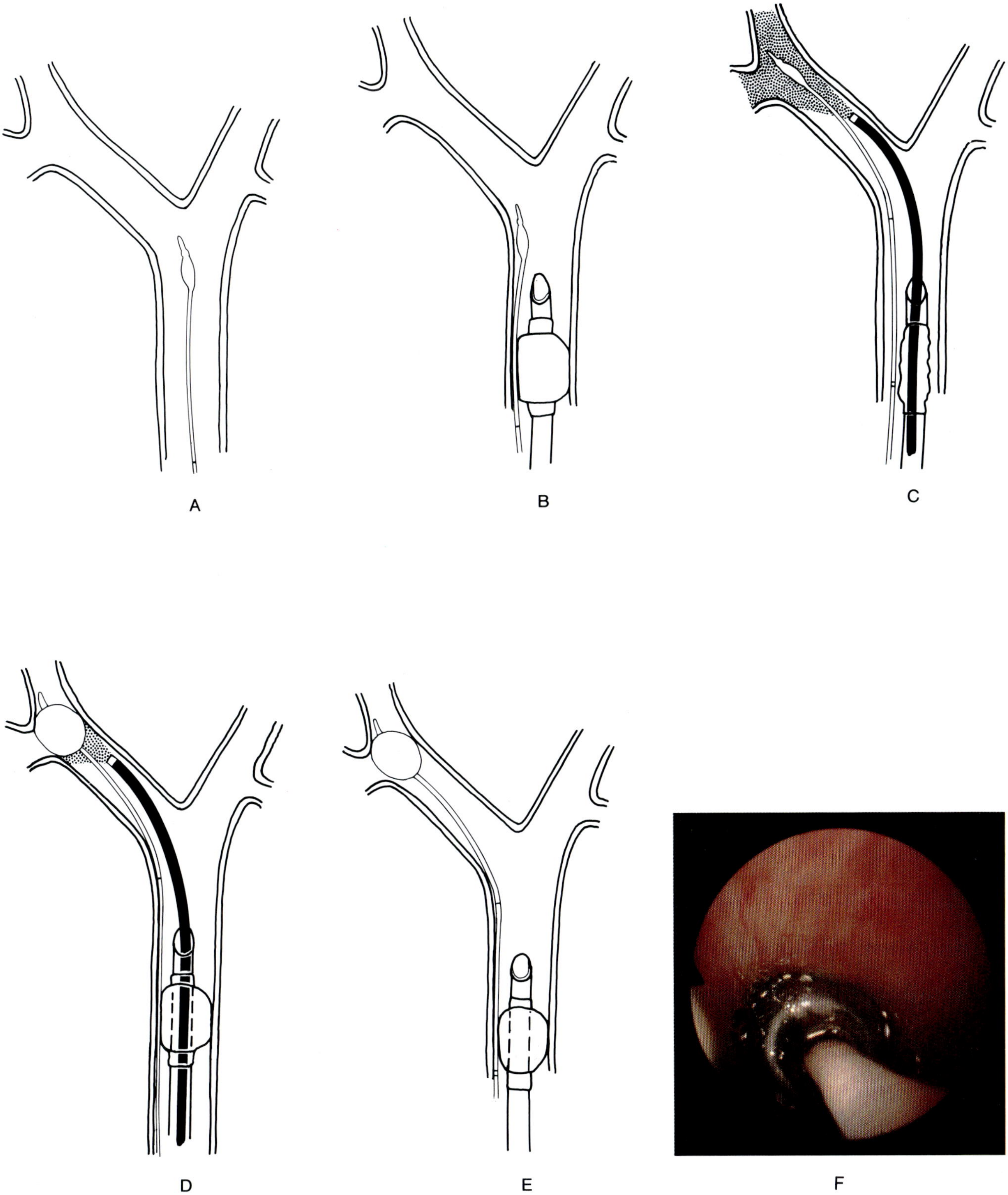

FIG. 25. *Continued.*

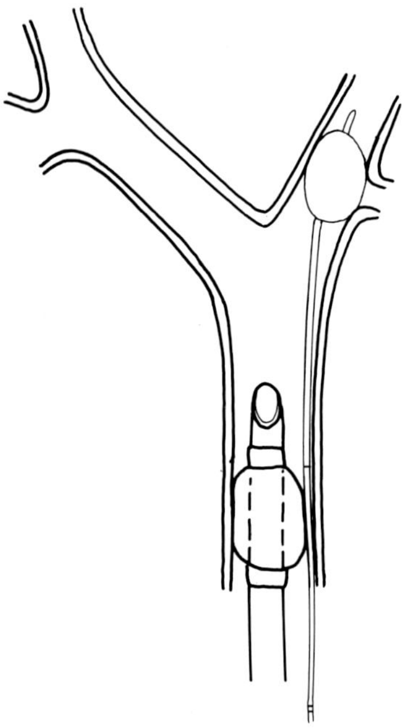

FIG. 26. Fogarty catheter in right main stem bronchus. The steps followed are similar to those in Fig. 25.

In children, a Fogarty catheter positioned in the bronchus of the diseased lung, with the tracheal tube placed in the opposite bronchus, serves the same objective as a DLT in the adult (87,88). If the Fogarty catheter fails to fully block the bronchus on the disease side, the dependent lung remains protected. The techniques utilized for selective bronchial intubation in infants and children include blind techniques, fluoroscopy, and direct visualization techniques by rigid and fiberoptic bronchoscopy.

Blind intubation of the right main stem bronchus includes a high incidence of right upper lobe collapse (89). This complication may be avoided by rotating the endotracheal tube 180°, so that its bevel faces laterally toward the orifice of the right upper lobe bronchus (89,90). The rotation of the bronchial tube after intubation may cause trauma. Fiberoptic bronchoscopy simplifies endobronchial intubation and allows the endoscopist to avoid blockade of the upper lobe bronchus.

ONE-LUNG ANESTHESIA

The performance of successful OLA is one of the more difficult and specialized skills that an anesthesiologist should develop when providing general anesthesia for intrathoracic operations. The technique must be performed in a safe and efficient manner, ensuring safety and control of the airway (78).

Monitoring during One-Lung Anesthesia

In addition to the routine anesthesia monitors, an arterial line is placed for continuous blood pressure and serial blood gas measurements. Sudden changes in arterial blood pressure, secondary to surgical manipulation or arrhythmias are common during thoracotomy. Routine and immediate arterial blood samples for gas and acid base analysis, along with measurements of hemoglobin and serum potassium, should be available.

The use of pulse oximetry, while of great value should not be substituted for arterial blood gas analysis. Changes in the partial pressure of arterial oxygen (PaO_2) provide early and concise quantitative data on arterial oxygen tension before changes are reflected in significant drops in hemoglobin oxygen saturation. The patient's acid-base status provides valuable data concerning alveolar ventilation, cardiac output, and fluid replacement. The technology for continuous monitoring of the arterial blood gases is now available and will provide continuous monitoring of oxygen tension, ventilation, and acid/base status of the patient. The usefulness of continuous monitoring of the arterial blood gases during OLV is described in a report by Greenblott (91).

Airway pressures require careful monitoring during intrathoracic operations. The peak and plateau airway pressures should be recorded during bilateral and single-lung ventilation in supine and lateral positions (3). Any major change in airway pressure should be evaluated and explained. Multiple factors may affect airway pressures. These factors include blockage of the upper lobe bronchus by the endobronchial tube, obstruction of the bronchial or tracheal tube lumen due to compression against the bronchial or tracheal walls, obstruction by secretions, patient biting on the tracheal tube, and bronchospasm. All may affect and change the peak and plateau airway pressures.

The recent use of on-line pressure and volume spirometry has proved useful for breath-to-breath measurement of airway pressure and resistance. The patient serves as their control, with subsequent patterns compared against the patient's baseline. Changes in generated pressure/volume loops may indicate malpositioning of the DLT (66,67). Bardoczky and colleagues could identify 66% of malpositioned DLTs by using pressure/volume loop data, and they utilized the spirometric loops to correct the malposition.

Measurements of central venous and pulmonary artery pressures are difficult to interpret during intrathoracic procedures and in laterally positioned patients (92). A central line, however, provides access for rapid blood replacement if needed. Placement of a central line on the operative side is useful should a pneumothorax develop. A pulmonary artery catheter should only be placed on the nonoperative side, with its position confirmed by radiography.

Ventilation during One-Lung Anesthesia

In the lateral decubitus position, the dependent lung's volume is reduced by the paralyzed, raised diaphragm and by the compressive effects of the mediastinum. This will contribute to atelectasis of the lower lung. To avoid atelectasis, relatively large tidal volumes (10 ml/kg) are essential during OLV.

If the minute ventilation during OLV is kept the same as during two-lung ventilation, the arterial carbon dioxide tension (P_aCO_2) will be maintained at a level similar to that of two-lung ventilation (93). However, since the compliance of the dependent lung is decreased and its tidal volume is almost doubled during OLV, the peak airway pressure is increased by approximately 50% when compared with two-lung ventilation. A larger proportion of the delivered tidal volume may be wasted because of increased airway pressure and compression effect and/or distension of the breathing circuit (94).

Oxygenation during One-Lung Anesthesia

Arterial oxygen tension (P_aO_2) decreases during OLA, primarily as a result of increased venous admixture (95–97). Various OLV studies have shown that the shunt (Qs/Qt), through the nonventilated lung is about 25–40% of cardiac output (95,97,98). This degree of shunt is less than one would expect from complete collapse of an entire lung. Several factors are responsible for this. The two most important factors are: the effect of gravity and hydrostatic pressure in the lateral decubitus position; and hypoxic pulmonary vasoconstriction (HPV) which shifts the distribution of the blood flow in favor of the dependent lung (99,100). The operative lung may also have decreased pulmonary blood flow, owing to the underlying pulmonary pathology. Surgical compression of the heart and major vessels, along with changes in cardiac output and oxygen consumption, are additional factors that will influence arterial oxygen tension.

The pulmonary circulation responds to acute hypoxia by vasoconstriction, leading to increases in pulmonary artery pressure and vascular resistance. The systemic circulation typically responds to hypoxia by vasodilation (101). Hypoxic pulmonary vasoconstriction initiates within seconds of pulmonary ventilation with an hypoxic gas mixture, peaks to a maximum within minutes, and can be sustained for hours (102,103).

The effect of time on the HPV was studied in six subjects during general anesthesia on mechanical ventilation. One-lung was ventilated with a mixture of 5% oxygen in nitrogen (104). A control lung was ventilated with 100% oxygen. The fractional perfusion of the hypoxic lung decreased from 53% to 25% of cardiac output within the first minute of unilateral hypoxia. The pulmonary artery mean pressure and pulmonary vascular resistance increased by 14% and 54%, respectively. Venous admixture increased from 21% to 39% of cardiac output while the true shunt was maintained at approximately 15%. The findings suggest that there is an immediate vasoconstrictive response to hypoxia in the human lung, with no further potentiation or diminution of the response, during a 60 min period of hypoxia (104).

The threshold for vasoconstriction occurs at alveolar oxygen tension (P_aO_2) of approximately 60 mm Hg. While alveolar hypoxia is the main cause of HPV, low mixed venous oxygen tension also contributes to the initiation of this response (105,106).

The small muscular pulmonary arteries at the level of the terminal respiratory bronchioles are the major site for HPV response (107,108). The pulmonary capillary bed and venous system also contribute, although much less, to this phenomenon (109).

The precise mechanism of HPV remains unproved. One hypothesis holds that it is induced by a vasoactive mediator released from a site within the hypoxic lung (101). A second theory suggests that hypoxia acts directly on the pulmonary vessel wall, causing vasoconstriction (110). Several factors may modify HPV, including inhalation of anesthetic agents, vasodilators, and vasoconstrictors, as well as deviation of the acid-base status of the blood (111).

High concentrations of inhalation anesthetics may inhibit HPV, increasing blood flow to the nonventilated lung and consequently decreasing PaO_2 (99,112). Halothane and isoflurane cause an insignificant change in the shunted blood volume when used in a concentration of up to 1 MAC (113,114). To avoid the possible inhibition of HPV by high concentrations of inhalation anesthetics and further minimize the respiratory depressant effect of high doses of narcotics, a combination of a narcotic and an inhalation anesthetic is recommended for intrathoracic operations and OLV.

Nitric oxide (NO), acts as a selective pulmonary vasodilator in patients with pulmonary hypertension. Vasodilation is limited to the pulmonary vasculature because inhaled NO is rapidly inactivated by hemoglobin as soon as it enters circulation (115). Nitric oxide inhaled at a concentration of 20 parts per million acts as a selective pulmonary vasodilator in patients undergoing one-lung ventilation with moderate pulmonary hypertension secondary to cardiac disease. Inhaled NO does not increase venous admixture or impair oxygenation (116). It is yet to be shown whether hypoxic thoracotomy patients undergoing OLV will benefit from inhaled NO.

Intravenous vasodilator prostacyclin, given to patients with ARDS, and sodium nitroprusside and nitroglycerine, used in patients with normal lung function, all increased pulmonary shunting by 25% and 20–70% respectively (117,118). The resultant decrease in P_aO_2 and the increase in shunting, secondary to intravenous vasodilation, result from the inhibition of HPV (119,120). Intravenous sodium nitroprusside used to lower patient's systolic blood pressure by 25% during OLV in the lateral decubitus position failed to produce increases in pulmonary shunt or lower arterial blood oxygen tension. The authors concluded that sodium nitroprusside, under these circumstances, increases cardiac index but fails to counteract the effects of HPV (121).

To guard against hypoxemia during OLV, oxygen at an FIO_2 of 1.0 should be used whenever possible. Patients treated with bleomycin, amiodarone, and mitomycin-C may suffer oxygen-induced pulmonary toxicity, and the use of 100% oxygen may not be desirable (122–125). In others P_aO_2 may remain suboptimal, even with 100% oxygen and an appropriately placed endobronchial tube. The application of various techniques to modify mechanical ventilation have been utilized in attempts to improve oxygenation during OLV. These techniques include:

1. The insufflation of oxygen at 2–4 l into the operative lung by a catheter placed inside the operative side tube lumen. Study results on the usefulness of this technique remain inconclusive (126–128).
2. The application of continuous positive airway pressure (CPAP). Nondependent lung CPAP has been shown to improve arterial blood oxygenation (127,129,130), and various devices for this purpose have been recommended (130–133). For CPAP to be effective, the nonventilated lung should be reinflated prior to application of CPAP (129). A self-assembled disposable CPAP device is available (Broncho-Cath CPAP System, Mallinkrodt Medical, Inc., St. Louis, Missouri). The device can deliver CPAP as low as 2 cm H_2O, with considerable improvement of P_aO_2 during OLV (133). CPAP will not be useful during bronchoplasty or in the presence of bronchopleural fistula or when the bronchial tree is obstructed with tumor.

While application of CPAP to the nonventilated lung improves arterial oxygenation, it also causes distension of the operative lung, which may interfere with surgical dissection. In one study, proper application of CPAP demonstrated overall improvement in oxygenation was possible without compromising the operative site (129). The use of CPAP applied to the operative lung during OLV with a Univent tube has been reported (134).

Patients treated with bleomycin may be at increased risk of developing pulmonary complications when exposed to oxygen concentration greater than 30% (136–138). Hughes and Benumof have described the use of air/O_2 mixture CPAP (FIO_2 0.3) applied to the nonventilated lung in a bleomycin-treated patient requiring OLV. The P_aO_2 was maintained between 79 to 130 mm Hg at an FIO_2 of 30% using this technique (135).

3. The application of positive end-expiratory pressure (PEEP) to the dependent lung. Positive end-expiratory pressure of the ventilated lung increases functional residual capacity and intra-alveolar pressure, diverting a higher proportion of pulmonary blood flow to the nonventilated lung. It also contributes to a reduction in cardiac output (96). Depending on the degree of increased intra-alveolar pressure, along with its effect on the pulmonary circulation and cardiac output, P_aO_2 may increase, decrease, or remain unchanged (139). It is best to apply PEEP to the dependent lung after CPAP has been applied to the nondependent lung.
4. Differential lung ventilation. Differential lung ventilation incorporating two separate ventilator systems, has been used in patients with severe unilateral lung disease (140). It has also been used to minimize shunting and improve oxygenation in patients undergoing surgery in the lateral decubitus position (141). A modified and simple technique of differential lung ventilation is described for thoracoscopic ligation of pulmonary bullae (142), as well as a means of improving oxygenation during thoracotomy (143).
5. The technique of intermittently reinflating the collapsed lung. During OLV, manual intermittent reinflation of the operative lung with 100% oxygen every 5 min helps to improve arterial oxygenation (144). This technique was initially recommended in 1950 by Bjork (145). The major drawback to the technique is its disturbance to the surgeon if not coordinated with the appropriate stage(s) of the surgical procedure.
6. Two lung, high-frequency positive pressure ventilation (HFPPV). High-frequency positive pressure ventilation has been used during thoracic surgery for maintaining good arterial oxygenation (146,147). The HFPPV compared favorably to one-lung ventilation with 5 cm CPAP (147).
7. Obstruction of the operative lung's pulmonary artery or its branches. Clamping or ligation of the pulmonary artery or its branches to the collapsed section of lung, will also reduce the shunt and improve arterial blood oxygenation.

COMPLICATIONS

Complications in the use of DLTs and endobronchial blockers are frequently associated with difficulties experienced in their passage and positioning. Dislodgement during patient positioning and during the operation also must be guarded against (Table 13). Problems resulting from improperly positioned bronchial tubes include incomplete isolation of the lungs, air entry into the wrong lung, difficulty in ventilating one or both lungs, air trapping, and unsatisfactory deflation of the lung (48,50).

If not recognized, airway obstruction will result in poor ventilation and hypoxemia. Additionally, air trapping may produce rupture of the lung and tension of the pneumothorax. If isolation is incomplete, potential soiling of the dependent lung may add to difficulties with ventilation and oxygenation, especially in the presence of bronchopleural fistula.

Because of the shape and size of DLTs, the incidence of difficult and failed tracheal intubation is high (24,48,50). The PVC tubes are easier to pass into the trachea and cause less mucosal damage than red rubber tubes (68,148).

Rupture of the tracheobronchial tree has been reported with all types and varieties of endobronchial tubes (50,148–154). In a series of 2700 thoracotomies using red rubber Carlens tubes, tracheobronchial rupture occurred in five patients (149). The site of laceration is usually the posterior membranous wall of the trachea or a main stem bronchus.

Tracheobronchial rupture has been attributed to direct trauma during intubation as a result of inappropriate tube size selection, advancing the tube with a stylet, or using undue force to advance the tube. Rapid overinflation of the bronchial cuff and respiratory tree pathology are other factors implicated in this complication (50,149,150).

TABLE 13. *Complications of bronchial intubation and one-lung ventilation*

- Technical
  - Unsuccessful or difficult intubation
  - Trauma of the airway
    - Minor trauma
    - Rupture of the tracheobronchial tree
  - Improper position of the bronchial tube
    - Tube not inserted far enough
    - Intubation of wrong bronchus
    - Tube inserted too far into the intended bronchus
  - Tube dislodgment
- Hypoxemia
  - One-lung ventilation—increased venous admixture
  - Alteration of hypoxic pulmonary vasoconstriction
  - Increased alveolar pressure
  - Decreased cardiac output
  - Atelectasis of the dependent lung

A number of suggestions to prevent bronchial rupture include inflation of the bronchial cuff with anesthetic gas mixture to prevent overdistension by nitrous oxide, periodic deflation of the bronchial cuff to prevent excessive pressure buildup (43), deflation of the bronchial cuff before placing the patient in the lateral decubitus position, and delaying inflation of the bronchial cuff until the onset of OLV (40,43). The deflation of the bronchial cuff, however, leaves the down lung unprotected and vulnerable to contamination or obstruction by secretions or necrotic tumor (155).

My routine practice is to inflate the bronchial cuff prior to positioning the patient, leaving it inflated until the operation is completed. The cuff is deflated only after careful suctioning and establishing that the lung is dry. In the presence of secretions and/or oozing of blood, the bronchial cuff should remain inflated until the patient is turned to the supine position. The cuff is deflated before reversal of muscle relaxants.

The presence of an air leak, subcutaneous emphysema, airway hemorrhage, pneumothorax, or cardiovascular instability should alert the practitioner to the possible existence of airway damage. The signs and symptoms of tracheobronchial injury may occur hours after the initial injury (154). Surgical correction and repair should be performed, as soon as possible after the diagnosis is made. The diagnosis of airway damage may be greatly aided by the use of fiberoptic bronchoscopy.

Malposition of the DLT may occur secondary to inadequate advancement of the tube, intubation of the wrong bronchus, or insertion of the endobronchial tube too far down the bronchus (48–50,54,156). Inadequate advancement of the endobronchial tube increases the chances of tube dislodgment, resulting in loss of separation of the lungs or ventilation of the wrong lung. In two separate case reports, the left-sided endobronchial tube repositioned itself into the unintended bronchus. In one case, this tube movement occurred during left lateral positioning. In the second case, the tube repositioned itself during surgical manipulation of the hilum of the lung (157, 158).

Obstruction of a DLT secondary to a manufacturing defect (159), torsion of the endobronchial tube (160), and design defects have all been reported (161). Anatomic variations, e.g., presence of tracheal bronchus, saber-sheath trachea, congenital tracheal stenosis and acute takeoff of the left main stem bronchus, have all been reported as potential obstructive problems (46,59,162).

The blind placement of a left-sided DLT producing

a torsion of its bronchial tube was implicated as causing a partial obstruction and inadequate ventilation of the left hemithorax. The retraction of the DLT back to the trachea with readvancment over a fiberscope into the left main bronchus corrected the problem. The author concluded that fiberoptic evaluation of both lumens of the DLT should be routinely performed to avoid this malpositioning problem (160).

The term "saber-sheath trachea" is used to describe a U-shaped tracheal lumen having a narrow coronal diameter and normal sagittal diameter (163). The saber-sheath trachea is often associated with chronic obstructive disease. The external diameter of a 37 Fr DLT is approximately 1.4 cm in the coronal plane, measured just above the opening of the tracheal lumen. The narrowed saber-sheath trachea may compress against the DLT's tracheal lumen opening, obstructing ventilation (162).

Two rare but potentially fatal complications reported in association with DLT use include the rupture of the pulmonary artery on extubation, due to inadvertent suturing of the pulmonary artery to the bronchial tube (41). In another case passage of an endobronchial tube in the presence of a large mediastinal mass led to displacement of the mass and resultant major vascular obstruction resulting in cardiac arrest (164).

Complications associated with the Univent® tube have included a failure to position the blocker in the intended bronchus (27,165), displacemnt of the blocker after positioning (83,165), dislodgment of the silicone cap covering the tip of the blocker (28), trauma to tracheobronchial mucosa (27), and pneumothorax (165). The Univent® tube bronchial blocker, because of its small diameter and stiffness, has the potential to penetrate into the pleural space or mediastinum during positioning. This danger is heightened during its blind placement.

CONCLUSION

Fiberoptic bronchoscopes are now used with greater regularity when an endobronchial tube or blocker is incorporated into the anesthesia procedure. However, their use is often limited to checking the position of the bronchial cuff after blind insertion of a left-sided DLT, or to evaluate difficulties encountered during the blind positioning of the tube. The discredited impression that fiberoptic techniques are too time consuming to allow for their full potential use for evaluation of the bronchial tree and endobronchial intubation continues to raise concern.

The full and greatest value of the fiberscope lies in its ability to enable the medical practitioner check out the anatomy of the lower airway and to direct the endobronchial tube or blocker to the proper bronchial position under direct vision. Such use of the fiberscope would completely eliminate the common error of incorrect bronchial placement of blind technique (Table 13).

Fiberoptic placement of bronchial tubes under direct vision represent a precise, highly successful technique. It is far less likely to intubate the wrong bronchus than the blind techniques, which currently result in a 20%–30% occurrence of wrong bronchial placement of left-sided tubes.

Anatomic abnormalities and pathologic conditions that may interfere with bronchial placement can also be recognized prior to bronchial intubation, thereby eliminating the possibility of a major complication developing in association with the use of these tubes. The ease with which the current generation of small-sized fiberscopes can be passed through the double-lumen tube allows for repeated examinations and therapeutic intervention when required, without impeding ventilation of the patient.

The technique of fiberoptic airway endoscopy is within the reach of every anesthesiologist in the United States. Every effort should be made to learn and develop the full potential of this tool for the insertion and positioning of bronchial tubes and blockers. There is a legitimate question as to whether blind instrumentation of the lower airway anatomy should take place with such a specific diagnostic instrument available. The documented discrepancies between auscultation and fiberoptic identification relative to appropriate placement and positioning of DLTs warn that traditional approaches to their placement should not be relied upon.

The fiberoptic approach is the only reliable technique available to accurately combat these problems. Its use should be mastered by all who provide anesthesia for intrathoracic operations.

REFERENCES

1. Coosemans W, Lerut TE, Van Raemdonk DE. Thoracoscopic surgery: the Belgian experience. *Ann Thorac Surg* 1993;56: 721–730.
2. Collard JM, Lendele B, Otte JB, Kestens PJ. En bloc and standard esophagectomy by thoracoscopy. *Ann Thorac Surg* 1993; 56:675–679.
3. Ovassapian A, Schrader SC. Fiberoptic-aided bronchial intubation. *Semin Anesthesia* 1987;6:133–142.
4. Benumof JL. *Anesthesia for thoracic surgery*. 2nd edition. Philadelphia: W.B. Saunders, 1955.
5. Marshall BE, Longnecker DL, Fairley HB. *Anesthesia for thoracic procedures*. Boston: Blackwell Scientific Publications, 1987.
6. Cohen E. The practice of thoracic anesthesia. Philadelphia: JB Lippincott, 1995.
7. Gothard JWW. *Anaesthesia for thoracic surgery*. 2nd ed. London: Blackwell Scientific Publication, 1993.
8. Selecky PA, Wasserman K, Benfield JR, Lippmann M. The clinical and physiological effect of whole-lung lavage in pulmo-

nary alveolar proteinosis: a ten year experience. *Ann Thorac Surg* 1977;24:451–461.

9. Stein JM, Lisbon A. Pulmonary hemorrhage from pulmonary artery catheterization treated with endobronchial intubation. *Anesthesiology* 1981;55:698–699.
10. Venus B, Pratap KS, Op'Tholt T. Treatment of unilateral pulmonary insufficiency by selective administration of continuous positive airway pressure through a double-lumen tube. *Anesthesiology* 1980;53:74–77.
11. White GMJ. Evolution of endotracheal and endobronchial intubation. *Br J Anaesth* 1960;32:235–246.
12. Poppin JC. The current practice of endobronchial intubation. *Anaesthesia* 1979;34:57–64.
13. Inoue H, Shohtsu A, Ogawa J, et al. New device for one-lung anesthesia: endotracheal tube with movable blocker. *J Thorac Cardiovasc Surg* 1982;83:940–941.
14. Vale R. Selective bronchial blocking in a small child. *Br J Anaesth* 1969;41:453–455.
15. Hogg CE, Lorhan PH. Pediatric bronchial blocking. *Anesthesiology* 1970;33:560–562.
16. Ginsberg RJ. New technique for one-lung anesthesia using an endobronchial blocker. *J Thorac Cardiovasc Surg* 1981;82: 542–546.
17. Carlens E. A new flexible double-lumen catheter for bronchospirometry. *J Thorac Surg* 1949;18:742–746.
18. Newman RW, Finer GE, Downs JE. Routine use of Carlens double-lumen endobronchial catheter: an experimental and clinical study. *J Thorac Cardiovasc Surg* 1961;42:327–336.
19. Bryce-Smith R. A double-lumen endobronchial tube. *Br J Anaesth* 1959;31:274–275.
20. White GMJ. A new double-lumen tube. *Br J Anaesth* 1960;32: 232–234.
21. Robertshaw FL. Low resistance double-lumen endobronchial tubes. *Br J Anaesth* 1962;34:576–579.
22. Hammond JE, Wright DJ. Comparison of resistances of double-lumen endobronchial tubes. *Br J Anaesth* 1984;56:299–301.
23. Chiaranda M, Rossi A, Manani G, et al. Measurement of the flow-resistive properties of double-lumen bronchial tubes *in vitro*. *Anaesthesia* 1989;44:335–340.
24. Burton NA, Watson DC, Brodsky JB, Mark JBD. Advantages of a new polyvinyl chloride double-lumen tube in thoracic surgery. *Ann Thorac Surg* 1983;36:78–84.
25. Slinger PD, Chripko D. A clinical comparison of bronchial cuff pressures in three different designs of left double-lumen tubes. *Anesth Analg* 1993;77:305–308.
26. Kamaya H, Krishna PR. New endobronchial tube (Univent tube) for selective blockade of one lung. *Anesthesiology* 1985; 63:342–343.
27. MacGillivray RG. Evaluation of a new tracheal tube with a movable bronchus blocker. *Anaesthesia* 1988;43:687–689.
28. Arai T, Hatano Y. Yet another reason to use a fiberoptic bronchoscope to properly site a double-lumen tube. *Anesthesiology* 1987;66:581–582.
29. Hannallah MS, Benumof JL. Comparison of two techniques to inflate the bronchial cuff of the Univent tube. *Anesth Analg* 1992;75:784–787.
30. Davis NJ. A new fiberoptic laryngoscope for nasal intubation. *Anesth Analg* 1973;52:807–808.
31. Prithvi Raj P, Forestner J, Watson TD, et al. Techniques for fiberoptic laryngoscopy in anesthesia. *Anesth Analg* 1974;53: 708–714.
32. Harrell JH, Spragg RG, Moser KM. Orotracheal intubation using the double-lumen tube. In: Nakhosteen JA, Maassen W, eds. *Bronchology: research, diagnostic and therapeutic aspect*. The Hague: Nijhoff, 1981;121–123.
33. Ovassapian A, Braunschweig R, Joshi CW. Endobronchial intubation using flexible fiberoptic bronchoscope. *Anesthesiology* 1981;55:A347.
34. Desira WR. The use of the fiberoptic bronchoscope for the passage of a double-lumen tube. *Anaesthesia* 1981;36:233.
35. Shinnick JP, Freedman AP. Bronchofiberscopic placement of a double-lumen endotracheal tube. *Crit Care Med* 1982;10: 544–546.
36. Shulman MS, Brodsky JB, Levesque PR. Fiberoptic bronchoscopy for tracheal and endobronchial intubation with a double-lumen tube. *Can J Anaesth* 1987;34:172–173.
37. Watson CB. Fiberoptic bronchoscopy for anesthesia. *Anesthesiol Rev* 1982;9:17–26.
38. Alfery DD, Benumof JL. Anesthesia for bronchopulmonary lavage. In: Kaplan J, ed. *Thoracic anesthesia*. New York: Churchill-Livingstone, 1982;403–419.
39. Smith GB, Hirsch NP, Ehrenwerth J. Placement of double-lumen endobronchial tubes. Correlation between clinical impressions and bronchoscopic findings. *Br J Anaesth* 1986; 58:1317–1320.
40. Wilson RS. Endobronchial intubation. In: Kaplan JA, ed. *Thoracic Anesthesia*. New York: Churchill-Livingstone, 1983; 389–402.
41. Dryden GE. Circulatory collapse after pneumonectomy. An unusual complication from the use of a Carlens catheter—case report. *Anesth Analg* 1977;56:451–452.
42. Benumof JL, Partridge BL, Salvatierra C, Keating J. Margin of safety in positioning modern double-lumen endotracheal tubes. *Anesthesiology* 1987;67:729–738.
43. Brodsky JB, Mark BD. A simple technique for accurate placement of double-lumen endobronchial tubes. *Anesthesiol Rev* 1983;10:26–30.
44. Saito S, Dohi S, Tajima K. Failure of double-lumen endobronchial intubation. *J Cardioth Vascul Anesth* 1990;4: 229–231.
45. Slinger PD. Fiberoptic bronchoscopic positioning of double-lumen tubes. *J Cardioth Vascul Anesth* 1989;3:486–496.
46. Ovassapian A. Fiberoptic-aided bronchial intubation. In: Ovassapian, A. ed. *Fiberoptic airway endoscopy in anesthesia and critical care*. New York: Raven Press, 1990;80–104.
47. Allliaume B, Coddens J, Deloof T. Reliability of auscultation in positioning of double-lumen endobronchial tubes. *Can J Anaesth* 1992;39:687–690.
48. Conacher ID, Herrema IH, Batchelor AM. Robertshaw double lumen tubes: a reappraisal thirty years on. *Anaesth Intens Care* 1994;22:179–183.
49. Hurford WE, Alfille PH. A quality improvement study of the placement and complications of double-lumen endobronchial tubes. *J Cardiothoracic Vasc Anesth* 1993;7:517–520.
50. Black AMS, Harrison GA. Difficulties with positioning Robertshaw double-lumen tubes. *Anaesth Intens Care* 1975;3: 299–311.
51. Cohen JA, Denisco RA, Richards RS, et al. Hazardous placement of a Robertshaw-type endobronchial tube. *Anesth Analg* 1986;65:100–101.
52. Dunne NM, Gillbe CE. Endobronchial apparatus and its intraoperative management. *Bailliere's Clin Anesthesiol* 1987;1: 79–98.
53. Burk WJ. Should a fiberoptic bronchoscope be routinely used to position a double-lumen tube? *Anesthesiology* 1988;68:826.
54. Watson CB. Fiberoptic bronchoscopy in thoracic anesthesia. *Bailliere's Clin Anesthesiol* 1987;1:33–60.
55. Cobley M, Kidd JF, Willis BA, Vaughan RS. Endobronchial Cuff Pressures. *Brit J Anaesth* 1993;70:576–578.
56. Hannallah MS, Benumof JL, Bachenheimer LC, Mundt DJ. The resting volume and compliance characteristics of the bronchial cuff of left polyvinyl chloride double-lumen endobronchial tubes. *Anesth Analg* 1993;77:1222–1226.
57. Barat M, Horst RK. Tracheal Bronchus. *Am J Otolaryngol* 1987;8:118–122.
58. Morrison SC. Case report: demonstration of a tracheal bronchus by computed tomography. *Clin Rad* 1988;39:208–209.
59. Stene R, Rose M, Weinger, MB, Benumof JL, Harrell J. Bronchial trifurcation at the carina complicating use of a double-lumen tracheal tube. *Anesthesiology* 1994;80:1162–1164.
60. Mori M, Chuma R, Kiichi Y, Masuda Y, Obara H. The anesthetic management of a patient with a thoracic aortic aneurysm that caused compression of the left main stem bronchus and the right pulmonary artery. *J Cardiothorac Vasc Anesth* 1993; 7:579–584.
61. Gorman RB, Merritt WT, Greenspun H, Greene PS, Williams

GM. Aneurysmal compression of the trachea and right main stem bronchus complicating thoracoabdominal aneurysm repair. *Anesthesiology* 1993;79:1424–1427.
62. Simpson PM. Tracheal intubation with a Robertshaw tube via a tracheostomy. *Br J Anaesth* 1976;48:373–374.
63. Brodskt JB, Tobler HG, Mark JBD. A double-lumen endobronchial tube for tracheostomies (letter). *Anesthesiology* 1991;74:387–388.
64. Saito S, Dohi S, Naito H. Alteration of double-lumen endobronchial tube position by flexion and extension of the neck. *Anesthesiology* 1985;52:696–697.
65. Shafieha MJ, Sit J, Kartha R, et al. End-tidal CO_2 analyzers in proper positioning of the double-lumen tubes. *Anesthesiology* 1986;64:844–845.
66. Bardoczky GI, Levarlet M, Engelman E, Defrancquen P. Continuous spirometry for detection of double-lumen endobronchial tube displacement. *B J Anesth 1993;70:499–502.*
67. Bardoczky G, D'Hollander A, Yernault JC, Van Meuylem A, Moures JM, Rocmans P. On-line expiratory flow-volume curves during thoracic surgery: occurrence of auto-PEEP. *Br. J Anaesth* 1994;72:25–28.
68. Read RC, Friday CD, Eason CN. Prospective study of the Robertshaw endobronchial catheter in thoracic surgery. *Ann Thorac Surg* 1977;24:156–161.
69. Brodsky JB, Shulman MS, Mark JB. Malposition of left-sided double-lumen endobronchial tubes. *Anesthesiology* 1985;62: 667–669.
70. Hirsch NP, Smith GB. Malposition of left-sided double-lumen endobronchial tubes. *Anesthesiology* 1985;63:563.
71. Greene ER, Gutierrez FA. Tip of polyvinyl chloride double-lumen endotracheal tube inadvertently wedged in left lower lobe bronchus. *Anesthesiology* 1986;64:406.
72. Ovassapian A. Fiberoptic positioning of right-sided double-lumen endobronchial tubes. *J of Bronchology* 1994;1:1–8.
73. Lewis JW, Serwin JP, Fathy, Gabriel FS, Bastanfar M, Jacobsen G. The utility of a double-lumen tube for one-lung ventilation in a variety of noncardiac thoracic surgical procedures. *J Cardiothorac Vascul Anesth* 1992;6:705–710.
74. Chui PT, Mainland P, Chung SCS, Chung DC. Anaesthesia for three-stage thoracoscopic oesophagectomy: an initial experience. *Anaesth Intens Care* 1994;22:593–596.
75. Patane PS, Sell BA, Mahla ME. Awake fiberoptic endobronchial intubation. *Journal of Cardiothoracic Anesthesia* 1990;4: 229–231.
76. Hultgren BL, Krishna PR, Kamaya H. A new tube for one-lung ventilation: experience with Univent tube. *Anesthesiology* 1986;65:A481
77. Doyle DJ. A simple technique for placement of the Univent bronchial blocker. *Anesthesiology* 1993;79:399.
78. Gayes JM. Con: The Univent tube is the best technique for providing one-lung ventilation. *J Cardiothor Vascul Anesth* 1993;7:103–107.
79. Inoue H, Suzuki I, Lwasaki M, Ogawa J, Koide S, Shohtsu A. Selective exclusion of the injured lung. *J of Trauma* 1993;34: 496–498.
80. Inoue H, Shotsu A, Ogawa J, et al. Endotracheal tube with movable blocker to prevent aspiration of intratracheal bleeding. *Ann Thorac Surg* 1984;37:497–499.
81. Slinger P. Con: The Univent tube is not the best method of providing one-lung ventilation. *J Cardiothorac Vascul Anesth* 1993;7:108–112.
82. Daugherty P, Hannallah M. A potentially serious complication that resulted from improper use of the Univent tube. *Anesthesiology* 1992; 77:835.
83. Karwande SV. A new tube for single lung ventilation. *Chest* 1987;92:761–763.
84. Badner NH. Lung isolation during thoracic aneurysmectomy. *J Cardiothorac Vascul Anesth* 1991;5:302–306.
85. Herenstein R, Russo JR, Moonka N, Capan LM. Management of one-lung anesthesia in an anticoagulated patient. *Anesth Analg* 1988;67:1120–1122.
86. Conacher LD. The urinary catheter as a bronchial blocker. *Anesthesia* 1983;38:475–477.
87. Rao CC, Krishna G, Grosfeld JL, et al. One-lung pediatric anesthesia. *Anesth Analg* 1981;60:450–452.
88. Lines V. Selective bronchial blocking in a small child. *Br J Anaesth* 1969;41:893.
89. Baraka A, Slim M, Dajani A, et al. One-lung ventilation of children during surgical excision of hydatid cysts. *Br J Anaesth* 1982;54:523–528.
90. Baraka A, Akel S, Muallem M, et al. Bronchial intubation in children: does the tube bevel determine the side of intubation? *Anesthesiology* 1987;67:869–870.
91. Greenblott GB, Tremper KK, Barker SJ, Gerschutz S, Gehrich JL. Continuous blood gas monitoring with an intraarterial optode during one-lung anesthesia. *J Cardiothorac Vasc Anesth* 1991;5:365–367.
92. Wittnich C, Trudel J, Zidulka A, Chu-Jeng Chiu, R. Misleading "pulmonary Wedge Pressure" after pneumonectomy: its importance in postoperatie fluid therapy. *Ann Thorac Surg* 1986; 42:192–196.
93. Kerr JH, Crampton Smith A, Prys-Roberts C, et al. Observation during endobronchial anaesthesia. I. Ventilation and carbon dioxide clearance. *Br J Anaesth* 1973;45:159–166.
94. Cote CJ, Petkau AJ, Ryan JF, et al. Wasted ventilation measured *in vitro* with eight anesthetic circuits with and without inlet humidification. *Anesthesiology* 1983;59:442–446.
95. Kerr JH, Crampton Smith A, Prys-Roberts C, et al. Observations during endobronchial anaesthesia. II. Oxygenation. *Br J Anaesth* 1974;46:84–92.
96. Khanam T, Branthwaite MA. Arterial oxygenation during one-lung anaesthesia. *Anaesthesia* 1973;28:280–290.
97. Torda TA, McCulloch CH, O'Brien HD, et al. Pulmonary venous admixture during one lung anesthesia. The effect of inhaled oxygen tension and respiratory rate. *Anaesthesia* 1974; 29:272–279.
98. Flacke JW, Thompson DS, Read RC. Influence of tidal volume and pulmonary artery occlusion on arterial oxygenation during endobronchial anesthesia. *South Med J* 1976;69:619–626.
99. Marshall BE, Marshall C. Continuity of response to hypoxic pulmonary vasoconstriction. *J Appl Physiol* 1980;59:189–196.
100. Benumof JL. Mechanism of decreased blood flow to atelectatic lung. *J Appl Physiol* 1980;59:189–196.
101. Cutaia A, Rounds S. Hypoxic pulmonary vasoconstriction. *Chest* 1990;97;706–718.
102. Hauge A. Conditions governing the pressor response to ventilation hypoxia in isolated perfused rat lungs. *Acta Physiol Scand* 1968;72:33–44.
103. Malik AB, Kidd BS. Time course of pulmonary vascular response to hypoxia in dogs. *Am J Physiol* 1973;224:1–6.
104. Carlsson JA, Bindslev L, Santesson J, Gottlieb I, Hedenstierna G. Hypoxic pulmonary vasoconstriction in the human lung: the effect of prolonged unilateral hypoxic challenge during anaesthesia. *Acta Anaesthesiol Scand* 1985:29;346–351.
105. Marshall BE, Marshall C, Benumof J, Saidman LJ. Hypoxic pulmonary vasoconstriction in dogs: effects of lung segment size and oxygen tension. *J Appl Physiol* 1981;51:1543–1551.
106. Marshall C, Marshall BE. Influence of perfusate PO_2 on hypoxic pulmonary vasoconstriction in rats. *Cir Res* 1983;52: 691–696.
107. Hirschmann JC, Bouncek RJ. Angiographic evidence of pulmonary vasomotion in the dog. *Br Heart J* 1963;25:375–381.
108. Kato M, Staub NC. Response of small pulmonary arteries to unilobar hypoxia and hypercapnea. *Cir Res* 1966;19:426–439.
109. Nagasaka Y, Bhattacharya F, Nanjo S, Gropper MA, Staube NC. Micropuncture measurement of lung microvascular pressure profile during hypoxia in cats. *Cir Res* 1984;54:90–95.
110. Madden JA, Dawson CA, Harder DR. Hypoxia-induced activation in small isolated pulmonary arteries from the cat. *J Appl Physiol* 1985;59:113–118.
111. Marshall C, Lindgren L, Marshall BE. Metabolic and respiratory hydrogen ion effects on hypoxic pulmonary vasoconstriction. *J Appl Physiol* 1984;57:545–550.
112. Ishibe Y, Gui X, Uno H, Shiokawa Y, Umeda T, Suekane K. Effect of sevofurane on hypoxic pulmonary vasoconstriction in the perfused rabbit lung. *Anesthesiology* 1993;79:1348–1353.

113. Rogers SN, Benumof JL. Halothane and isoflurane do not decrease P_aO_2 during one-lung ventilation in intravenously anesthetized patients. *Anesth Analg* 1985;64:946–954.
114. Benumof JL, Augustine SD, Gibbons JA. Halothane and isoflurane only slightly impair arterial oxygenation during one-lung ventilation in patients undergoing thoracotomy. *Anesthesiology* 1987;67:910–915.
115. Gibson QH, Roughton FJW. The kinetics of equilibration of the reactions of nitric oxide with sheep hemoglobin. *J Physiol* [London] 1957;136:507–526.
116. Rich GF, Lowson SM, Johns RA, Daugherty MO, Uncles DR. Inhaled nitric oxide selectively decreases pulmonary vascular resistance without impairing oxygenation during one-lung ventilation in patients undergoing cardiac surgery. *Anesthesiology* 1994;80:57–62.
117. Rossaint R, Falke KJ, Lopez F, Slama K, Pison U, Zapol WM. Inhaled nitric oxide for the adult respiratory distress syndrome. *N Engl J Med* 1993;328:399–405.
118. Casthely PA, Lear S, Cottrell JE. Intrapulmonary shunting during induced hypotension. *Anesth Analg* 1982;61:231–235.
119. Hill AB, Sykes MK, Reyes MK. A hypoxic pulmonary vasoconstrictor response in dogs during and after infusion of sodium nitroprusside. *Anesthesiology* 1979;50:484–488.
120. Colley PS, Cheney FW. Sodium nitroprusside increases Qs/Qt in dogs with regional atelectasis. *Anesthesiology* 1977;47: 338–341.
121. Friedlander M, Sandler A, Kavanagh B, Winton T, Benumof J. Is hypoxic pulmonary vasoconstriction important during single lung ventilation in the lateral decubitus position. *Can J Anaesth* 1994;41:26–30.
122. Ingrassia TS III, Ryu JH, Trastek VF, Rosenow EC III. Oxygen-exacerbated bleomycin pulmonary toxicity. *Mayo Clin Proc* 1991;66:173–178.
123. Van Mieghem W, Coolen L, Malysse I, Lacquet LM, Deneffe GJD, Demedts MGP. Amiodarone and the development of ARDS after lung surgery. *Chest* 1994;105:1642–1645.
124. Morrow B, Shorten GD, Sylvester W. Postoperative amiodarone pulmonary toxicity. *Anaesth Intens Care* 1993;21:361–362.
125. Thompson CC, Bailey, MK, Conroy JM, Bromley HR. Postoperative pulmonary toxicity associated with mitomycin-C therapy. *South Med J* 1992;85:1257–1259.
126. Rees DI, Wansbrough SR. One-lung anesthesia: percent shunt and arterial oxygen tension during continuous insufflation of oxygen to the nonventilated lung. *Anesth Analg* 1982;61: 507–512.
127. Capan LM, Turndorf H, Patel C, et al. Optimization of arterial oxygenation during one-lung anesthesia. *Anesth Analg* 1980; 59:847–851.
128. Alfery DD, Benumof JL, Trousdale FR. Improving oxygenation during one-lung ventilation: the effects of PEEP and blood flow restriction to the nonventilated lung. *Anesthesiology* 1981; 55:381–385.
129. Slinger P, Triolet W, Wilson J. Improving arterial oxygenation during one-lung ventilation. *Anesthesiology* 1988;68:291–295.
130. Baraka A, Sibai AN, Muallem M, et al. CPAP oxygenation during one-lung ventilation using an underwater seal assembly. *Anesthesiology* 1986;65:102–103.
131. Thiagarajah S, Rao A. A device for applying CPAP to the nonventilated upper lung during one-lung ventilation. *Anesthesiology* 1984;60:253–254.
132. Hannenberg AA, Satwicz PR, Dienes RS Jr, O'Brien JC. A device for applying CPAP to the nonventilated upper lung during one-lung ventilation. *Anesthesiology* 1984;60,254–255.
133. Hogue CW. Effectiveness of low levels of nonventilated lung continuous positive airway pressure in improving arterial oxygenation during one-lung ventilation. *Anesth Analg* 1994;79: 364–367.
134. Benumof JL, Gaughan SD, Ozaki GT. Operative lung constant positive airway pressure with the Univent bronchial blocker tube. Anesth. *Analg* 1992;74:406–410.
135. Hughes SA, Benumof JL. Operative lung continuous positive airway pressure to minimize FIO_2 during one-lung ventilation. *Anesth Analg* 1990;71:92–95.
136. Toledo CH, Ross WE, Hood CI, Block ER. Potentiation of bleomycin toxicity by oxygen. *Cancer Treat Rep* 1982;66: 359–362.
137. Hulbert JC, Grossman JE, Cummings KB. Risk factors of anesthesia and surgery in bleomycin treated patients. *J Urol* 1983; 130:163–164.
138. Tryka AF, Skornik WA, Godleski JJ, Brain JD. Potentiation of bleomycin-induced lung injury by exposure to 70% oxygen. *Am Rev Respir Dis* 1992;126:1074–1079.
139. Katz JA, Laverner RG, Fairley HB, et al. Pulmonary oxygen exchange during endobronchial anesthesia: effects of tidal volume and PEEP. *Anesthesiology* 1982;56:164–171.
140. Gallagher TJ, Banner MJ, Smith RA. A simplified method of independent lung ventilation. *Critic Care Med* 1980,8:396–399.
141. Hedenstierna G, Bachrendtz S, Klingstedt C, Santesson J, Soderborg B, Dahlborn M, Bindslev L. Ventilation and perfusion of each lung during ventilation with selective PEEP. *Anesthesiology* 1984;61:369–376.
142. Millar FA, Hutchison GL, Wood RAB. Anaesthesia for thoracoscopic pleurectomy and ligation of bullae. *Anaesthesia* 1992; 47:1060–1062.
143. Baraka A. Differential lung ventilation as an alternative to one-lung ventilation during thoracotomy. *Anaesthesia* 1994;49: 881–882.
144. Malmkvist G. Maintenance of oxygenation during one-lung ventilation. Effect of intermittent reinflation of the collapsed lung with oxygen. *Anesth Analg* 1989;68:763–766.
145. Bjork VO, Carlens E. The prevention of spread during pulmonary resection by the use of a double-lumen catheter. *J Thorac Surg* 1950;20:151–157.
146. Godet G, Bertrand M, Rouby JJ, et al. High frequency jet ventilation versus continuous positive airway pressure for differential long ventilation in patients undergoing resection of thoracoabdominal aortic aneurym. *Acta Anaesthesiol Scand* 1994; 38:562–568.
147. Tsue SL, Chan CS, Chan AS, Wong SJ, Lam CS, Jones RD. A comparison of two-lung high frequency positive pressure ventilation and one-lung ventilation plus 5 cm H_2O non-ventilated lung CPAP in patients undergoing anaesthesia for oesophagectomy. *Anaesth Intens Care* 1991;19:205–212.
148. Clapham MCC, Vaughan RS. Bronchial intubation. A comparison between polyvinyl chloride and red rubber double lumen tubes. *Anaesthesia* 1985;40:1111–1114.
149. Guernelli N, Bragaglia RB, Briccoli A, et al. Tracheobronchial ruptures due to cuffed Carlens tube. *Ann Thorac Surg* 1979; 28:66–68.
150. Foster JMG, Lau OJ, Alimo EB. Ruptured bronchus following endobronchial intubation. *Br J Anaesth* 1983;55:687–688.
151. Wagner DL, Gammage GW, Wong MI. Tracheal rupture following the insertion of a disposable double—a lumen endotracheal tube. *Anesthesiology* 1985;63:698–700.
152. Burton NA, Fall SM, Lyons T, Graeber GM. Rupture of the left main stem bronchus with a polyvinylchloride double-lumen tube. *Chest* 1983;83:928–929.
153. Heiser M, Steinberg JJ, McVaugh H III, Klineberg PL. Bronchial rupture. A complication of use of the Robertshaw double-lumen tube. *Anesthesiology* 1979;51:88.
154. Kumar SM, Sujit PK, Cohen PJ. Tracheal laceration associated with endotracheal anesthesia. *Anesthesiology* 1977;47: 298–299.
155. Maguire DP, Spiro AW. Bronchial obstruction and hypoxia during one-lung ventilation. *Anesthesiology* 1987;66:830–831.
156. Oakes DD, Cohn RB, Brodsky JB. Lateral thoracotomy and one-lung anesthesia in patients with morbid obesity. *Ann Thorac Surg* 1982;34:572–580.
157. Riley RH, Marples IL. Relocation of a double-lumen tube during patient positioning. *Anesth Analg* 1992;75:1071.
158. Yazigi A, Madi-Jebara S, Haddad F, Antakly MC. Relocation of a double-lumen tube during surgical dissection. *Anesth Analg* 1993;77:1303.
159. Campbell C, Viswanathan S, Riopelle JM, Naraghi M. Manufacturing defect in a double-lumen tube. *Anesth Analg* 1991; 73:825–826.

160. Asai T. Torsion of a double-lumen tube in the left bronchus. *Anesthesiology* 1992;76:1064–1065.
161. Desal FM, Rocke DA. Double-lumen tube design fault. *Anesthesiology* 1990;75:576–577.
162. Bayes J, Slater EM, Hedberg PS, Lawson D. Obstruction of a double-lumen endotracheal tube by a saber-sheath trachea. *Anesth Analg* 1994;79:186–188.
163. Greene R, Lechner GL. "Saber-sheath" trachea: a clinical and functional study of marked coronal narrowing of the intrathoracic trachea. *Radiology* 1975;115:265–268.
164. Wells DG, Zeleer J, Padolakin W, et al. Cardiac arrest from pulmonary outflow tract obstruction due to a double-lumen tube. *Anesthesiology* 1987;66:422–423.
165. Schwartz DE, Yost CS, Larson MD. Pneumothorax complicating the use of a Univent[R] endotracheal tube. *Anesth Analg* 1993;76:443–445.

CHAPTER 9

Fiberoptic Airway Endoscopy in Critical Care

Andranik Ovassapian, M.D.

The value of the fiberoptic bronchoscope in the care of the critically ill patient was recognized by clinicians (1–3) shortly after its introduction into clinical practice (4). Fiberoptic bronchoscopy is now widely utilized in a variety of clinical situations in the treatment of the critically ill (Table 1) (5–11). Bellomo et al., in their study on the diagnostic and therapeutic uses of fiberoptic bronchoscopy, showed it to be an effective, safe diagnostic and therapeutic tool (12).

When one considers the many applications of the fiberscope as well as its safety and ease of use, in the hands of the trained endoscopist the record is impressive. The widespread use of the instrument deserves encouragement. The operating room, intensive care unit, and emergency room should be equipped with these instruments, and their access for immediate use encouraged (13).

A number of sophisticated diagnostic and therapeutic procedures may be performed with the fiberoptic bronchoscope. The procedures however require appropriate training and expertise (Tables 2 and 3). The reader should refer to a number of excellent textbooks and review articles in this area (14–16). This chapter emphasizes the use of fiberoptic bronchoscopy in the management of patients with upper and lower airway problems that are commonly encountered by anesthesiologists and critical care physicians (5,6,11,13).

EVALUATION AND MANAGEMENT OF THE COMPROMISED AIRWAY

The condition of the upper airway can be evaluated by fiberoptic pharyngolaryngoscopy (PL), without distorting the anatomy or physiology of the airway. The technique is simple, safe, and well tolerated by the awake patient. It is associated with minimal hemodynamic change and can be performed with the patient in any position (13,17–19).

When airway evaluation is combined with the possibility of a tracheal intubation, the fiberscope is mounted with an endotracheal tube prior to the examination. This allows an option for immediate tracheal intubation, after the application of topical anesthesia through the working channel of the fiberscope (20–22).

Fiberoptic PL can be used to evaluate and manage upper airway obstruction secondary to a variety of conditions (Fig. 1) (Table 4) and postextubation laryngeal spasm and stridor (Table 5). Stridor is a high-pitched respiratory sound produced by a partial obstruction of

TABLE 1. *Indications for fiberoptic airway endoscopy*

Evaluating and managing the compromised airway
Upper airway obstruction
Vocal cord palsy
Epiglottitis
Smoke inhalation
Obstructive sleep apnea
Bedside bronchoscopy
Diagnosis and treatment of acute hypoxemia
Treatment of atelectasis
Tracheobronchial toilet
Securing the airway
Tracheal and bronchial intubation
Positioning endobronchial tubes and blockers
Checking the endotracheal tube
Checking the patency of the endotracheal tube
Verifying the endotracheal tube position
Repositioning the endotracheal tube
Changing the endotracheal tube
Evaluating for optimal time of extubation
Major head and neck operations
Edema of upper airway
Epiglottitis
Checking and placement of a nasogastric tube

TABLE 2. *Uses of diagnostic fiberoptic bronchoscopy*

Pulmonary infections
Mass lesions
Persistent atelectasis
Mediastinal and hilar abnormalities
Diffuse parenchymal lung disease
Follow-up of patients with bronchogenic carcinoma
Chronic cough and wheezing

TABLE 3. *Advanced fiberoptic bronchoscopic procedures*

Transbronchial biopsy
Removal of foreign bodies from distal bronchial tree
Brachytherapy (localized radiation therapy)
Laser bronchoscopy
Photodynamic therapy
Electrocautery
Cryotherapy

TABLE 4. *Common causes of upper airway obstruction*

Airway polyps, cysts, and tumors
Laryngeal edema
Vocal cord palsy
Tracheal stenosis and compression
Epiglottitis and other airway infectious process
Obstructive sleep apnea
Smoke inhalation
Airway trauma
Tracheomalacia and laryngomalacia

the airway in the trachea, larynx, or pharynx. Inspiratory stridor usually suggests airway obstruction in the supraglottic larynx or pharynx. Lesions producing airway obstruction in the glottic or subglottic region produce stridor during inspiration and expiration. Expiratory stridor alone indicates an obstructive lesion(s) in the intrathoracic tracheobronchial tree. In infants, lar-

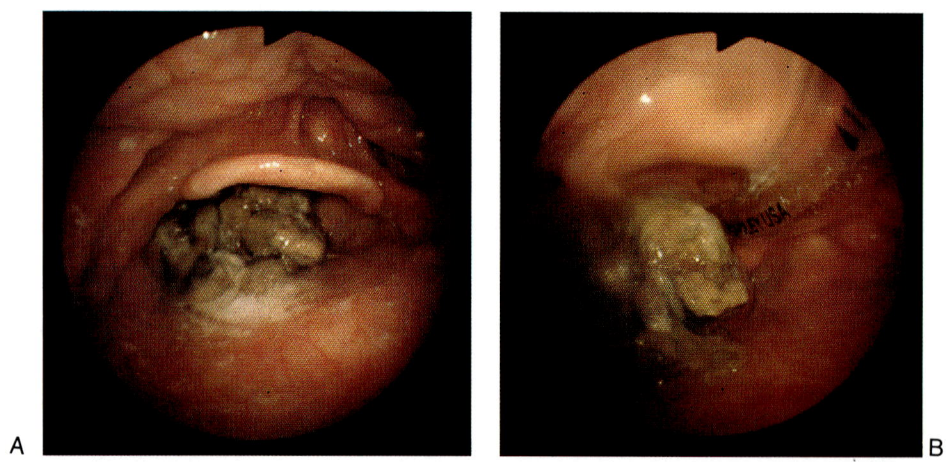

FIG. 1. Laryngeal carcinoma in a 65-year-old man with long-standing history of smoking. The tumor originated from left false vocal folds and blocks the view of the glottic opening. Patient had no stridor and could lie supine without getting short of breath. **A:** Epiglottis and the tumor beneath it. Glottis opening not visible. **B:** After awake fiberoptic intubation with 6-mm endotracheal tube. The endotracheal tube is on the right upper quadrant of the picture. Smooth intubation with no trauma to the lesion.

TABLE 5. *Postextubation stridor*

Laryngeal edema
Traumatic intubation and extubation
Allergic reactions to medications (angioneurotic)
Large-volume fluid replacement
Steep Trendelenburg position
Vocal cord palsy
Thyroidectomy
Carotid endarterectomy
Esophagectomy
Laryngeal placement of endotracheal tube cuff
Nasogastric tube (delayed pseudoparalysis)
Existed but undiagnosed prior to surgery
Vocal cord polyps (unknown preoperatively)
Redundant supraglottic tissue
Obstructive sleep apnea
Obesity
Edema of tissues
Hematoma

yngomalacia, congenital subglottic stenosis, vocal cord paralysis, and airway compression (usually by a vascular ring defect) may produce stridor immediately after birth (20–23). Auscultation is useful in determining the principal location producing the stridor.

Tracheal Stenosis

Obstructive tracheal lesions secondary to a prior tracheostomy include tracheal stenosis (Fig. 2), tracheomalacia, or granuloma formation (Fig. 3) at the tracheal stoma. Post-tracheostomy tracheal granuloma is very common and causes significant airway obstruction. It is easily removed with laser surgery (24). If the patient is not tolerating progressive closure of a tracheostomy, PL may help to identify the cause. Figure 3 shows granuloma formation secondary to a tracheostomy, requiring surgical removal before the patient could tolerate decannulation.

The incidence of tracheal stenosis varies depending on the defining criteria and method of airway evaluation. Tracheal stenosis, defined as bronchoscopic observation of concentric tracheal narrowing greater than 20%, was reported as occurring 16% of the time in patients with prolonged tracheostomy (24). In another prospective study, the incidence of tracheal stenosis defined as 10% narrowing or greater was reported at 20% (25). Woo reported the incidence of tracheal stenosis at 26%, but did not separate the conditions of tracheomalacia and tracheal granuloma from stenosis (26).

The reported predisposing factors that contribute to tracheal stenosis include shock (27); infection (25,28); steroid therapy (26,27); patient movement (29); cuff pressures (30); duration of intubation (31); type of surgery (32); and chronic lung disease (33). These factors have not been substantiated however by careful clinical studies.

The early recommendation that fiberoptic intubation be utilized in tracheal intubation of all patients with a prior history of previous tracheostomy or prolonged intubation was based on the high incidence of tracheal stenosis in these patients. Fiberoptic intubation conducted awake or asleep will identify such tracheal stenosis before an endotracheal tube is advanced. This diagnostic precaution will prevent repeated attempts at intubation of the stenotic airway and the associated trauma (34). A narrowed trachea, if traumatized, may

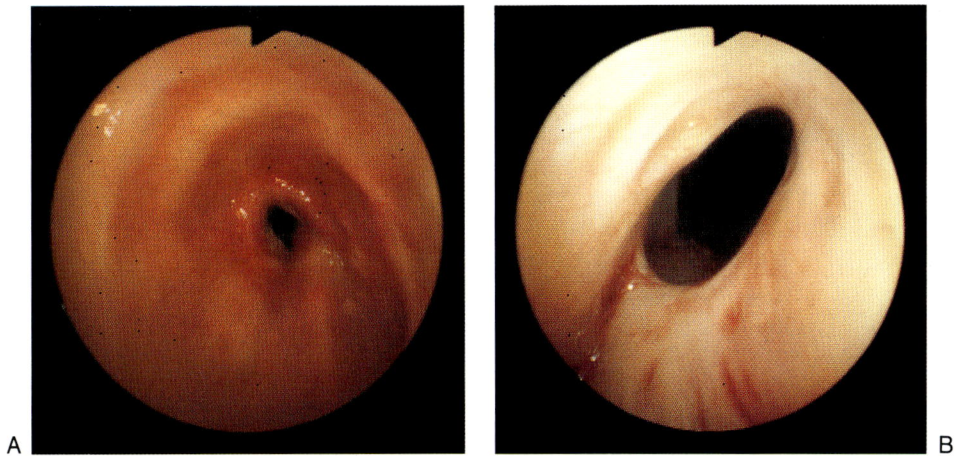

FIG. 2. Tracheal stenosis. Patient had tracheostomy in 1988, following which he had developed tracheal stenosis. He was asymptomatic, but his physical activities were limited. After induction of anesthesia and complete muscle paralysis, an 8-mm endotracheal tube was passed easily through the cords but could not be advanced into the trachea. Fiberoptic examination through the endotracheal tube identified the problem. **A:** Stenotic trachea seen from distance. **B:** Closer view of stenosis shows scar tissues. The lumen at stenotic area was limited to 6 mm.

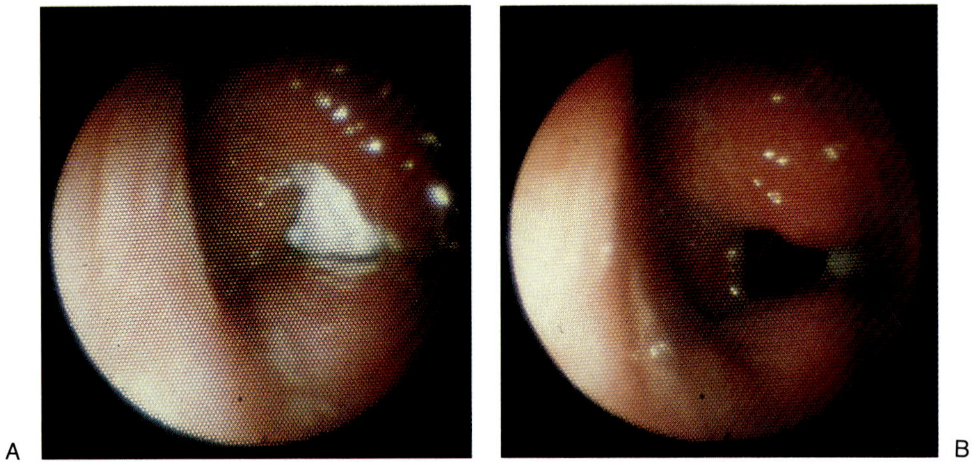

FIG. 3. Granuloma at tracheostomy site causing tracheal stenosis. The patient would not tolerate closure of the tracheostomy. The fiberscope was introduced through the right nostril, with the tip of it positioned about 10 mm above the lesion. **A:** White cuff of Shiley tracheostomy tube in view. Upper half of the tracheal lumen is blocked by granulation tissue. **B:** Tracheostomy tube removed. The tracheal lumen is narrowed by granulation tissue to less than 40% of its lumen.

develop a severe airway obstruction necessitating another tracheostomy.

Tracheopathia osteochondroplastica is a rare disease that is associated with accumulation of bony and cartilaginous nodules in the trachea and bronchial mucosa, causing tracheal stenosis. It is often diagnosed at autopsy (35), and less frequently during routine bronchoscopic examination (36,37). It has also been identified with unexpected tracheal intubation problems (38).

Vocal Cord Palsy

Unilateral vocal cord palsy (2,39) may be asymptomatic in an awake patient. It may present as an acute airway obstruction during recovery from general anesthesia (Fig. 4). During inspiration, the vocal cords abduct and open the glottis. During expiration, the vocal cords return to their normal passive position. When this normal vocal cord motion is lost, secondary to paralysis, the inspiratory resistance to airflow is increased. While this condition may not be clinically obvious at rest, it limits the individual's ability to hyperventilate (40).

Upon emerging from anesthesia, an agitated and restless patient who is breathing deep and rapidly may increase negative airway pressure, retracting laryngeal and pharyngeal tissue into the airway. This action may produce an acute airway obstruction with stridor. Treatment of this condition consists of mild sedation and patient reassurance, while encouraging the patient to breathe slowly (13).

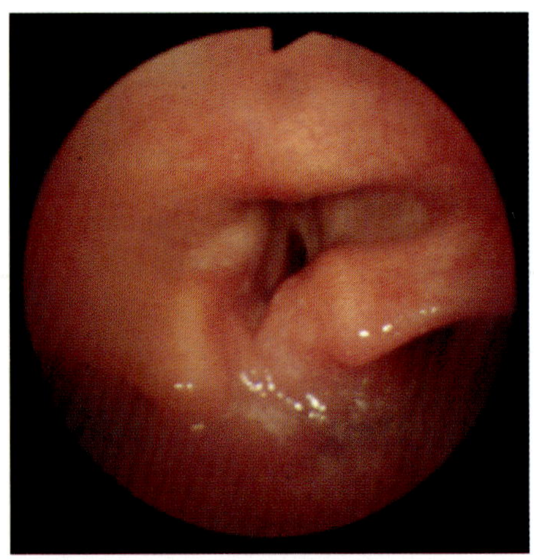

FIG. 4. Right vocal cord palsy. Left arytenoid hypertrophied to compensate for right-sided palsy. This patient had agitation and stormy recovery from general anesthesia. He had stridor and complained of difficult breathing. Fiberoptic laryngoscopy showed right vocal cord palsy unknown to the patient and the managing service. Management was sedation and assurance. Recovery was uneventful. Consultation with ear, nose, and throat service confirmed the diagnosis.

Over the past 15 years we have used the fiberscope in the immediate postoperative period in patients with upper airway obstruction or stridor. Four patients were identified with unilateral vocal cord palsy unknown to us preoperatively. All four patients were managed with sedation and reassurance, avoiding reintubation or racemic epinephrine therapy (13).

Surgical trauma to the recurrent laryngeal nerve may occur during neck surgery and left-sided thoracotomy (41). Vocal cord paralysis may also be a feature of the uncommon Shy-Drager syndrome (42). In these circumstances the anesthesiologist should consider the possibility of bilateral vocal cord palsy as a possible cause of postoperative upper airway obstruction.

Several cases of bilateral vocal cord palsy secondary to tracheal intubation are also reported (41,43–45). Shortly after extubation these patients presented with signs of stridor, and in some cases severe airway obstruction. Tracheal intubation or tracheostomy may be needed to save the patient's life (Fig. 5).

Paradoxical vocal cord adduction may also present a similar but even more severe picture. Treatment may on occasion require prolonged ventilatory support (46,47). Paradoxical vocal cord adduction is an uncommon condition that produces signs of wheezing, and may be mistakenly diagnosed as asthma (47). It is characterized by paradoxical vocal cord adduction during inspiration (48). Typically the patient is female, under 40 years of age. The patient typically presents with episodes of wheezing, shortness of breath, and stridor.

Patterson and his colleagues in 1974 were the first to describe this upper airway obstruction in patients free of any known organic abnormalities (49). This functional upper airway obstruction, while usually secondary to paradoxical vocal cord adduction, has recently been seen in functional pharyngeal constriction and abnormal motion of the arytenoid region (50,51).

Epiglottitis

Acute epiglottitis is an infectious disease with a great potential for airway obstruction in both children and adults (52–54). Since the introduction of Hemophilus influenza type b vaccine, the incidence of acute epiglottitis in the pediatric community has decreased significantly. The incidence of acute epiglottitis in adults has remained essentially unchanged at 1.8 cases per 100,000 population (55).

A lateral neck soft tissue roentgenogram along with rigid laryngoscopy are used to confirm the diagnosis. Radiographic examination is time consuming and may not be diagnostic, delaying therapeutic intervention (56). Direct rigid laryngoscopy in the awake state may precipitate laryngeal spasm and airway obstruction. The laryngoscopic examination is therefore usually performed in the operating room under general anesthesia (57). This is especially true in children. However, this viewpoint is under challenge. Awake rigid and fiberoptic laryngoscopic examination and tracheal intubation have been performed successfully in adults and children with acute epiglottitis (20,21,54,58).

Fiberoptic PL can confirm the diagnosis and assist in tracheal intubation (59). If the diagnosis of epiglottitis is confirmed, a decision on airway management needs to be made. Some have recommended tracheal intubation or tracheostomy in all adult patients (52). Other practitioners feel that adult patients with acute epiglottitis, without signs or symptoms of upper airway

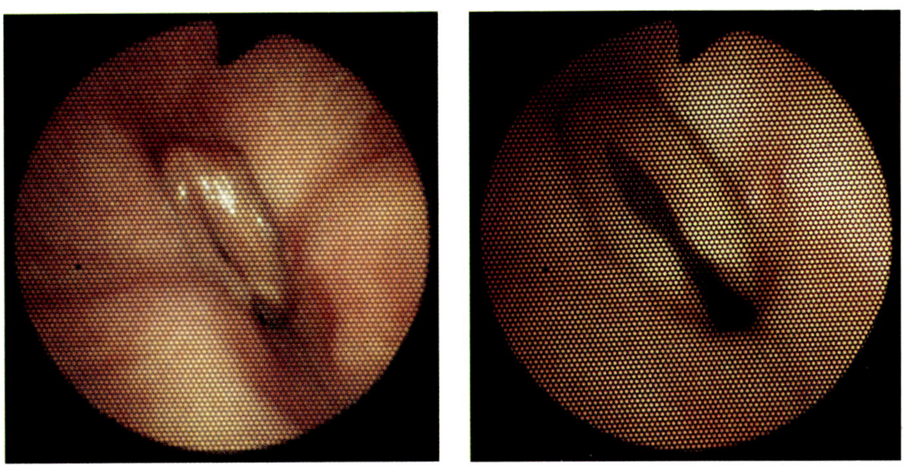

A B

FIG. 5. Bilateral partial recurrent laryngeal nerve palsy. Patient had esophagectomy and gastric pull-up 2 years ago. He was brought to the emergency room because of severe difficulty in breathing. He was rushed to the operating room for a tracheostomy, suspecting bilateral partial recurrent laryngeal nerve palsy due to compression by a malignant tumor. Fiberoptic laryngoscopy confirmed the diagnosis, and the trachea was intubated after application of topical anesthesia to secure the airway and make tracheostomy safer and easier. **A:** During inspiration cords are adducted, causing almost complete airway obstruction. **B:** During expiration vocal cords open passively.

obstruction, can be treated conservatively in an intensive care setting. The patients are closely monitored for signs of airway compromise, with prompt airway intervention available if needed (55,60).

In adults who present with airway obstruction requiring tracheal intubation, the patient is placed in a sitting position and topical anesthesia applied to the nasal passage. A lubricated fiberscope mounted with an endotracheal tube is inserted through the prepared nostril into the oropharynx. With careful advancement, the epiglottis is exposed without being contacted by the fiberscope. Prior to advancement through the vocal cords, 2% or 4% lidocaine is sprayed through the working channel of the fiberscope to produce topical anesthesia of the larynx. The fiberscope is then advanced into the trachea, followed by the endotracheal tube. Two adult patients with acute epiglottitis were managed with this approach with ease and without complication (R. Pyatetsky, M.D., *personal communication*).

Fiberoptic PL has also been used to assess the early resolution of epiglottic edema in this condition after intubation (20,58,61). Nussbaum (61), using fiberoptic PL airway assessment, was able to extubate 12 of 16 patients with epiglottitis within 12 to 24 hr of intubation.' Early extubation minimizes laryngotracheal damage and shortens the stay in the intensive care unit. Fiberoptic airway endoscopy has been suggested as the technique of choice for the diagnosis and airway management of acute adult epiglottitis (59). Shortcomings include difficulty in passing the fiberscope through the glottis on occasion and temporary airway obstruction upon entrance into the larynx (62,63).

Smoke Inhalation

Acute airway obstruction in smoke inhalation may occur secondary to laryngeal and pharyngeal tissue edema or acute retention of secretions and necrotic debris. Fiberoptic PL can be used to diagnose the cause of the airway obstruction, locate and suction secretions, or to place an endotracheal tube (64,65). In severe cases, the normal anatomy of the hypopharynx and larynx may be markedly distorted, making visualization of the glottis extremely difficult (66). The presence of stridor, hoarseness, and tachypnea all signal a developing airway obstruction, which may require emergency intervention. Tracheal intubation is preferred over tracheostomy in the burn patient since a prolonged artificial airway is usually not needed. Furthermore, tracheostomy is associated with increased morbidity and contamination of the airway in these patients (67).

Obstructive Sleep Apnea

Obstructive apnea is caused by upper airway obstruction while respiratory movement of the diaphragm continues (68). Partial collapse of the pharyngeal airway during sleep produces snoring, and complete collapse causes obstruction of the airway. Davies and Straddling reported that 17% of normal British men snore, and 1 in 300 have severe obstructive sleep apnea (69). The characteristic symptoms of sleep apnea are snoring, morning tiredness, excessive daytime sleepiness, fatigue, headaches, and nausea.

Various techniques have been utilized for assessment of upper airway patency in sleep apnea patients. These techniques include study of flow-volume curves, radiographic techniques, magnetic resonance imaging, acoustic reflection techniques, and direct observation by fiberoptic endoscopy. Fiberoptic PL has been used in adults, children, and infants with obstructive sleep apnea to help establish the site and mechanism of obstruction.

The continuous observation of the airway while a patient is breathing spontaneously is best done with the fiberscope. The technique is extremely valuable in evaluating the dynamics of the supraglottic and pharyngeal structures in these patients (Fig. 6). Endoscopic findings have confirmed obstruction at various sites including the velopharyngeal sphincter and tongue, the midpharynx, hypopharynx, and larynx (70–73). Rubinstein et al. described patients with severe obstructive sleep apnea who had paradoxical movements of the vocal cords (74).

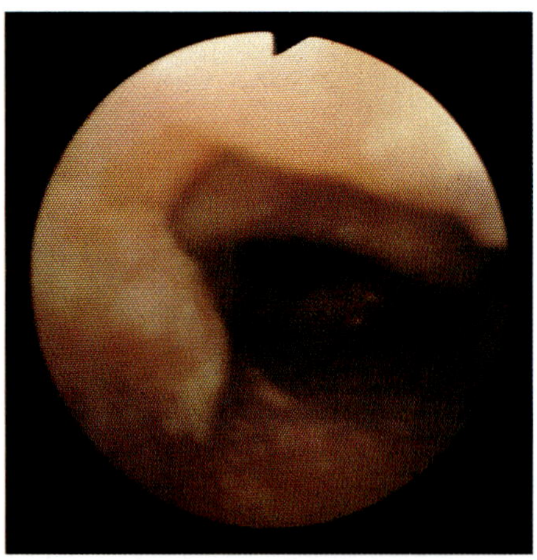

FIG. 6. Endoscopy view of the hypopharynx and larynx in a 285-lb man with sleep apnea syndrome. Redundant tissues contributed to the difficulty of mask ventilation and tracheal intubation. Fiberoptic intubation can also be difficult in these patients. Abundant soft tissues are seen in supraepiglottic and left pharyngeal wall. The tip of the epiglottis as well as right arytenoid are visible.

BEDSIDE FIBEROPTIC BRONCHOSCOPY

The indications for the use of the fiberoptic bronchoscope in the practice of anesthesia and critical care are summarized in Table 1. Limited fiberoptic bronchoscopy is a bedside procedure and is frequently used to identify causes and treatment of hypoxemia (Table 6), e.g., atelectasis and malpositioned endotracheal or endobronchial tubes. Limited fiberoptic bronchoscopy is defined as the use of a bronchoscope for observation, evaluation, and management of airway related problems limited to the trachea and first generation bronchial tree.

Fiberoptic bronchoscopy can be used to rule out bronchial intubation and/or tracheal tube obstruction by secretions or compression. Obstruction of the airway by secretions and mucus plugs, causing acute atelectasis, is a good indication for fiberoptic bronchoscopy and therapeutic pulmonary toilet (75). Fiberoptic bronchoscopy is also indicated for diagnosis and treatment in witnessed or suspected cases of gastric aspiration (76,77). Traumatic injuries to the airway are also easily evaluated by this technique.

In awake patients, the fiberscope is introduced either orally or nasally. The disadvantages of the transoral approach include the patient biting and damaging the instrument, difficulty in suppressing the gag reflex in some patients, and the need for gaining patient cooperation.

The passage of the fiberscope through the nose may cause bleeding, and the fiberscope may be contaminated with nasal secretions. The repeated removal and reinsertion of the fiberscope through the nose may cause trauma and pain. The use of a soft nasopharyngeal airway will minimize nasal trauma and limit contamination of the distal tip of the fiberscope. However, a nasopharyngeal airway reduces the diameter of the nasal passage. In critically ill patients, or where repeated withdrawal and reinsertion of the fiberscope is required, a laryngeal mask airway or an orotracheal tube should be placed to provide easy airway access.

Mild sedation may be used in addition to topical airway anesthesia, based upon the patient's condition. Good topical anesthesia is essential for patient comfort, blocking of the cardiovascular responses to airway stimulation, and providing optimal working conditions for the endoscopist (78).

When the patient is intubated, or has a tracheostomy in place, a swivel adapter with bronchoscopy port is used. This adapter permits bronchoscopy while the patient is being ventilated. If the fiberscope fits too tightly in the tracheal tube, however, the increase in airway resistance will be substantial. This can result in unreliable gas delivery, excessive airway pressure, and barotrauma. The larger the fiberscope, the smaller the effective internal diameter of the endotracheal tube (79). A small increase in the size of the fiberscope will produce a substantial increase in airway resistance and increase the work of breathing (79). The size of the fiberscope should be 2–3 mm smaller than the inner diameter of the endotracheal tube used for conducting a safe bronchoscopy (80).

The patient is monitored continuously during the procedure, with EKG, pulse oximeter and blood pressure cuff. Pulse oximetry provides an excellent monitoring system for early detection of hypoxemia. Supplemental oxygen is administered during and immediately after completion of the procedure. In debilitated, poor risk, and immunocompromised patients, sterility should be observed.

The bronchoscopy is performed with the endoscopist at the head of the bed with the patient supine. The trachea, carina, and nonpathologic bronchi are inspected before the fiberscope is advanced into the affected side. Saline lavage with aspiration through the fiberscope suction channel is utilized to mobilize and remove thick secretions. To avoid hypoxemia, suctioning through the fiberscope should be intermittent and of short duration. Awake patients can be encouraged to cough, helping to mobilize secretions.

TABLE 6. *Causes of hypoxemia during and after anesthesia*

Intraoperative period
Bronchial intubation
Acute atelectasis—inspissation of secretions
Endotracheal tube blocked by secretions
Malposition of double-lumen endobronchial tube and/ or blocker
Pneumothorax
Mechanical compression of endotracheal tube
Immediate postoperative period
Acute atelectasis
Laryngeal closure and stridor
Aspiration of gastric contents

Complications of Fiberoptic Bronchoscopy

Prospective studies on this technique show higher complication rates (80,81) than retrospective studies (82,83). The complications may be produced by premedication, intravenous sedation, local anesthetic drugs, as well as from the procedure itself (Table 7). Most reported complications are minor in nature, but major life-threatening complications may be encountered. The elderly and patients in poor general health are at the greatest risk. It should be kept in mind that many of these high-risk patients will tolerate fiberoptic

TABLE 7. *Complications of bedside fiberoptic bronchoscopy*

Premedication and/or sedation
Respiratory depression
Hypoxemia
Hyperexcitement
Ventilatory failure
Cardiac arrhythmias
Circulatory depression
Hypotension
Bradycardia
Local anesthetic agents
Toxic reactions
Excitability
Seizures
Cardiorespiratory collapse
Inadequate topical anesthesia
Coughing and retching
Gagging
Laryngospasm
Bronchospasm
Bronchoscopy
Hypoxemia
Tachycardia and hypertension
Cardiac arrhythmias
Trauma to airway
Postbronchoscopy fever and pneumonia
Barotrauma

endoscopy with minimal or no sedation. The appropriate and judicious use of local anesthetic agents will minimize toxic reactions.

Laryngospasm, bronchospasm, and coughing are common if topical anesthesia is inadequate. Patients with bronchospastic disease may develop severe bronchospasm, sometimes with a fatal outcome (84). Cardiovascular responses include tachycardia, hypertension, and concomitant increase in the cardiac index. These hemodynamic changes, alone or combined with hypoxemia, may cause myocardial ischemia, manifested by ST-T segment changes (85).

Many factors such as underlying respiratory disease, excessive suctioning, hypoventilation, laryngospasm, and bronchospasm may contribute to a drop in arterial oxygen tension during bronchoscopy (81,84). In adult patients, the average decline in P_aO_2 has been reported to be 15–20 mm Hg, with individual variations as high as 61 mm Hg (86). Due to these potential complications, bedside fiberoptic bronchoscopy should be undertaken with extreme caution, and only when absolutely essential in patients with severe hypoxemia, serious arrhythmia, unstable angina pectoris, recent myocardial infarction, poorly controlled bronchospastic disease, or low cardiac output state.

CHECKING THE ENDOTRACHEAL TUBE

Endotracheal Tube Patency

The patency of an endotracheal tube can be easily checked with a fiberscope. The fiberscope is advanced into the endotracheal tube while ventilation continues to be performed. Obstruction of the tracheal tube by secretions, external compression, overdistended cuff, or foreign body is easily identified.

Endotracheal Tube Position

When the trachea is intubated by conventional methods, the exact position of the tip of the endotracheal tube in relation to the carina is not known. If the tube is placed too far into the trachea, bronchial intubation results. If the tube is not advanced far enough, accidental extubation may occur. Therefore, in intensive care units, it is common practice to obtain a portable chest X-ray to document the position of the tube (87). A portable chest X-ray has several disadvantages including an unavoidable waiting period, difficulty in identifying the tip of the endotracheal tube, movement of the patient that causes discomfort, increased risk of disconnection or extubation, and unnecessary exposure to radiation (88,89).

The fiberscope has been used for confirmation of tracheal tube position in adults, infants, and children (39,90,91). Fiberoptic measurement of the distance between the carina and endotracheal tube tip in adults and neonates was compared with radiologic measurement (88,91). In both studies, bronchoscopic measurements were found to be rapid and accurate, with excellent correlation with radiologic measurement. In infants, transcutaneous oxygen tension dropped during both bronchoscopic measurement and radiography of the chest, but was more marked in the latter (91).

To perform the procedure, advance the fiberscope through the endoscopy port of the swivel adapter into the trachea until the tip of the fiberscope touches the ridge of the carina. The insertion cord is then firmly held by the thumb and index finger at the level of the adapter, and the fiberscope slowly withdrawn until the tip of the endotracheal tube comes into view. The distance between the fingers holding the insertion cord (marking the carinate level) and the level of the adapter (marking the tip of the endotracheal tube) is noted. This represents the distance of the tip of the endotracheal tube above the carina.

The carina moves caudad during inspiration, therefore its position is verified during exhalation, when the carina is in the most cephalad position (Fig. 7). The

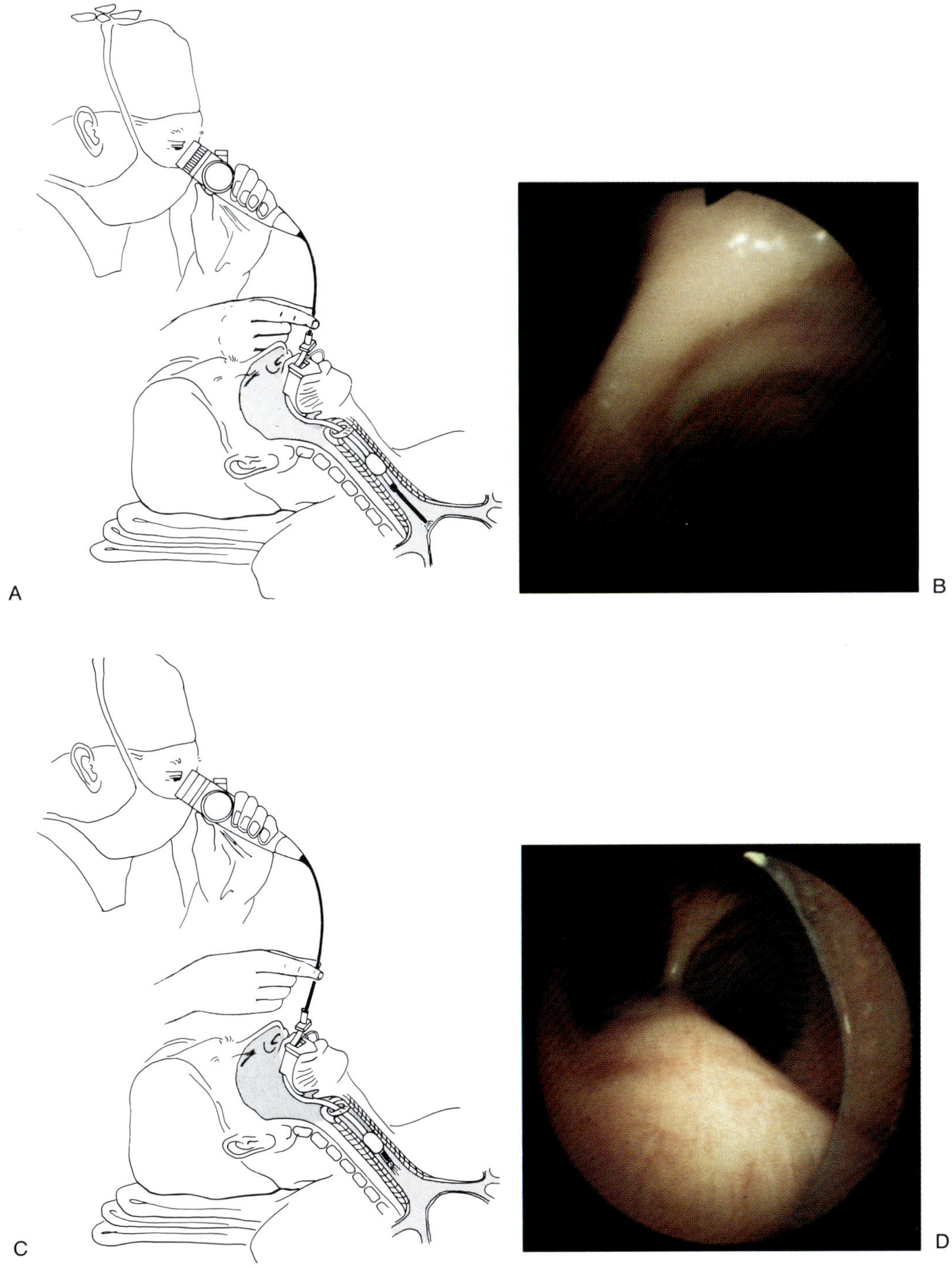

FIG. 7. Checking endotracheal tube position. **A:** The fiberscope is advanced through the swivel adapter and endotracheal tube into the distal trachea until the tip of the fiberscope is within 1–2 mm of the carina. **B:** Endoscopic view showing close-up of the carina. **C:** The insertion cord of the fiberscope is held by the thumb and index finger at the level of the tracheal tube adapter (marking the carinal level), and the fiberscope is slowly withdrawn until the tip of the endotracheal tube is visualized (marking the tip of the endotracheal tube). The distance between the fingers holding the insertion cord and the adapter of the endotracheal tube represents the distance from the tip of the endotracheal tube to the carina. **D:** Endoscopic view of the distal end of the endotracheal tube positioned 3 cm above the carina.

distance between the carina and tip of the endotracheal tube should be between 2.5 and 4 cm in adults. In the newborn, it is recommended that the tip of the tracheal tube be 2 cm above the carina and 1–1.5 cm below the vocal cords (92). This recommendation is based on the fact that the tracheal tube moves cephalad and caudad with extension and flexion of the head, respectively, and adequate space must be available to accommodate this movement (92,93).

A problem encountered in infants when using the fiberscope for tracheal confirmation involves secretions. The small suction channel of the pediatric fiberscope lacks a suction channel, requiring scope removal to allow for direct suctioning.

In adults and children, if the tracheal tube is resting in a main stem bronchus, the secondary bifurcation of the bronchial tree may be misidentified as carina.

The practitioner should also be aware of the increased airway resistance that the spontaneously breathing patient must overcome when the fiberscope is positioned inside of the endotracheal tube. The airway resistance, depending on the respective diameters of the tracheal tube and fiberscope, may be substantial. In premature infants and unstable patients, the examination time for the procedure should be limited to 30 seconds to avoid untoward respiratory distress.

Repositioning the Endotracheal Tube

If an endotracheal tube is advanced into a main stem bronchus, it can be withdrawn under direct vision to the desired location, with the help of the fiberscope (94). This minimizes potential accidental extubation and provides an element of safety. This is especially true when the patient is in an inaccessible position, such as the prone or sitting position.

The fiberscope is advanced inside the endotracheal tube until its tip is positioned at the distal end of the tube (Fig. 8). The cuff is deflated, and the fiberscope and endotracheal tube are slowly pulled back as a single unit until the carina is visualized. The tube is then positioned 2–4 cm above the carina.

CHANGING THE ENDOTRACHEAL TUBE

Replacing an endotracheal tube may be necessary when the cuff is damaged, the tube becomes ob-

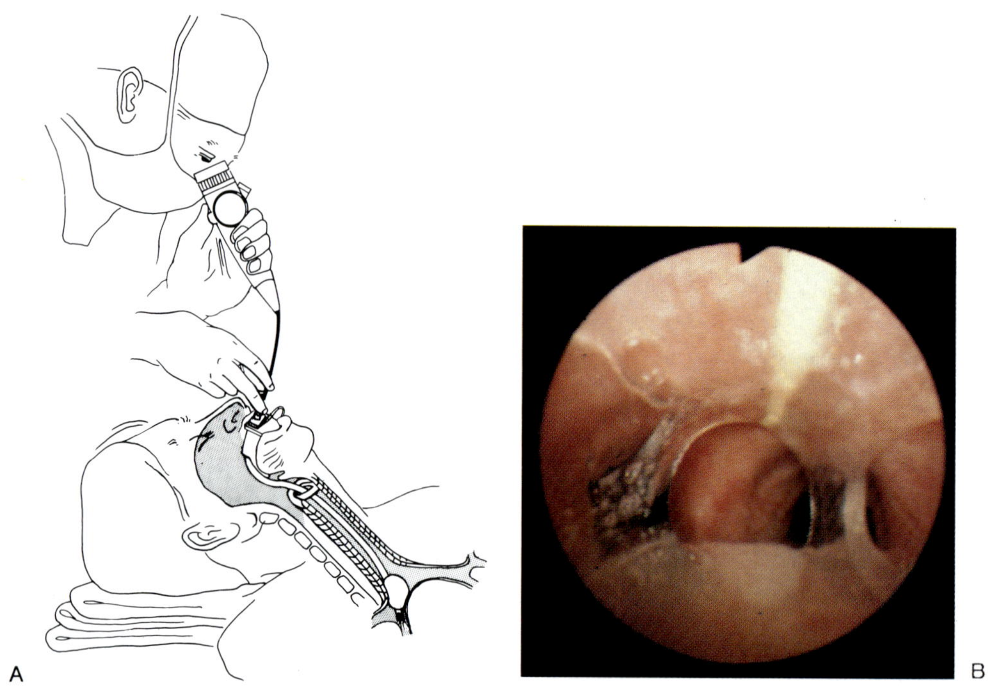

FIG. 8. Repositioning of the endotracheal tube. **A:** The endotracheal tube has been advanced too far into the right main stem bronchus. **B:** Endoscopic view of the distal tip of the tube. The medial wall of the right main stem bronchus is visualized. **C:** The tip of the fiberscope is positioned at the distal end of the endotracheal tube. The tracheal cuff is deflated, and both fiberscope and tube are pulled out together slowly until the carina is seen. **D:** Endoscopic view of the carina just beyond the tip of the endotracheal tube. **E:** The fiberscope and tube are pulled back farther until the tip of the tube is 2.5–4 cm above the carina. **F:** Endoscopic view of the carina 3 cm beyond the tip of the endotracheal tube.

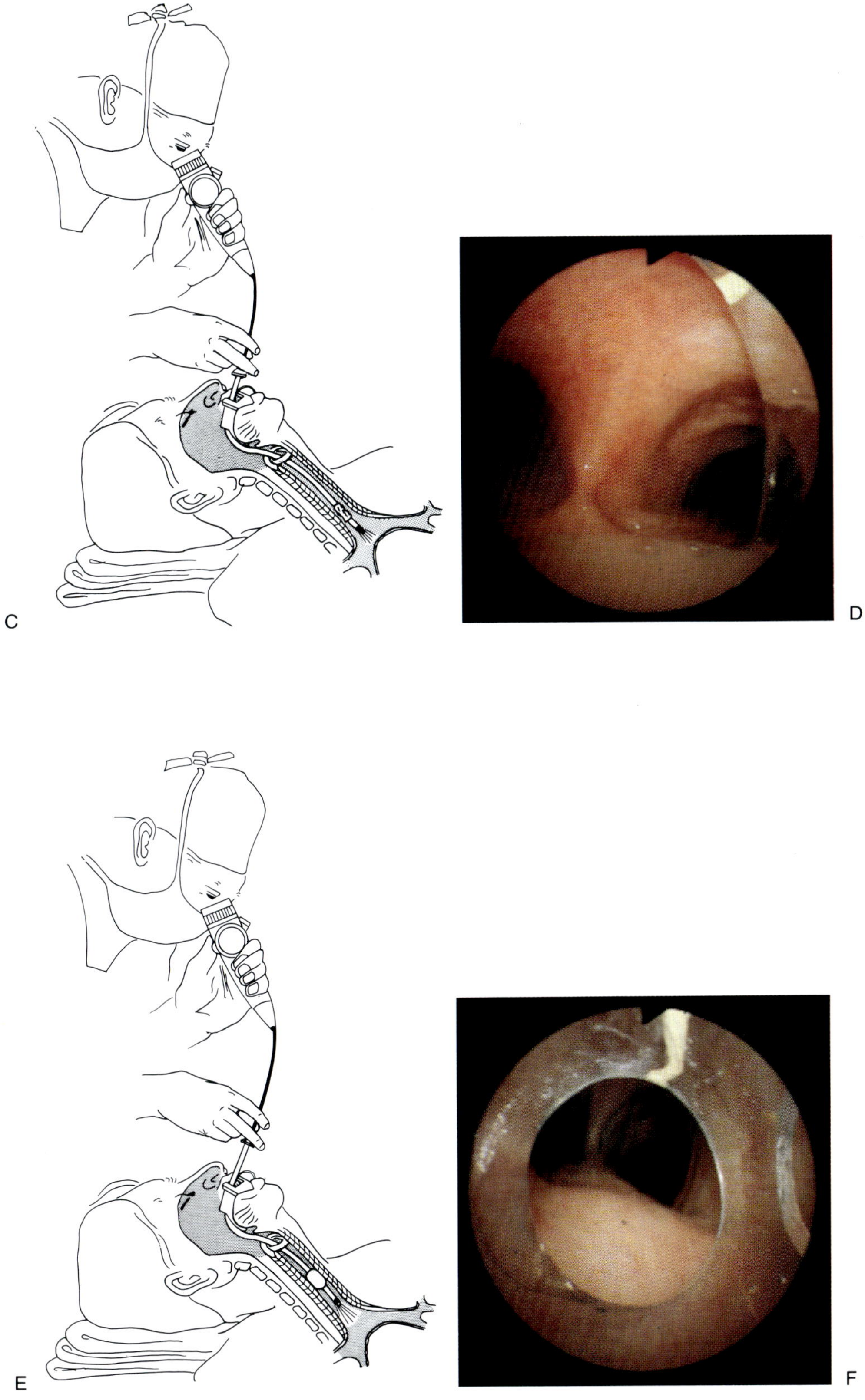

FIG. 8. *Continued.*

structed, or a larger tube is required. It may be necessary to change from an oral to a nasal tube for prolonged ventilatory support, or from a nasal tube to an oral or contralateral nasal tube due to developing sinusitis.

Guides or stylets have been used for replacing endotracheal tubes, without changing the orifice used for intubation (95). When the route of intubation is to be changed, however, guides or stylets cannot be used. The choice is then be between rigid or fiberoptic laryngoscopy. Fiberoptic laryngoscopy should be considered when the initial intubation was difficult. Other indications for its consideration include a patient on mechanical ventilation requiring high positive end expiratory pressure (PEEP), or a patient with an unstable cervical fracture (96,97).

Changing an Orotracheal Tube to a Nasotracheal Tube

If conscious, the procedure is first explained to the patient. Small doses of midazolam (1–2 mg) and fentanyl (50–100 μg) are administered intravenously to provide sedation and suppress the pharyngeal and laryngeal reflexes.

In the anesthetized and paralyzed patient, a jaw thrust maneuver is required to assist in exposure of the glottis. The administration of an antisialagogue drug is very important to combat the abundant secretions in these patients.

The nasal mucosa is treated with cocaine, and the endotracheal tube inserted into the nose (Fig. 9A). The pharynx is thoroughly suctioned, and the fiberscope advanced through the nasal tube into the oropharynx. To assure a safe and fast exchange of endotracheal tubes, it is best to advance the fiberscope alongside the existing orotracheal tube into the midtrachea (Fig. 9B).

The orotracheal tube lies in the larynx posteriorly against the arytenoids and posterior commissure, thereby leaving the anterior one-third of the glottis open (Fig. 9C). The fiberscope should be directed toward the anterior commissure, making passage of the fiberscope into the trachea possible (13,98). To assist anterior commissure exposure, it may be necessary to move the existing orotracheal tube from one side of the mouth to the other. Usually to the side of the mouth away from the nostril through which the fiberscope is being passed.

The orotracheal tube may also be pushed backward against the posterior pharyngeal wall to assist passage of the fiberscope anterior to the existing orotracheal tube. It is often necessary to rotate the fiberscope 90° and flex the tip anteriorly to expose the anterior commissure of the larynx. In awake patients and anesthetized patients breathing spontaneously, topical anesthesia (4–5 ml, 4% lidocaine) is sprayed on the larynx through the fiberscope. This prevents laryngeal spasm and resistance to tube advancement. Most of the local anesthetic sprayed onto the vocal cords is suctioned after 2 or 3 min of contact to minimize systemic absorption.

The fiberscope is then advanced anterior to the existing tube into the larynx (Fig. 9D). The cuff of the orotracheal tube is deflated, and the fiberscope further advanced into the trachea until the tracheal bifurcation is identified (Figs. 9E and F). The orotracheal tube is removed, and the nasotracheal tube threaded over the fiberscope into the trachea (Figs. 9G and H).

In some cases, the fiberscope cannot be advanced into the trachea alongside the existing orotracheal tube. In such cases, the tip of the fiberscope is positioned on top of the vocal cords, and the existing oral tube withdrawn slowly under direct vision (Figs. 10A–F). As soon as the oral tube leaves the glottis, the fiberscope is advanced into the trachea followed by the nasotracheal tube (Figs. 10G–J).

A major disadvantage of this approach is that accumulated secretions enter into the pharynx as soon as the orotracheal tube cuff is deflated, and the tube is pulled back. These secretions may obscure the view through the fiberscope, delaying or causing failure of fiberscope placement into the trachea. To overcome this problem, the following modification of the technique is recommended.

Modified Technique

After placement of the nasal tube, the fiberscope is positioned proximal to the glottis as described above (Figs. 11A–C). Under fiberoptic observation, positive pressure ventilation is applied, and the cuff of the existing orotracheal tube deflated and reinflated immediately (13). The secretions accumulated above the endotracheal tube cuff are pushed up into the oropharynx. Ventilation is continued until all secretions are suctioned. The orotracheal tube cuff is deflated again, and the tube slowly withdrawn until the cuff is located between the vocal cords. The cuff is reinflated between the vocal cords (Figs. 11D and E). The secretions are again suctioned thoroughly through the fiberscope.

If necessary, the fiberscope may be removed, cleaned, and reinserted. When all secretions have been thoroughly suctioned and a clear view obtained, the orotracheal tube cuff is deflated for a final time and the tube removed from the larynx (Figs. 11F and G). The fiberscope is immediately advanced into the trachea, followed by the nasotracheal tube (Figs. 11H and I).

The advantages of using the fiberscope for endotracheal tube changes include minimal required sedation

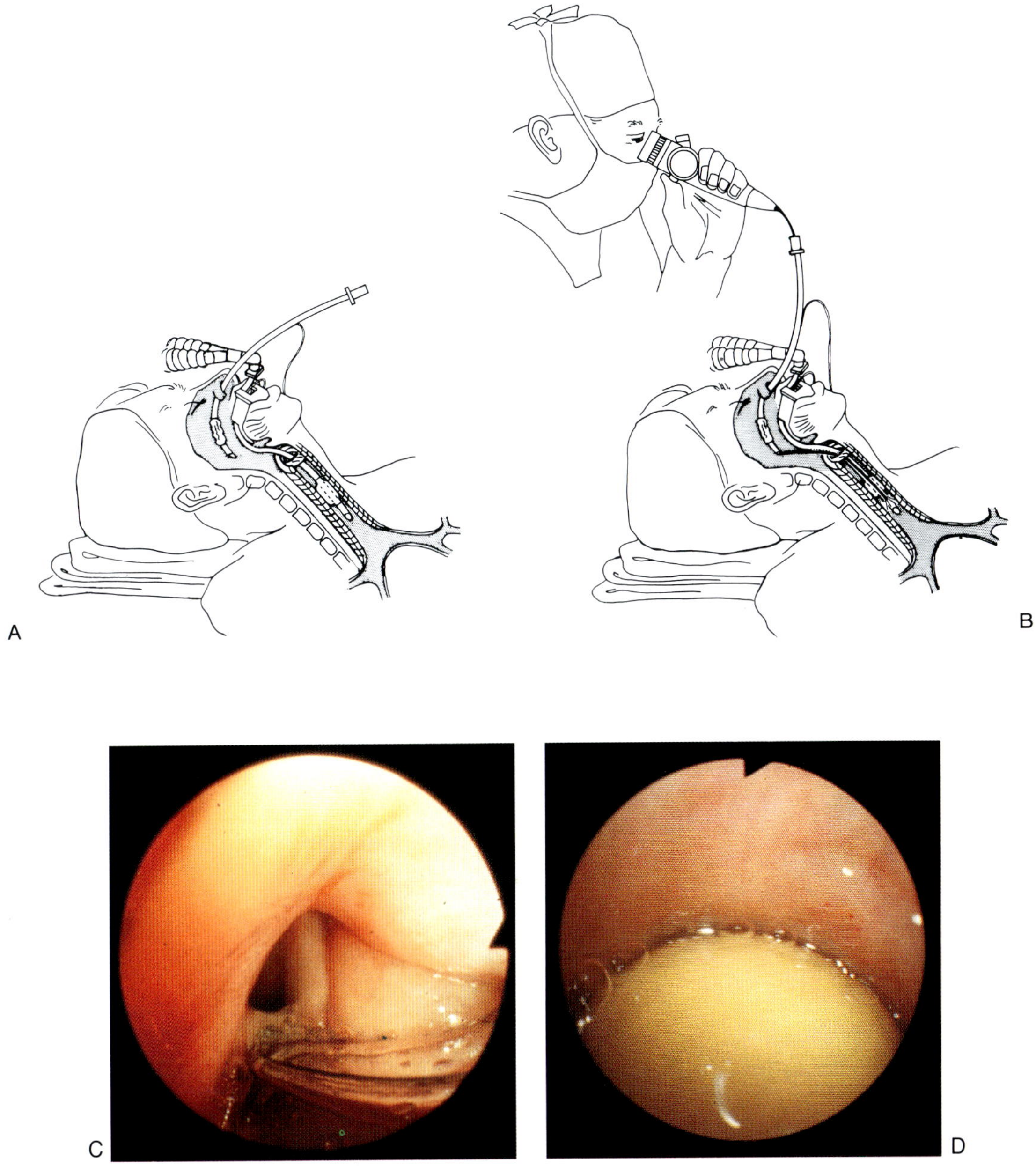

FIG. 9. Changing an orotracheal tube to a nasotracheal tube. **A:** The nasotracheal tube is advanced into the oropharynx, and secretions are suctioned thoroughly. **B:** The fiberscope is passed through the nasal tube into the oropharynx and is advanced alongside the existing orotracheal tube into the larynx. The tracheal cuff of existing orotracheal tube is deflated to allow advancement of the fiberscope to the lower trachea. **C:** Endoscopic view of the orotracheal tube. The anterior commissure is unoccupied. The fiberscope is rotated 90° to the left, and the tip of the fiberscope is positioned above the tube. **D:** Endoscopic view of the larynx and yellow inflated cuff of the existing orotracheal tube. The tip of the fiberscope is just beyond the vocal cords.

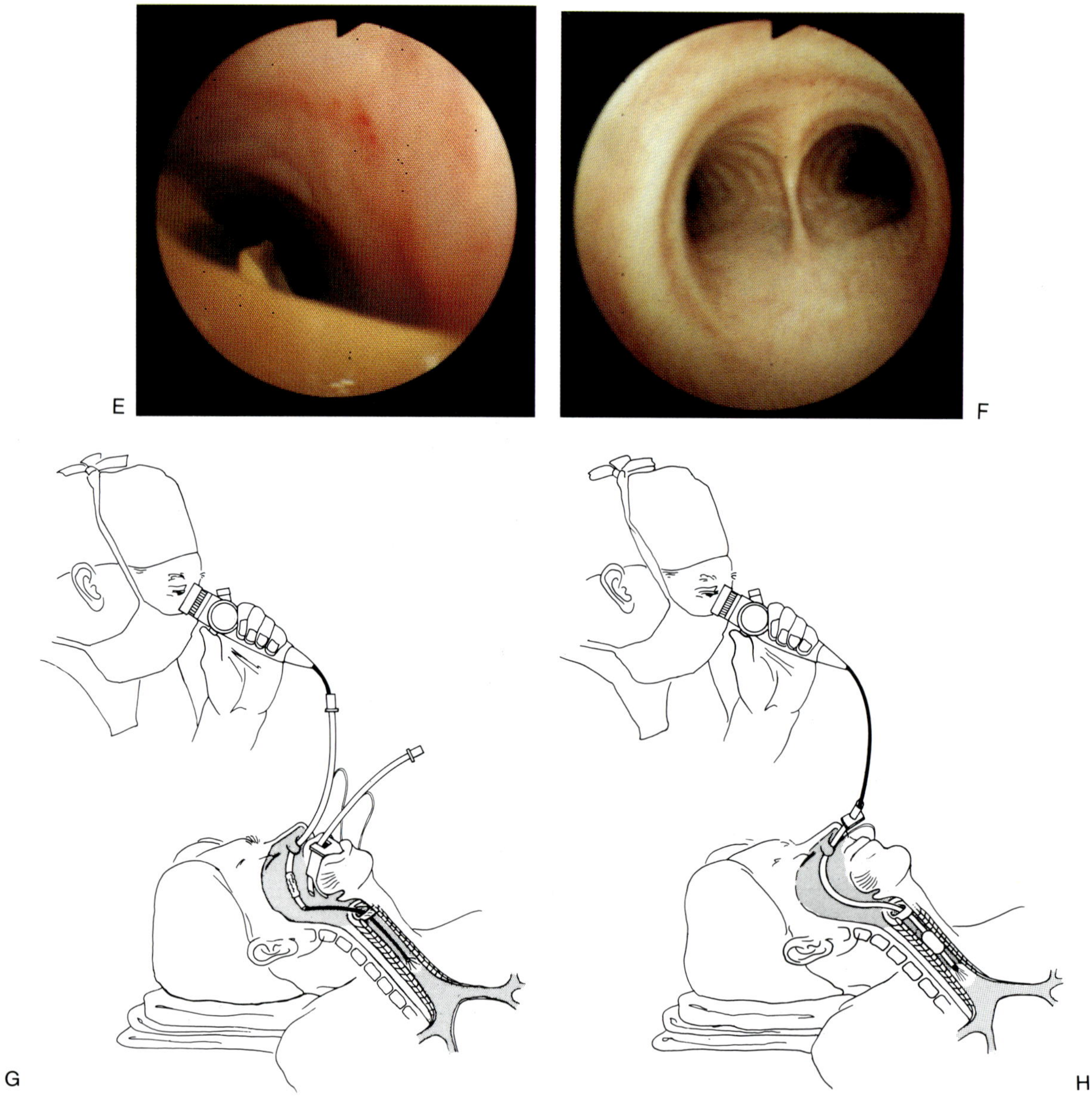

FIG. 9. *Continued.* **E:** Endoscopic view of deflated cuff. **F:** The fiberscope can now be advanced beyond the cuff to expose the carina. **G:** The existing orotracheal tube is removed. **H:** The nasotracheal tube is advanced over the fiberscope into the trachea.

in awake patients, short interruption of mechanical ventilation in patients on high PEEP, and facilitation of a known difficult tracheal intubation (13,96,98). The major disadvantage is having secretions or blood obscure the fiberscope tip, increasing the time it may take to complete the procedure.

In a series of 15 such intubations in adult patients the failure rate was reported to be 20% (96). In another report, the technique was successful in 27 of 29 attempts in patients ranging from 20 months to 90 years of age (99). Although our initial attempts to replace orotracheal tubes with a nasotracheal tubes were associated with a high failure rate, it was later successful in 13 consecutive tube changes in 1988 and 1989.

The author has used the technique(s) described to change a single-lumen orotracheal tube to a double-lumen endobronchial tube on three patients. In two patients, where orotracheal intubation failed with rigid laryngoscopy, the fiberscope was used for tracheal placement of a single-lumen endotracheal tube for fiberoptic bronchoscopy prior to thoracotomy (13). The fiberscope (Olympus LF-1) was then used to replace the single-lumen endotracheal tube with a 39 French (Fr) double-lumen endobronchial tube.

On one occasion, a double-lumen endobronchial tube was fiberscopically replaced with another double-lumen tube after a difficult rigid laryngoscopy and intubation had damaged the original tracheal cuff. On two

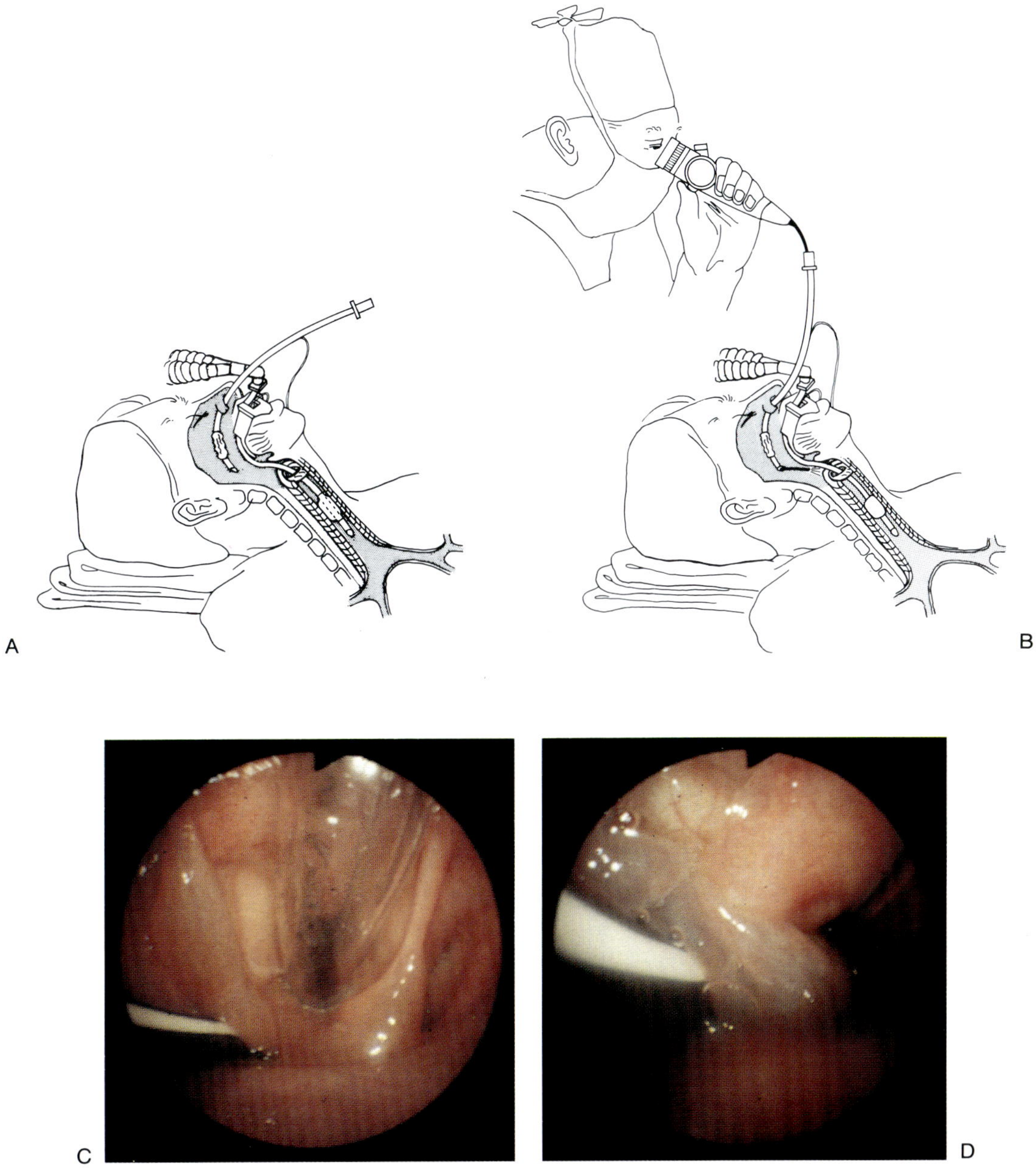

FIG. 10. Changing an orotracheal to a nasotracheal tube. Second approach. **A:** The nasotracheal tube is advanced into the oropharynx, and secretions are suctioned thoroughly. **B:** The tip of the fiberscope is advanced through the nasal tube and positioned proximal to the glottis, which is occupied by the orotracheal tube. **C:** Endoscopic view of the larynx with jaw thrust. The base of the tongue and pharyngeal tissues are moved up showing clear view of the nasogastric tube on the left side. The clear endotracheal tube is between the cords with arytenoids posterior to the tube. **D:** Same endoscopic view as in **C** without a jaw thrust. Loose laryngopharyngeal tissues block exposure of the orotracheal tube and arytenoids.

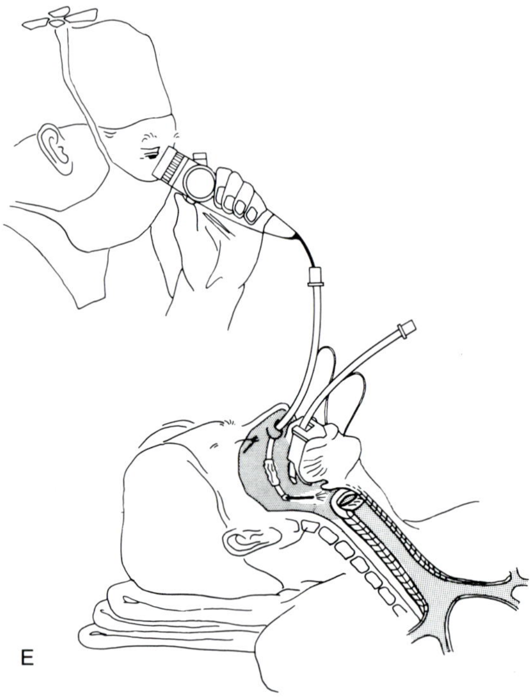

E

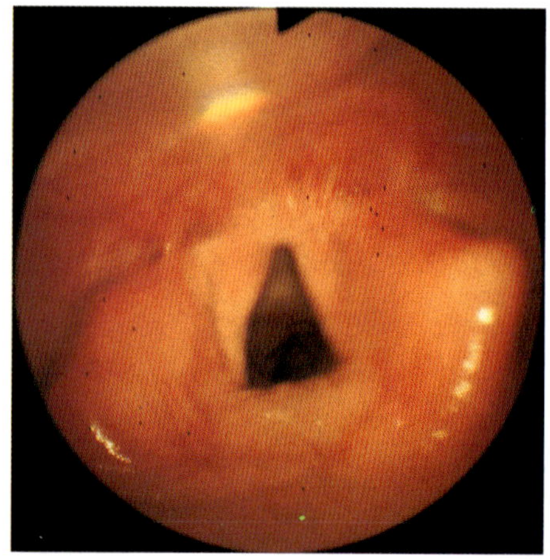

F

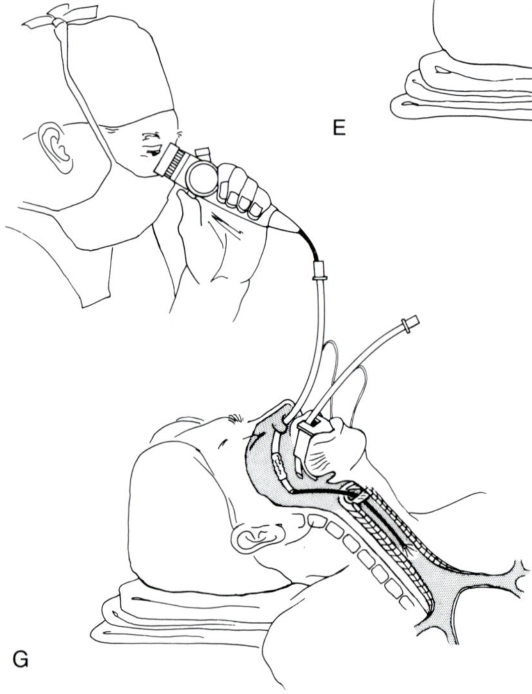

G

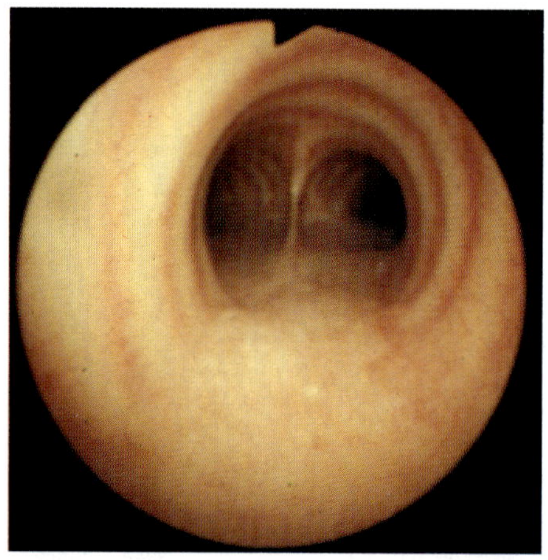

H

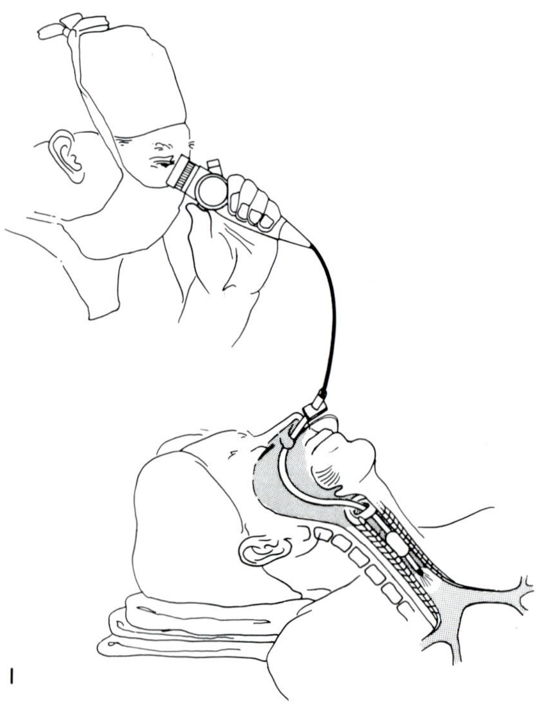

I

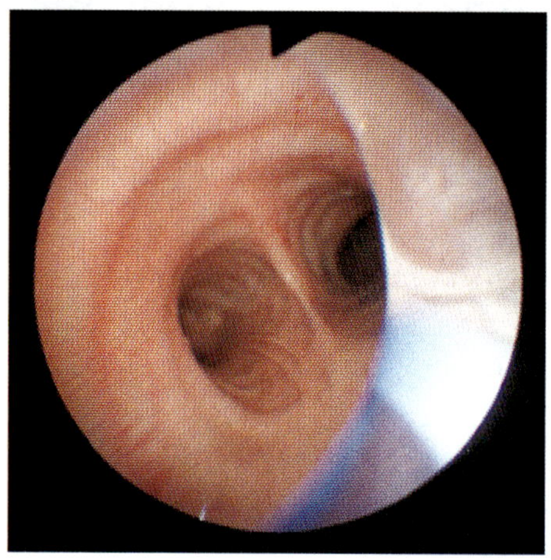

J

FIG. 10. *Continued.* **E:** The existing orotracheal tube is removed under visualization. **F:** Endoscopic view of the open glottis after extubation. **G:** The fiberscope is immediately advanced into the trachea. **H:** Endoscopic view of carina. **I:** The nasotracheal tube is advanced into the trachea over the fiberscope. **J:** Endoscopic view of the carina and the tip of the tube.

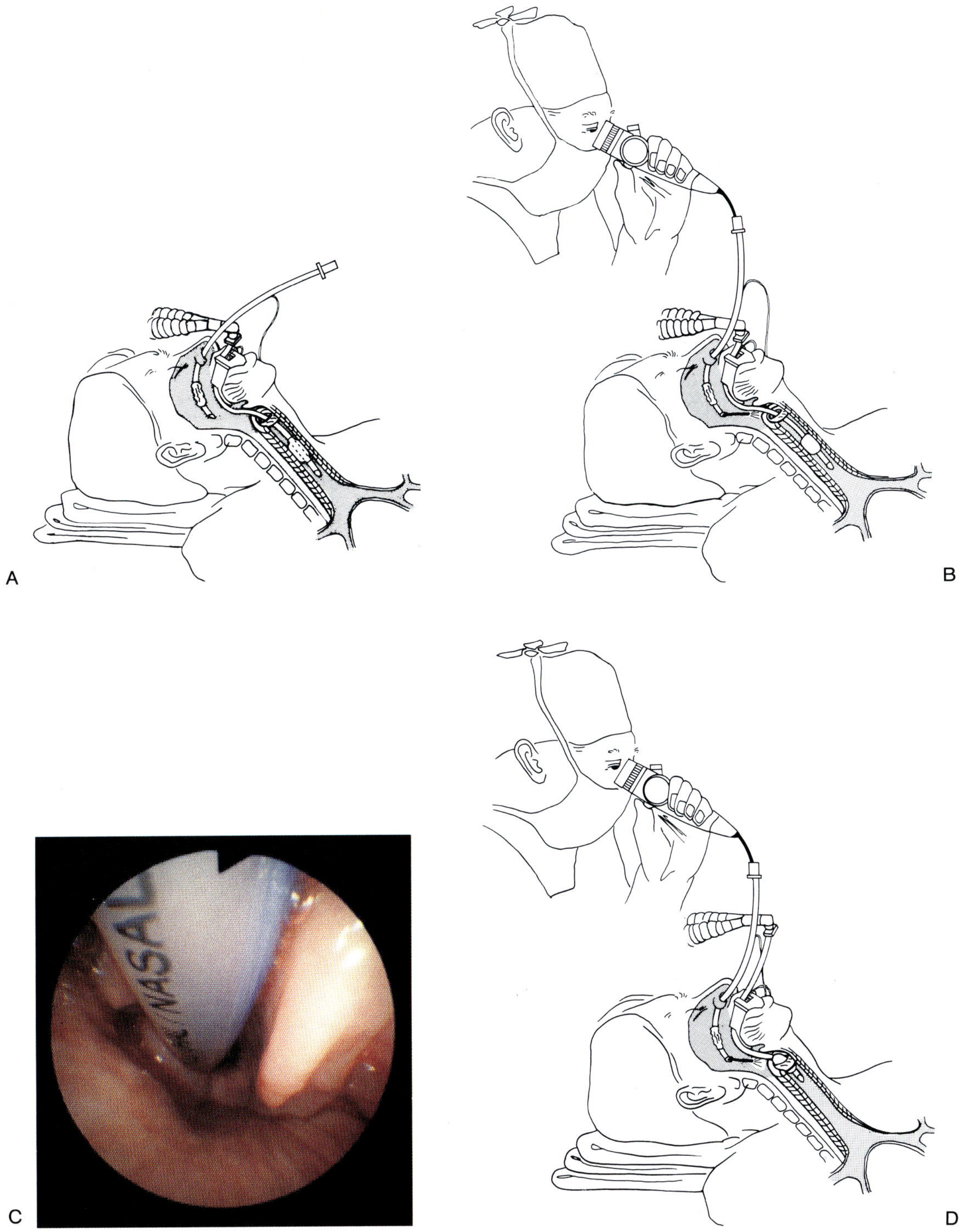

FIG. 11. Changing an orotracheal to a nasotracheal tube. A modified technique of the second approach. **A:** The nasotracheal tube is advanced into the oropharynx, and secretions are suctioned thoroughly. **B:** The tip of the fiberscope, which is advanced through the nasal tube, is positioned proximal to the glottis, which is occupied by the orotracheal tube. The secretions are suctioned through the fiberscope. The tracheal tube cuff is deflated while positive pressure is applied momentarily to push secretions that have accumulated on top of the cuff into the pharynx and are suctioned again. **C:** Endoscopic view of the orotracheal tube and the larynx. **D:** Under visual observation, the orotracheal tube is pulled back slowly, until the cuff lies between the vocal cords. The cuff is inflated and ventilation continued, while the secretions remaining in the pharynx are suctioned.

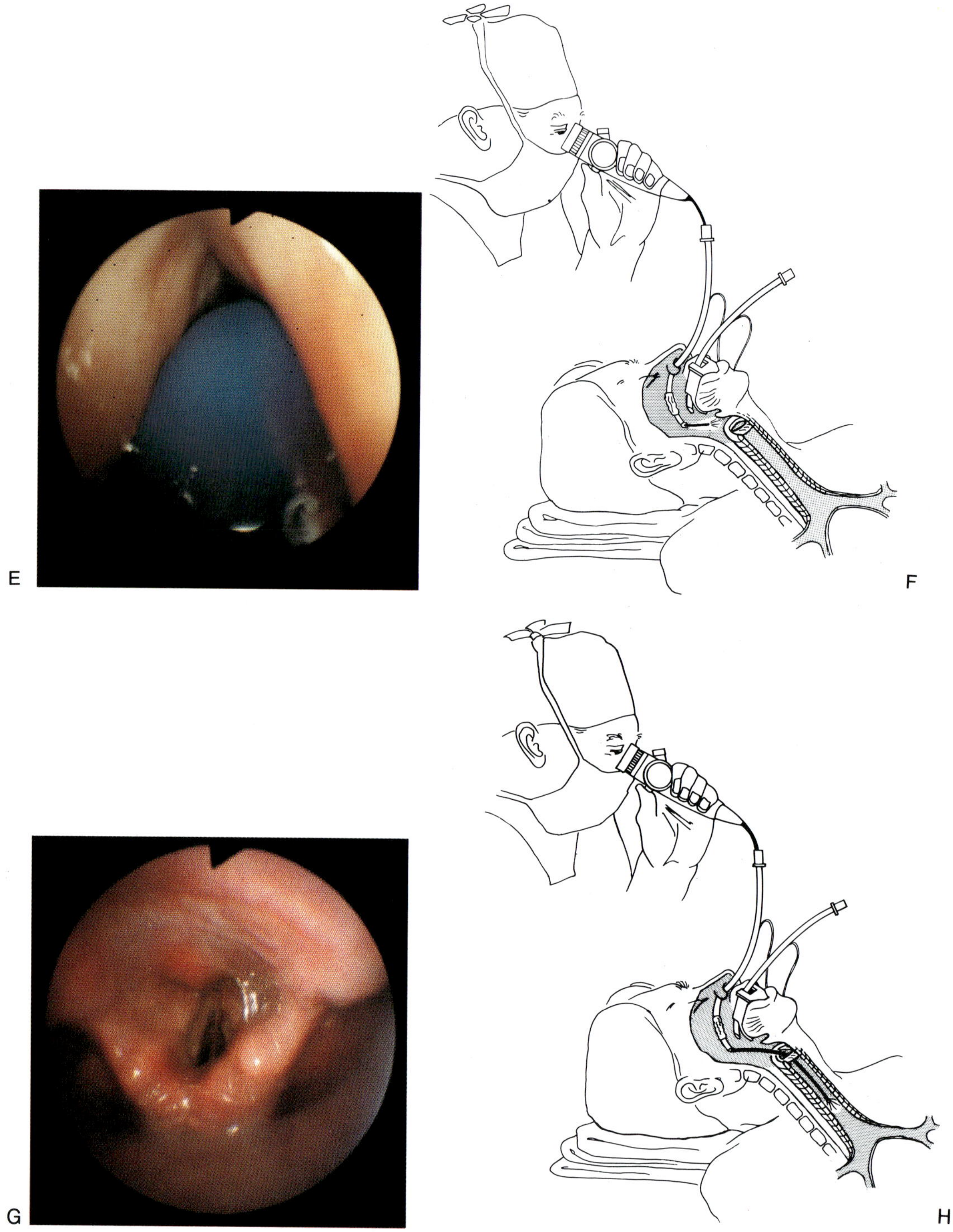

FIG. 11. *Continued.* **E:** Endoscopic view of inflated blue cuff between the vocal cords. All secretions have been cleared. **F:** Cuff is deflated and the existing tube is pulled out. **G:** Endoscopic view of the glottis after removing the tube. **H:** The fiberscope is advanced into the trachea immediately. **I:** The nasotracheal tube is threaded into the trachea.

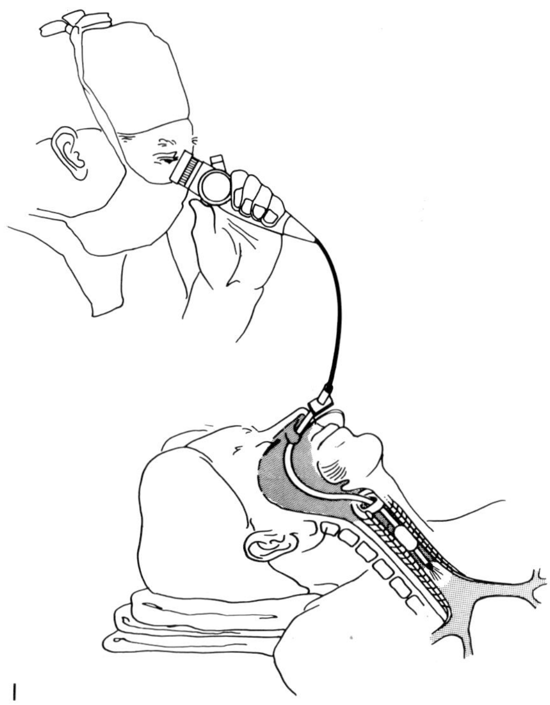

FIG. 11. *Continued.*

occasions, at the conclusion of surgery a double-lumen endobronchial tube was changed by fiberscope to a single-lumen endotracheal tube for postoperative ventilatory support (13). The techniques require considerable experience, and the equipment necessary for alternative approaches should be readily available should they fail.

TRACHEAL AND BRONCHIAL INTUBATION

Awake fiberoptic tracheal intubation offers many advantages for the critically ill patient, including patients with impending ventilatory failure (100), unstable neck, nasal packs, and Sangstaken-Blakemore tubes equipped with helmet traction (Fig. 12) (13).

Double-lumen endobronchial tubes have been used for independent lung ventilation in patients with pulmonary pathology primarily confined to one lung (Table 8) (101). In such cases, the compliance of one lung may be markedly different from the other. Thus, the application of positive pressure breathing through a single-lumen endotracheal tube shall be preferentially directed to the normal lung. Blood flow may also be shifted to the unaffected lung, producing further deterioration of arterial oxygenation (102). This problem may be reversed by selectively ventilating each lung by use of a double-lumen tube, and by selective application

TABLE 8. *Nonsurgical indications for separation of the lungs*

Bronchoalveolar lavage
Alveolar proteinosis
Atelectasis
Hemoptysis
Differential lung ventilation
Severe unilateral lung pathology
Contusion
ARDS
Large emphysematous cyst
Large bronchopleurocutaneous fistula

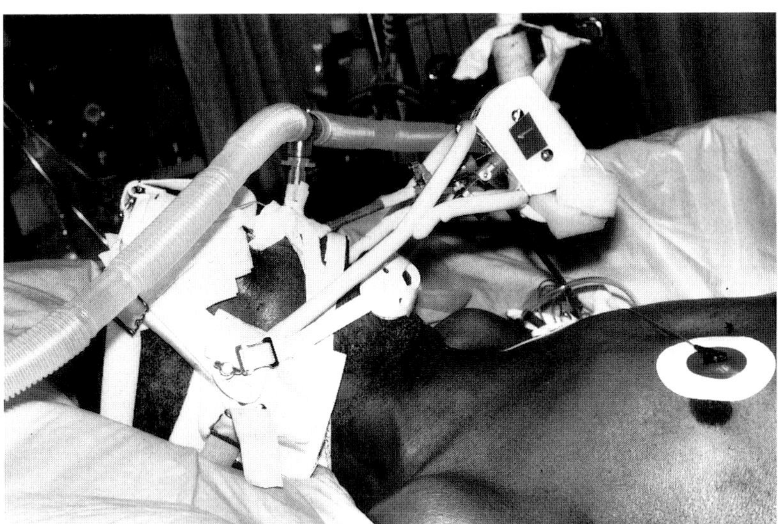

FIG. 12. Patient with esophageal bleeding. Sangstaken-Blakemore tube with helmet traction applied to control esophageal bleeding. Ventilatory failure necessitated tracheal intubation. Fiberoptic nasotracheal intubation was easily performed without interfering with Sangstaken-Blakemore tube traction.

of PEEP or continuous positive airway pressure (CPAP) to the diseased lung.

Double-lumen endobronchial tubes have also been used for the management of pulmonary hemorrhage (103). Placement of a double-lumen endobronchial tube provides complete separation of the lungs and prevents blood from entering the unaffected lung. The ability to either selectively ventilate or suction both lungs facilitates the management of patients with pulmonary hemorrhage. The double-lumen endobronchial tube is also used for lung lavage in patients suffering from pulmonary alveolar proteinosis (104).

CHECKING AND PLACEMENT OF THE NASOGASTRIC TUBE

A nasogastric (NG) tube is commonly placed to aspirate stomach contents and supplement nutrition in the critically ill patient (Table 9) (105). Nasogastric tubes are larger in size and stiffer than nasoenteric tubes. Nasoenteric tubes are thin plastic catheters with a balloon tip, which is filled with mercury prior to placement.

INSERTION OF THE NASOGASTRIC TUBE

Passage of an NG tube is usually attempted with the patient awake in the sitting position. To minimize discomfort, the selected nostril is anesthetized with lidocaine spray before the lubricated NG tube is introduced into the nose. The tube is advanced firmly but gently. As soon as it enters the oropharynx, the patient is asked to swallow to facilitate the tube's entrance into the esophagus (105).

Placement of an NG tube is often required in an unconscious or anesthetized patient. In the absence of patient cooperation, the NG tube has a tendency to coil in the pharynx, making its insertion more difficult (106,107). Passage of an NG tube may also be impeded by esophageal narrowing secondary to an overinflated endotracheal tube cuff, inadequate relaxation of the cricopharyngeus muscle, and a variety of anatomic abnormalities (108).

Many techniques and maneuvers have been described to assist with the insertion of an NG tube (Table 10) (106–110). When these measures fail, the fiberscope may be used to place an endotracheal tube or guide wire into the esophagus to help guide the NG tube into the stomach.

Fiberoptic-Aided Nasogastric Intubation

A 7-mm internal diameter (ID) endotracheal tube is cut along its length, and passed through a nostril into the oropharynx (Fig. 13). The fiberscope is inserted through the endotracheal tube, into the oropharynx, and passed into the esophagus. The endotracheal tube is then advanced over the fiberscope into the esophagus, and the fiberscope removed. A lubricated NG tube is then threaded through the endotracheal tube into the stomach. The endotracheal tube is then removed, leaving the NG tube in place.

If for any reason insertion of an endotracheal tube via the nose is not desirable or possible, the split endotracheal tube is placed into the esophagus via the oral route (Fig. 14). A lubricated NG tube is then passed through the nose into the oropharynx, and the tip drawn out of the mouth. The NG tube is threaded through the orotracheal tube into the stomach. The split tracheal tube is then removed (106).

Another approach advances the fiberscope through the nose into the esophagus, and a guide wire is then inserted through the suction channel of the fiberscope (111). The NG tube is then advanced over the guide wire into the stomach (Fig. 15).

TABLE 9. *Indications for placing a nasogastric tube*

Aspiration of gastric contents
Diagnostic
Gastric juice analysis
Upper gastrointestinal bleeding
Therapeutic
Decompression
Evacuation
Lavage
Gastric feeding

TABLE 10. *Facilitating nasogastric tube placement*

Tube-related
Lubricating nasogastric (NG) tube
Increasing stiffness of NG tube
Placing in ice water
Using stylet
Patient-related
Have patient swallow small amount of water
Turn the patient's head from one side to another
Displace the larynx forward
Placing finger into the mouth to guide advancement of the NG tube in an anesthetized patient
Placing endotracheal tube in the esophagus and using it as a conduit
Fiberoptic-guided
Rigid laryngoscopy-aided
Blind technique
Placement of a guide wire in the esophagus through the working channel of the fiberscope to help guide the NG tube into the esophagus
Palpation by surgeon during intraabdominal surgery

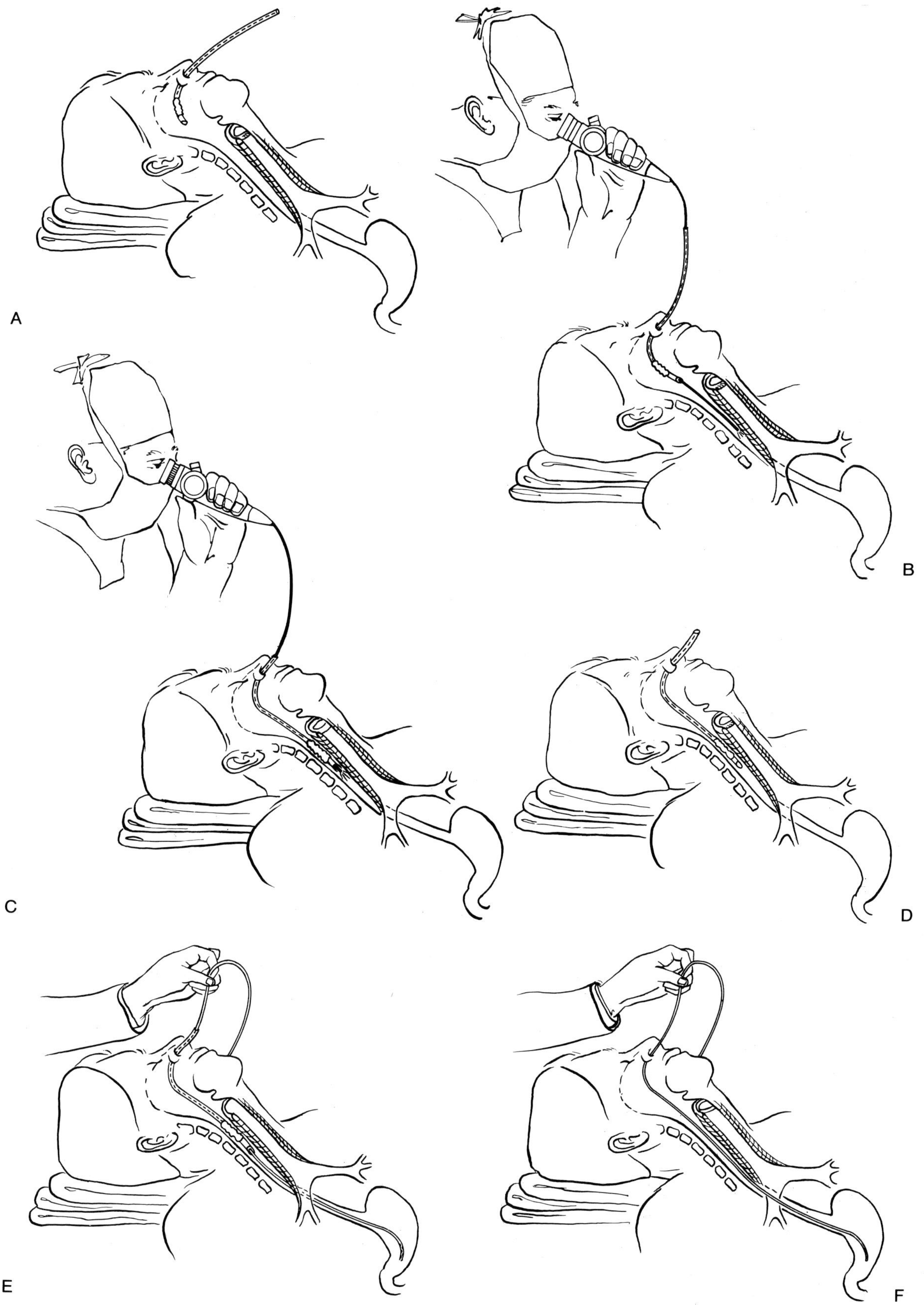

FIG. 13. Fiberoptic-aided nasogastric intubation. **A:** A longitudinally cut tracheal tube without an adapter is placed in the prepared nostril. **B:** The fiberscope is advanced through the tracheal tube into the esophagus. **C:** The tracheal tube is threaded over the fiberscope into the esophagus. **D:** The fiberscope is removed, leaving the tracheal tube in the esophagus. **E:** The NG tube is advanced through the tube into the stomach. **F:** The tracheal tube is removed, leaving the NG tube in the stomach.

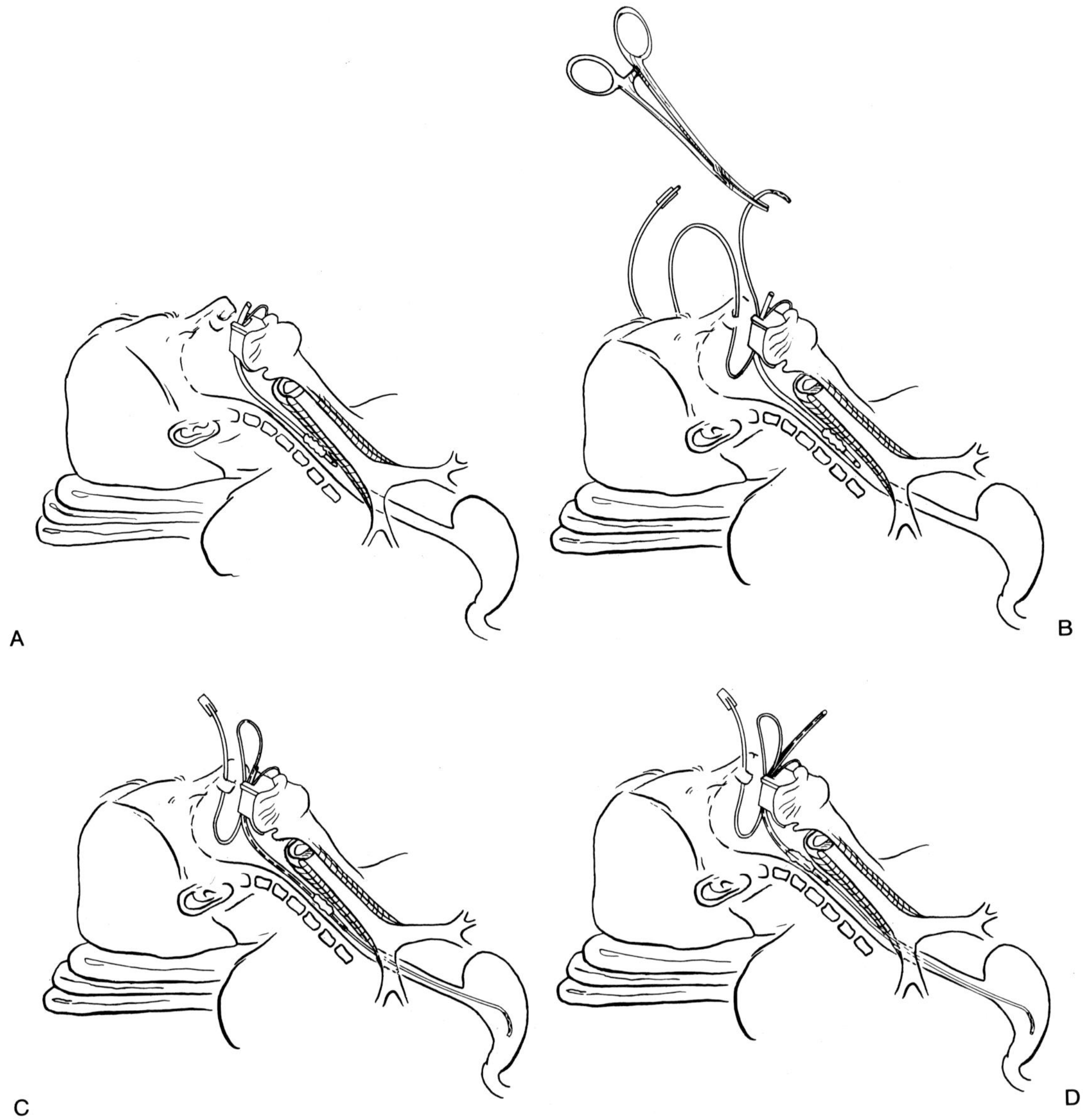

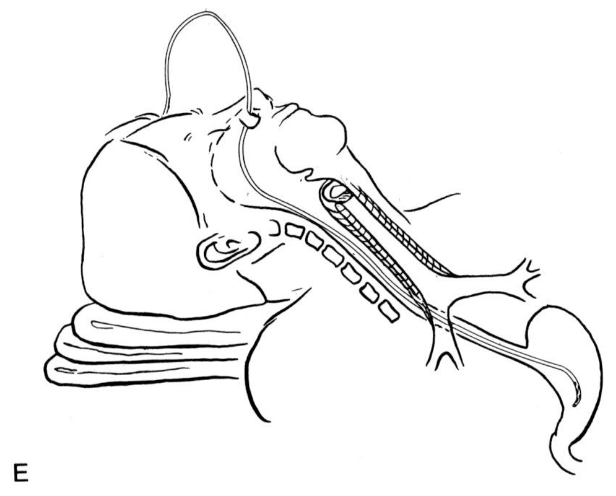

FIG. 14. Fiberoptic-aided nasogastric (NG) intubation. Second approach. **A:** A longitudinally cut tracheal tube is placed inside the esophagus orally with the help of the fiberscope. **B:** The lubricated NG tube is advanced through the nose into the pharynx. The tip of the NG tube is drawn out of the mouth. **C:** The NG tube is fed through the tracheal tube into the stomach. **D:** The tracheal tube is removed. **E:** The NG tube in place.

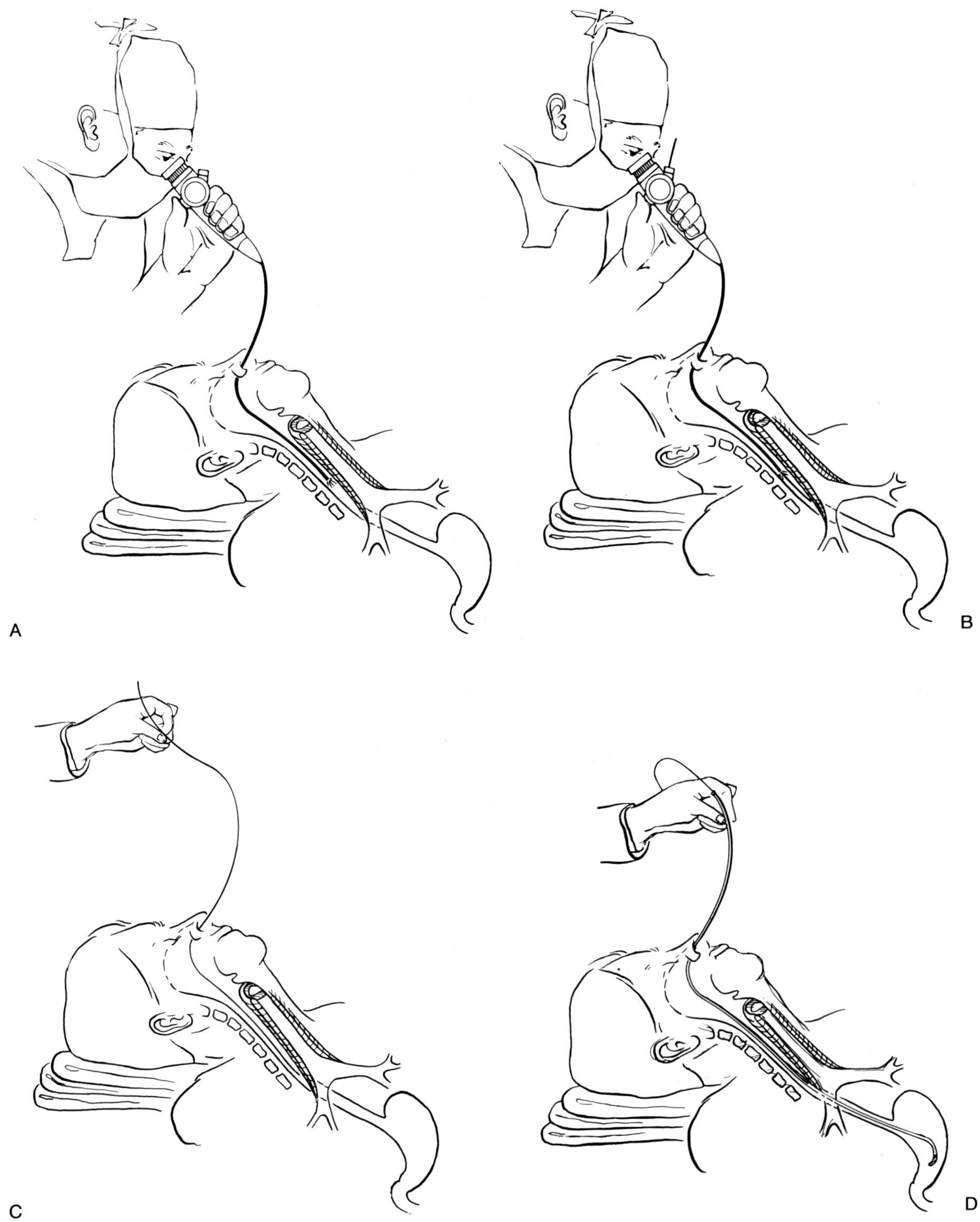

FIG. 15. Fiberoptic-aided nasogastric intubation. Third approach. **A:** The fiberscope is passed through the nose into the esophagus. **B:** The guide wire is inserted through the working channel of the fiberscope into the esophagus. **C:** The fiberscope is removed, leaving the guide wire in the esophagus. **D:** The nasogastric (NG) tube is threaded over the guide wire into the stomach.

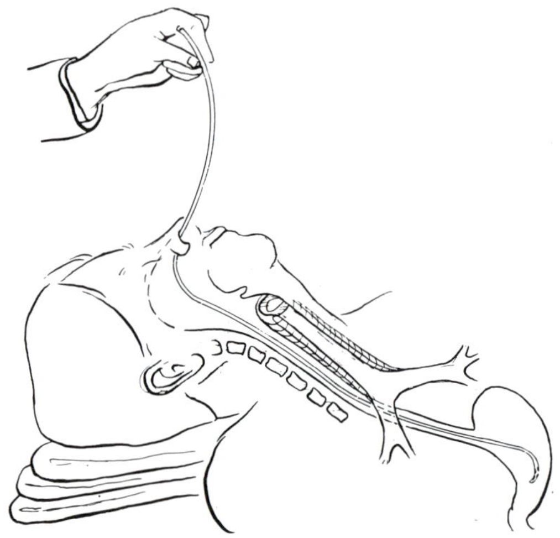

E

FIG. 15. *Continued.* **E:** The guide wire is removed, leaving the NG tube in the stomach.

Fiberoptic Confirmation of Nasogastric Tube Placement

The nasogastric tube may enter the tracheobronchial tree instead of the esophagus. This is especially common in patients with obtunded airway reflexes. It is critical to make sure that the NG tube is passed into the esophagus before any feeding is started. Fiberoptic PL may easily be utilized for this purpose.

The fiberscope is introduced nasally or orally through an intubating airway. Visualization of the NG tube entering the esophagus and an empty rima glottidis confirms the proper passage of the NG tube (Fig. 16).

To identify the exact location of the tip of the NG or feeding tube, an X-ray examination may still be needed. The conventional method for confirming NG tube position is the aspiration of gastric contents and auscultation over the epigastrium while air is being injected through the tube. Aspiration of fluid with an acidic pH confirms the proper placement of the tube and is a good method of differentiating gastric contents from fluids obtained from the pleural space or cranium (112).

It is not always possible to obtain fluid when an NG tube is in the stomach, and auscultation over the epigastrium may on occasion be misleading. Sounds may be transmitted from the pharynx, esophagus, the left bronchus, and pleural space to the epigastric area through a misplaced NG tube (113–115).

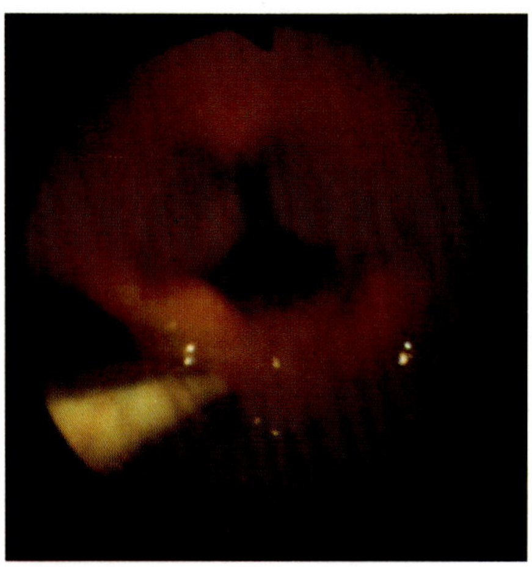

FIG. 16. Endoscopic view of the larynx. The nasogastric tube passes into the esophagus to the left of the larynx.

Complications of Nasogastric and Nasoenteric Tubes

Complications associated with the use of the NG and nasoenteric tubes include pain and trauma during insertion, tissue irritation with long-term use, and complications resulting from misplaced tubes (Table 11).

Pain, epistaxis, and mucosal laceration can be minimized by applying topical anesthesia to the nasal mucosa, lubricating the tube generously, and advancing the tube gently along the correct anatomic pathway. More serious complications include pharyngeal dissection and esophageal perforation, with the tube entering the pleural space (112–114). Ulceration of the esophagus, reduction in cardioesophageal sphincter competency, and perforation of the stomach have all been reported (116).

A rare but severe complication of the NG tube is development of vocal cord fixation, leading to concomitant airway obstruction (117–119). The NG tube, as it rests between the cervical spine and cricoid cartilage, may cause postcricoid ulceration. Inflammation and edema may extend to the arytenoids and posterior cricoarytenoid muscles, causing fixation of the vocal cords and airway obstruction.

TABLE 11. *Complications of nasogastric and nasoenteric tubes*

Trauma
Pain and epistaxis during insertion
Irritation of tissues
Perforation of pharynx, esophagus, and stomach
Airway obstruction
Misplaced
Tracheobronchial tree
Hemoptysis
Atelectasis
Mediastinum and pleural space
Pneumothorax
Hydrothorax
Intracranial cavity

Case reports and an experimental study in dogs substantiate the clinical impression that a midline-positioned NG tube is a precipitating factor in laryngeal injuries (120). However, midline tube position is uncommon, occurring in only 6% of 100 consecutive patients evaluated roentgenographically (120). Most laryngeal complications develop after several days of NG intubation. The duration of esophageal intubation does not correlate directly with the severity of symptoms. One case of bilateral cord paralysis was reported only 24 hr after placement of an NG tube (121). Although laryngeal injury secondary to NG tube placement is rare, it is important to recognize the problem early. Aggressive management is indicated to prevent long-term sequelae.

Complications of NG tubes may also result from misplacement in the tracheobronchial tree, mediastinum, or cranium. Misplacement of an NG tube into the trachea is more likely to occur in elderly patients with poor gag and cough reflexes (122), in seriously ill patients (123), in chronically ill and malnourished patients (112,113,115,124), in patients with altered mental status (114,124), and in patients under heavy sedation and/or general anesthesia (125) (Figs. 17 and 18). An alert patient may also have weak gag and cough reflexes, and their reaction to tracheal placement of a NG tube not appreciated.

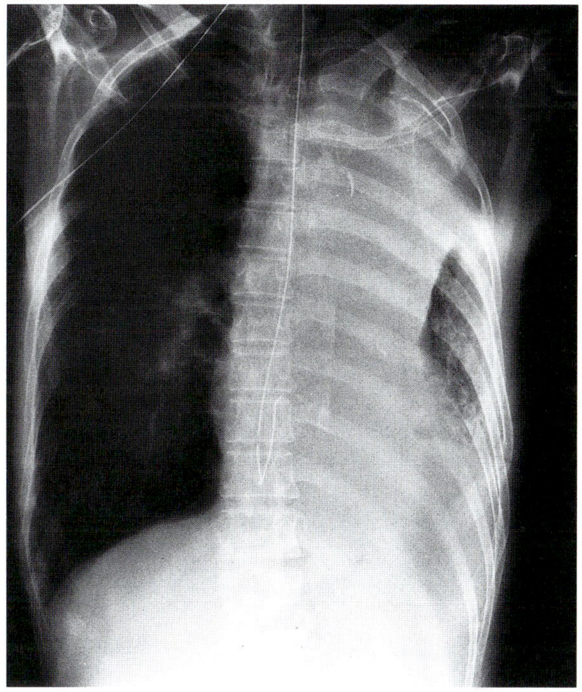

FIG. 18. Chest X-ray 1 hr after administration of a colonoscopy preparation solution into the left lung. Opacity of the left lung is caused by administration of the solution through the nasogastric tube.

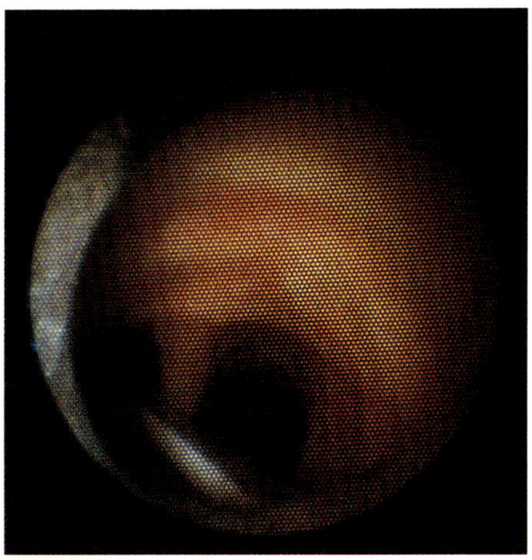

FIG. 17. Misplaced nasogastric (NG) tube in the left main stem bronchus. An NG tube was inserted in a 60-year-old patient, and 35 ml of colonoscopy preparation solution was administered through the NG tube. A few minutes later, the patient developed severe respiratory distress. After mask ventilation, the trachea was intubated with an 8-mm internal diameter (ID) endotracheal tube. There were many secretions, and exposure of larynx was less than satisfactory. A cuff leak could not be corrected on mechanical ventilation. It was suspected that the NG tube may be in the trachea. Fiberoptic endoscopy through a swivel adapter while ventilation was continued showed the NG tube in the left main stem bronchus. It was clear that acute respiratory distress was iatrogenic and was caused by putting a large volume of irritating solution into the lungs. The NG tube was removed, and the cuff leak was abolished. The tip of the endotracheal tube is also in view.

The clinical signs associated with placement of an NG tube in the respiratory tract include coughing, breath holding, agitation, hypertension, and tachycardia. If the patient is intubated and on mechanical ventilation, air leak, decreases in peak airway pressure, and difficulty maintaining adequate tidal volumes should alert the clinician to the possibility of NG tube passage into the trachea (Table 12) (125).

Complications reported as a result of inadvertent placement of NG and nasoenteric tubes in the tracheo-

TABLE 12. *Signs and symptoms of the tracheally placed nasogastric tube*

Coughing, breath holding, and laryngeal spasm
Agitation, hypertension, and tachycardia
Unexplained hypoxemia
Unexpected atelectasis
Development of air leak in the intubated patient
Difficulty in maintaining tidal volume in patients on mechanical ventilation
Decrease in peak airway pressure during mechanical ventilation
Bronchospasm and increase in peak airway pressure during mechanical ventilation
Condensation of water vapor in the nasogastric tube during expiration

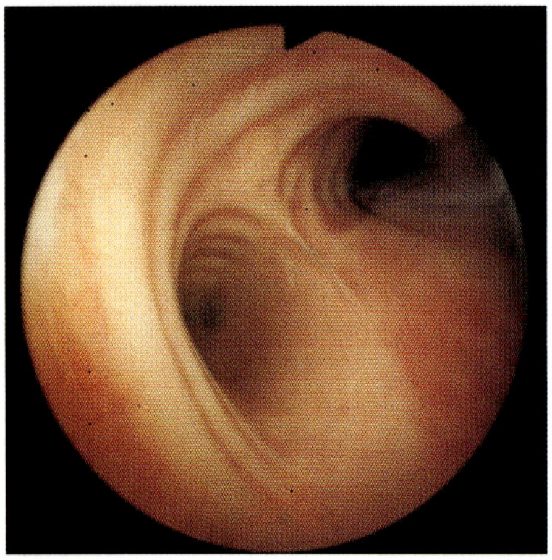

FIG. 19. Esophageal stethoscope inadvertently placed in the right main stem bronchus.

bronchial tree include pulmonary hemorrhage (126), atelectasis (125), pneumothorax (113,123), empyema, and bronchopleural fistula (115).

Esophageal monitoring devices such as esophageal stethoscopes and temperature probes may also be misplaced in the tracheobronchial tree (Fig. 19). These devices may interfere with mechanical ventilation of the patient. A falsely low or high temperature may be reflected by an esophageal temperature probe placed in the trachea, contacting cool or heated inspired gases (125).

The presence of a cuffed endotracheal tube does not always protect the tracheobronchial tree. If resistance is met on removal of an esophageal stethoscope at the conclusion of anesthesia, one should think about this possibility. Deflating the endotracheal tube cuff will allow easy removal if the esophageal stethoscope is in the trachea. Forceful removal of an esophageal stethoscope in one of our patients, operated upon for open reduction and fixation of the mandible, resulted in premature partial extubation of the endotracheal tube.

In trauma patients with basilar skull fractures, the NG tube may pass from the nasopharynx into the intracranial cavity (127,128). To avoid intracranial intubation, several suggestions have been made. The NG tube should be directed along the floor of the nose, not in a cephalad direction (128). In addition, NG tube intubation can be performed through the mouth. NG intubation may also be performed with the aid of X-ray imaging (128). A nasopharyngeal airway can be used as a conduit for the NG tube facilitating placement.

REFERENCES

1. Lindholm CE, Ollman B, Snyder J, Millen E, Grenvik A. Flexible fiberoptic bronchoscopy in critical care medicine: diagnosis, therapy and complications. *Crit Care Med* 1974;2:250–261.
2. Sackner MA. State of the art. Bronchofiberscopy. *Am Rev Resp Dis* 1975;111:62–88.
3. Milledge JS. Therapeutic fiberoptic bronchoscopy in intensive care. *Br Med J* 1976;2:1427–1429.
4. Ikeda S. *Atlas of flexible bronchofiberscopy*. Baltimore: University Park Press, 1974.
5. Marini JJ, Pierson DJ, Hudson L. Acute lobar atelectasis: a prospective comparison of fiberoptic bronchoscopy and respiratory therapy. *Am Rev Respir Dis* 1979;119:971–978.
6. Olopade CO, Prakash UBS. Bronchoscopy in the critical care unit. *Mayo Clin Proc* 1989;64:1255–1263.
7. Tsao TC, Tsai YH, Lan RS, Shieh WB, Lee CH. Treatment for collapsed lung in critically ill patients—selective intra bronchial air insufflation using the fiberoptic bronchoscope. *Chest* 1990;97:435–438.
8. Phillip Delinger R. Fiberoptic bronchoscopy in adult airway management. *Crit Care Med* 1990;18:882–887.
9. Zupan J. Fiberoptic bronchoscopy in anesthesia and critical care. In: Benumof J, ed. *Procedures in anesthesia and intensive care*. New York: Lippincott, 1990, 253–273.
10. Meduri GU, Baselski V. The role of fiberoptic alveolar lavage in diagnosing non opportunistic bacterial pneumonia. *Chest* 1991;100:179–190.
11. Ovassapian A, Randel GI. The role of the fiberscope in the critically ill patient. *Crit Care Clin North Am* 1995;11:29–51.
12. Bellomo R, Tai E, Parkin G. Fiberoptic bronchoscopy in the critically ill: a prospective study of its diagnostic and therapeutic value. *Anaesth Intens Care* 1992;20:464–469.
13. Ovassapian A. *Fiberoptic airway endoscopy in anesthesia and critical care*. New York: Raven Press, 1990.
14. Prakash UBS. *Bronchoscopy*. New York: Raven Press, 1994.
15. Ono R. Bronchoscopy. *Practical methods and case reports*. Tokyo: Nakayama-Shoten, 1994.
16. Oho K, Amemiya R. *Practical fiberoptic bronchoscopy*, 2nd ed. Tokyo: Igaku-Shoin, 1984.
17. Lindholm CE. Flexible fiberoptic bronchoscopy in the critically ill patient. *Ann Otol* 1974;83:786–794.
18. Wood RE. Spelunking in the pediatric airways: explorations with the flexible fiberoptic bronchoscope. *Pediatric Clin North Am* 1984;31:785–799.
19. Nussbaum E. Pediatric flexible bronchoscopy and its application in infantile atelectasis. *Clin Pediatr* 1985;24:379–382.
20. Vauthy PA, Reddy R. Acute upper airway obstruction in infants and children. Evaluation by the fiberoptic bronchoscope. *Ann Otol* 1980;89:417–418.
21. Guidice JC, Komansky H, Gordon R, Kaufman JL. Acute upper airway obstruction—fiberoptic bronchoscopy in diagnosis and therapy. *Crit Care Med* 1981;9:878–879.
22. Fan LL, Sparks LM, Dulinski JP. Applications of an ultrathin flexible bronchoscope for neonatal and pediatric airway problems. *Chest* 1986;89:673–676.
23. Baxter MRN. Congenital laryngomalacia. *Can J Anaesth* 1994; 41:332–339.
24. Law JH, Barnhart K, Rowlett W, de la Rocha O, Lowenberg S. Increased frequency of obstructive airway abnormalities with long-term tracheostomy. *Chest* 1993;104:136–138.
25. Aass AS. Complications to tracheostomy and long term intubation: a follow-up study. *Acta Anaesthesiol Scand* 1975;19: 127–133.
26. Woo T, Kelly G, Kirshner P. Airway complications of head injury. *Laryngoscope* 1989;99:725–731.
27. Stiles PJ. Tracheal lesions after tracheostomy. *Thorax* 1965; 20:517–522.
28. Westgate HD, Rou KL. Tracheal stenosis following tracheostomy. *Anesth Analg* 1970;49:393–401.
29. Dunham MC, LaMonica C. Prolonged tracheal intubation in the trauma patient. *J Trauma* 1984;24:120–124.
30. Cooper JD, Grillo HC. The evolution of the tracheal injury due to ventilatory assistance through cuffed tubes: a pathologic study. *Ann Surg* 1969;169:334–348.
31. Klingbeil GEG. Airway problems in patients with traumatic brain injury. *Arch Phys Med Rehabil* 1988;69:493–495.
32. Friman L, Hedenstierna G, Schildt B. Stenosis following tracheostomy. *Anaesthesia* 1976;31:479–493.
33. Andrews MJ. The incidence and pathogenesis of tracheal injury

following tracheostomy with cuff tube and assisted ventilation. *Br J Surg* 1971;58:749–755.

34. Ovassapian A. Fiberoptic tracheal intubation. In: Ovassapian A, ed. *Fiberoptic airway endoscopy in anesthesia and critical care*. New York: Raven Press, 1990;57–79.
35. Martin CJ. Tracheopathia osteochondroplastica. *Arch Otolaryngol* 1974;100:290–293.
36. Lundgren R, Stjernberg NL. Tracheobronchopathia osteochondroplastica. A clinical bronchoscopic and spirometric study. *Chest* 1981;80:706–709.
37. Magnusson P, Rotemark G. Tracheobronchopathia osteocondroplastica. *J Laryngol Otol* 1974;88:159–164.
38. Smith DC, Pillai R, Gillbe CE. Tracheopathia osteochondroplastica. A cause of unexpected difficulty in tracheal intubation. *Anaesthesia* 1987:42:536–538.
39. Amikam B, Landa J, West J, Sackner MA. Bronchofiberscopic observations of the tracheobronchial tree during intubation. *Am Rev Resp Dis* 1972;105:747–755.
40. Kuna ST, Remmers JE. Neural and anatomic factors related to upper airway occlusion during sleep. *Med Clin North Am* 1985;69:1221–1242.
41. Cheong KF, Chan MYP, Sin-Fai-Lam KN. Bilateral vocal cord paralysis following endotracheal intubation. *Anaesth Intens Care* 1994;22:206–208.
42. Drury PME, Williams EGN. Vocal cord paralysis in the Shy-Drager syndrome. A cause of postoperative respiratory obstruction. *Anaesthesia* 1991;46:466–468.
43. Holey HS, Gildea JE. Vocal cord paralysis after tracheal intubation. *JAMA* 1971;215:281–284.
44. Cavo JW. True vocal cord paralysis following intubation. *Laryngoscope* 1985;95:1352–1359.
45. Brandwein M, Abramson AL, Shikowitz MJ. Bilateral vocal cord paralysis following endotracheal intubation. *Arch Otolaryngol Head Neck Surg* 1986;112:877–882.
46. Hammer G, Schwinn D, Wollman H. Postoperative complications due to paradoxical vocal cord motion. *Anesthesiology* 1987;66:686–687.
47. Hayes JP, Nolan MT, Brennan N, FitzGerald MX. Three cases of paradoxical vocal cord adduction followed up over a 10-year period. *Chest* 1993;104:678–679.
48. Goldman J, Muers M. Vocal cord dysfunction. *Thorax* 1991; 46:401–404.
49. Patterson R, Schatz M, Horton M. Munchausen's stridor: non-organic laryngeal obstruction. *Clin Allergy* 1974;4:307–310.
50. Nagai A, Yamaguchi E, Sakomoto K, Takashi E. Functional upper airway obstruction: psychogenic pharyngeal constriction. *Chest* 1992;101:1460–1561.
51. Nagai A, Kanemura T, Konno K. Abnormal movement of the arytenoid region as a cause of upper airway obstruction. *Thorax* 1992;47:840–841.
52. Baxter FJ, Dunn GL. Acute epiglottitis in adults. *Can J Anaesth* 1988;35:428–435.
53. Rothstein P, Lister G. Epiglottitis—duration of intubation and fever. *Anesth Analg* 1983;62:785–787.
54. MayoSmith MF, Hirsch PJ, Wodzinski SF, Schiffman FJ. Acute epiglottitis in adults. An eight-year experience in the state of Rhode Island. *N Engl J Med* 1986;314:1133–1139.
55. Frantz TD, Rasgon BM, Quesenberry CP. Acute epiglottitis in adults: analysis of 129 cases. *J Am Med Assoc* 1994;272: 1358–1360.
56. Diaz JH, Lockhart CH. Early diagnosis and airway management of acute epiglottitis in children. *South Med J* 1982;75: 399–403.
57. Burns JE, Hendley JO. Epiglottitis. In: Mandell GL, Douglas RG, Bennett JE, eds. *Infectious diseases,* 2nd ed. New York: John Wiley, 1985;372–375.
58. Guidice JC, Komansky HJ. Acute epiglottitis—the use of the fiberoptic bronchoscope in diagnosis and therapy. *Chest* 1979; 75:211–212.
59. Warshawski J, Havas TE, McShane DP, Gullane PJ. Acute epiglottitis. *J Otolaryngol* 1986;15:362–365.
60. Crosby E, Reid D. Acute epiglottitis in the adult: is intubation mandatory? *Can J Anaesth* 1991;38:914–918.
61. Nussbaum E. Fiberoptic laryngoscopy as a guide to tracheal extubation in acute epiglottitis. *J Pediatr* 1983;102:269–270.
62. Warner JA, Finlay WEI. Fulminating epiglottitis in adults: report of three cases and review of the literature. *Anaesthesia* 1985;40:348–352.
63. Phelan DM, Love JB. Adult epiglottitis: is there a role for the fiberoptic bronchoscope? *Chest* 1984;86:783–784.
64. Haponik EF, Meyers DA, Munster AM, et al. Acute upper airway injury in burn patients. Serial changes of flow—volume curves and nasopharyngoscopy. *Am Rev Respir Dis* 1987;135: 360–366.
65. Clark CJ, Reid WH, Telfer ABM, Campbell D. Respiratory injury in the burned patient. The role of flexible bronchoscopy. *Anaesthesia* 1983;38:35–39.
66. Hunt JL, Agee RN, Pruitt BA. Fiberoptic bronchoscopy in acute inhalation injury. *J Trauma* 1975;15:641–649.
67. Moylan JA. Smoke inhalation and burn injury. *Surg Clin North Am* 1980;60:1533–1540.
68. Hoffstein V, Zamel N. Sleep apnea and the upper airway. *Br J Anaesth* 1990;65:139–150.
69. Davies RJO, Straddling JR. Acute effects of obstructive sleep apnea. *Br J Anaesth* 1993;71:725–729.
70. Haponik EF, Smith PL, Bohlman ME, et al. Computerized tomography in obstructive sleep apnea. Correlation of airway size with physiology during sleep and wakefulness. *Am Rev Resp Dis* 1983;127:221–226.
71. Brouillette RT, Fernback SK, Hunt CE. Obstructive sleep apnea in infants and children. *J Pediatr* 1982;100:31–40.
72. Rojewski TE, Schuller DE, Clark RW, et al. Synchronous video recording of the pharyngeal airway and polysomnograph in patients with obstructive sleep apnea. *Laryngoscope* 1982; 92:246–250.
73. Fan LL. Transnasal fiberoptic endoscopy in children with obstructive apnea. *Crit Care Med* 1984;12:590–592.
74. Rubenstein I, Slutsky AS, Zamel N, Hoffstein V. Paradoxical glottic narrowing in patients with severe obstructive sleep apnea. *J Clin Invest* 1988;81:1051–1055.
75. Barrett CR Jr, Vecchione JJ, Loomis Bell AL Jr. Flexible fiberoptic bronchoscopy for airway management during acute respiratory failure. *Am Rev Respir Dis* 1974;109:429–434.
76. Campinos L, Duval G, Couturier M, et al. The value of early fiberoptic bronchoscopy after aspiration of gastric contents. *Br J Anaesth* 1983;55:1103–1105.
77. Wolfe JE, Bone RC, Ruth WE. Diagnosis of gastric aspiration by fiberoptic bronchoscopy. *Chest* 1976;70:458–459.
78. Reed A. Preparation of the patient for awake flexible fiberoptic bronchoscopy. *Chest* 1992;101:244–253.
79. Baier H, Begin R, Sackner MA. Effect of airway diameter, suction catheters, and the bronchofiberscope on airflow in endotracheal and tracheostomy tubes. *Heart Lung* 1976;5: 235–238.
80. Pereira W, Kovnat DM, Snider GL. A prospective cooperative study of complications following flexible fiberoptic bronchoscopy. *Chest* 1978;73:813–816.
81. Katz AS, Michelson EL, Stawicki J, Halford FD. Cardiac arrhythmias—frequency during fiberoptic bronchoscopy and correlation with hypoxemia. *Arch Intern Med* 1981;141: 603–606.
82. Credle WF, Smiddy JF, Elliott RC. Complications of fiberoptic bronchoscopy. *Am Rev Resp Dis* 1974;109:67–72.
83. Sturatt PM, Smiddy JF, Gruber B. Deaths and complications associated with fiberoptic bronchoscopy. *Chest* 1976;69: 747–751.
84. Sahn SA, Scoggin C. Fiberoptic bronchoscopy in bronchial asthma. A word of caution. *Chest* 1976;69:39–42.
85. Lundgren R, Haggmark S, Reiz S. Hemodynamic effects of flexible fiberoptic bronchoscopy performed under topical anesthesia. *Chest* 1982;82:295–299.
86. Ghows MB, Rosen MJ, Chuang MT, et al. Transcutaneous oxygen monitoring during fiberoptic bronchoscopy. *Chest* 1986;89: 543–544.
87. Ovenfors CO, Hedgecock MW. Intensive care unit radiology: problems of interpretation. *Radiol Clin North Am* 1978;16: 407–439.
88. O'Brien D, Curran J, Conroy J, Bouchier-Hayes D. Fiberoptic assessment of tracheal tube position. A comparison of tracheal

tube position as estimated by fiberoptic bronchoscopy and by chest X-ray. *Anaesthesia* 1985;40:73–76.
89. Yezerski J, Arnold BL, Sachatello CR. Technique to locate the end of an endotracheal tube. *Crit Care Med* 1984;12:600–601.
90. Whitehouse AC, Klock LE. Evaluation of endotracheal tube position with the fiberoptic intubation laryngoscope. *Chest* 1975;68:848.
91. Vigneswaran R, Whitfield JM. The use of a new ultra-thin fiberoptic bronchoscope to determine endotracheal tube position in the sick newborn infant. *Chest* 1981;80:174–177.
92. Todres ID, deBros F, Kramen SS, et al. Endotracheal tube displacement in the newborn infant. *J Pediatr* 1976;89:126–127.
93. Goodman LR, Conrardy PA, Laing F, Singer MM. Radiographic evaluation of endotracheal tube position. *Am J Roentgenol* 1976;127:433–434.
94. Moyers J, Gregory GA. Use of fiberoptic bronchoscopy to reposition an endotracheal tube intraoperatively. *Anesthesiology* 1975;43:685.
95. Finucane BT, Kupshik HL. A flexible stylet for replacing damaged tracheal tubes. *Can Anaesth Soc J* 1978;25:153–154.
96. Watson CB, Prough DS, Balestrieri FJ. Bronchoscopic tube change in critically ill patients [abstr]. *Crit Care Med* 1980;8: 246.
97. Rosenbaum SH, Rosenbaum LH, Cole RP, et al. Use of the flexible fiberoptic bronchoscope to change endotracheal tube in critically ill patients. *Anesthesiology* 1981;54:169–170.
98. Watson CB. Fiberoptic bronchoscopy for anesthesia. *Anesthesiol Rev* 1982;9:17–26.
99. Halebian P, Shires T. A method for replacement of the endotracheal tube with continuous control of the airway. *Surg Gynecol Obstet* 1985;161:285–286.
100. Delaney KA, Hessler R. Emergency flexible fiberoptic nasotracheal intubation: a report of 60 cases. *Ann Emerg Med* 1988; 17:919–926.
101. Venus B, Pratap KS, Op'Tholt R. Treatment of unilateral pulmonary insufficiency by selective administration of continuous positive airway pressure through a double lumen tube. *Anesthesiology* 1980;53:74–77.
102. Carlon GC, et al. Criteria for selective positive end expiratory pressure and independent synchronized ventilation of each lung. *Chest* 1978;74:501–507.
103. Stein JA, Lisbon A. Pulmonary hemorrhage from pulmonary artery catheterization treated with endobronchial intubation. *Anesthesiology* 1981;55:698–699.
104. Benumof JL. *Anesthesia for thoracic surgery*. 2nd ed. Philadelphia: W. B. Saunders, 1995;548–554.
105. Tucker A, Lewis J. Passing a nasogastric tube. *Br Med J* 1980; 281:1128–1129.
106. Cohen DD, Fox RM. Nasogastric intubation in the anesthetized patient. *Anesth Analg* 1963;42:578–580.
107. Rosenberg H. A new technique for inserting nasogastric tubes during anesthesia. *Anesthesiology* 1975;42:632.
108. Perel A, Ya'ari Y, Pizov R. Forward displacement of the larynx for nasogastric tube insertion in intubated patients. *Crit Care Med* 1985;13:204–205.
109. Tahir AH, Adriani J. A method of inserting a nasogastric tube in anesthetized or comatose patient. *Anesth Analg* 1971;50: 179–180.
110. May M, Nellis KJ. Nasogastric intubation: avoiding complications. *Resident Staff Physician* 1984;30:60–62.
111. Lee TS, Wright BD. Flexible fiberoptic bronchoscope for difficult nasogastric intubation. *Anesth Analg* 1981;60:904–905.
112. James RH. An unusual complication of passing a narrow-bore nasogastric tube. *Anaesthesia* 1978;33:716–718.
113. Siemers PT, Reinke RT. Perforation of the nasopharynx by nasogastric intubation: a rare cause of left pleural effusion and pneumomediastinum. *Am J Roentgenol* 1976;127:341–343.
114. Lind LJ, Wallace DH. Submucosal passage of a nasogastric tube complicating attempted intubation during anesthesia. *Anesthesiology* 1978;49:145–147.
115. Torrington KG, Bowman MA. Total hydrothorax and empyema complicating a malpositioned nasogastric tube. *Chest* 1981;79:240–242.
116. Feinberg GL, Ravin MB. Multiple general anesthesias, gastroesophageal reflux and spontaneous esophageal rupture. *Anesthesiology* 1967;28:782–784.
117. Iglauer S, Molt WF. Severe injury to the larynx resulting from the indwelling duodenal tube. *Ann Otol Rhinol Laryngol* 1939; 48:886–904.
118. Foster CA, Meyerhoff WL. Cricoid chondritis. *Ear Nose Throat J* 1980;59:106–109.
119. Sofferman RA, Hubbell RN. Laryngeal complications of nasogastric tubes. *Ann Otol Rhinol Laryngol* 1981;90:465–468.
120. Friedman M, Baim H, Stobricki M. Laryngeal injuries secondary to nasogastric tubes. *Ann Otol Rhinol Laryngol* 1981;90: 469–474.
121. Brand JB, Emerson CW, Wilson RS. Acute laryngeal edema 24 hours after passage of a nasogastric tube. *Anesthesiology* 1976;45:555–557.
122. Aronchick JM, Epstein DM, Gefter WB, Miller WT. Pneumothorax as a complication of placement of a nasogastric tube. *JAMA* 1984;252:3287–3288.
123. Nakao MA, Killam D, Wilson R. Pneumothorax secondary to inadvertent nasotracheal placement of a nasoenteric tube past a cuffed endotracheal tube. *Crit Care Med* 1983;11:210–211.
124. Theodore AC, Frank JA, Ende J, et al. Errant placement of nasoenteric tubes. A hazard in obtunded patients. *Chest* 1984; 86:931–933.
125. Sweatman AJ, Tomasello PA, Loughhead MG, et al. Misplacement of nasogastric tubes and oesophageal monitoring devices. *Br J Anaesth* 1978;50:389–392.
126. McDanal JT, Wheeler DM, Ebert J. A complication of nasogastric intubation: pulmonary hemorrhage. *Anesthesiology* 1983; 57:356–358.
127. Seebacher J, Nozik D, Mathieu A. Inadvertent intracranial introduction of a nasogastric tube, a complication of severe maxillofacial trauma. *Anesthesiology* 1975;42:100–102.
128. Borovich B, Braun J, Yosefovich T, et al. Intracranial penetration of nasogastric tube. *Neurosurgery* 1981;8:245–247.

CHAPTER 10

The Difficult Airway

Andranik Ovassapian, M.D.

The difficult airway features anatomic or pathologic characteristics that make mask ventilation and/or tracheal intubation difficult (1). The difficulties experienced may be due to upper or lower airway features.

The treatise *Guidelines for Management of the Difficult Airway*, developed by the Task Force on Management of the Difficult Airway of the American Society of Anesthesiologists (ASA), defines difficult mask ventilation as a condition where " . . . it is not possible for the unassisted anesthesiologist to prevent or reverse signs of inadequate ventilation during positive pressure mask ventilation." Difficult rigid laryngoscopy is further defined as a circumstance where " . . . it is not possible to visualize any portion of the vocal cords with conventional laryngoscopy." A circumstance in which proper insertion of an endotracheal tube, with conventional laryngoscopy, requires more than three attempts, or greater than 10 min is considered a difficult intubation under the ASA guidelines (2).

The reported incidence of difficult intubation associated with rigid laryngoscopy ranges from 0.5% to 13.6% (3–9). In the parturient, 2.7% of rigid intubations were found to be difficult (3). The incidence of difficult intubation reported by Savva (10) is 4.9% and is similar to the findings of Frerk in an earlier report (11). Four of the 350 patients in Savva's study had laryngoscopy grades of III or IV (1.14%) and are similar to previously reported findings (11–13). A prospective study in 1200 patients revealed a 3.6% incidence of difficult intubation (8).

The varying differences in the calculated incidence of difficult intubation probably relate to differences in defining a difficult intubation. Most reports on difficult intubations are based on retrospective studies, and few large-scale prospective studies have been reported (4,5). Most published reports also lack specific information about the number of intubation attempts required to intubate, or the nature and severity of complications caused by a difficult intubation.

The frequency of failed intubation in the general surgical population is reported to be 1 in every 2230 patients (14), while the incidence of failed intubation in the parturient is reported as 1 in every 280 patients (14). A more recent study by Rocke et al. in obstetric patients reported the failure rate of intubation as 1 in every 750 patients (15).

While the features that produce difficult mask ventilation and difficult tracheal intubation may coexist, they are often not present simultaneously (16). The frequency of difficult mask ventilation concurrently present with a difficult or failed intubation is unknown. A recent report from Australia indicated that 15% of difficult intubations were associated with difficult mask ventilation (17).

The degree of difficulty encountered performing mask ventilation during a difficult intubation can worsen due to the trauma and associated tissue edema produced by repeated intubation attempts (18). This is one of the main reasons to discourage the practice of multiple repeated intubation attempts (2,19).

Prior to performing a tracheal intubation, the patient should be ventilated and oxygenated, using a bag-valve mask device. If ventilation by face mask proves easy, then a few atraumatic attempts to insert an endotracheal tube should not cause significant trauma that might further complicate airway management.

TABLE 1. *Causes of the difficult airway*

Common anatomic factors	
	Short, muscular neck with full set of teeth
	Protruding upper incisors
	Long, high arched palate with narrow mouth
	Limited mobility of cervical spine at C1 and C2 levels
	Receding lower jaw
	Small opening of the mouth
Tumors and cysts	
	Oropharyngeal
	Laryngeal
	Head and neck
	Anterior mediastinal
	Laryngeal polyps
Infection	
	Ludwig's angina
	Retropharyngeal abscess
	Epiglottitis
Congenital anomalies	
	Pierre Robin syndrome
	Treacher Collins syndrome
	Goldenhar's syndrome
	Temporomandibular joint dysfunction
Scarring of tissues	
	Postsurgical
	Burn
	Radiation
Trauma	
	Facial
	Cervical spine
	Laryngeal
	Hematoma
Arthritis and ankylosing spondylosis	
	Cervical spine
	Temporomandibular joint
	Subluxation of cervical vertebrae
	Laryngeal/arytenoid involvement
Allergic and angioneurotic edema	
	Tongue and palate
	Epiglottis
Endocrine diseases	
	Obesity
	Acromegaly
	Myxedema
	Enlarged thyroid
Technical	
	Poor technique
	Poor equipment
	Inexperience
Miscellaneous	
	Halo traction
	Body cast
	Masseter spasm due to hyperthermia and succinylcholine

If a failure to intubate is associated with the inability to mask ventilate, the patient's life is in serious danger. Therefore, to prevent airway catastrophes, our clinical attention should be directed not to the difficult intubation per se, but more importantly to the difficulties inherent in mask ventilation and patient oxygenation. Unfortunately this is too frequently not the focus of concern.

When intubation of the trachea proves unsuccessful and mask ventilation is compromised, the immediate priority is to select a rapidly applicable technique to establish effective ventilation. Tracheal intubation is a secondary issue under these circumstances. However, any selected technique should be applied prior to the time that hypoxemia becomes a severe problem. All alternative airway techniques (e.g., the laryngeal mask airway, Combitube, percutaneous transtracheal jet ventilation, or tracheostomy) take time to perform; they may not immediately prove successful and may themselves fail. Therefore, their application should be initiated relatively early in the decision-making process.

Total and accurate prediction of a difficult intubation is not possible with the tests presently available (Table 1). In addition, even when a difficult intubation is anticipated, the prediction of coexisting problems with mask ventilation are problematic.

One way to minimize airway-related complications is to accept the high rate of false positive predictors associated with current tests of evaluating airway status. All patients identified as possible difficult intubations are thereby treated accordingly.

The loss of consciousness on induction of anesthesia, and the concomitant relaxation of the oropharyngeal tissues, may aggravate a difficult mask ventilation (20). Therefore, securing of the airway prior to induction of anesthesia, in selected patients, should be exercised more frequently. The development of the fiberoptic bronchoscope has made awake tracheal intubation a simple, atraumatic, and relatively easy technique to perform. There should be little hesitation in the mind of the anesthesiologist trained in its use to apply this airway technique frequently and effectively in such cases.

AIRWAY PATENCY DURING UNCONSCIOUSNESS

The state of unconsciousness produced by general anesthesia, trauma, or systemic disease often interferes with upper airway patency and gas exchange.

Undue delay in overcoming an airway obstruction will contribute to complications secondary to hypoxemia and lead to possible loss of life. The establishment and maintenance of airway patency is the cornerstone of safe anesthesia.

Upper airway obstruction can occur anytime, during or after induction of general anesthesia. Most commonly this occurs as the base of the tongue falls posteriorly, as the genioglossus and geniohyoid muscles relax. The epiglottis itself can also produce airway obstruction at this time (20–23).

The Tongue and Pharyngeal Soft Tissues

The oropharyngeal passage has a rigid posterior wall formed by the cervical vertebrae, with collapsible anterior and lateral walls formed by the tongue and pharyngeal muscles.

Three variables are important in the development of upper airway obstruction: decreased activity of the muscles that dilate the pharyngeal airway, a negative pressure generated within the upper airway during inspiration, and the structural anatomy of the airway itself.

While awake, the patency of the upper airway is maintained by phasic contraction of the muscles of the tongue, pharynx, and larynx. This is required to resist the collapsing effect of the negative intraluminal pressure produced by inspiration (21–24). When the patient is unconscious, the neuromuscular control of the upper airway muscles is diminished or lost. This factor allows the tongue and structures attached to the hyoid bone to gravitate toward the posterior pharyngeal wall, causing varying degrees of airway obstruction (20,25–28).

Patient effort to breathe in the presence of this partial obstruction, only aggravates the situation, by pulling the tongue and pharyngeal soft tissues posteriorly toward the glottis. Roentgenographic studies (21,29–31), as well as spirometry and clinical observation (32), demonstrate that head and neck extension opens the airway by stretching the genioglossus muscles, pulling the tongue forward and away from the posterior pharyngeal wall. The muscle stretching is further increased by closing the mouth and displacing the mandible forward (30,33).

The average pharyngeal clearance in awake subjects, with the head held in a neutral position, is approximately 10.5 mm (range, 4.5–14 mm). In the anesthetized subject, the clearance decreases to 5 mm (range, 0–10.5 mm). The distance between the epiglottis and posterior pharyngeal wall is significantly reduced or eliminated. Upon hyperextension of the head and forward displacement of the mandible pharyngeal clearance increases to 17 mm (range, 5.5–23 mm) (29).

The Epiglottis

In some patients, despite a clear pharyngeal passageway, the airway may become obstructed and ventilation difficult. The epiglottis has been suspected as a major cause of this airway obstruction. While applying roentgenographic examination of the pharynx, Fink (34) observed that the epiglottis often sags into the laryngeal aditus. More recently, radiographic (20) and bronchofiberscopic (35) study of the epiglottis and tongue in spontaneously breathing anesthetized patients has shown that posterior movement of the soft palate and epiglottis were the main causes of upper airway obstruction.

In clinical practice, when oro- or nasopharyngeal airways or appropriate maneuvers of the head and jaw fail to clear the airway, the epiglottis should be suspected as being involved in the obstruction.

Supraepiglottic cysts or tumors have long been recognized as being associated with difficult mask ventilation and intubation (36–38). These cysts are rare, and the majority are asymptomatic, or cause mild symptoms, such as voice change and snoring in adults, mild stridor in infants, dysphagia, or the vague feeling of something in the throat (39). Supraepiglottic cysts are potentially dangerous since they may completely obstruct the airway following induction of anesthesia, and may further interfere with rigid laryngoscopy and tracheal intubation (36,40). Scientific papers based on prospective clinical or laboratory studies of this problem are lacking. However, case reports leave little doubt, that a supraepiglottic cyst or mass can cause difficult mask ventilation and failure of intubation.

When a 55-year-old patient was anesthetized for repair of an inguinal hernia, mask ventilation proved to be difficult. Rigid laryngoscopy revealed a large cyst arising from the vallecula, completely obstructing the view of the epiglottis and underlying vocal cords. The epiglottis could not be lifted out of the way with the rigid laryngoscope blade (40). Upon the return of spontaneous ventilation, the otolaryngologist performed a rigid laryngoscopy and aspirated 20 ml of clear serous fluid. The anesthesiologist was then able expose the epiglottis and vocal cords and easily performed tracheal intubation.

An unsuspected supraepiglottic cyst, or a mass on the base of the tongue, represents a potential danger when rapid sequence induction and intubation of the trachea are attempted (37,41).

VENTILATION BY FACE MASK

A properly positioned face mask and a maintained patent airway are essential for positive pressure pulmonary ventilation. The mask must fit well over the bridge of the nose and chin, producing an airtight seal. Without a tight seal, positive pressure ventilation is difficult, anesthetic agents escape to contaminate the room air, and inspired anesthetic gases are diluted.

Various maneuvers may be applied to reduce air leakage around the face mask. The hypothenar eminence can serve as a base to draw the soft tissue of the left cheek against the cushion of the mask. The mask strap positioned under the patient's occiput can be utilized to perform a similar function on the right side.

The mask strap also helps to maintain a snug mask fit. Undue pressure must be avoided over the area of the bridge of the nose, or facial trauma may result.

The last three fingers of the left hand maintain the jaw in a forward (jaw thrust) position. The seal of the face mask is maintained against the face by the thumb and the index finger, positioned below the mask connector. Clear disposable face masks designed with a large soft cushions better fit patients with flat noses. The masks also allow a view of the mouth to observe for secretions, vomitus, or cyanosis.

In the anesthetized patient, use of an oral airway, or the placing of moistened gauze packing into the buccal cavities, may enhance mask fit (42). The oropharyngeal airway also improves airway patency in the unconscious patient. It should be used during prolonged mask ventilation, even when mask ventilation proves easy (43). An oropharyngeal airway may be inserted when partial or complete airway obstruction is encountered and the mandible is relaxed. Severely depressed, comatose, or anesthetized patients will usually tolerate the stimulation induced by the airway.

The mouth is opened and the base of the tongue lifted with a tongue blade to permit proper placement of the airway behind the tongue. Improper placement of an oral airway may force the tongue backward, aggravating soft tissue obstruction. The use of an oversized airway may press the epiglottis against the posterior pharyngeal wall, obstructing the larynx.

The nasopharyngeal airway is frequently used when a patient requires relief of soft tissue airway obstruction and a preserved gag reflex or clenched mouth prevents the use of a oropharyngeal airway. The possibility of epistaxis resulting from its insertion may be reduced by applying a mucosal vasoconstrictor to the nasal passage, along with generous lubrication and gentle insertion of the airway.

In the anesthetized patient, airway obstruction is usually avoided by positioning the head in a "sniffing" position (that is, extending the head at the atlanto-occipital joint and thrusting the jaw forward) and by using artificial airways as described. The application of moderate positive pressure to the airway may serve to overcome slight soft tissue obstruction of the upper airway. However, excessive airway pressures may produce distension of the stomach.

In some patients, adequate mask pulmonary ventilation may require the help of an assistant. While one person maintains the mask fit using both hands, the assistant provides ventilation by squeezing on the anesthesia reservoir bag. In two-person mask ventilation, there is a tendency to produce overly large tidal volumes. There is also a tendency to create high airway pressures, predisposing to gastric distension. This can be prevented by utilizing small tidal volumes supplemented with 100% oxygen and monitoring the epigastrium by stethoscope.

BREATHING AGAINST THE OBSTRUCTED AIRWAY

Vigorous spontaneous attempts to breathe against an obstructed airway produces hypoventilation and hypoxemia and increases the danger of gastric regurgitation and the development of pulmonary congestion and edema. The severity and rapidity of developing hypoxemia depends on the degree of airway obstruction, the inspired oxygen concentration, and the patient's physical condition.

In order for gastric regurgitation to occur, several conditions must usually be present. There needs to be fluid in the stomach, the cardioesophageal junction must prove incompetent, the pressure within the stomach exceeds that in the esophagus, and the cricopharyngeus muscle allows material to pass into the oropharynx (44). In addition, the airway reflexes must be impaired for foreign material to passively enter the tracheobronchial tree.

The reduction in intrathoracic pressure, produced by breathing against an obstructed airway, increases the pleuroperitoneal and gastroesophageal pressure gradients (45,46). These pressure changes open the cardioesophageal junction, permitting gastric fluid to enter the esophagus (45,46). This phenomenon was directly observed and reported during esophagoscopy by Sinclair (47).

Anesthetics and muscle relaxants relax the cricopharyngeus muscle, allowing regurgitated gastric contents to easily enter the oropharynx. All premedicant drugs, especially anticholinergics and opioids, decrease the competence of the esophageal sphincter. Superimposed on the administration of a potent inhalational anesthetic agent, this fact heightens the importance of maintaining a patent airway (48).

The mechanism producing noncardiac pulmonary edema during airway obstruction is unclear and probably relates to a combination of factors. Forced inspiratory breathing against a closed airway increases intrapleural negative pressure, raising the transpulmonary pressure gradient. This results in the lowering of pulmonary capillary perivascular pressures, thus favoring the hydrostatic transudation of fluid from the pulmonary capillaries into the interstitial space. In addition, elevated left ventricular afterload and associated hypoxemia increase pulmonary venous volume and pulmonary arterial pressure. Hypoxemia serves to damage pulmonary capillary walls, further increasing their permeability.

Three key factors combine to favor movement of fluid from the pulmonary capillaries into interstitial areas, producing congestion and edema (49,50). These factors are a decreased capillary perivascular pressure, raised pulmonary arterial pressure, and increased pulmonary capillary permeability. Obstructive noncardiac pulmonary edema usually resolves rapidly and spontaneously on relief of the airway obstruction.

AIRWAY PRESSURE AND GASTRIC DISTENSION

Positive mask airway pressure in excess of 20 cm H_2O (15 mm Hg) forces air into the stomach, raising intragastric pressure and predisposing the patient to regurgitation and cardiopulmonary compromise. Factor(s) that increase intragastric-esophageal or pleuroperitoneal pressure differences predispose to regurgitation of stomach contents. Factors that elevate intragastric pressure include inflation of the stomach with air, steep head-down positioning, and raised intra-abdominal pressure due to distended bowel or intra-abdominal mass (51).

The average intragastric pressure in anesthetized spontaneously breathing subjects is 11 cm H_2O (range, 9–16) (52). In paralyzed anesthetized patients, the average intragastric pressure required to cause reflux has been reported to be 23 cm H_2O (range, 13–28) in one study (53), and 35 cm H_2O (range, 16–77) in another (54).

The relationship between the airway pressure required to ventilate the lungs and that required to force air into the stomach has been studied in adults, children, and infants (55–59). Ruben and associates (56) found that pressures below 15 cm H_2O rarely caused stomach inflation, whereas those exceeding 25 cm H_2O did so in most patients. Moynihan and colleagues demonstrated that muscle paralysis in children significantly decreased the median airway pressure required to force air into the stomach. The application of cricoid pressure was 100% effective in preventing gas insufflation of the stomach, up to 40 cm H_2O peak inspiratory pressure, with or without muscle paralysis present (59).

Lawes and co-workers (55), studying anesthetized adults without cricoid pressure applied, found the minimum airway pressure required to push air into the stomach was 20 cm H_2O. The mean inflation pressure required to adequately move the chest wall was 16.5 cm H_2O, with an average peak inflation pressure of 31.2 cm H_2O. Peak inflation pressure was defined as the pressure at which gas would enter the stomach or, conversely, the maximum pressure reached during mask ventilation without air entering the stomach. The application of cricoid pressure increased the mean peak inflation pressure to 44.7 cm H_2O (range, 30–60) (55).

Complete airway obstruction can result from inappropriately applied cricoid pressure. This is more likely in infants and children due to the reduced rigidity of the trachea in these subjects. The appropriate application of cricoid pressure, as described by Sellick, consists of firm pressure applied to the cricoid cartilage. The pressure exerted should not obstruct the trachea in any clinically notable way (59,60).

Cricoid pressure should not interfere with pulmonary ventilation. If airway resistance increases and pulmonary ventilation becomes more difficult, the degree of cricoid pressure should be decreased or the position of the fingers applying pressure changed (59). In general, the application of cricoid pressure is a safe maneuver. One case of esophageal rupture has been reported in an 81-year-old patient during cricoid pressure application (61). The correct application of cricoid pressure will prevent gastric inflation and regurgitation of fluids into oropharynx (55,58–65).

Gastric distension during mask ventilation can be minimized by maintaining proper patient head position, application of the jaw thrust maneuver, the insertion of an oro- or nasopharyngeal airway, and small tidal volumes to ventilate the patient. All of these factors have been previously discussed. While the maintenance of an appropriate level of oxygenation is important under these circumstances, hypoventilation of brief duration is unlikely to prove of detrimental clinical significance. Stomach distension, however, may pose a significant clinical risk.

PREDICTING THE DIFFICULT INTUBATION

A careful preoperative evaluation to identify patients in whom tracheal intubation and mask ventilation may prove difficult should be a routine part of the anesthetic assessment. This is especially important in patients already at high risk for gastric aspiration being considered for a rapid sequence induction. The failure to identify the potential difficult intubation through inadequate patient assessment has contributed to significant morbidity and mortality in this area.

The series of reports *Confidential Enquiries into Maternal Deaths in England and Wales* reports that 41% of maternal deaths due to anesthesia from 1973 to 1984 were secondary to difficulties encountered during tracheal intubation. In another communication, approximately one-third of all anesthetic deaths are attributed to the inability to manage a difficult airway (66). If a difficult intubation is anticipated, precautionary measures can be undertaken and special techniques applied to properly secure the airway.

The Expected Difficult Intubation

Numerous pathologic and anatomical factors that produce a difficult airway have been extensively reviewed (Table 1) (67,68). The mechanisms by which pathologic or congenital anomalies contribute to the difficulties of airway management can be grouped into six categories (Table 2)

The tissues of the oral cavity, pharynx, and larynx can be swollen and expanded, due to inflammation, edema, hematoma, or tumor limiting the airway opening (69–72). Further, an expanding hematoma or tumor of the neck, anterior mediastinal mass, or vascular anomaly can compress the tracheobronchial tree, interfering with mask ventilation and tracheal intubation (69–72).

A swollen epiglottitis is a common cause of airway obstruction in young children. Airway compromise due to retropharyngeal or intraoral abscesses (e.g., Ludwig's angina) is often seen in older children and adults (72). Patients with congenital malformations associated with micrognathia, retrognathia, and macroglossia and patients with obstructive sleep apnea have a smaller oropharyngeal open space and are therefore prone to soft tissue upper airway obstruction (73–75).

When tissues of the head and neck, oral cavity, pharynx, or larynx are fixed by tumor, surgical, or radiation scars, sufficient mouth opening, or head and neck positioning to allow for exposure of the glottic area, is compromised. A supraepiglottic mass can severely limit mobility of the epiglottis, causing complete airway obstruction after induction of anesthesia. This problem can be extremely difficult to overcome, since the mass may prevent any forward displacement of the epiglottis from the posterior pharyngeal wall (39,40,76,77).

Tumors not only decrease the size of the airway and cause tissue fixation, but also distort the anatomy. Burns of the airway, inflammation of laryngeal structures, laryngeal trauma, bleeding, and hematoma all can distort the airway and significantly interfere with airway management.

A history of difficult intubation or mask ventilation given by the patient or through a Medic Alert warning bracelet is a strong indication of difficult airway, and these patients should be treated as such.

TABLE 2. *Mechanisms by which various conditions contribute to the difficulty of the airway*

Limiting the head and neck mobility
Limiting the mouth opening
Limiting mandibular subluxation
Decreasing the airway open space
Fixing the tissues of the airway
Distorting the airway anatomy

The Potentially Difficult Intubation

A number of preoperative assessment techniques have been recommended, to detect a potentially difficult intubation (Table 3). These clinical examinations are easy to perform at the bedside, with the patient in a sitting or supine position. However, these tests are imprecise and associated with a high incidence of false positive and false negative outcomes (Table 4).

External Physical Features

The assessment of physical features, including head, neck, and other body measurements, was made by Wilson and co-workers (5) to predetermine difficult rigid laryngoscopy. The difficulty of laryngeal exposure,

TABLE 3. *Tests applied to predict the difficult intubation*

External anatomical features
Head and neck movement (atlanto-occipital joint)
Jaw movement (temporomandibular joint)
Mouth opening
Subluxation of the mandible
Receding mandible
Protruding maxillary incisors
Obesity
Thyromental distance
Sternomental distance
Visualization of the oropharyngeal structures
Anterior tilt of the larynx
Combined factors of airway predictability
Radiographic assessment

TABLE 4. *Shortcomings of tests predicting difficult intubation*

High incidence of false positives
High incidence of false negatives
Do not address lower airway problems
Do not address mask ventilation difficulties
Miss lingual tonsil as cause of failed intubation

employing a Macintosh laryngoscope, was recorded on a scale of 1 to 5. Grade 1 represented full exposure of the larynx; grade 2, exposure of one-half of the vocal cords; grade 3, only arytenoid exposure; grade 4, only epiglottis exposure; and grade 5, inability to expose the epiglottis itself.

Five risk factors contributing to the difficulty of laryngoscopy were selected for additional scoring values (Table 5). Each risk factor was given three possible scores, ranging from zero to two. A score greater than two predicted 75% of the difficult intubations but had a high incidence of false positives. Increasing the limit of scores greater than four reduced the number of false positives, but increased a number of false negatives. In Wilson's prospective study of 778 patients, 1.5% of rigid laryngoscopies were considered "difficult."

In a recent paper by Oates et al., Mallampati classification scores were compared to Wilson's five risk factors (78). The predictive value of both tests were found to be similar. Both tests had a high incidence of false positives as well as false negatives. There was less interobserver variability, however, with Wilson's scoring system.

Head and Neck Movement (Atlanto-occipital joint)

The mobility of the head and neck at the atlanto-occipital joint, combined with adequate opening of the mouth, are essential elements in the alignment of the oral, pharyngeal, and laryngeal axes. The proper alignment of these axes allows for the visualization of the glottis during rigid laryngoscopy (79–84) (Fig. 5, Chapter 11). The optimal neck position in rigid laryngoscopy maintains the cervical region in a neutral or slightly flexed position, with extension of the head at the atlanto-occipital joint (81–83).

Disease processes, such as cervical spine arthritis, cervical spine trauma, congenital abnormalities, burn or radiation scars, tumors, infection, scleroderma, or a thick short neck, limit cervical mobility, thus limiting visualization of the glottic opening. Decreased neck mobility also limits the maneuvers that can be applied to keep the airway open, and thereby predispose to difficult mask ventilation (84).

The greater the atlanto-occipital distance in the neutral position, the greater the degree of head extension possible. If the posterior tubercle of the atlas is in contact with the occiput in the neutral position, attempts to extend the head shall result in the anterior bowing of the cervical spine with forward displacement of the larynx (85,86). While limitations in head extension may occur secondary to pathological conditions (e.g., rheumatoid arthritis), it may also occur secondary to anatomical variations of the atlanto-occipital gap in people who appear otherwise normal (85).

If the degree of atlanto-occipital extension is reduced by one-third or more, it will contribute to difficulties in tracheal intubation (87). Bedside evaluation of atlanto-occipital extension is performed by having the patient sit up straight, extending their head while maintaining the cervical spine in a neutral position (87).

Other anatomical factors may also interfere with the line of vision from mouth to vocal cords. These factors include protruded maxillary incisors (buck teeth), receding mandible, limited mandibular movement, mandibular subluxation and obesity.

TABLE 5. *Five risk factors of difficult intubation*

Risk factor	Level	
Weight	0	<90 kg
	1	90–110 kg
	2	>110 kg
Head and neck movement	0	>90°
	1	~90°
	2	<90°
Jaw movement	0	IG[a] > 5 cm or SLux[b] > 0
	1	IG < 5 cm and SLux = 0
	2	IG < 5 cm and SLux < 0
Receding mandible	0	Normal
	1	Moderate
	2	Severe
Buck teeth	0	Normal
	1	Moderate
	2	Severe

[a] IG, interincisor gap measured with mouth fully open.
[b] SLux, subluxation (maximal forward protrusion of the lower incisors beyond the upper incisors).
(From ref. 5.)

Jaw Movement

Limited movement of the mandible is a well-recognized factor in some difficult intubations (83,88,89). The hinge-like movement of the temporomandibular joint controls the interincisor gap (mouth opening). The horizontal gliding movement of the joint allows for subluxation of the jaw and determines the maximal forward protrusion of the lower incisors. Mandibular subluxation allows additional anterior displacement of the tongue during rigid laryngoscopy, further opening the line of vision.

A mouth opening limited to 3.5 cm or less (measured between the incisors) will contribute to intubation difficulty (90). A compromised mouth opening produces difficulty with laryngoscope insertion and passage of the endotracheal tube. In addition to temporomandibular joint dysfunction(s), tissue contractures around the mouth, facial trauma, and trismus limit mouth opening. Trismus induced by pain associated with infection, usually relaxes under general anesthesia. However, this cannot be relied upon, if the infection has been long- standing or involves the pterygoid space (90).

The relationship between mouth opening and difficulty of rigid laryngoscopy has recently been challenged (10). In this study 259 of 350 patients had interincisor gaps between 1.5 to 3.4 cm. One patient with an interincisor gap of less than 2 cm proved an easy intubation. A small mouth opening may not create difficulty with intubation if mandibular subluxation is zero or greater (5).

Receding Mandible

The presence of a receding mandible has been associated with difficult intubation (87,88). The tongue is displaced into the mandibular space during rigid laryngoscopy, opening the line of vision from mouth to the larynx. A small mandibular space accommodates tongue displacement poorly, thus interfering with visualization of the larynx.

Protruded Maxillary Incisors (Buck Teeth)

Protruded maxillary incisors interfere with laryngoscope placement and passage of the endotracheal tube, adding to the difficulty of intubation (5,88,90). Some authors have failed to identify "buck teeth" as a risk factor in predicting difficult intubation (87,91).

Obesity

There is general agreement that airway management is more difficult in the morbidly obese patient. Wilson et al. regarded obesity as an aggravating factor (5). In their intubation scoring system, a body weight of 95–110 kg was given a risk factor of one, and a weight in excess of 110 kg was given a risk factor of two. Of the five factors identified by multivariate analysis, obesity was considered the weakest. Buckley et al. reported a 13% incidence of difficult intubations using a rapid sequence technique in the obese patient (92).

Rocke et al. excluded obesity as a risk factor in their study on parturients (15). Bond's study on 26 obese and 14 non-obese patients failed to demonstrate a correlation between body mass index and difficulty of laryngoscopy (93).

Large scale, well-planned studies are needed to determine whether obesity per se is a risk factor, contributing to the incidence of difficult intubation. Weight alone may not be as important as where the excess weight is. Patients with massive weight in their lower abdomen and hip region may behave differently than patients with obese upper body and neck areas. A short, thick, immobile neck produced by cervical spine fat pads will interfere with rigid laryngoscopy, irrespective of the patient's total body weight. The presence of redundant soft tissue structures inside the oropharyngeal and supralaryngeal area also make visualization of the laryngeal structures more difficult (94).

Other airway-related factors to consider in the morbidly obese patients include difficulties with face mask ventilation, the need for high positive pressure to ventilate a noncompliant heavy chest wall, higher risk of regurgitation and aspiration, and more rapid oxygen desaturation during periods of apnea. Other techniques of intubation, including fiberoptic techniques, may be more challenging and difficult to perform. Access to the neck for transtracheal jet ventilation or tracheostomy shall also be more difficult.

In recognition of all of the factors discussed, securing the airway in most morbidly obese patients will be safer if performed prior to induction of general anesthesia. The fiberscope has made awake intubation a relatively easy, highly successful technique. It is without doubt the technique of choice in our group when securing the airway of most morbidly obese patients. Where mask ventilation and intubation have failed, the laryngeal mask airway may provide a unique backup capability in the obese patient (95,96).

McIntyre's statement in 1968 that "The anatomical structure of the obese patient is an intimidating sight in the operating room" remains equally valid today (97). Of all the potential problems posed by the morbidly obese patient, none contributes more to the anxiety of the anesthesiologist than their airway management.

Thyromental Distance

The thyromental distance is measured between the bony point of the mentum of the mandible and the thyroid notch, with the head fully extended. If the thyromental distance is short, the laryngeal axis makes a more acute angle with the pharyngeal axis and interferes with their alignment. Patil (98) reported that the thyromental distance in the adult usually exceeds 6.5 cm and that visualization of the larynx by rigid laryngoscopy may be impossible if the distance is less than 6.0 cm.

A recent study of 22 patients with known intubation difficulties, reported that a thyromental distance of less than 6 cm and a horizontal mandibular length of less than 9 cm correlated well with a Mallampati class III airway. Similar measurements in 22 patients rated as easy intubations showed thyromental distances greater than 6.5 cm and mandibular lengths greater than 9 cm. These patients correlated well with Mallampati class I or II airways (99). A distance of less than three finger breadths thyromental distance is considered indicative of a receding mandible (15,99).

Lewis et al. recommended measuring the distance from the thyroid cartilage to the inner border of the mentum, with the patient in the sitting and the head in sniffing position. The recommendation is based on their study of 213 adult patients in which measurements in multiple body positions were evaluated (100).

Sternomental Distance

The sternomental distance is measured with the head in full extension and the mouth closed. Proponents of this measurement claim it is more sensitive and specific in predicting difficult rigid laryngoscopy than other measuring techniques. It is argued that the sternomental distance better reflects maximum head extension, allowing a more accurate assessment (10). The predictive value of sternomental distance regarding the difficult intubation has not been studied or verified by other investigators.

Visualization of Oropharyngeal Structures

The ease of visualization of the soft palate, uvula, and faucial pillars was described by Mallampati as an easy reliable approach to predicting the difficult intubation (6). The key feature of this examination relates to the degree of concealment of the faucial pillars and uvula by the base of the tongue.

The evaluation is performed with the patient in the sitting position. The patient is asked to open his mouth as wide as possible and maximally protrude his tongue. The airway is then graded into three classes according to the visibility of the faucial pillars, soft palate, and uvula. In class I the faucial pillars, soft palate, and uvula are all visualized. In class II the faucial pillars and soft palate are visualized, but the uvula is masked by the base of the tongue. In class III, only the soft palate can be visualized (Fig. 1).

In the class III airway, visualization of the glottis by rigid laryngoscopy is expected to be difficult (6). This classification was evaluated prospectively in 210 patients undergoing orotracheal intubation,using a #3 Macintosh blade. The class III group patients were then graded according to difficulty of glottic exposure. Grade 1 represented full exposure of the glottis, including the anterior commissure. In grade 2 only the posterior commissure could be visualized. In grade 3 the glottis could not be seen, but the corniculate cartilage was visible; and in grade 4 neither glottis nor corniculate cartilage could be seen. Grades 1 and 2 were considered examples of adequate exposure. Grades 3 and 4 were considered inadequate.

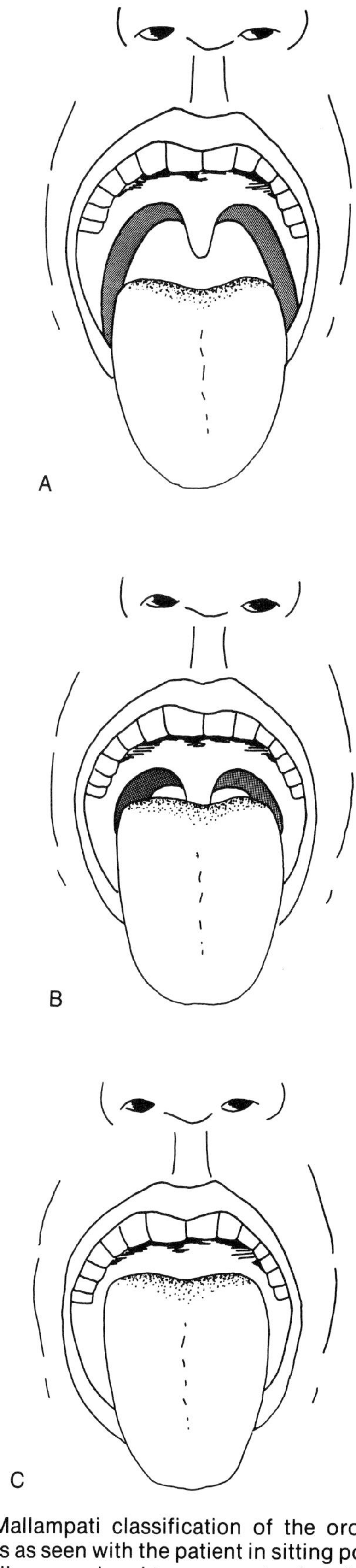

FIG. 1. Mallampati classification of the oropharyngeal structures as seen with the patient in sitting position, with mouth fully opened and tongue protruded: **A:** Class I; **B:** Class II; **C:** Class III.

In the 210 patients studied, 155 (73.8%) were Mallampati class I. All were graded as a 1 or 2 on laryngoscopy. Forty (19%) had been classified as Mallampati class II. Twenty-six of these patients were graded 1 or 2 on laryngoscopy, with four of the group graded as 3 or 4. Of the 210 patients, 15 (7.1%) were judged to have Mallampati class III airways. Fifteen of these patients were graded as 2, and 14 were graded either a 3 or 4 during laryngoscopy. The data from this study suggests significant false-negative and false-positive findings in the use of the Mallampati classification technique.

Samsoon and Young (14) in their retrospective study of 13 failed intubations found that in 12 of these patients there was a good correlation between the degree of intubation difficulty and the of visibility of the oropharyngeal structures. In the one patient with a Mallampati class II airway, a failed intubation was attributed to the presence of tracheal stenosis.

Bellhouse and Dore have shown that a combination of reduced atlanto-occipital extension, reduced chin protrusion, and increased tongue size influence the difficulty of intubation (87). They found no consistent evidence of a relationship between the difficulty of intubation, depth of the mandible, degree of mouth opening, or length of the upper incisor teeth. Other investigators consider the Mallampati classification too subjective, and not a useful predictor of intubation difficulty (101,102).

The Mallampati airway evaluation is simple and easy to perform and has become a popular test of airway evaluation. However, the classification method predicts only about 50% of difficult intubations accurately and has a high incidence of false positive results. The high incidence of false positives, as well as false negative evaluations, has prompted a number of investigators to modify Mallampati's original evaluation technique.

The presence of phonation may be a cause of error when the Mallampati classification evaluation is performed (103,104). During the oral evaluation, the patient phonates by saying "ah" while the tongue is protruded. This action seems to increase the specificity of the test in that it better correlates with predicting a difficult intubation. However, it also results in an increase in false negative results.

Tham et al. showed that phonation provided a significant systematic improvement in viewing the oropharyngeal structures (105). Airway evaluation in the supine position produced a small but insignificant worsening of the view. Lewis and associates studied Mallampati's airway classification in the sitting and supine position, with three different head positions (neutral, sniff, and full extension) and two tongue positions, with and without phonation (100). His group recommended that the oropharyngeal evaluation be conducted with the patient phonating in the sitting position with full head extension and the tongue protruding.

In his editorial on predicting difficult intubation, Wilson summarized a number of tests currently utilized as predictors. He concluded that no ideal test exists and encouraged investigators to develop more reliable predictive test models (106). He also emphasized the importance of all anesthesiologists to be well trained and versed in dealing with the unexpected failed intubation.

The Anteriorly Tilted Larynx

The explanation "high anterior larynx" is often used as a descriptive term, designating a difficult or failed intubation associated with rigid laryngoscopy. Usually no other obvious anatomical or pathological causes are evident. Despite the term's common usage in the anesthesia literature, no clinical reports or studies defining the entity of an "anterior larynx" exists.

Roberts et al., measuring the degree of anterior tilt of the thyroid cartilage, showed a relationship between the degree of the thyroid cartilage tilt and the difficulty of laryngeal exposure (107). The laryngeal tilt is easily and directly measured using a bubble inclinometer (Fig. 2). When the tilt of the anterior surface of the thyroid cartilage is greater than 20° rigid laryngoscopy proved to be difficult.

This test showed a sensitivity of 70%, with a 95% specificity, and a positive predictive value of 80%. The value of this test has not been studied by other investigators. Anterior laryngeal tilt is reduced by manual depression of the thyroid cartilage, but is further exaggerated by cricoid pressure.

Combined Factors of Airway Predictability

No single factor is reliably predictive of a difficult laryngoscopy or intubation (5,87,108). Investigators in this area have attempted to improve the predictive value of difficult intubation by looking at a combination of factors or tests.

Bellhouse and Dore have shown that measurements of atlanto-occipital extension, chin protrusion, and tongue size, increase the sensitivity of preoperative prediction of difficult intubation (87). Frerk studied the usefulness of combining the Mallampati and thyromental distance measurements as predictors of intubation difficulty. They studied 244 patients of which 11 (4.9%) proved to be difficult to intubate. The Mallampati classifications used alone showed a sensitivity of 81.2% and a specificity of 81.5% as predictors of difficult intubation. Measurements of thyromental distance showed a sensitivity of 90.9% and a specificity of 81.5%, re-

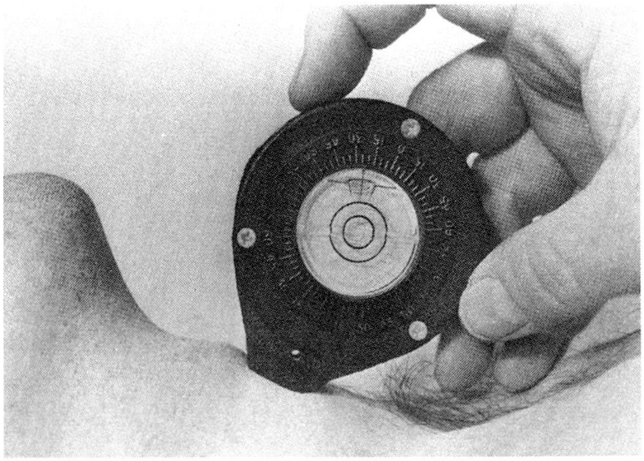

FIG. 2. Measuring the laryngeal tilt with bubble inclinometer. The flat surface of the bubble inclinometer is placed against the anterior surface of the thyroid cartilage with the patient's head in a neutral position without pillows. An anterior tilt of the larynx greater than 20° was associated with grade 3 rigid laryngoscopy (i.e., vocal cords not visualized). (With permission, ref. 107.)

spectively, when used as a predictor. The predictive value combining the two tests improved specificity to 97.8% (low false positive rate), but did not improve sensitivity, which remained at 81.2% (11).

Rocke and his associates studied 1500 patients, subjected to elective or emergency cesarean section under general anesthesia (15). In addition to the Mallampati classification, patients were evaluated for eight other potential risk factors, which included short neck, obesity, missing maxillary incisors, protruding maxillary teeth, a single maxillary tooth, receding mandible, facial edema, and enlarged tongue. An assessment was made of the laryngoscopic exposure of the larynx, as well as the ease of tracheal intubation. The various factors described were compared as predictors of difficult intubation.

Only 6.6% of Mallampati class IV airway cases were associated with very difficult tracheal intubation, and none were failed (low specificity). Of the two failed intubations (1 in 750), one had Mallampati airway class II with no other risk factors. The second failed intubation had Mallampati airway class III with the esophageal intubation performed by a resident. After recognition, tracheal intubation was performed by the senior anesthesiologist.

Rocke et al. have calculated the probability of various risk factors contributing to the difficult intubation. They concluded that the presence of a Mallampati class III airway is associated with a risk of a difficult intubation 7.58 times greater than class I. A class IV airway was found to have a risk factor 11.2 times greater than class I. The probability of predicting a difficult intubation combining the Mallampati airway classification with the factors of a short neck, protruding maxillary incisors, and receding mandible is presented in Fig. 3.

Radiographic Assessment

Lateral X-rays of the head and neck region, combined with distance measurements between bony landmarks, have been used to identify factors predictive of difficult rigid laryngoscopy (85,87,88,90,108,109). In the study conducted by White and Kander (89), a ratio of less than 3.6 between mandibular length and posterior mandibular depth was associated with difficult intubation. Other predictive measurements utilized included measurements of atlanto-occipital distance and the C1-C2 interspinous gap.

A number of studies have confirmed that limitation of extension of the atlanto-occipital joint is a factor in the difficult intubation (85–87,109). Nichol and Zuck stressed the importance of the atlanto-occipital gap in allowing for head extension during rigid laryngoscopy (85). Reduction of the atlanto-occipital gap has been demonstrated in otherwise normal patients.

A study by Horton et al. that reviewed lateral cervical radiographs in healthy volunteers undergoing laryngoscopy showed a mean C1-C2 extension of 25°. There was also a progressive increase in extension from C4 to C1 (110). Any limitation of this extension may interfere with rigid laryngoscopy and glottic exposure.

Radiographic assessment is expensive, time consuming, and not practical for routine airway evaluation. However, radiological studies may prove of considerable value in evaluating the known difficult airway patient.

Hidden Causes of a Difficult Airway

On rare occasion, a patient with no external physical findings or features indicative of difficult intubation is found to have an airway that proves extremely difficult. These patients are at increased risk for major airway related complications, especially under emergency circumstances.

A lack of information regarding internal anatomy (e.g., the shape of the epiglottis, valleculae, lingual tonsils, and so on) certainly contributes to the difficulty of predicting airway probems. In our institution patients with a unexpected failed intubation were examined carefully over the past five years for possible causes of difficult intubation. In several patients the only positive finding that contributed to the failed intubation or mask ventilation technique was the presence of large lingual tonsils.

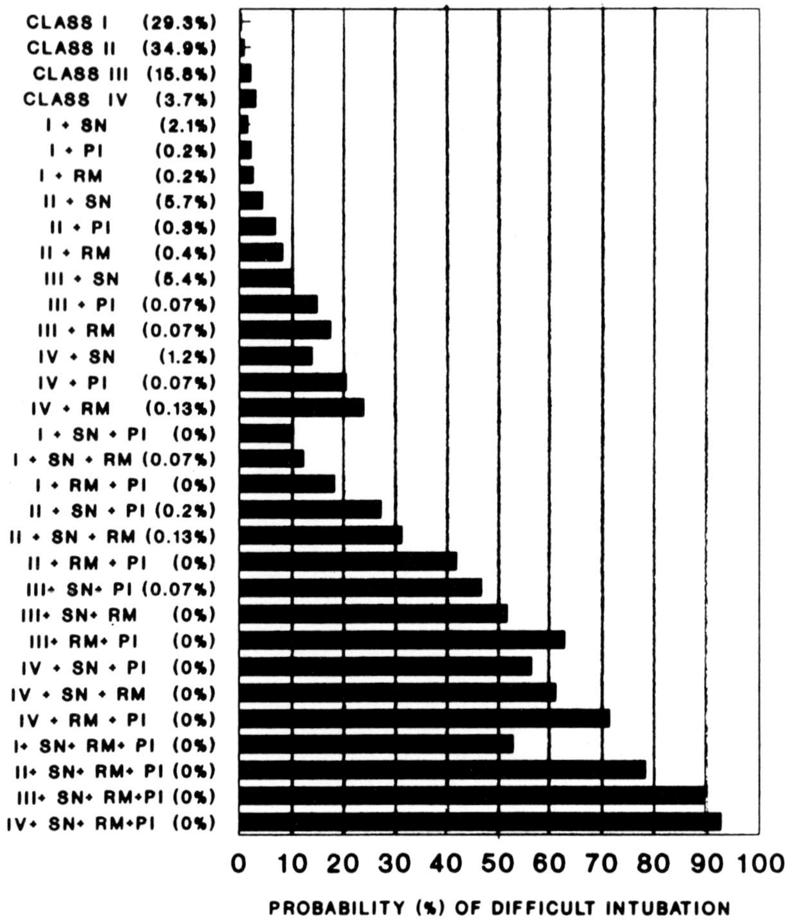

FIG. 3. Combined factors of airway predictability. Demonstrates the probability of experiencing difficult intubation for various combinations of risk factors and the observed incidence of these combinations in Rocke et al.'s study. (With permission, ref. 15.) SN: short neck; PI: protruding maxillary incisors; RM: receding mandible; Class I–IV: Mallampati classification of the visibility of the oropharyngeal structures.

Lingual tonsillar hypertrophy has been reported as a cause of difficult or failed intubation during anesthesia (41,111,112). Difficulties with mask ventilation are not uncommon in these patients and have resulted in death due to an inability to secure or support the airway under anesthesia (41). Lingual thyroidal tissue and infected laryngocele may also contribute to airway support problems after the induction of anesthesia (40,113,114).

SUMMARY

Patients experiencing difficulty during rigid orotracheal intubation fall into two main groups: (a) those with obvious pathologic conditions or anatomic variations affecting the airway, and (b) those without obvious signs of an impending difficult intubation.

Attempts have been made to identify factors predictive of a difficult intubation in the second group of patients. All methods have shortcomings, including a high incidence of false positives and an inability to detect intrathoracic airway problems, such as tracheal stenosis, and other hidden findings.

In addition, no method addresses the critical issue of predicting difficult mask ventilation. It is this technique that must usually support the patient until definitive securing of the airway takes place. Physicians involved in airway management should be aware of the weaknesses inherent in the various tests used to predict a difficult intubation (106). In addition, they must be trained and prepared to use specific strategies to manage unanticipated difficulties in intubation.

A difficult airway cart equipped with necessary supplies should be ready for immediate use. The development of skillful proficiency in the use of the fiberoptic bronchoscope is becoming a routine necessity for those involved in airway management.

Airway complications of hypoxia and aspiration increase if repeated attempts at intubation become unduly prolonged. Cormack and Lehane have suggested that in obstetric patients, no more than three intubation attempts should be made before starting a failed intubation procedure. In cases where the epiglottis is not identified on the initial attempt a new approach should be initiated (3).

The ASA algorithm on the difficult airway recommends limiting multiple attempts at intubation to minimize airway trauma. It encourages proceeding to alternative techniques to establish ventilation and oxygenation. The skill and judgment of the physician is critical in preventing anesthetic deaths as a result of a failure to secure the airway. A significant number of reported major airway related complications are due to a lack of experience. Anesthesia trainees require close supervision until they have mastered various methods of airway management particularly relevant to the difficult intubation (66).

REFERENCES

1. Gupa B, McDonald JS. The difficult airway. *Hospital Physician* 1986; January:65–74.
2. Practice guidelines for management of the difficult airway. A report by the American Society of Anesthesiologists Task Force on management of the difficult airway. *Anesthesiology* 1993;78:597–602.
3. Cormack RS, Lehane J. Difficult tracheal intubation in obstetrics. *Anaesthesia* 1984;39:1105–1111.
4. Bellhouse CP. An angulated laryngoscope for routine and difficult tracheal intubation. *Anesthesiology* 1988;69:126–129.
5. Wilson ME, Spiegelhalter D, Robertson JA, Lesser P. Predicting difficult intubation. *Br J Anaesth* 1988;61:211–216.
6. Mallampati SR, Gatt SP, Gugino LD, et al. A clinical sign to predict difficult tracheal intubation: a prospective study. *Can Anaesth Soc J* 1985;32:429–434.
7. Aro L, Takki S, Aromaa U. Technique for difficult intubation. *Br J Anaesth* 1971;43:1081–1083.
8. Latto IP. Management of difficult intubation. In: Latto IP, Rosen M, eds. *Difficulties in tracheal intubation*. London: Bailliere Tindall, 1985;99–141.
9. Lyons G. Failed intubation. Six years experience in a teaching maternity unit. *Anaesthesia* 1985;40:759–766.
10. Savva D. Prediction of difficult tracheal intubation. *Br J Anaesth* 1994;73:149–153.
11. Frerk CM. Predicting difficult intubation. *Anaesthesia* 1991; 46:1005–2008.
12. Wilson ME, Spiegelhalter D, Robertson JA, Lesser P. Predicting difficult intubation. *Br J Anaesthesia* 1988;61:211–216.
13. Butler PJ, Dhara SS. Prediction of difficult laryngoscopy: an assessment of the thyromental distance and Mallampati predictive tests. *Anaesth Intens Care* 1992;20:139–142.
14. Samsoon GLT, Young JRB. Difficult tracheal intubation: a retrospective study. *Anaesthesia* 1987;42:487–490.
15. Rocke DA, Murray WB, Rout CC, Gouws E. Relative risk analysis of factors associated with difficult intubation in obstetric anesthesia. *Anesthesiology* 1992;77:67–73.
16. Williamson R. Endotracheal intubation in temporomandibular ankylosis. *Anesth Analg* 1988;67:602–603.
17. Williamson JA, Webb RK, Szekely S, Gillies ERN, Dreosti AV. Difficult intubation: An analysis of 2000 incident reports. *Anaesth Intens Care* 1993;21:602–607.
18. Utting JE. Pitfalls in anaesthesia practice. *Br J Anaesth* 1987; 59:877–890.
19. Ovassapian A. Fiberoptic tracheal intubation. In: Ovassapian A, ed. *Fiberoptic airway endoscopy in anesthesia and intensive care*. New York: Raven Press, 1990;57–79.
20. Nandi PR, Charlesworth CH, Taylor SJ, Nunn JF, Dore CJ. Effect of general anaesthesaia on the pharynx. *Br J Anaesth* 1991;66:157–162.
21. Mark JD, Brooks JG. Sleep-associated airway problems in children. *Ped Clin North Am* 1984;31:907–918.
22. Kuna ST, Kemmers JE. Neural and anatomic factors related to upper airway reclusion during sleep. *Med Clin North Am* 1985;69:1221–1242.
23. Remmers JE, deGroot WJ, Sauerland EK. Pathogenesis of upper airway occlusion during sleep. *J Appl Physiol* 1978;44: 931–938.
24. Lunteren EV, Van De Graaff WB, Parker DM, et al. Nasal and laryngeal reflex responses to negative upper airway pressure. *J Appl Physiol* 1984;56:746–752.
25. Ochiai R, Guthrie RD, Motoyama EK. Effects of varying concentrations of halothane on the activity of the genioglossus, intercostalis, and diaphragm in cats: an elctromyographic study. *Anesthesiology* 1989;70:812–816.
26. Nishino T, Honda Y, Kohchi T, Shirahata M, Yonezawa T. Comparison of changes in the hypoglossal and phrenic nerve activity in response to increasing depth of anesthesia in cats. *Anesthesiology* 1984;60:19–24.
27. Brouillette RT, Thach BT. A neuromuscular mechanism maintaining extrathoracic airway patency. *J Appl Physiol* 1979;46: 772–779.
28. Orr WC. Sleep and breathing: an overview. *Ear Nose Throat J* 1984;63:191–198.
29. Morikawa S, Safar P, DeCarlo J. Influence of the head—jaw position upon airway patency. *Anesthesiology* 1961;22: 265–270.
30. Safar P, Escarraga LA, Chang F. Upper airway obstruction in the unconscious patient. *J Appl Physiol* 1959;14:760–764.
31. Rubin HM, Elam JD, Ruben AM, Greene DG. Investigation of upper airway problems in resuscitation. Studies of pharyngeal X-rays and performance by laymen. *Anesthesiology* 1961; 22:271–279.
32. Asmussen E, Hahn-Petersen A, Rosenthal TH. Air passage through hypopharynx in unconscious patients in prone position. *Acta Anaesth Scand* 1958;3:123.
33. Elam JO, Greene DG, Schneider MA, et al. Head-tilt method of oral resuscitation. *JAMA* 1960;172:812.
34. Fink BR. Roentgenographic studies of oropharyngeal airway. *Anesthesiology* 1957;18:711.
35. Boidin MD. Airway patency in the unconscious patient. *Br J Anaesth* 1985;57:306–310.
36. Asherson N. Large cysts of the epiglottis: a classification and case records. *J Laryngol* 1957;71:730–743.
37. Padfield A. Epiglottic cysts. A case report and review. *Anaesthesia* 1972;27:84–88.
38. Chang-Lo N. Laryngeal involvement in Von Recklinghausen's disease: a case report and review of the literature. *Laryngoscope* 1977;87:435–442.
39. Henderson LT, Denneny JC, Teichgraeber J. Airway-obstructing epiglottic cyst. *Ann Otol Rhinol Laryngol* 1985;94:473–476.
40. Mason DG, Wark KJ. Unexpected difficult intubation. Asymptomatic epiglottic cysts as a cause of upper airway obstruction during anesthesia. *Anaesthesia* 1987;42:407–410.
41. Jones DH, Cohle SD. Unanticipated difficult airway secondary to lingual tonsillar hyperplasia. *Anesth Analg* 1993;77: 1285–1288.
42. Coleman DL, Cohen NH. Airway management of the nonintubated patient. *J Intens Care* 1987;2:354–362.
43. Gold MI, Helrich M. Mechanics of breathing during anesthesia. II. The influence of airway adequacy. *Anesthesiology* 1965;26: 751.
44. Dinnick OP. Hiatus hernia. An anesthetic hazard. *Lancet* 1961; 1:470–473.
45. Marchand P. Gastro-oesophageal sphincter and mechanisms of regurgitation. *Br J Surg* 1955;42:504.
46. O'Mullane EJ. Vomiting and regurgitation during anaesthesia. *Lancet* 1954;ii:1209.
47. Sinclair RN. The oesophageal cardia and regurgitation. *Br J Anaesth* 1959;31:15.
48. Cotton BR, Smith G. The lower oesophageal sphincter and anaesthesia. *Br J Anaesth* 1984;56:37–46.

49. Lorch DG, Sahn SA. Postextubation pulmonary edema following anesthesia induced by upper airway obstruction. Are certain patients at increased risk? *Chest* 1986;90:802–805.
50. Price SL, Hecker BR. Pulmonary oedema following airway obstruction in a patient with Hodgkin's disease. *Br J Anaesth* 1987;59:518–521.
51. Stevens J. Anesthetic problems of intestinal obstruction in adults. *Br J Anaesth* 1964;36:438–450.
52. Roe RB. The effect of suxamethonium on intragastric pressure. *Anaesthesia* 1962;17:179–181.
53. Clark CG, Riddoch ME. Observations on the human cardia at operation. *Br J Anaesth* 1962;34:75.
54. Greenan J. The cardio-oesophageal junction. *Br J Anaesth* 1961;33:432–439.
55. Lawes EG, Campbell I, Mercer D. Inflation pressure, gastric insufflation and rapid sequence induction. *Br J Anaesth* 1987; 59:315–318.
56. Ruben H, Krudsen EJ, Carngati G. Gastric inflation in relation to airway pressure. *Acta Anaesth Scand* 1961;5:107–114.
57. Vyas H, Milner AD, Hopkin IE. Face mask resuscitation: does it lead to gastric distention? *Arch Dis Child* 1983;58:373–375.
58. Admani M, Yeh TF, Jain R, et al. Prevention of gastric inflation during mask ventilation in newborn infants. *Crit Care Med* 1985;13:592–593.
59. Moynihan RJ, Brock-Utne JG, Archer JH, Kreitzman TR. The effect of cricoid pressure on preventing gastric insufflation in infants and children. *Anesthesiology* 1993;78:652–656.
60. Sellick BA. Cricoid pressure to control regurgitation of stomach contents during induction of anesthesia. *Lancet* 1961;ii: 404–406.
61. Ralph SJ, Wareham CA Rupture of the esophagus during cricoid pressure. *Anaesthesia* 1991; 46:40–41.
62. Petito SP, Russell WJ. The prevention of gastric inflation. A neglected benefit of cricoid pressure. *Anaesth Intens Care* 1988;16:139–143.
63. Wraight WJ, Chamney AR, Howells TH. The determination of an effective cricoid pressure. *Anaesthesia* 1983;38:461–466.
64. Lawes EG, Duncan PW, Bland B, et al. The cricoid yoke—a device for providing consistent and reproducible cricoid pressure. *Br J Anaesth* 1986;58:925–931.
65. Lawes EG. Cricoid pressure with or without the "Cricoid Yoke." *Br J Anaesth* 1986;58:1376–1379.
66. King TA, Adams AP. Failed tracheal intubation. *Br J Anaesth* 1990;65:400–414.
67. McIntyre JWR. The difficult tracheal intubation. *Can J Anaesth* 1987;34:204–213.
68. Jones AEP, Pelton DA. An index of syndromes and their anaeathesia implications. *Can Anaesth Soc J* 1976;23:207–226.
69. Schwartz HC, Bauer RA, Davis NJ, Guralnick WC. Ludwig's angina: use of fiberoptic laryngoscopy to avoid tracheostomy. *J Oral Surg* 1974;32:608–611.
69. Filstom HC, et al. Airway obstruction by vascular anomalies. Importance of telescopic bronchoscopy. *Ann Surg* 1987;205: 541–549.
70. Heindel DJ. Deep neck abscesses in adults: management of a difficult airway. *Anesth Analg* 1987;66:774–776.
71. Ovassapian A, Doka JC, Romsa DE. Acromegaly—use of fiberoptic laryngoscopy to avoid tracheostomy. *Anesthesiology* 1981;54:429–430.
72. Baxter FJ, Dunn GL. Acute epiglottitis in adults. *Can J Anaesth* 1988;35:428–435.
73. Handler SD, Keon TP. Difficult laryngoscopy intubation: the child with mandibular hypoplasia. *Ann Otol Rhinol Laryngol* 1983;92:401–404.
74. Heaf DP, Helms PJ, Dinwiddie R, et al. Nasopharyngeal airways in Pierre-Robin syndrome. *J Pediatr* 1982;100:698–703.
75. Roa NL, Moss KS. Treacher-Collins syndrome with sleep apnea: anesthetic considerations. *Anesthesiology* 1984;60: 71–73.
76. Crozier WC. Upper airway obstruction in neurofibromatosis. *Anaesthesia* 1987;42:1209–1211.
77. McKiernan EP, Meakin G. Vallecular cysts. *Anaesthesia* 1988; 43:808–809.
78. Oates JDL, MacLeod Ad, Oates PD et al. Comparison of two methods for predicting difficult intubation. *Br J Anaesth* 1991; 66:305–309.
79. Brechner VL. Unusual problems in the management of airways. I. Flexion-extension mobility of the cervical vertebrae. *Anesth Analg* 1968;47:362–373.
80. Horton WA, Fahy L, Charters P. Defining a standard intubating position using "angle finder." *Br J Anaesth* 1989;62:6–12.
81. Banister FB, MacBeth RG. Direct laryngoscopy and tracheal intubation. *Lancet* 1994;2:651–654.
82. Cobley M, Vaughan RS. Recognition and management of difficult intubation. *Br J Anaesth* 1992;68:90–97.
83. Murrin KR. Intubation procedure and causes of difficult intubation. In: Latto IP, Rosen M, eds. *Difficulties in tracheal intubation*. London: Balliere Tindall, 1987;75–89.
84. D'arcy EJ, Fell RH, Ansell BM, Arden GP. Ketamine and juvenile chronic polyarthritis (Still's disease). *Anaesthesia* 1976;31: 124.
85. Nichol HC, Zuck D. Difficult laryngoscopy—the "anterior" larynx and the atlanto-occipital gap. *Br J Anaesth* 1983;55: 141–143.
86. Skues M. Anatomical factors complicating direct laryngoscopy. *Anaesthesia Points West* 1984;17:31–33.
87. Bellhouse CP, Dore C. Criteria for estimating likelihood of difficulty of endotracheal intubation with the Macintosh laryngoscope. *Anaesth Intens Care* 1988;16:329–337.
88. Cass NM, James NR, Lines V. Difficult direct laryngoscopy complicating intubation for anesthesia. *Br Med J* 1956;1: 488–489.
89. White A, Kander PL. Anatomical factors in difficult direct laryngoscopy. *Br J Anaesth* 1975;47:468–473.
90. Block C, Brechner VL. Unusual problems in airway management. II. The influence of the temporomandibular joint, the mandible, and associated structures in endotracheal intubation. *Anesth Analg* 1971;50:114–123.
91. Zuck D. Factors in difficult direct laryngoscopy. *Br J Anaesth* 1976;48:395–396.
92. Buckley FP, Robinson NB, Simonowitz DA, Dellinger EP. Anesthesia in the morbidly obese. A comparison of anesthetic and analgesic regimens for upper abdominal suegery. *Anaesthesia* 1983;38:840–851.
93. Bond A. Obesity and difficult intubation. *Anaesth Intens Care* 1993;21:828–830.
94. Trempy GA, Rock P. Anesthetic management of a morbidly obese woman with a massive ovarian cyst. *J Clin Anesth* 1993; 5:62–68.
95. Meyer RJ. Obesity and difficult intubation (letter). *Anaesth Intens Care* 1994;22:314–315.
96. Bond A. Obesity and difficult intubation—a reply. *Anaesth Intens Care* 1994;22:316.
97. McIntyre JWR. Problems for the anesthetist in the care of the obese patient. *Can J Anaesth* 1968;15:317–324.
98. Patil VU, Stehling LC, Zauder HL. Predicting the difficulty of intubation utilizing an intubation guide. *Anesthesiol Rev* 1983; 10:32–33.
99. Mathew M, Hanna LS, Aldrete JA. Pre-operative indices to anticipate difficult tracheal intubation. *Anesth Analg* 1989;68: S187.
100. Lewis M, Keramati S, Benumof JL, Berry CC. What is the best way to determine oropharyngeal classification and mandibular space length to predict difficult laryngoscopy. *Anesthesiology* 1994;81:69–75.
101. Charters P, Perera S, Horton WA. Visibility of pharyngeal structures as a predictor of difficult intubation. *Anaesthesia* 1987;42:1115.
102. Arora RD, Patterson L, Hagen JF, Pinchak AC. Prediction of difficult intubation. *Anesthesiology* 1987;67:A472.
103. Wilson ME, John R. Problems with the Mallampati sign. *Anaesthesia* 1990;45:486–487.
104. Oates JDL, Oates PD, Pearsall EJ, et al. Phonation affects Mallampati class. *Anaesthesia* 1990;45:984.

105. Tham EJ, Gildersleve CD, Sanders LD, et al. Effects of posture, phonation and observer on Mallampati classification. *Br J Anaesth* 1992;68:32–38.
106. Wilson ME. Predicting difficult intubation. *Br J Anaesth* 1993; 71:333–334.
107. Roberts JT, Ali HH, Shorten GD. Using the bubble inclinometer to measure laryngeal tilt and predict difficulty of laryngoscopy. *J Clin Anesth* 1993;5:306–309.
108. Van der Linde JC, Roelofse SA, Steenkamp EC. Anatomical factors relating to difficult intubation. *S Afr Med J* 1983;63: 976–977.
109. Levack ID, Masson AHB. Difficult tracheal intubation in obstetrics. *Anaesthesia* 1985;40:384.
110. Horton WA, Fahy L, Charter P. Disposition of cervical vertebrae, atlanto-axial joint, hyoid and mandible during x-ray laryngoscopy. *Br J Anaesth* 1989;63:435–438.
111. Biro P, Shahinian H. Management of difficult intubation caused by lingual tonsillar hyperplasia. *Anesth Analg* 1994;79:389.
112. Johnson CA, Mehdiabadi RJ, Ruff T. Infection and hypertrophy of the lingual tonsil as a cause of airway obstruction. *Tex Med* 1986;82:29–31.
113. Fogarty D. Lingual thyroid and difficult tracheal intubation. *Anaesthesia* 1990;45:251.
114. Rashid J, Warltier B. Awake fiberoptic intubation for a rare cause of upper airway obstruction: an infected laryngocoele. *Anaesthesia* 1989;44:834–836.

CHAPTER 11

Management of the Difficult Airway

Andranik Ovassapian, M.D.

In 1985, the American Society of Anesthesiologists Committee on Professional Liability began to review and analyze closed claims malpractice files of several insurance companies to assess the types, outcomes, and amount of monetary awards for anesthesia-related events. Several publications have summarized the findings of the committee. Approximately one-third of all adverse anesthetic outcomes are related to respiratory problems (1). The three common mechanisms of these adverse outcomes were related to inadequate ventilation (38%), esophageal intubation (18%), and difficult tracheal intubation (17%). In the *Report on Confidential Enquiries into Maternal Deaths in England and Wales, 1973–1984,* approximately 41% of anesthetic deaths were related to difficulties encountered with tracheal intubation (2).

Analysis of anesthetic mishaps that have led to medical liability claims reveals that difficult tracheal intubation (DI) and aspiration of gastric contents are two major causes of death or brain damage in anesthetized patients (3–6). In one report airway misadventures constituted 69% of anesthesia-related deaths (5). In another study, faulty techniques of tracheal intubation were responsible for 50 (14.4%) of 348 cases of death or severe cerebral damage attributed to anesthesia (6). Difficult intubation and aspiration of gastric contents allegedly have been the main causes of anesthesia-related maternal deaths (7–10).

Under normal circumstances tracheal intubation is a simple, highly successful procedure. However, the consequences of a failed intubation in the face of deteriorating oxygenation and difficult or impossible mask ventilation remain a major cause of patient morbidity and mortality.

In 1992, the American Society of Anesthesiologists (ASA) established the Task Force on Management of the Difficult Airway. The ASA task force produced guidelines for Management of the Difficult Airway

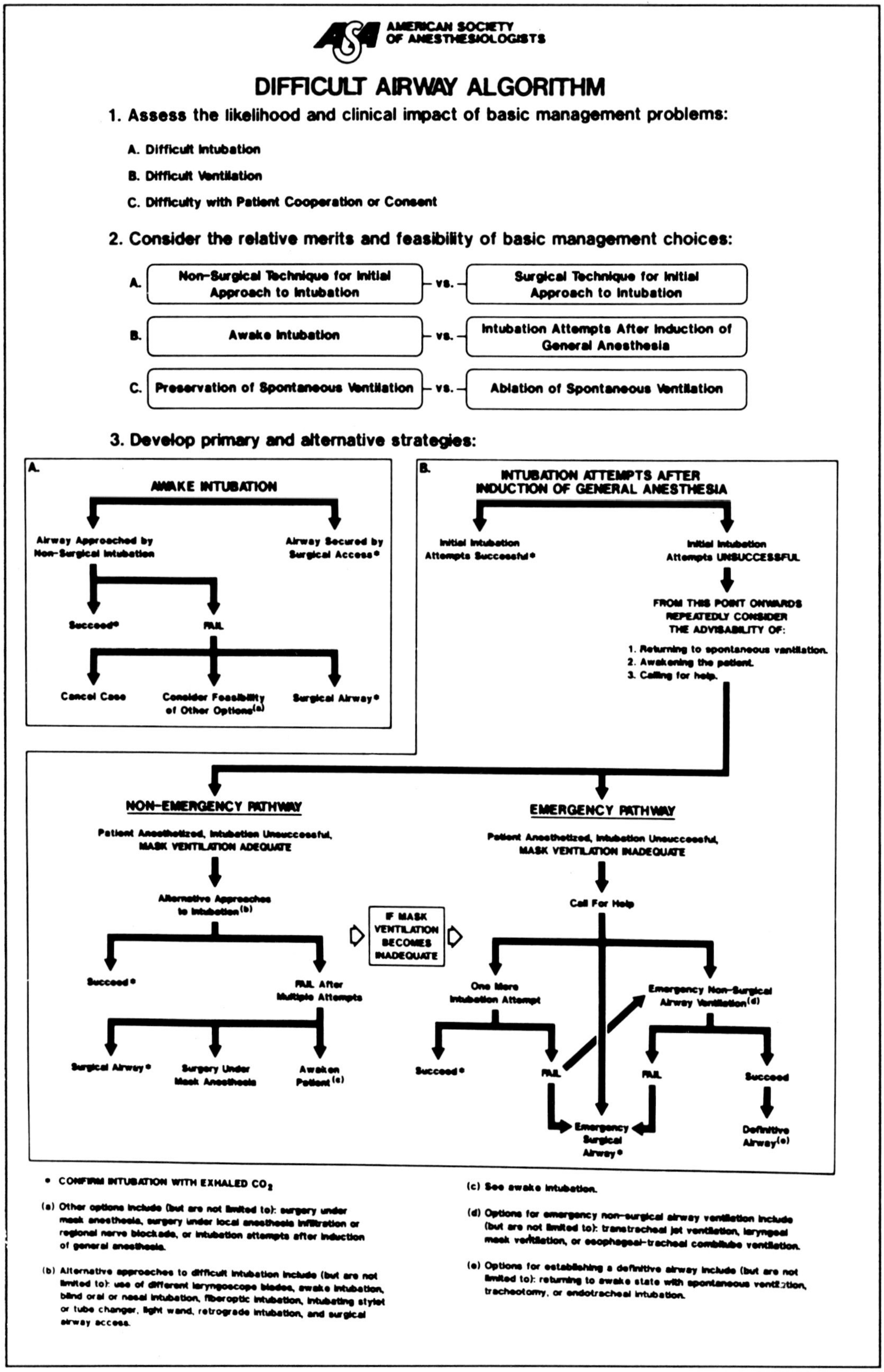

FIG. 1. ASA difficult airway algorithm. (With permission, ref. 11.)

which included "A Difficult Airway Algorithm" (Fig. 1) (11).

The algorithm begins by helping to define and recognize the presence of a difficult airway. To recognize the potential problem of a difficult airway, careful patient evaluation is essential. Proper planning of and preparation for airway management is critical in helping to prevent untoward complications. Successful airway management further requires skillful application of the various techniques to be employed.

PATIENT EVALUATION

In most patients, the difficult airway is easily recognized either by anatomic features, or signs and symptoms related to a compromised airway. However, in a small group of patients, a difficult intubation may not be easily discerned. To avoid an airway-related disaster in this group of patients, careful evaluation and planning of airway management is essential. This includes obtaining a detailed history, thorough review of prior anesthetic records and laboratory data, as well as performing a careful physical examination of the airway.

History

The medical history should include questioning the presence of diseases or syndromes known to be associated with difficult airway problems (12). Any history of difficulty with tracheal intubation should be noted. A history of difficult intubation is a strong indicator of repeat difficulties, even if external physical signs do not indicate a reason to suspect a difficult intubation. It is important to remember that the features that predict a difficult intubation are not very specific, while a history of difficult intubation is.

The list of diseases and syndromes associated with difficult intubation is extensive (12). A list might be maintained in the anesthesia office for immediate review. Patients with a compromised airway may have few indicative signs and symptoms. General questions should be asked about signs and symptoms suggestive of airway abnormalities, such as hoarseness or shortness of breath. The onset and progress of the symptoms, changes in voice quality, dysphagia, difficulty with secretions, exercise intolerance, or the effect of body position on breathing are all important findings. Changes in the character of voice may indicate the site of a lesion and progressive disease. A coarse, scratchy voice suggests a glottic origin, whereas a muffled voice is characteristic of a supraglottic source (13). A history of obstructive sleep apnea (OSA) is important, especially in patients without obvious anatomic abnormalities (14). Hidden causes such as a vallecular cyst can contribute to obstructive sleep apnea and may make mask ventilation and tracheal intubation difficult.

Patients who have difficulty breathing in the supine position, preferring to sleep on their side or prone, should be carefully examined; this history may suggest presence of an anterior mediastinal, pharyngeal, or neck mass (15). Anesthetizing these patients in the supine position without first securing the airway may lead to severe airway obstruction.

If a patient has been previously hospitalized, it is important to review any anesthetic records from those admissions. If an anesthetic was administered at another institution, such data may be obtained. When further history is needed, it is wise to contact the referring or previously treating physician.

It is important to clearly document airway-related information in the anesthesia record. The anesthesia record should specifically reflect whether the patient could be easily ventilated by face mask or not, the difficulty of the intubation, and any advice or suggestions for future airway management. This information will prove of considerable help in future airway management and in developing an anesthetic plan (16).

Concurrent medical conditions may complicate or dictate a special airway management approach (17). Hypertension and tachycardia, often seen with tracheal intubation, may not be tolerated by patients with serious valvular or coronary artery disease. Patients with a history of asthma, allergies, or heavy smoking may have a highly reactive airway. The placement of an endotracheal tube into a reactive airway in a lightly anesthetized or poorly topicalized patient, may provoke severe bronchoconstriction.

Tracheal stenosis may be mistaken for chronic obstructive pulmonary disease or asthma. A prior tracheostomy, tracheal trauma, or prolonged intubation causing tracheal stenosis, contributes to respiratory distress and may complicate tracheal intubation (18).

Special precautions may need to be taken in patients with neurologic disease, coagulopathy, or those at increased risk of aspiration.

Physical Examination

The physical examination of the patient, and particularly the airway, should be systematic and thorough. The head and neck should be inspected in both profile and frontal planes to recognize micrognathia, prognathia, and overbite. The presence of micrognathia, protruding teeth, and overbite are best appreciated from the lateral aspect. A short, thick muscular neck may predict difficult mask ventilation (DMV) and DI; the patient should be asked to extend the head as far as possible. The degree of motion of the cervical spine and atlanto-occipital joint should be noted.

Rigid laryngoscopy involves displacing the soft tissues of the oropharynx, thus clearing a line of vision from the teeth to the epiglottis and larynx. Decreased cervical spine mobility and masses of the neck (e.g., goiter, tumor, abscess, hematoma, or cyst), tracheal deviation, or tracheal and laryngeal immobility, may interfere with laryngoscopy and intubation.

The neck should be palpated to detect any masses, and the midline position of the larynx and trachea verified. Any lateral airway deviation is indicative of abnormal airway anatomy, and the cause should be identified.

To assess temporomandibular joint mobility, have the patient open the mouth wide and measure the distance between the upper and lower incisors. In most adults, this should be 4–6 cm (2.5–3 finger-breadths). The ability to open the mouth reflects temporomandibular joint (TMJ) rotational movement. The mouth must also be opened widely to demonstrate the forward gliding action of the mandibular condyle, necessary for protrusion of the mandible and for rigid laryngoscopy. Limitations of this gliding motion of the TMJ reflect the first evidence of arthritis in this joint (19).

When mouth opening is reduced to 3.0 cm, significant joint disease is present which shall diminish the effectiveness of rigid laryngoscopy. Ankylosis of the temporomandibular joint is seen in patients with rheumatoid arthritis. Trismus from masseter spasm often presents after mandibular or maxillary fractures; infections of the mouth or neck will severly limit mouth opening. The cause of any joint dysfunction must be determined.

The shape and size of the teeth, missing teeth, the presence of loose or diseased teeth, or extensive dental work, can all contribute to a DI. A high arched, narrow palate reduces the space available for rigid laryngoscopy, adding to the difficulty of tracheal intubation. A relatively large tongue can interfere with mask ventilation and tracheal intubation, while a fixed tongue, regardless of its size, can interfere with rigid laryngoscopy.

The tongue and pharyngeal soft tissue are displaced anteriorly into a potential space during laryngoscopy. An alteration in the shape or size of the bony structures of the mouth, such as a small mandible, may result in decreasing the space into which the soft tissues can be displaced.

An increased amount of soft tissue (e.g., large tongue, redundant pharyngeal tissues, or tumors of the oropharynx) will interfere with laryngeal exposure and successful tracheal intubation. Anatomically, the larynx is "anterior" to the line of vision during rigid laryngoscopy.

The patency of each nostril should be tested by occluding each side alternately while asking the patient to breathe through the other. This is important should unplanned nasotracheal intubation or use of a nasopharyngeal airway become necessary.

Patients with partial upper airway obstruction should be observed for substernal and intercostal retraction, dyspnea, tachycardia, ability to swallow, changes in mental status, or limitations in maintaining a given posture (Table 1). Patients with dyspnea often assume an upright posture to get mechanical assistant from gravity to keep the tongue and other tissues of the hypopharynx forward and dependent. Auscultation of the larynx, trachea, and chest may reveal stridor, wheezing, or absence of breath sounds.

Stridor occurs secondary to an increase in airflow through a narrow passage, and is pathognomonic of partial airway obstruction. Inspiratory stridor is usually associated with an obstructive lesion at or above the vocal cords. Expiratory stridor suggests obstruction of a major bronchus. Biphasic inspiratory and expiratory stridor can be heard in subglottic or tracheal obstructive lesions (17).

Assessment of the patient's mental status and ability to cooperate during the airway evaluation is important, should awake tracheal intubation with topical anesthesia be indicated. Careful examination of the chest and lungs by inspection, auscultation, and percussion is essential for evaluation of adequate air exchange or for the discovery of a major pathology, such as pneumothorax, pleural effusion, etc.

Fiberoptic endoscopy is useful in identifying potential upper and lower airway abnormalities and assessing their functional significance prior to the induction of general anesthesia (20). This applied skill can provide information about the location and extent of a lesion, mobility of the vocal cords, presence of inflammation or edema of the glottis, and encroachment on the airway by tumor or edema.

TABLE 1. *Signs and symptoms and possible causative factors of ventilatory distress*

Mental status	
Alert and distressed	Anxious
Obtunded	Fatigue, respiratory failure, drug effect
Breathing pattern	
Tachypnea	Nonspecific hypoxemia
Paradoxical respiration	Airway obstruction
Asymmetrical chest wall movement	Splinting, pneumothorax, atelectasis of one lung
Prolonged slow expiration	Lower airway obstruction, bronchoconstriction
Prolonged inspiration	Upper airway obstruction
Stridor	Severe narrowing of the airway
Cardiovascular response	
Hypertension, tachycardia	Hypoxemia, hypercarbia
Hypotension, bradycardia	Severe hypoxemia
Subcutaneous emphysema	Airway disruption
Voice characteristics	
Coarse, scratchy	Glottic origin
Muffled	Supraglottic lesion

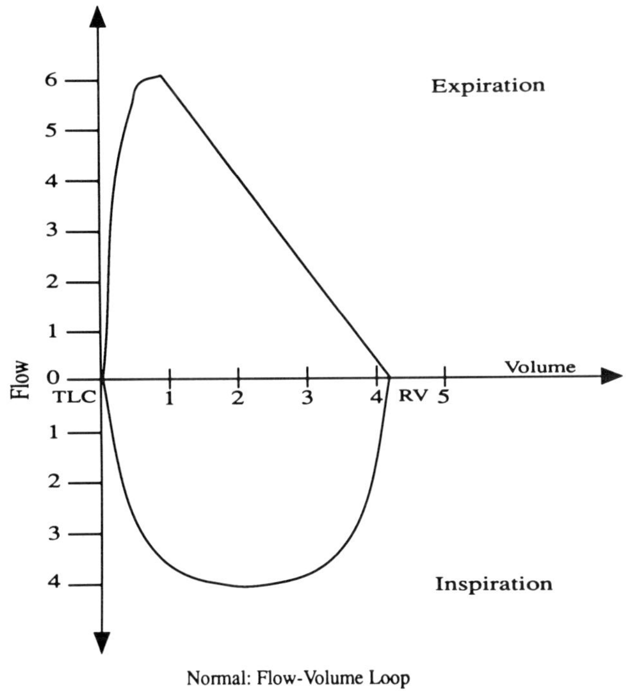

FIG. 2. Flow-volume loops demonstrating normal pattern.

Laboratory Assessment

Radiography of the chest, head, and neck, arterial blood gas analysis, and pulmonary function tests are all helpful in evaluating the complicated airway. A review of such data may be useful in evaluating the degree of airway compromise and in the selection of a given technique for tracheal intubation.

Radiographic studies provide information about airway diameter, tracheal deviation, extrinsic compression of the trachea, and the extent of pathology. X-rays also provide critical information in patients who have sustained head and neck trauma, and cervical spine fractures. The latter is of great importance because it may dictate the use of certain precautions during airway management. These X-rays should be reviewed with the radiologist and surgeon.

Arterial blood gas analysis is helpful in assessing acid base status, hypoventilation, and hypoxemia. Severe hypoxemia should be corrected, if possible, before intubation is attempted.

A flow-volume loop is a study of pulmonary function in which forced expiratory flow (FEF) and forced inspiratory flow (FIF) are recorded against volume. Flow is recorded on the vertical axis and volume on the horizontal axis. The inspiratory loop is obtained after maximum patient exhalation to residual volume (Fig. 2). Flow-volume loops are useful in distinguishing the location of airway obstruction and whether the obstruction is fixed or variable.

Peak inspiratory flow rates are sensitive to upper airway obstruction. Peak expiratory flow rates are sensitive to lower (tracheal and bronchial) airway obstruction (Fig. 3).

Fixed airway obstruction diminishes both the inspiratory and expiratory flow-volume loops equally. Maximal expiratory and maximal inspiratory flow at midvital capacity is nearly 1.0. A variable intrathoracic

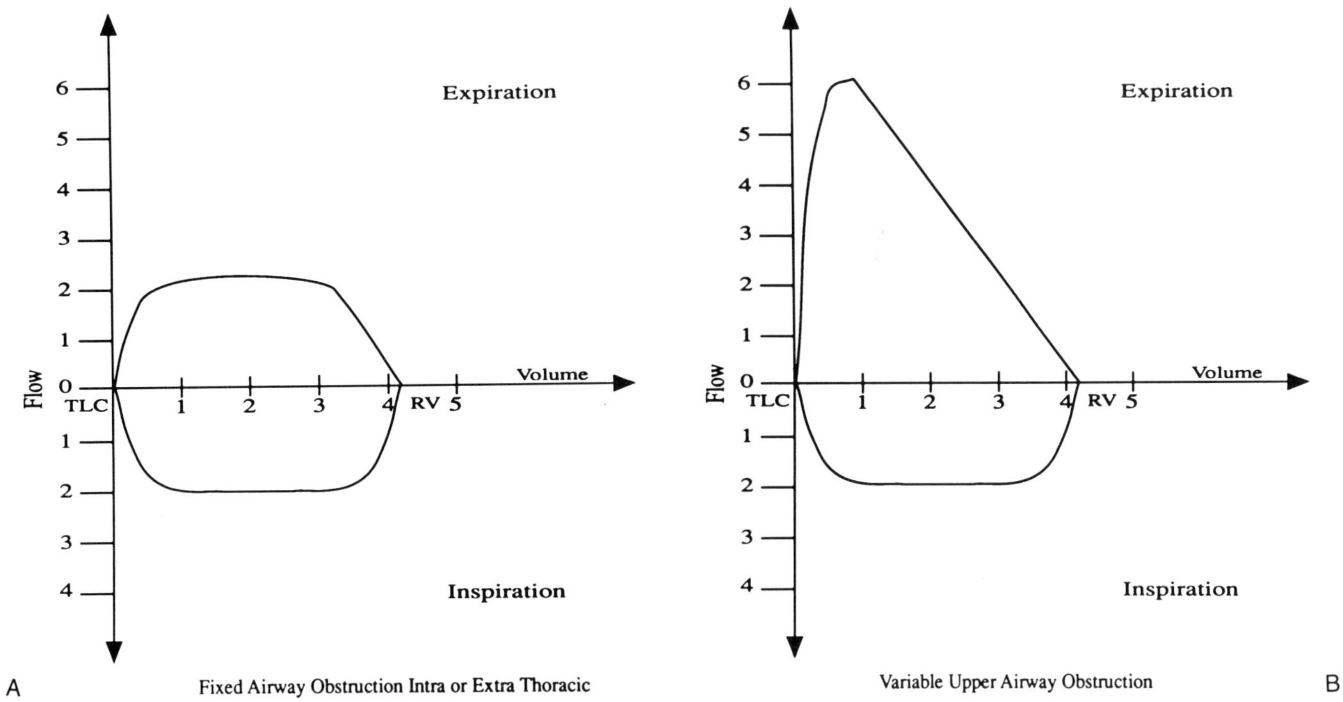

FIG. 3. A: Characteristic flow-volume curve in a fixed upper or lower airway obstruction. **B:** Characteristic flow-volume curve in a variable upper airway obstruction.

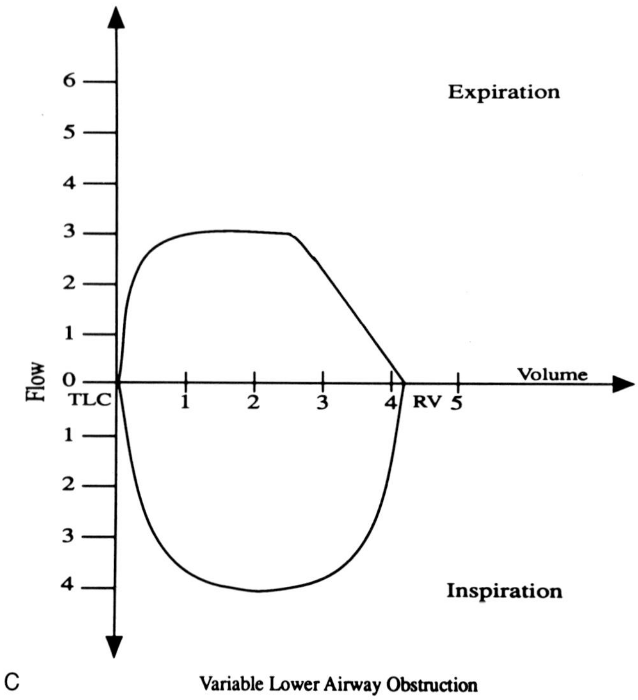

FIG. 3. *Continued.* **C:** Characteristic flow-volume curve in a variable lower airway obstruction.

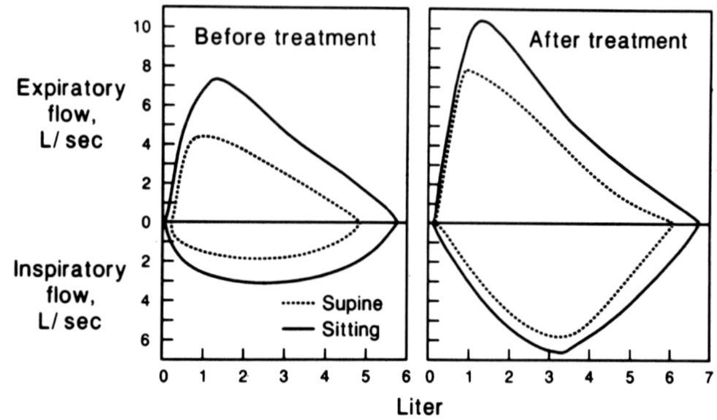

FIG. 4. Flow-volume curves obtained in upright and supine position before (left) and four weeks after (right) two courses of chemotherapy in patient with Hodgkin's lymphoma. (With permission, ref. 22.).

obstruction diminishes the expiratory loop. The ratio of maximal expiratory to maximal inspiratory flow at midvital capacity becomes closer to 0.3. Variable extrathoracic lesions distort and diminish the inspiratory loop, making the expiratory-inspiratory ratio about 2.

Comparison of flow-volume loops obtained in the upright and the supine position may demonstrate flow-volume configuration changes indicating susceptibility to airway obstruction. This susceptibility may produce serious airway obstruction in the heavily sedated or anesthetized patient (Fig. 4) (21,22).

A sawtooth pattern noted on the flow-volume loop may be produced secondary to fluttering tissue in the upper airway in patients with obstructive sleep apnea (23) or following neck surgery (24).

CIRCUMSTANCES OF A DIFFICULT AIRWAY

Patients with the potential for a difficult intubation may be divided into four groups: known, expected, suspected, and unanticipated (Table 2). However, from the management point of view, difficult airways fall into two basic categories: those in whom difficulty is anticipated, allowing the physician time to study and make preparations (circumstances 1–3), and those in whom difficulty is unanticipated and discovered during attempted intubation (circumstance 4). The difficulty may become apparent, even though the vocal cords are visualized, when the endotracheal tube cannot be advanced due to subglottic or tracheal stenosis. Five basic principles of managing the difficult intubation are summarized in Table 3.

TABLE 2. *Circumstances of a difficult airway*

1. Known. Patient has a history of difficult or failed intubation and/or mask ventilation.
2. Expected. Patient has a disease process or anatomic features known to be associated with difficult airway management.
3. Suspected. Patient has some signs or symptoms suggestive of a difficult airway.
4. Unanticipated. Patient presents with no evidence for difficult airway, but intubation and/or mask ventilation fails after induction of anesthesia.

TECHNIQUES OF DIFFICULT INTUBATION

Over the years, various techniques have been developed to secure the airway in difficult situations (Table 4) (25–29). Some of these techniques are used infrequently, while others are invasive and carry the potential for major complications. These techniques vary greatly in their levels of sophistication and application.

Studies comparing the application and usefulness of these various intubation techniques under varying situations are few. It remains difficult, therefore, to specifically recommend a particular technique for use under a given circumstance. While generic recommendations are possible, each case merits special consideration and judgment relative to overall management and selection.

TABLE 3. *Principles to apply in the difficult intubation*

1. The difficult intubation cart is checked and ready.
2. Awake intubation is performed when mask ventilation is suspected to be difficult.
3. Spontaneous breathing is maintained when mask ventilation may be difficult and awake intubation is not an option.
4. The technique most likely to succeed is tried first.
5. Visually guided intubation is preferable to blind intubation.

TABLE 4. *Difficult intubation techniques*

Visual techniques
Fiberoptic bronchoscope (indirect)
Rigid laryngoscope (direct)
Bullard laryngoscope (indirect)
Rigid bronchoscope (direct)
Guided blind techniques
Retrograde percutaneous insertion
Light wand
Laryngeal mask
Magnetic guide
Bougie
Blind techniques
Blind nasal
Tactile oral
Combination techniques
Surgical techniques
Cricothyrotomy
Tracheostomy

The expertise of the anesthesiologist and other practitioners dealing with airway management and their skill and familiarity with different intubation techniques vary considerably. Physicians trained one or two decades ago may not be familiar with some of the techniques introduced in recent years. On the other hand, most recent trainees in anesthesia would not have the extensive experience in the use of earlier techniques, such as blind nasal intubation.

In the selection of a given technique one should look at its desirable features, its applicability, and the possibility and incidence of technique-related complications. The ideal characteristics by which a technique may be judged are summarized in Table 5.

VISUAL TECHNIQUES

Fiberoptic Bronchoscope

As a tool and technique for management of the difficult airway, the fiberoptic bronchoscope scores high.

TABLE 5. *Proposed ideal features of an intubation technique*

Primary features
High success rate in the difficult airway
Useful for both upper and lower airway problems
Useful for oral and nasal intubations
Allows ventilation during intubation
Performed under visual guidance
Allows application of topical anesthesia
Devoid of technique-specific complications
Head and neck manipulation not crucial for success
Useful in combination with other techniques
Blood/secretions do not interfere with its use
Secondary features
Avoids dental trauma
Equipment easily cleaned and stored
Portable
Easily learned and mastered
Cost effective

It possesses nine out of ten of the primary ideal features of an intubation technique. The only major shortcoming of the fiberoptic bronchoscope is visualization difficulties encountered in the presence of large amounts of blood and secretions. Other more minor shortcomings of the fiberoptic bronchoscope are its relatively high cost, the bulky size of its ancillary equipment, and the time needed for cleaning and storage.

The fiberoptic bronchoscope has revolutionized the management of the difficult intubation. It has been successfully applied to complex upper and lower airway problems and in the evaluation and follow-up of patients with airway problems. Due to its high success rate in the hands of the trained practitioner, fiberscopic intubation is recommended as the technique of choice under these circumstances (30–34).

Tracheal intubation aided by a fiberscope was compared to conventional methods in 44 patients with advanced rheumatoid arthritis of the cervical spine scheduled for cervical spine fusion (31). Compared to conventional techniques, fiberoptic intubation was shown to significantly diminish the number of complicated intubations and related trauma.

Northwestern Experience

Our experience with fiberoptic intubation at the Veterans Affairs Lakeside Medical Center (VALMC) and Northwestern Memorial Hospitals removes any doubt that fiberoptic intubation is highly successful in patients who present a difficult or conventionally impossible intubation.

As mentioned in Chapter 6, a special data collection form was used for each patient having a fiberoptic intubation since 1978. Patient data collected included the indication, route of intubation, time required to complete intubation, success or failure of the procedure, and complications encountered. A total of 2031 fiberoptic intubations were performed between 1978 and 1989 (34). Within this group, there were 302 patients (14 female and 288 male), all with anatomic and/or pathologic conditions rendering use of rigid laryngoscopy difficult or impossible. On these 302 patients, 338 tracheal intubations were performed (Table 6).

All patients were visited postoperatively, with patient recall of the experience documented. Over 100 residents and eight staff anesthesiologists were involved. Initially, the fiberoptic technique was applied only after conventional methods had failed. As experience and confidence in the technique was gained, it was routinely chosen for most potentially difficult intubations.

In 194 of these 338 intubations, difficulty with rigid laryngoscopy was expected because of the presence of special anatomic features and/or disease processes affecting the airway (Table 7). Patients presenting with

TABLE 6. *Causes of difficult intubation*

Cause	*N*
1. Common causes[a]	144
2. Compromised airway[b]	
Tumor	66
Arthritis/spondylosis	47
Anatomic deformity (surgical and burn)	40
Facial trauma	24
Infection	10
Morbid obesity	2
Acromegaly	1
Scleroderma	1
Supraglottic cyst or mass	3
Total	338

[a] Combination of features such as short, thick neck; limited neck extension; protruding upper incisors; large tongue; or narrow mouth opening.

[b] Pathology involving head, neck, oral cavity, and larynx.

any combination of short, thick neck; protruding upper incisors; overbite; receding mandible; marked obesity; small mouth opening; narrow and high arched palate; and/or limited ability to extend the head were classified as potential problems.

Patients with anatomic abnormalities of the head, neck, or upper airway, resulting from surgery, radiation or burn scars, tumors, trauma, infection, arthritis, ankylosing spondylosis of the cervical spine and larynx, and diseases such as scleroderma and acromegaly, were considered patients with a "compromised airway."

In 111 of the 338 cases, difficult tracheal intubation was also expected because of a history of previous difficult or failed intubation. In the remaining 33 cases, tracheal intubation using the rigid technique had failed unexpectedly during general anesthesia, and fiberoptic intubation was required (Table 7) (34).

Fiberoptic intubation was attempted on 287 occasions with the patient awake but sedated, with local anesthetic applied to the airway. In 51 patients, the airway was intubated after induction of general anesthesia. Two hundred twenty-four intubations were performed orally, and 114 were performed nasally (Table 8).

Fiberoptic intubation was successful in 334 of the 338 attempts (98.8%). In two of the four failed intubations, the patients had advanced laryngeal carcinoma and severely compromised airways. They were scheduled to have an emergency tracheostomy using local anesthesia. While the patients were being prepped and draped, awake fiberoptic laryngoscopy was attempted briefly, with the intention of intubating the trachea if possible. Due to the extensive nature of the airway lesions, the glottis could not be visualized, and tracheostomy was performed as scheduled under local anesthesia.

The third failure was in a 53-year-old patient scheduled for carotid endarterectomy in which airway difficulty was not anticipated. Several attempts at both rigid and fiberoptic intubation under general anesthesia were unsuccessful.

The fourth failure was a 35-year-old male scheduled to have a craniotomy. Attempts at rigid laryngoscopy and tracheal intubation failed due to the presence of a short, thick neck; small mouth opening; and limited ability to extend the head. Mask ventilation was possible but difficult. Several attempts at fiberoptic intubation were also unsuccessful; secretions were abundant but there was no bleeding. The trachea was finally intubated nasally with great difficulty, using a rigid laryngoscope and Magill forceps.

The low intensity of the fiberoptic light contributed

TABLE 7. *Categories of difficult intubation (DI)*

Category	Common causes	Compromised airway	Total
Anticipated DI			
Physical findings	47	147	194
History of difficult and/or failed intubation[a]	69	42	111
Unanticipated DI			
Failed rigid intubation followed by fiberoptic intubation attempts	28	5	33
Total	144	194	338

[a] History of failed rigid laryngoscopy and tracheal intubation in a previously anesthetized patient, resulting in canceling the operation and rescheduling.

TABLE 8. *Fiberoptic approach to 338 difficult intubations (DI)*

	Awake		Anesthetized	
Category	Oral	Nasal	Oral	Nasal
Anticipated DI				
Physical findings	120[a]	64	9	2
History of difficult and/or failed intubation	62	41	7	0
Unanticipated DI	0			
Failed rigid intubation followed by fiberoptic attempt		0	26[a]	7
Total	182	105	42	9

[a] Fiberoptic technique failed in two patients (see text).

TABLE 9. *Patients with difficult intubation also considered at high risk for aspiration*

Category	N
Emergency	
Miscellaneous nonabdominal operations	12
Acute abdomen	9
Ludwig's angina/peritonsillar abscess	6
Bowel obstruction	5
Upper gastrointestinal bleeding	2
Nonemergency	
Presence of hiatal hernia	6
Intermittent bowel obstruction	1
Esophageal diverticulum	1
Total	42

TABLE 11. *Complications of fiberoptic intubation in 319 difficult intubations*

Complication	N
Coughing during intubation[a]	34
Laryngeal spasm	9
Epistaxis (mild)	9
Esophageal intubation by fiberscope or endotracheal tube[b]	4
Laceration of lips, mouth, or pharynx	2
Pain at translaryngeal injection site	5
Small hematoma at translaryngeal injection site	2
Vomiting	1

[a] Does not include coughing during application of topical anesthesia.
[b] All recognized and corrected at the time of intubation.

to failure of laryngeal exposure in the presence of secretions. The poor light was thought to be due to a malfunction of the fiberscope. It was later noticed that the universal cord adapter of the fiberscope had not been seated properly into the light source socket resulting in the low light intensity. The same patient underwent another operation 3 months later, with the trachea easily intubated orally using a fiberscope; the patient was awake, sedated, and the airway topicalized.

In the group of 338 DIs, 42 were in patients who were also considered to be at high risk for aspiration of gastric contents (Table 9). All 42 patients were intubated successfully with the patients awake.

Intubation times and the degrees of difficulty of fiberoptic visualization of the vocal cords in 307 DIs are presented in Table 10. Ninety percent of all difficult and failed intubations using conventional techniques became easy intubations using the fiberoptic technique.

Complications encountered during fiberoptic intubation are summarized in Table 11. Most were minor in nature without lingering consequences. In nine patients, nasotracheal intubation resulted in minor nasal bleeding requiring no special treatment. In one patient, yellowish secretions similar to gastric contents were noted in the trachea after successful fiberoptic intubation. This patient was difficult to ventilate by mask and could not be intubated despite repeated attempts at rigid laryngoscopy. One attempt resulted in esophageal intubation, which may have caused regurgitation and aspiration. The patient's surgery was canceled. No signs or symptoms of aspiration pneumonitis appeared, and he was rescheduled 5 days later when awake fiberoptic orotracheal intubation was easily accomplished.

Postoperative interviews with 238 patients revealed that 84 (35.3%) had recall of the intubation and 15 (6.3%) considered the recall unpleasant. Most of the patients with unpleasant recall had a compromised airway and were given little or no sedation.

Rigid Laryngoscope

In the author's experience, fiberoptic intubation is the technique of choice in the patient known or expected to be a difficult intubation. If a difficult intubation is unanticipated and initial attempts at rigid laryngoscopy have failed, various maneuvers may be applied to improve the chance of successful intubation. Repeated attempts at rigid laryngoscopy should be limited and performed as atraumatically as possible (35).

If intubation proves difficult, do not persist in an intubation attempt for more than 30–40 sec unless oxygen saturation is monitored continuously. Clinical signs of oxygen desaturation (e.g., cyanosis) are unreliable and occur late. Mask ventilation and oxygenation

TABLE 10. *Ease of fiberoptic laryngeal exposure in 307 difficult intubations*

	Not difficult	Moderately difficult	Difficult
Conscious patients (*N* = 275)	155 (56.4%)	87 (31.6%)	33 (12%)
Anesthetized patients (*N* = 32)	20 (62.5%)	9 (28.1%)	3 (9.4%)
Intubation time (min)[a]	2.6	3.75	6.85
Total intubation time (min)[b]	13.6	14.0	18.7

[a] Average time from insertion of the fiberscope to completion of intubation in conscious patients.
[b] Average time from beginning of sedation to completion of intubation in conscious patients.
Intubation times include resident and staff participation. In experienced hands, the average intubation time in the not difficult group is <30 sec; in the moderately difficult group, 30–60 sec; and in the difficult group, 2–4 min.

should be resumed before cyanosis is noticed, or as soon as oxygen saturation (pulse oximeter) starts to decline. One should not wait until the saturation falls below 90% because oxygen saturation will not improve immediately upon commencing mask ventilation (36). It often takes 1–2 min of ventilation with 100% oxygen before oxygen saturation, measured by pulse oximetry, starts to rise. Obese and pregnant patients, with their lowered lung functional residual capacity (FRC), tend to desaturate rapidly and take longer to respond to reoxygenation.

If the initial attempts at intubating with rigid laryngoscopy prove unsuccessful, various maneuvers can be applied to improve glottic exposure and assist in passage of the endotracheal tube. These measures include repositioning the head and neck, changing to a different laryngoscope blade, and using the Howland lock adapter, stylets, and introducers.

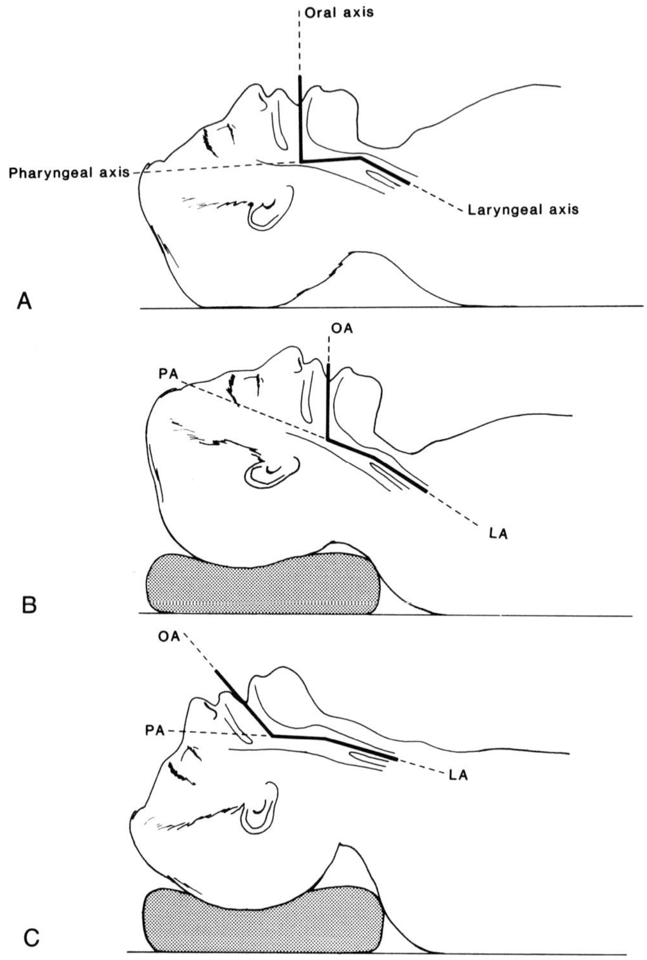

FIG. 5. Intubating position during rigid laryngoscopy. **A:** Supine patient without head rest. **B:** Head elevation and neck flexion bring the pharyngeal and laryngeal axes into line. **C:** Extension of head at occiputocervical joint aligns the oral axis with other two. (With permission, ref. 38.)

Improving Exposure of the Larynx

Common technical difficulties that interfere with visualizing the glottis during rigid laryngoscopy include improper positioning of the patient's head, inadequate opening of the mouth, selection of the wrong laryngoscope blade, improper insertion of the blade into the oral cavity, applying leverage rather than traction with the blade, and obscuring the line of vision during insertion of the tube into the trachea (25,37). The importance of correct positioning of the head and neck during rigid laryngoscopy to achieve alignment of the axes of the mouth, pharynx, and larynx should be emphasized (Fig. 5) (2,25,37,38).

The careful positioning of the patient's head into the sniffing position is frequently helpful. The patient's occiput should be elevated on a pad or pillow. In adults, flexion of the neck and extension of the head at the atlanto-occipital joint will better align the axes of the mouth, pharynx, and larynx. Pregnant or obese patients may require a pad under the shoulders with an extra pad under the head. External pressure over the thyroid cartilage, pushing the larynx back and cephalad, will further improve exposure (25). In small children and infants, the larynx is situated relatively higher, and the sniffing position is not helpful. External pressure on the thyroid cartilage is more effective (25,39).

Opening the mouth widely makes it easier to insert the laryngoscope blade and pass the endotracheal tube. This is easily accomplished by using the thumb and third finger to pry the mouth open. An undersized endotracheal tube is easier to maneuver than a large tube, leaving more room to see the tube enter the larynx.

Adequate exposure of the larynx is achieved with a forward and upward lifting movement of the laryngoscope blade, elevating the mandible and epiglottis.

The laryngoscope blade must not be used as a lever with the teeth as a fulcrum. Normally the laryngoscope blade is inserted in the right corner of the mouth, the tongue pushed to the left, and the tip of the curved blade positioned in the midline in the vallecula. In this position, the tip of the laryngoscope blade will be able to lift the epiglottis maximally. If the epiglottis is not visualized the laryngoscope blade may be inserted too far, thus lifting the entire larynx anteriorly.

If this is felt to be the case, pull the laryngoscope blade back slowly until the epiglottis drops into view. It should be remembered that an extended cervical spine can push the larynx anteriorly and away from the axes of the mouth and pharynx, increasing the difficulty of laryngeal exposure.

Different Laryngoscope Blades

Various kinds of straight and curved blades, with and without prism attachments, and laryngoscope adapters have been designed to manage the DI (40–44). Sometimes the difficulty is simply related to selection of too short a laryngoscope blade which does not allow the tip to reach the base of the epiglottis. A blade of different shape or size may provide better exposure (45). If a curved blade is unsuccessful, a straight blade may be tried. Recently, an angulated straight blade, similar to a Siker blade, has been introduced with initial reports indicating a high rate of success in DIs (46,47).

Factors to consider in the selection of the laryngoscope blade include the distance from teeth to the base of the tongue, the need to avoid prominent upper incisors, ability to maneuver the blade in a small mouth, and control of anatomic structures (e.g., a large tongue and redundant pharyngeal soft tissue) (48).

Stylets

A malleable stylet can be used to create a desired curvature to the distal end of the endotracheal tube. This curvature can assist passage of the tube between the vocal cords when the epiglottis or arytenoid cartilages are seen but the glottis is not visualized. In this case, the stylet is inserted in the endotracheal tube and its distal end bent into a hockey stick configuration. The tube is positioned underneath the epiglottis. As the tube passes through the vocal cords, an assistant removes the stylet and the tube is advanced into the trachea.

While a stylet is simple to use and often helpful, serious complications with its use have been reported (49–54). The tip of the stylet should remain inside the endotracheal tube to avoid airway trauma such as perforation of the pharynx or trachea (49,50). A stylet which is used repeatedly may fracture during intubation; part of the stylet may be sheared off during removal from the tube, further complicating the technique (51–54).

Introducers

Various introducers have been designed to facilitate a DI. With the aid of a rigid laryngoscope, an introducer can be guided into the trachea and the tracheal tube threaded over it. The Macintosh gum-elastic bougie has been used successfully this way and is highly recommended (26,55,56). The Salem-Resce intubation guide (Flexiguide Division, Scientific Sales International, Inc., Highland Park, Illinois) is an introducer with a flexible distal tip that can be manipulated anteriorly or posteriorly by operating a control knob on the proximal handle (25,57). Passed through the tracheal tube, the tip is guided into the trachea and the tube threaded over it.

Howland Lock

The Howland lock fits between the handle and blade of the laryngoscope and is often used with a straight blade. It changes the angle of the blade in reference to the laryngoscope handle. It may be advantageous in the patient with a receding mandible, an anterior larynx, or decreased jaw mobility (40).

The Bullard Laryngoscope

The Bullard laryngoscope is a rigid laryngoscope blade with two fiberoptic bundles (light and image transmission bundles) positioned behind the blade close to the distal tip (58–60). The unique shape of the blade, combined with its long axis, allows it to be easily moved from the horizontal position (during insertion into the mouth) to the vertical position (during laryngeal exposure). A minimal mouth opening is required for introducing the blade.

The shape of the blade combined with the objective lens located on its tip makes exposure of the vocal cords possible without alignment of the oral, pharyngeal, and tracheal axes. Two sizes are available, one for children up to 8–10 years of age and one for adults (Fig. 6).

The blade is at a 90° angle to the handle. Between the handle and viewing arm are two channels (suction and stylet) that extend to the tip of the blade. The small suction channel has a Luer-Lok fitting which may be used for suctioning of secretions, insufflation of oxygen, or adminstration of local anesthetics. The larger channel accepts the intubation stylet. The source of illumination for the Bullard laryngoscope can be either a standard laryngoscope battery handle, or a fiberoptic light source.

The intubating stylet loaded with the endotracheal tube, with its 15-mm adapter removed, is attached to the Bullard laryngoscope. The endotracheal tube is positioned to allow the distal end of the stylet to project through the Murphy eye of the tube. The blade is inserted midline in the mouth, with the shaft of the laryngoscope held parallel to the body of the patient. As the blade is advanced inside the mouth, the laryngoscope handle is moved from horizontal to a vertical position, sliding the blade around the base of the tongue and into the hypopharynx. When the laryngoscope handle reaches the vertical position, the scope and blade are allowed to drop to the posterior pharynx. The tongue

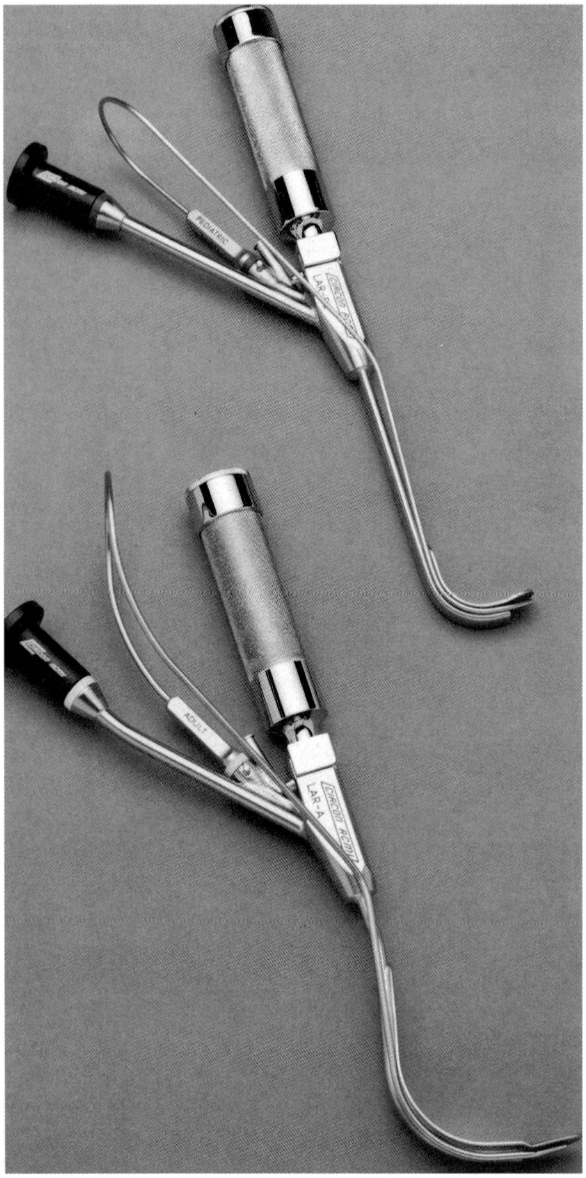

FIG. 6. Pediatric and adult Bullard(R) intubating laryngoscope. (Courtesy of Circon Corp., Santa Barbara, California.)

and epiglottis are then elevated to reveal the vocal cords. The epiglottis must be retracted by the blade to allow passage of the endotracheal tube into the trachea. If the epiglottis is not retracted, the blade is repositioned to place the tip of the blade under the epiglottis.

With the vocal cords exposed, the tip of the stylet is pointed directly at the glottic opening. The endotracheal tube is advanced off the stylet toward the glottic opening and into the trachea. The laryngoscope is then removed while the endotracheal tube is held in position by the other hand.

In a nasotracheal intubation, the laryngoscope is inserted orally to visualize the glottis. The nasotracheal tube is inserted and advanced, under fiberoptic observation, toward the glottis (61,62). This technique is helpful when the mouth opening is limited and the use of a Magill forceps is not possible. The directional tip tube (Endotrol(TM)) was found superior to other tubes for quick and atraumatic intubation with this technique (62).

The Bullard laryngoscope has been used successfully in awake and anesthetized patients. Its value in the management of the difficult intubation, and in patients with cervical spine disease, has been emphasized (63–65). Borland and Casselbrant reported 17 successful awake intubations in infants (59). Saunders and Geisecke found it difficult to introduce the blade in three awake patients under topical anesthesia (66).

As with other fiberoptic methods, secretions and fogging of the lens contribute to failure of the technique. Adminstration of a antisialagogue is important, and application of antifog solution to the objective lens is critical to avoid difficulties.

Training and experience is needed for effective use of this device. The intubation technique may seem easy, but it requires considerable practice before one can rely on it for routine management of the difficult intubation. Dyson and associates demonstrated that the Bullard laryngoscope was not easier to use than the fiberoptic bronchoscope when attempting to master the technique on an intubation model (60). Although exposure of the vocal cords was easily achieved with either the fiberoptic bronchoscope or Bullard laryngoscope, the passage of the endotracheal tube was technically more difficult and time consuming with the Bullard laryngoscope.

GUIDED BLIND INTUBATION TECHNIQUES

Light Wand

The technique uses a lighted stylet to transilluminate the tissues of the neck, helping to guide placement of the endotracheal tube. Orotracheal intubation using a lighted stylet was first used in the management of a difficult tracheal intubation in 1957 (67). The first nasotracheal intubation using a lighted stylet was reported in 1959 (68). Originally a laryngoscope light bulb attached to a copper wire was used as a lighted stylet. A small surgical flashlight (Flexi-lum Surgical Light, Concept Corporation, Clearwater, Florida) was used in the seventies as a rigid light wand. Since then, various modifications of the technique and equipment have been utilized. The lighted stylet has also been used as a guide over which the endotrachael tube is threaded after the stylet has passed into the trachea (69).

One new design (Trachlight(TM)), includes a brighter light, and longer stylet to be used along with an uncut endotracheal tube. A side clip holds the endotracheal tube in place. The retractable inner wire stylet can be removed, converting the light wand to a flexible instrument suitable for nasal intubation (Fig. 7) (70,71). The Trachlight™ has been used successfully in patients with difficult airways in oral and nasotracheal intubation.

The light wand can also be used to confirm endotracheal tube position at midtrachea after intubation has been achieved by rigid laryngoscopy (72). A study in adult cadavers demonstrated 96% accuracy in determining tracheal tube position in the trachea, esophagus, or upper airway (72). In adult patients with a thin body habitus, or in infants, determination between tracheal and esophageal placement of the tube may be difficult. The success of determining tube position with the lighted stylet technique in obese patients is not addressed in the literature. One can anticipate that redundant neck tissue may interfere with light transmission.

The Technique

The light wand is lubricated and inserted inside an endotracheal tube with the light just short of its distal tip. The distal end of the tube is then bent with a distal angle of slightly greater than 90° into a "hockey stick" shape. The patient's head is maximally extended and the occiput supported on a pillow (71,73). After induction of anesthesia and muscle relaxation, the tongue is grasped with a gauze bandage and pulled forward. The loaded light wand is introduced into the mouth and passed over the tongue in the midline position.

The operating room lights are dimmed for better visibility of the transilluminated light in the neck. When light is seen in the anterior neck, the tip of the tube is in the vallecula. If the tube enters the esophagus, the light is invisible or markedly diminished. When the tip of the tube enters the larynx, the light becomes visible below the cricoid cartilage, at which time the tube is threaded over the light wand into the trachea and the light wand removed (71).

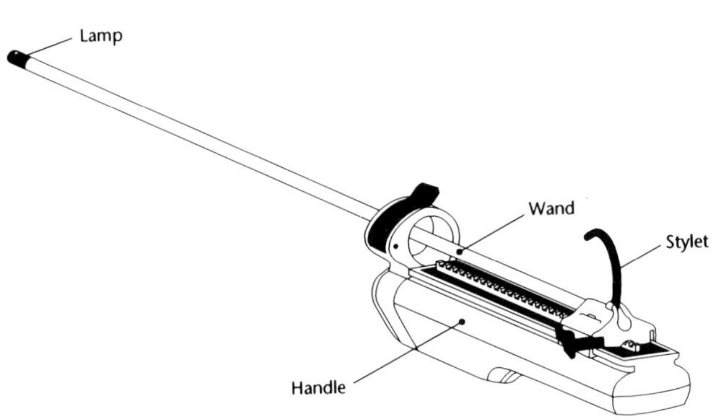

FIG. 7. Trachlight®. (Courtesy of Laerdal Medical Corp., Armonk, New York.)

Two reports have compared the light wand with other techniques: one with the rigid laryngoscope for orotracheal intubation in the anesthetized patient, and the other with blind nasotracheal intubation in the conscious patient (74,75). All 50 light wand orotracheal intubations were successful in one to three attempts, with 72% successful on the first attempt. Rigid laryngoscopy was successful in 98% of patients on the first attempt. Compared with blind nasotracheal intubation in the conscious patient, light wand orotracheal intubation was associated with less trauma and required significantly fewer attempts (75). A randomized prospective study comparing blind nasotracheal intubation with the light wand technique, reported by Verdile and associates, showed that the success rate for either technique was better with a regular endotracheal tube than when an RAE tube was used (76).

The light wand orotracheal intubation technique has been used successfully in patients with unstable cervical vertebrae, burn stricture of the neck, and congenital airway problems such as Treacher Collins' and Pierre Robin syndromes. There are several reports about the effectiveness of the technique in difficult intubations (75,77). The light wand is a useful, alternative approach after failed routine laryngoscopic intubation (71,74–79). It is less traumatic than blind nasal intubation and may be applied after failed intubation using rigid laryngoscopy. Common causes of failure include improper curving at the distal end of the tube, unfamiliarity with the technique, poor topical anesthesia or relaxation in the anesthetized patient, and anatomical features of the patient.

Retrograde Intubation

Retrograde intubation involves passage of a guide wire in a retrograde direction usually through a needle percutaneously inserted into the larynx. The guide wire tip is delivered through the mouth or nose and serves as a guide for passage of a tracheal tube (80,81).

The first reported case of retrograde-guided tracheal intubation describes passing a red rubber catheter through an existing tracheostomy stoma cephalad into the oropharynx. The tip of the catheter was then sutured to the tip of an endotracheal tube. Traction on the catheter brought the end of the tracheal tube through the tracheostomy stoma. The suture was cut to allow the endotracheal tube to be positioned inside the trachea (80).

The idea of percutaneous guide insertion through the cricothyroid membrane was developed by Waters in 1963 (81). He used a Tuohy needle to pass a plastic tube through the cricothyroid membrane into the oropharynx; the plastic tube was then used to guide the endotracheal tube into the trachea. Guides such as Seldinger wire and epidural, pulmonary artery, or central venous catheters have been used for this purpose (82–85). Various needles, such as Tuohy, 17-gauge intracath, or 20-gauge Angiocath, have also been used. Most recently, special retrograde intubation sets (Cook Retrograde Intubation Set, Bloomington, Indiana) have been introduced for pediatric and adult use.

The Technique

The head of the awake supine patient is placed in the sniffing position. The oropharynx, larynx, and trachea are topically anesthetized. A Tuohy needle attached to a syringe containing 2 ml of 2% lidocaine is inserted through the cricothyroid membrane in a slightly cephalad direction into the larynx. Aspiration of air confirms correct placement of the needle, and the local anesthetic is injected. A guide wire is threaded through the needle into the pharynx, with the tip delivered through the mouth. If nasotracheal intubation is desired, a suction catheter is inserted through the nostril into the oropharynx. The tip of the guide wire and suction catheter are pulled out of the mouth, tied together, and recovered through the nostril (86). The needle is removed from the neck and a clamp applied to the guide wire near the puncture site on the neck. With tension applied to both ends of the wire, an endotracheal tube is threaded over it into the trachea. The wire is then cut near the skin. The remaining wire is removed from above, and the tube advanced as necessary (Fig 8).

The tube may catch the larynx and fail to enter the trachea. Various maneuvers such as relaxing the tension on the guide wire, using a smaller tube, or pulling the tube back and readvancing it with a counterclockwise rotation may prove helpful. The displacement of the larynx posteriorly by manual pressure and neck flexion may help overcome this problem (87,88).

Another approach to assist the passage of the endotracheal tube into the trachea is to thread a plastic sheath (89) or various catheters, such as a modified Eschman (90) or a specially designed multilumen catheter (91), over the wire to increase its rigidity and external diameter. With less gap between the endotracheal tube and the guide wire there is a better chance for the tube to enter the trachea (92).

If the guide wire is passed through the side hole of the endotracheal tube, it allows an extra 1 cm of the tube to rest below the vocal cords prior to removal of the guide wire.

A slipknot tied at the tip of the tube (93), or sewing the retrograde nylon through the sidewall of the tube (94–95), provides the option of pulling the tube into the trachea.

Entering the airway through the cricotracheal membrane allows more room for advancing the tube before the retrograde guide entry site is reached (95,96). In addition, it avoids the cricothyroid arteries that cross the cricothyroid membrane at its proximal section (95,96).

If the size of the endotracheal tube permits, an antegrade guide or a fiberscope may be advanced through the endotracheal tube parallel to the retrograde guide wire into the trachea to aid passage (88).

Lechman and associates (97) have described a technique in which a guide wire is passed retrograde into the suction channel of a fiberscope, over which a tracheal tube has been mounted. The fiberscope is guided over the wire into the trachea, the tracheal tube threaded into the trachea, and the wire and fiberscope withdrawn. The described technique of retrograde-assisted fiberoptic intubation subsequently has been applied by others in adults, children, and neonates (98,99).

The retrograde technique has been used in patients with trismus (81), ankylosis of the jaw (82,87), cervical arthritis (82), tumors of the mouth (81,82), and in head and neck trauma (97). Barriot and Riou used retrograde intubation successfully in 19 patients with maxillofacial trauma and/or cervical spine fracture (100). In 13 patients, conventional intubation techniques had failed. In 6 patients, difficulty was expected with conventional techniques. Successful use of the retrograde intubation technique in infants and children with congenital anomalies has been described (99,101–103).

The most common complication in the retrograde technique is bleeding in and around the airway. Bleeding is usually minor in nature and does not require special treatment. In a series of 25 retrograde-guided tracheal intubations in patients subjected to open heart procedures, one case of peritracheal hematoma was reported (104). Subcutaneous emphysema is common. Recently one case of severe symptomatic pneumomediastinum was reported after elective retrograde- guided fiberoptic intubation (105). Severe crushing chest pain necessitated intensive care unit admission and urgent workup to rule out acute myocardial infarction. The recovery was complete and the patient was discharged on the seventh postoperative day.

Practice of the technique on the intubation model, and if possible, on other simulators, is a sensible prerequisite before performing the technique clinically.

In experienced hands, retrograde intubation can be lifesaving. A bloody and traumatized airway can be secured with this approach when techniques that rely on visualization of the airway are ineffective.

The Augustine Guide

The Augustine guide is a device designed for blind orotracheal intubation in adults. It consists of a dispos-

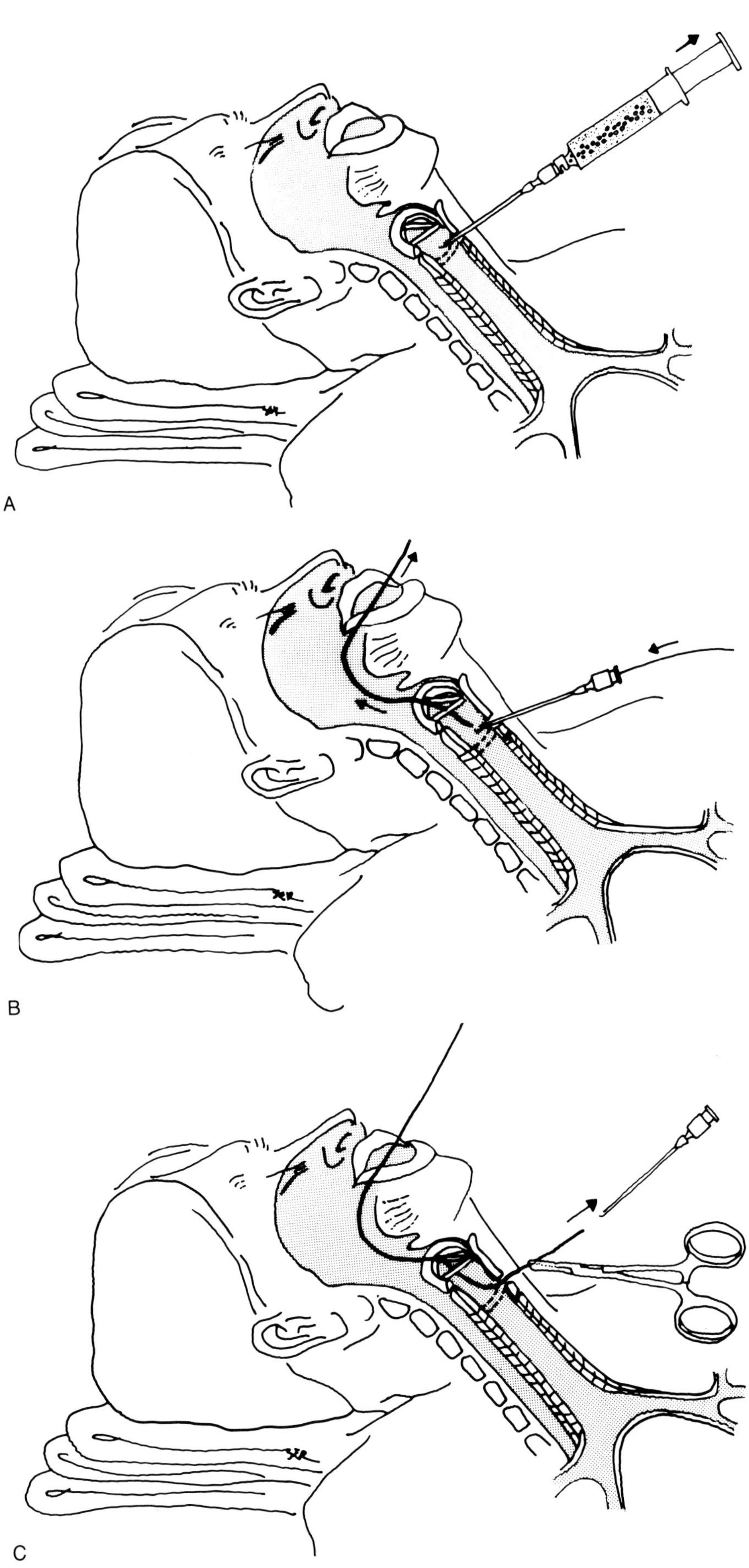

FIG. 8. Retrograde intubation. **A:** The needle attached to the syringe filled with lidocaine is passed through the cricothyroid membrane into the larynx. Free aspiration of air confirms correct placement of the needle. Lidocaine is injected to provide topical anesthesia of the airway. **B:** The guide wire is passed into the needle, retrograde through the larynx, and up into the oropharynx. The guide wire is retrieved through the mouth using a hook or a forceps. **C:** Once the needle is removed, the distal portion of the wire is held in position at the exit site of the neck by placing a clamp on wire.

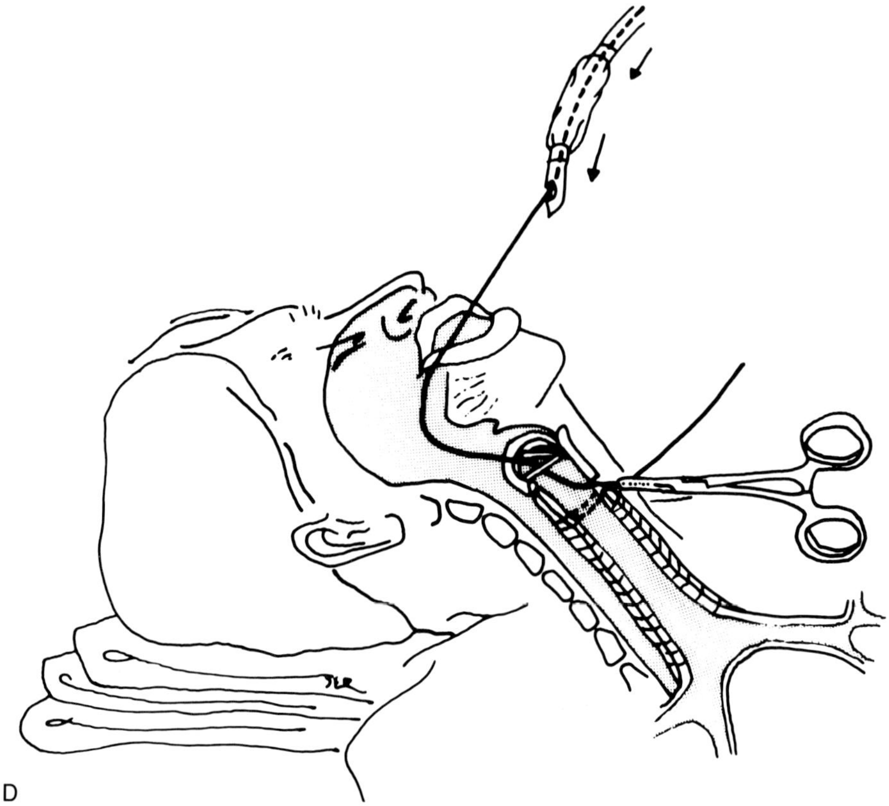

D

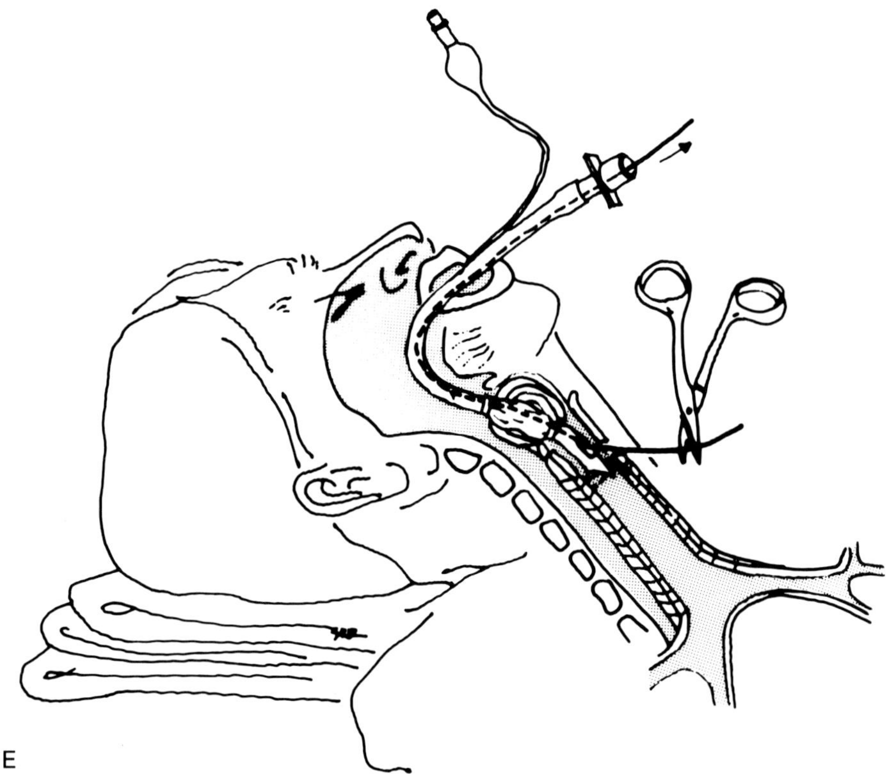

E

FIG. 8. *Continued.* **D:** The guide wire is passed through the Murphy eye of the endotracheal tube. **E:** The endotracheal tube is advanced over the guide wire into the trachea.

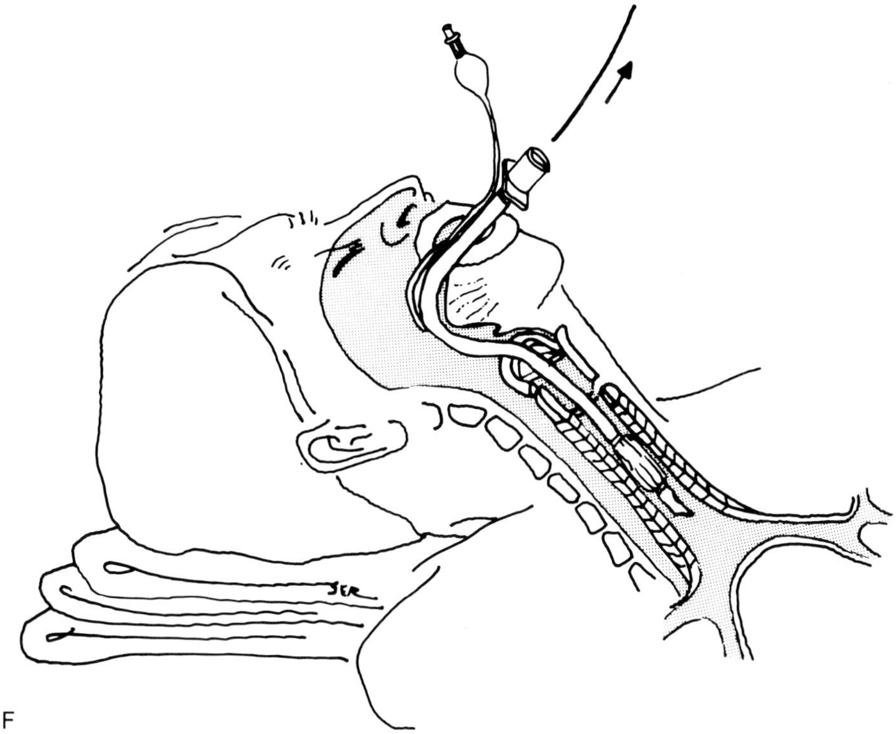

F

FIG. 8. *Continued.* **F:** The guide wire is cut at the neck close to its entrance site. The guide wire is pulled out of the endotracheal tube, leaving the tube in the trachea.

able plastic channel guide and a specially designed stylet (Fig. 9). The channel guide is used to direct the stylet into the trachea, which in turn is used to guide an endotracheal tube blindly into position.

The Augustine stylet has two special features. It is a hollow tube allowing air aspiration to confirm its tracheal placement. The tip of the stylet is also angulated to assist passage beneath the epiglottis into the trachea. The device combines the features of a pharyngeal airway, intubation stylet, bougie, and esophageal detector device (106).

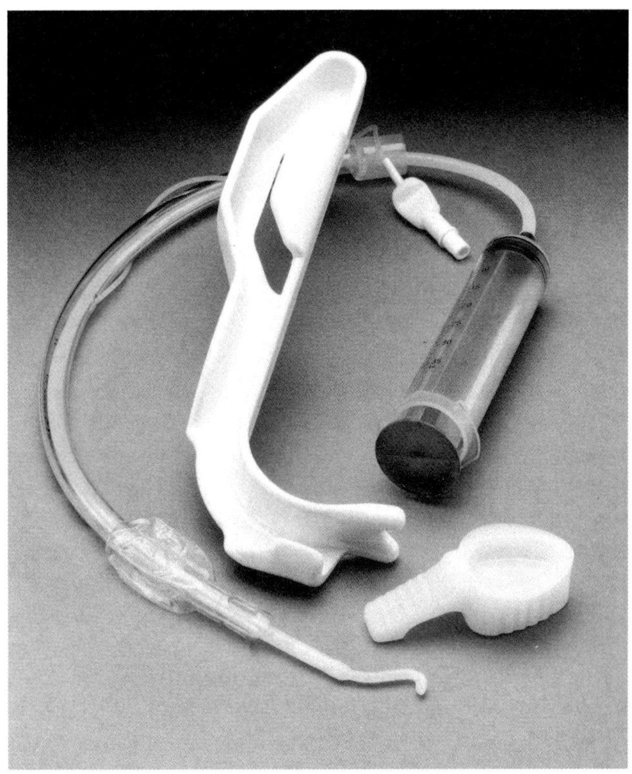

FIG. 9. Augustine Guide(R). (Courtesy of Augustine Medical, Inc., Eden Prairie, Minnesota.)

Technique

The mouth is opened with the patient's head in a neutral position. A bite block is placed between the molar teeth to keep the mouth open. The tongue is then held with gauze, and withdrawn out of the mouth. The Augustine guide, preloaded with the stylet and endotracheal tube, is placed inside the mouth and advanced toward the larynx until it stops advancing at the base of the tongue. The stylet is then advanced through the guide into the trachea. Free and easy aspiration of air by the 35 ml syringe attached to the stylet confirms intratracheal placement of the stylet. The endotracheal tube is detached from the guide and advanced over the stylet and into the trachea. If the stylet enters the esophagus, aspiration of a large volume of free air is not possible and the stylet is withdrawn and redirected.

The largest reported series of orotracheal intubations with the guide consisted of 100 orotracheal intubations in surgical patients undergoing general anesthesia. The success rate was 94%, with 75% of intubations considered easy and achieved on first attempt. In 25%, repositioning of the guide was necessary because the stylet had either entered the esophagus or could not be advanced into the trachea (107).

Complications consisted of 18 minor injuries to the mucosa of the oral cavity and the tongue. Retraction of the tongue is an essential step in this intubation technique and caution should be exercised in patients with sharp lower teeth.

False positive and false negative results from aspiration of air through the stylet are likely. Free aspiration of air with the stylet in the esophagus (false positive) is possible if air is pushed into the stomach and esophagus during ventilation by bag and mask. Failure to aspirate air with the stylet in the trachea (false negative) is possible when secretions occlude the holes in the tip of the stylet (107).

The Augustine guide has been used successfully for difficult and failed tracheal intubations. It may be applied with less movement of the cervical spine than rigid laryngoscopy, and it is easy to learn and master (108–110). The Augustine guide may be used to aid fiberoptic intubation (111). The preloaded fiberoptic bronchoscope is passed through the guide toward the larynx. The guide then acts like a laryngoscope by keeping the tongue and soft tissues away from the tip of the fiberoptic bronchoscope.

Magnetic-Guided Intubation

Patil and her colleagues have described a new orotracheal intubation technique that uses a magnet and a ferrous stylet. The tip of the epiglottis is exposed using a rigid laryngoscope, and a magnet is held over the thyroid cartilage. A catheter with stylet is placed behind the tip of the epiglottis. The magnetic power pulls the stylet and the catheter close to the glottic opening. The catheter is advanced into the trachea. This special catheter has an extension that is connected to the catheter before the endotracheal tube is advanced over the catheter into the trachea. This technique can be used when exposure of the glottis is difficult and other means of intubation are not available. The presence of blood and secretions does not affect magnetic intubation. The magnet should not be used when either the patient or the physician has a pacemaker (112).

Blind Nasal Intubation

Blind nasal intubation is a valuable technique in obtaining access to the airway in an uncooperative patient, a patient unable to open the mouth widely, or one with significant secretions or blood in the airway (113–116). The technique can be used with the patient supine or sitting.

Technique

Expertise in blind nasotracheal intubation requires an understanding of the anatomy of the upper airway, good patient preparation, and mastery of the maneuvers necessary to direct the tip of the tube.

Topical anesthesia is applied using cotton-tipped applicators soaked with 4% cocaine, or a mixture of 4% lidocaine and 1% neosynephrine (3 ml of 4% lidocaine with 1 ml of 1% neosynephrine). The head is placed in the sniffing position and a lubricated tracheal tube is advanced gently into the oropharynx. If resistance is encountered in entering the oropharynx, the tube is pulled back about 2 cm, rotated 90° to the right or left and readvanced. If still unsuccessful, a suction catheter or a nasogastric tube passed through the endotracheal tube into the oropharynx can be used as a guide (117–120).

The practitioner must sense the position and location of the tip of the tube as it is advanced. The intensity of breath sounds and bulging produced at the anterior neck by the tip of the tube help guide maneuvering of the tube. As the tube is advanced toward the larynx, the breath sounds become louder. To help passage of the tube through the vocal cords, the patient is encouraged to breathe deeply and rapidly, and the tube is advanced quickly during inspiration. Successful intubation is confirmed with continued breath sounds through the tube, loss of ability to phonate, and coughing.

If the breath sounds are lost, the tube has not entered the trachea. It may enter the esophagus, vallecula, or one of the pyriform sinuses. The loss of breath sounds without resistance to passage indicates esophageal placement. If this is the case, the tube is withdrawn and readvanced while further elevating and extending the patient's head.

If these maneuvers are unsuccessful, inflate the tracheal tube cuff with 15 ml of air when good breath sounds are noted (121). Inflation of the cuff will displace the tip of the tube away from the posterior pharyngeal wall. Advance the tube 1–3 cm, deflate the cuff, and advance further, making sure that the airway is not obstructed by the inflated cuff (121–122). The epiglottis can also be elevated by pulling the mandible forward or applying traction on the tongue (123). A hook may be used to direct the tube toward the glottis. The hook can be used in patients where rigid laryngoscopy is impossible and access to the mouth is limited (124,125).

Ketamine and propanidid have been used to induce general anesthesia to facilitate blind nasal intubation. Propanidid causes hyperventilation, while ketamine allows maintenance of a good airway with spontaneous ventilation (126,127).

The success rates of blind nasal intubation have been reported between 86% to 97% (114,115,126,127). Success rates in emergency rooms have been reported as approximately 90% (128–130). Blind nasal intubation is less successful in the hands of paramedics (131), and will be even less successful when the larynx is distorted by a mass, edema, or prior surgery.

Complications of blind nasal intubation include trauma to the nasopharyngeal mucosa, entering the submucosal plane of the pharynx, dislodging nasal polyps, pushing foreign bodies into the larynx, and nasal bleeding (117,118,132–134). Difficulty in advancing the tracheal tube into the oropharynx may be due to septal deviation, a turbinate spur, hypertrophied inferior turbinates, or nasopharyngeal lymph nodes. A smaller tube or use of the other nostril may remedy these problems.

Intubation through a Laryngeal Mask Airway

Successful tracheal intubation using the laryngeal mask airway (LMA) as a conduit has been reported in awake and anesthetized patients (Chapter 12).

Combination Techniques

The fiberscope can be used with almost all intubation techniques to overcome a difficult intubation. The fiberscope can be combined with rigid laryngoscopy in patients with abundant oropharyngeal soft tissues, or combined with blind nasal intubation in patients with a distorted upper airway (see Chapters 6 and 7).

TECHNIQUES FOR EMERGENCY VENTILATION

When tracheal intubation has failed and mask ventilation is deteriorating or failing entirely, one should not persist in further intubation attempts. In such a case, ventilation must be established as quickly as possible to avoid anoxic brain damage or death. The laryngeal mask airway (Chapter 12), esophageal-tracheal Combitube® (Chapter 13), percutaneous transtracheal jet ventilation, cricothyrotomy, or tracheostomy are procedures that can establish emergency ventilation without the need for tracheal intubation. The choice of the technique will depend on the cause of difficult ventilation, the expertise of the operator, availability of the equipment, the location, and possible complications of the technique.

Percutaneous Transtracheal Ventilation

Placement of a large bore catheter through the cricothyroid membrane (needle cricothyrotomy) into the trachea provides easy and rapid access to the airway and can be lifesaving when mask ventilation and tracheal intubation have failed. Percutaneous transtracheal ventilation may be the only option short of surgical intervention when difficulty with ventilation/intubation is due to upper airway pathology.

Percutaneous transtracheal ventilation was tried in 1949 when Whitehead et al. studied diffusion ventilation (oxygenation) through a transtracheal needle (135). A few years later, percutaneous transtracheal positive pressure ventilation was attempted in patients with compromised airways and partial upper airway obstruction (136,137). Jacoby and associates inserted 14-gauge needles into the tracheas of five patients in which intubation had been unusually difficult (136,137). Positive pressure ventilation, using an anesthesia machine–breathing circuit, maintained oxygenation sufficient to gain time to perform a tracheostomy or intubation. In these patients, while adequate oxygenation was maintained, carbon dioxide levels continued to rise because alveolar ventilation proved inadequate due to the small size of the 14-gauge needle.

In 1967, Sanders introduced the technique of jet ventilation, which proved to be an effective means of maintaining ventilation during rigid bronchoscopy and laryngoscopy (138). Numerous investigators have demonstrated the effectiveness of transtracheal jet ventilation through a catheter placed distal to a rigid laryngoscope or bronchoscope (139,140).

Percutaneous transtracheal jet ventilation has been successfully applied in human and animal studies through 16- and 14-gauge catheters (141–144). It has been used in patients under total intravenous anesthesia for surgical procedures involving the airway (139,140,145,146). Percutaneous transtracheal ventilation has been used in emergency resuscitation and as an interim means of ventilation during a difficult intubation (147–151).

Technique and Equipment

Angiocatheters, sized 16 or 14 gauge, can be used to establish transtracheal ventilation in extremely urgent circumstances. A 14-gauge over-the-needle catheter is attached to 5-ml syringe filled with lidocaine and inserted through the cricothyroid membrane into the larynx. The needle is advanced caudally at a 45° angle while gentle negative pressure is applied to the syringe. The free flow of air bubbles into the syringe, indicating correct placement of the needle inside the trachea. The needle is held stationary, while the catheter is advanced into the trachea until its hub is resting on the skin of the neck. The needle is then removed and the catheter hub is taped to the patient's neck. The jet ventilation device is attached, and the patient is ventilated.

The high incidence of malfunctioning of these catheters, due to kinking, misplacement, or dislodgment, can cause major complications. A recently introduced Arndt emergency cricothyrotomy catheter set (Cook Critical Care, Bloomingdale, Indiana) may minimize these problems (Fig. 10). The set features a 3-mm nonkinkable catheter with both a 15-mm and Luer-Lok connector. A hollow, tapered tip dilator is provided to assist the placement of the catheter into the trachea. In addition, the set contains an 18-gauge introducer needle with a stiff wire guide, a retaining plastic bag, and side tubing attached together as one piece. A sterile water vial, scalpel, syringe, and tape strip for fixation of the airway catheter are also included. The set allows for an effective way of entering the airway. Its similarities to central catheter sets in design and application provide a structured and familiar environment for application by the acute care practitioner.

Once in place, the airway catheter and its 15-mm adapter may be connected to the common gas outlet of the anesthesia machine, Ambu bag, or directly to a jet ventilator through the Luer-Lok adapter. The relatively large-size tracheal catheter permits effective high pressure jet ventilation. Bag valve manual ventilation provides oxygenation but ineffective ventilation, owing to a progressive increase in carbon dioxide concentration.

An Ambu bag or anesthesia breathing circuit can be used for oxygenation via the tracheal catheter by materials usually on hand. In one design, a 7.5-mm internal diameter (ID) tracheal tube adapter fitted into the barrel of a 3-ml syringe can be connected to an anesthesia machine or Ambu bag (Fig. 11) (152). A connector can also be fashioned by inserting the cuffed end of a precut endotracheal tube into the barrel of a 10-ml syringe with the plunger removed. The cuff is inflated and the syringe connected to the hub of the catheter. The attached 15-mm endotracheal tube adapter may be connected to an anesthesia machine or bag valve device to allow ventilation of the patient (Fig. 12) (153).

Optimal ventilation can be provided by an intermittent flow of high-pressure oxygen administered through a Sanders venturi apparatus or similar device. In general, this equipment consist of a jet injector powered by high oxygen pressure (50 psi from a piped wall oxygen, or oxygen tank regulator), a pressure adjustment valve, a hand-operated release valve, and high pressure tubing with Luer-Lok adapter (154). The advantage of an oxygen tank is that it is mobile and easily attached to a difficult airway cart (Fig. 13).

Oxygen delivered under high pressure must exit from the lungs to prevent barotrauma. Most airway obstructions that occur during anesthesia are inspiratory in nature. Positive pressure ventilation, applied through a catheter below the vocal cords, tends to open the airway, allowing oxygen and secretions to be blown out through the mouth (147,154). Air bubbles leaking through the larynx may aid tracheal intubation by identifying the location of the glottis. Expansion of the chest wall and audible airflow on exhalation noted in the oral cavity indicate airflow is occurring during percutaneous tracheal jet ventilation. Auscultation of the

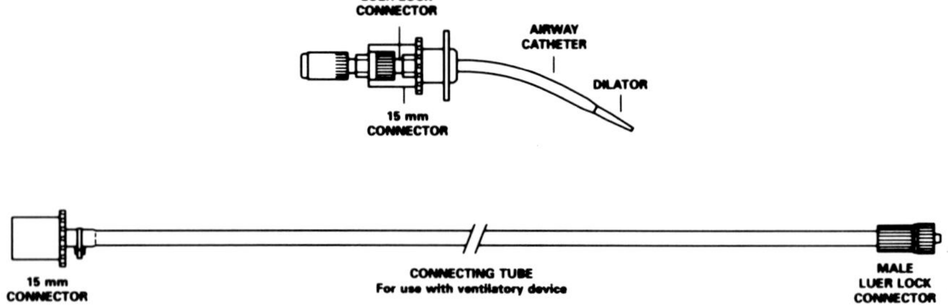

FIG. 10. Arndt emergency cricothyrotomy catheter set. (Courtesy of Cook Critical Care, Bloomington, Indiana.)

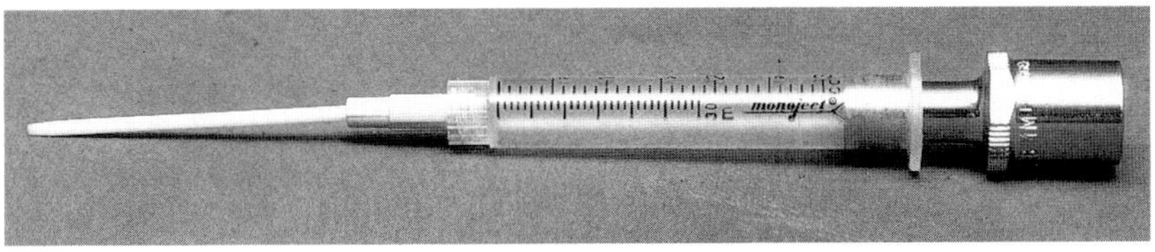

FIG. 11. A 7-mm tracheal tube adapter is fitted into the barrel of a 3-ml syringe. The syringe is connected to the catheter hub, while the adapter is connected to an Ambu bag or anesthesia machine for delivering oxygen or positive pressure ventilation.

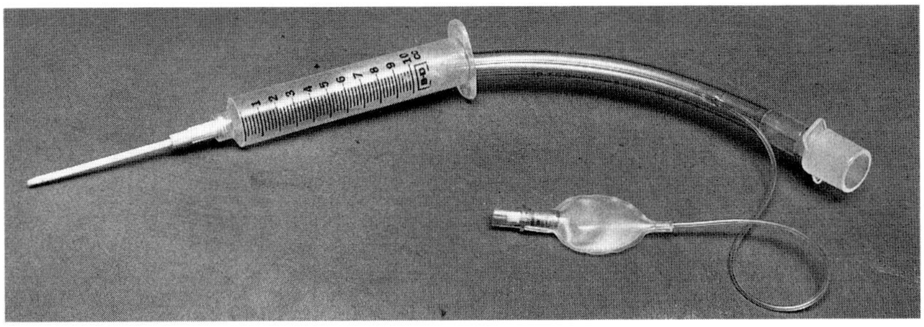

FIG. 12. Distal end of a cuffed endotracheal tube is inserted into the barrel of a 10-ml syringe barrel. The cuff is inflated, the syringe is connected to the hub of the catheter, and the tracheal tube is connected to an anesthesia machine or Ambu bag.

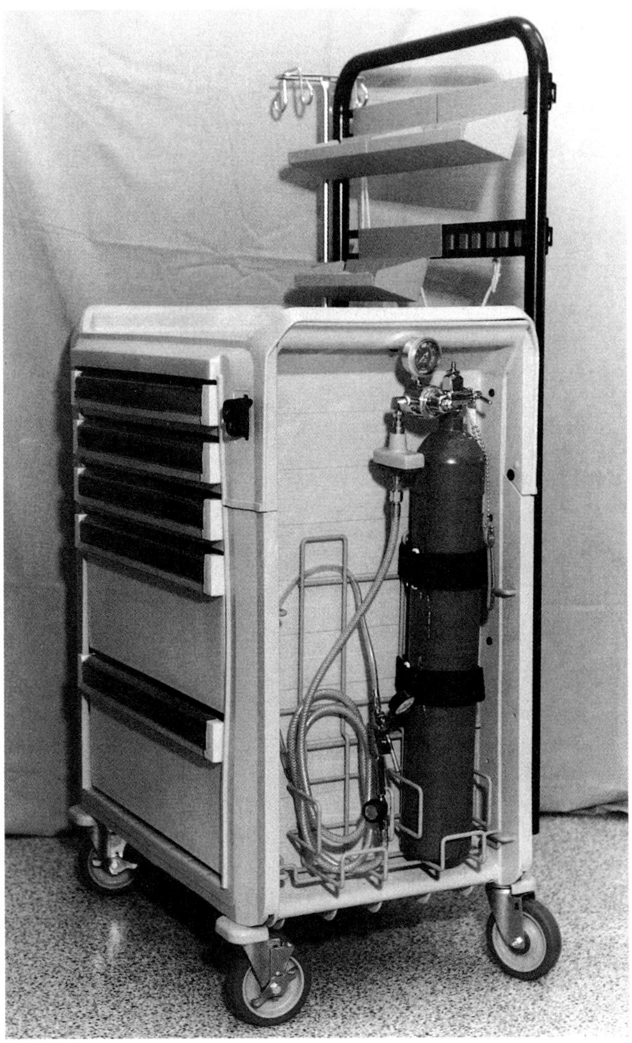

FIG. 13. Jet ventilator with portable oxygen tank setup with difficult airway cart.

chest usually does not provide a clear indication of airflow.

If a jet ventilator is not available, the anesthesia machine flush valve can be used as a jet injector (154). High pressure oxygen tubing, mounted with a 15-mm endotracheal tube adapter at one end and Luer-Lok connector at the other, is required. This tubing will replace the anesthesia machine's fresh gas delivery tube. It is directly connected to the tracheal catheter. Intermittently pushing the anesthesia machine oxygen flush valve will deliver oxygen to the patient and maintain good oxygenation and reasonable alveolar ventilation. Again, the possibility of barotrauma exists if there is obstruction to exhalation.

Complications

Reported complications of transtracheal jet ventilation are summarized in Table 12. Severe mediastinal emphysema, producing airway obstruction and necessitating surgical drainage and chest tube placement, has been reported (155).

Intravenous catheters used for transtracheal ventilation are thin walled and easily bent, causing obstruction of the catheter. This problem is more likely to happen with an awake, struggling patient. The catheter

TABLE 12. *Complications of transtracheal jet ventilation*

Hemorrhage and hematoma from needle puncture site
Pulmonary barotrauma
Kinking and blockade of the catheter
Airway outlet obstruction
Inadequate ventilation

should be held in position while jet ventilation is being delivered. A kinked or displaced catheter should be removed and replaced.

Rupture of the lungs may produce a pneumomediastinum, pneumothorax, or other major complication (142,154). In the event of total upper airway obstruction, percutaneous transtracheal jet ventilation requires that an exit airway be established. The placement of a second 14-gauge catheter in the trachea has been suggested (147). An experimental study suggests that a 10-gauge needle may be sufficient as an expiratory airway (142).

Effective ventilation by transtracheal jet ventilation in the presence of large amounts of distal airway secretions may not be possible (142).

In the hand of the inexperienced, the technique can cause major injury to the lungs. It is prudent to practice the technique initially on mannequins, gaining further expertise under controlled patient care conditions before applying it to emergency situations (142).

Cricothyrotomy and Tracheostomy

In cases of upper airway obstruction or difficulty and when the airway cannot be established with oronasotracheal intubation, surgical entrance into the trachea through the anterior neck is indicated (Table 13).

Surgical cricothyrotomy involves entering the larynx through a surgical incision of the cricothyroid membrane, allowing passage of a tracheostomy tube or endotracheal tube into the trachea. Cricothyrotomy is preferred to tracheostomy when an airway needs to be established promptly. Cricothyrotomy is faster, easier to perform, safer, and is farther away from the mediastinum than tracheostomy. The Melker® cricothyrotomy system (Cook Critical Care, Bloomington, Indiana), Nu-Trake® (International Medical Devices, Inc., Northridge, California), and Pertrach® (Pertrach Inc., Bridgeton, West Virginia) are kits created for this purpose (Fig. 14).

TABLE 13. *Indications for cricothyrotomy*

Maxillofacial trauma
Upper airway obstruction
Foreign body
Infection (Ludwig's angina, epiglotittis)
Angioneurotic edema
Tumor, hematoma, mass
Failed tracheal intubation
Expected difficult intubation

These preassembled kits can be carried easily and placed in various airway management carts or locations for easy access. Applying the Seldinger technique for cricithyrotomy is easy for nonsurgeons faced with a difficult airway (156). The Seldinger technique is used frequently for vascular access by physicians involved in critical care. The Melker® cricothyrotomy and Pertrach® systems are based on this principle and under difficult conditions should be considered as the first choice by clinicians not experienced in surgical cricothyrotomy or tracheostomy (156).

Technique

The procedure can be performed with the head and neck in the neutral position. If there is no suspicion of cervical spine injury, neck extension will facilitate the exposure.

The skin is prepared and the incision line infiltrated with 1% lidocaine. A vertical incision is made over the cricothyroid membrane. The skin and inferior border of the thyroid cartilage is retracted anteriorly by a skin hook. A 1 cm horizontal incision is made with a #11 blade above the cricoid cartilage in a perpendicular or slightly caudal direction to avoid damaging the vocal cords. The incision is widened with a hemostat or tracheal dilator to accept a size 5 or 6 mmID tracheostomy tube or a cuffed endotracheal tube. The skin hook is used to retract the superior border of the incised membrane and thyroid cartilage to assist passage of

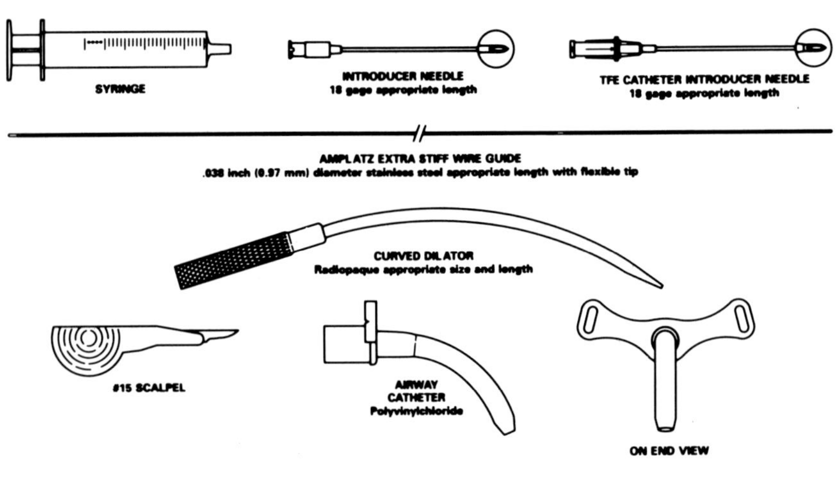

FIG. 14. Melker emergency cricothyrotomy set. (Courtesy of Cook Critical Care, Bloomington, Indiana.)

TABLE 14. *Contraindications to cricothyrotomy*

Coagulopathy
Subglottic stenosis
Laryngeal and tracheal trauma
Infection and tumor at incision site

TABLE 15. *Categories of compromised airway*

Patient with no airway obstruction
Patient with partial airway obstruction
Patient in respiratory distress
Patient in acute ventilatory failure

the tube through the incision. The tracheostomy or endotracheal tube cuff is inflated. The correct position of the tube is verified, and ventilation begun.

Cricothyrotomy is usually performed under emergency situations and under less than optimal conditions, increasing the chances for laryngeal injury. Once the patient is stabilized, the wound and the larynx should be examined. If there is any sign of significant injury or if long-term intubation is expected, the cricothyrotomy should be converted to a formal tracheostomy. Contraindications to cricothyrotomy are summarized in Table 14.

Tracheostomy is often performed to establish an adequate airway, either as an elective procedure or as an emergency measure. Tracheal intubation is always preferable to an emergency tracheostomy as the initial means of securing the airway. Once the airway is secured by endotracheal tube placement, the tracheostomy becomes elective, better tolerated, and safer to perform (113). Certain conditions (e.g., facial or tracheal injuries) may prevent the insertion of a endotracheal tube prior to tracheostomy.

Patients with severe upper airway obstruction who are to have a tracheostomy performed under local anesthesia should be fully monitored and given oxygen. It is often possible to intubate these patients with the aid of a fiberscope prior to beginning a tracheostomy. The fiberoptic intubation is attempted in the operating room with the surgeon gowned and the patient draped. The success rate with this approach has been high, but should it not prove successful, the patient's condition usually remains unchanged (34). The surgeon may then proceed as planned.

MANAGEMENT OF THE ANTICIPATED DIFFICULT INTUBATION

There are many causes of difficult intubation. The management of this problem is frequently complex. Patient management is based on the cause of the difficulty, the patient's general condition, the availability of equipment, and the familiarity of the physician with the chosen techniques.

The difficult intubation can be placed in four categories (Table 2). These patients may present with or without evidence of airway compromise (Table 15) by history or on physical examination. The selection of an intubation technique and whether intubation should be done awake, with or without sedation, or under general anesthesia are influenced by the degree and nature of airway compromise.

Patients with No Airway Obstruction

With an elective patient presenting with a known or suspected difficult intubation, the practitioner has ample time to perform a complete preoperative evaluation and develop a plan for airway management. The evaluation should include a detailed history, complete physical examination, appropriate laboratory tests, as well as consultation with other physicians. Patients with a history of failed intubation and those with conditions such as acromegaly, scleroderma, obesity, temporomandibular joint dysfunction, and tumors of the neck and oropharynx fall into this category. The clinical challenge is to recognize the existing problems, identify the extent and location of the pathology, and avoid reducing a manageable airway to an unmanageable one.

Patients with Partial Airway Obstruction

Airway management in this group of patients is similar to the group just described. The presence of partial airway obstruction leaves less room for mistakes in judgment and limits the time available for preparation and decision making. Close observation and monitoring of the patient is critical during evaluation and preparation since the condition can change from an elective or semielective circumstance to an immediate emergency state.

Preoperative medication to sedate and relax these patients should be avoided unless monitored by expert nursing or medical staff. When given, such medications should be carefully titrated, and the patient's response ascertained before increasing the dosage.

Patients in Respiratory Distress

These patients are usually conscious of their dyspnea and obstructive breathing. They may prefer sitting or lying on their side with the head elevated, rather than the supine position. The signs of partial airway obstruction, such as labored breathing, stridor, intercostal retraction, difficulty lying down, and difficulty clearing secretions, are evident. The available time for preparation and planning the airway management of these patients is limited. Delay in intervention and treatment in favor of further laboratory testing needs to be weighed relative to the risk and value of further test results.

The plan for securing the airway should be comprehensive, with an alternate plan ready to be implemented should the initial approach fail. The technique that the practitioner feels shall provide the best chance for securing the airway under the given circumstances should be tried initially. Consultation and appropriate support from other medical disciplines should be obtained without delay.

Patients in Acute Ventilatory Failure

These patients present with severe airway obstruction, usually associated with hypercarbia, hypoxemia, and mental confusion, which if untreated, shall rapidly deteriorate to cardiac arrest. Severe airway obstruction may present as an acute event after extubating a difficult airway, airway trauma, infection, or smoke inhalation injury, and in angioneurotic edema. Some patients with upper or lower airway tumors seek help only when an airway problem deteriorates to the point of almost complete obstruction.

These patients may be unconscious and exhibit no resistance to airway manipulation, or they may prove combative and totally uncooperative. The latter condition greatly complicates medical intervention and the establishment of a secured airway. The primary goal, in this extreme situation, is to rapidly establish ventilation and oxygenation.

GENERAL PRINCIPLES FOR MANAGEMENT OF PATIENTS WITH COMPROMISED AIRWAY

Basic general principles to be considered in patients who present with a compromised airway are:

1. Avoid premedication, especially narcotics. Even a small dose of morphine can change partial airway obstruction into complete obstruction. The use of an antisialagogue may be beneficial to decrease copious airway secretions and in aiding fiberoptic intubation. In severe airway obstruction, antisialagoges should be avoided since the drying of inspissated secretions may further deteriorate the airway condition.
2. Do not abolish spontaneous ventilation until the airway is secured.
3. In severe and difficult cases, the surgeon should be present and ready to immediately perform a tracheostomy.
4. Securing the airway by intubation, when possible, is desirable and associated with less morbidity than tracheostomy.
5. A trained physician should accompany the patient with an unresolved airway obstruction during transportation.
6. Oxygen, preferably by high-flow humidity face mask, should be provided.
7. Transport the patient in the sitting or semisitting position. Do not force the patient to lie in an uncomfortable position.

When a general anesthetic is required and tracheal intubation is expected to be very difficult, the options of percutaneous transtracheal jet ventilation or tracheostomy using local anesthesia may be considered.

The author believes that intubation of the trachea, after obtaining light sedation and topical anesthesia using the fiberoptic bronchoscope, is the safest and most versatile approach available. It further allows dynamic airway evaluation to be performed with minimal discomfort and interruption of airflow in the awake patient as part of the airway management process. At our institution, the advancement in fiberscope intubation techniques has made the truly difficult intubation a very rare occurrence.

Most difficult, rigid laryngoscopic intubations are easily accomplished using a fiberoptic bronchoscope. In patients at high risk for aspiration, sedatives and narcotics are given cautiously, and topical anesthesia of the vocal cords and trachea is applied through the fiberscope after progressive exposure of those structures. The administration of an H-2 blocker, metoclopramide, and oral antacid will minimize the risk of and potential lung injury secondary to aspiration.

If direct fiberoptic intubation fails, then fiberoptic intubation through a laryngeal mask airway may be attempted, or a guided blind tracheal intubation technique considered. Final remaining options include the establishment of transtracheal ventilation or tracheostomy.

If awake intubation is impractical or undesirable and the ease of mask ventilation unsure, a slow induction of general anesthesia by inhalational agents, supplemented with small doses of intravaneous induction agents, should be considered in the spontaneously breathing patient. The details of the induction technique are explained to the patient. The patient should not be asked to take deep breaths, which could increase airway discomfort, irritation, and possible coughing or spasm. During induction, the anesthesiologist should quietly talk to the patient giving positive reinforcement. The operating room environment must be quiet and controlled, any kind of stimulation of the patient should be avoided to help promote a smooth induction.

Face mask positioning and placement of airway devices should be smooth and timely. A nasopharyngeal airway should only be used if absolutely essential, as it can cause bleeding and add to airway problems. Muscle relaxants should be avoided until the ability to ventilate the lungs by bag and mask has been demonstrated. The use of a rapid sequence induction in a patient with an expected difficult intubation and poor mask ventilation status can result in catastrophe.

If the ability to mask ventilate is confirmed, the anesthetic technique, along with muscle relaxation, may proceed as usual, followed by tracheal intubation. At our institution, the fiberoptic bronchoscope intubation technique is tried first. In experienced hands, it provides the best success rate and is virtually atraumatic, with very few failures.

If fiberoptic exposure of the larynx proves difficult or requires extra time, the use of an endoscopy mask provides the option of ventilating the patient during fiberoptic intubation. The ability to ventilate the patient during the intubation attempt is an extremely valuable option that is lacking in most other intubation techniques.

The ability to suction airway secretions and apply topical anesthesia to the larynx and trachea are other valuable options of the fiberoptic technique. The intubation of a difficult airway under light general anesthesia in a spontaneously breathing patient is facilitated by spraying topical anesthesia on the vocal cords and trachea before advancing the endotracheal tube.

When a patient has severe upper airway obstruction, or has suffered major trauma to the airway with bleeding, a tracheostomy performed under local anesthesia is usually the preferred technique. Many of these patients will benefit from securing the airway prior to tracheostomy. This should only be attempted, with the patient surgically prepared and the surgeon ready.

MANAGEMENT OF THE UNANTICIPATED FAILED INTUBATION

The discovery of an unanticipated difficult intubation usually occurs after initial attempts at intubation by rigid laryngoscopy have failed, with the patient anesthetized and paralyzed. These patients frequently do not have obvious anatomical or pathologic conditions that would strongly indicate a potentially difficult intubation.

Difficult mask ventilation may also be discovered after induction of anesthesia and failed intubation attempts. Avoidance of positive pressure mask ventilation during rapid sequence induction will delay discovery of this important finding for 3 min or longer. The incidence of coexisting difficult mask ventilation and difficult intubation has been reported to be 15% (157). To minimize the incidence of this dangerous situation, all airways that are suspect for possible difficulties should be assumed as such and approached with caution.

Unanticipated failed intubation is a relatively common clinical phenomenon chiefly for two reasons:

1. The criteria used to identify the difficult intubation are imprecise.
2. Inadequate attention is given to the preoperative airway evaluation.

Should an unanticipated failed intubation occur, the steps required for effective management include recognition of the degree of difficulty of rigid laryngoscopy, trauma resulting from persisting in repeated unsuccessful rigid laryngoscopy attempts, selection of alternative techniques, and awakening of the patient.

The course of action depends largely on the ability to ventilate the patient by mask. If mask ventilation is easy, anesthesia and muscle relaxation can be maintained, the oropharynx suctioned, and asleep fiberoptic orotracheal intubation performed through an intubating airway. If the equipment is readily available, the trained practitioner should have little difficulty in atraumatically intubating the vast majority of these patients. In patients at risk for aspiration, an assistant should apply gentle cricoid pressure until the airway is secured. Undue persistence at rigid laryngoscopy or attempted nasal intubation may lead to laryngeal edema and bleeding, making fiberoptic intubation difficult.

Combining rigid and fiberoptic laryngoscopic techniques may be extremely helpful. An assistant should try to expose the tip of the epiglottis using the rigid laryngoscope. One endoscopist, looking directly into the mouth, can then place the tip of the fiberscope next to or under the tip of the epiglottis. Then, while looking through the fiberscope, the second endoscopist advances the fiberscope through the visualized vocal cords into the trachea. Combining these techniques serves to minimize the time required to identify the epiglottis fiberoptically. This approach may also be helpful to the endoscopist of limited experience in the use of the fiberscope.

If fiberoptic intubation is unsuccessful, a guided, blind orotracheal intubation technique may be used. If the patient regains spontaneous ventilation, fiberoptic intubation attempts should be repeated since exposure of the larynx with the fiberscope is often improved by spontaneous ventilation. If still unsuccessful, other options (e.g., laryngeal mask airway, Combitube™, transtracheal jet ventilation, or simply allowing the patient to regain consciousness) should be considered. If surgery is urgent, a regional technique may be substituted. A controlled tracheostomy under local anesthesia remains an option if surgery must proceed.

If mask ventilation is extremely difficult or impossible, and the patient is still paralyzed, irreversible hypoxic brain damage or death may occur. At this time, attention should be directed to techniques that can restore oxygenation rather than persisting with tracheal intubation. Laryngeal mask airway, esophageal intubation with a Combitub™, transtracheal jet ventilation, or surgical cricothyrotomy should be considered.

AIRWAY MANAGEMENT OF PATIENTS WITH TRACHEAL STENOSIS OR COMPRESSION

Difficulty in advancing a tracheal tube after it has passed between the vocal cords is usually due to subglottic or tracheal stenosis, often a late complication of tracheostomy or prolonged tracheal intubation (158). Other intrinsic causes of tracheal stenosis are trauma and surgical repair of the trachea, congenital tracheal stenosis (159,160), tumors invading the tracheal lumen, and tracheopathia osteochondroplastica (161,162).

Extrinsic causes of tracheal stenosis include a large aortic arch (163,164), thoracic aortic aneurysm (165), congenital vascular anomalies (166), substernal thyroid, mediastinal masses (Fig. 15), and paratracheal lymph nodes (22).

The signs and symptoms of severe tracheal stenosis (lumen reduced to 3–4 mm in diameter) include inspiratory and expiratory stridor, low exercise tolerance, and inability to raise sputum (158). Less severe degrees of stenosis are often asymptomatic. A careful history and physical examination supplemented by radiologic studies, flow-volume loop measurement (Fig. 3), and fiberoptic airway endoscopy, are useful for assessing the degree and extent of stenosis.

Patients with a mediastinal mass, especially noted in

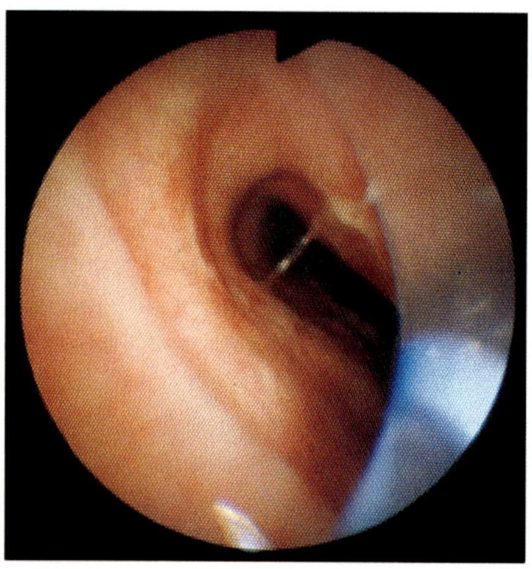

FIG. 15. Endoscopic view of a tracheal compression.

Hodgkin's disease, are likely to develop acute severe airway obstruction especially if anesthetized in the supine position (167,168). Piro and associates (168) reported a 10% incidence of life-threatening airway complications in 25 patients with mediastinal Hodgkin's disease undergoing staging laparotomy. Many of these patients were asymptomatic prior to induction of anesthesia.

The acute airway obstruction seen on induction of anesthesia is attributed to the loss of spontaneous ventilation and negative intrathoracic pressure on inspiration. This negative pressure helps to dilate intrathoracic airways during spontaneous ventilation. Other contributing factors include the loss of bronchial smooth muscle tone, decreases in thoracic air volume, and cephalad displacement of the dome of the diaphragm (169).

Studies of patients with mediastinal Hodgkin's disease should include upright and supine flow-volume loop studies. A change in severity of obstruction, as shown by a flow-volume loop obtained in the supine position compared with the upright study, may indicate a propensity for this problem after induction of anesthesia (Fig. 4) (22,169).

A thoracic aortic aneurysm and enlarged aortic arch may compress the tracheal lumen and prevent passage of a tracheal tube. Forceful attempts to advance a tube may cause tracheal trauma and even rupture a dissecting aneurysm. In one patient with a prominent aortic arch, complete airway obstruction occurred when the patient was placed in the right decubitus position prior to extubation. Turning the patient back to the supine position cleared the obstruction immediately (163).

A prominent aortic arch or aneurysm is easily recognized from a routine preoperative chest X-ray; the trachea is deviated to the right and its diameter reduced. Fiberoptic endoscopy reveals an indentation in the tracheal wall and aortic pulsation is often visible. The left main stem bronchus may not be visible on bronchoscopy until the fiberscope passes the point of compression. Tracheopathia osteochondroplastica is a progressive benign dysplasia which causes gradual tracheal stenosis. It has been described as a cause of difficulty with tracheal intubation (161,162).

Patients with an anterior mediastinal mass also remain at high risk of acute airway obstruction following surgery; edema, bleeding, and hematoma are potential contributing factors. Resection of a tumor may cause tracheomalacia leading to acute respiratory distress. Other complications associated with mediastinal masses include, massive hemorrhage, superior vena cava syndrome, pericardial restriction or tamponade, and vocal cord paralysis. All patients with a narrowed airway should be monitored carefully after extubation. Even a small degree of edema at the stenotic site can cause airway obstruction. Prophylactic steroid therapy and the use of racemic epinephrine inhalation may be considered.

In all of these cases, fiberoptic tracheal intubation using topical anesthesia in the sedated awake patient is the technique of choice. This technique allows for examination of the airway, selection of an appropriately sized tube, and precise placement of the endotracheal tube in relation to the stenotic area. The scope acts as a guide to pass the tube beyond the compression. If the endotracheal tube cannot be advanced beyond the compression site, the tip of the tracheal tube may, alternatively, be positioned just above the stenotic area (161–163).

In patients with a history of tracheostomy or prolonged tracheal intubation, induction of anesthesia should always proceed with caution. However, tracheal intubation aided by a fiberscope provides the advantage of permitting examination of the airway prior to insertion of a tube and induction of anesthesia, thus avoiding undue trauma and delays.

Recent reports have recommended the use of the laryngeal mask airway (LMA) for administration of general anesthesia in patients with tracheal stenosis (170,171). Since the LMA does not enter the trachea, airway trauma and mucosal edema at the stenotic site is avoided. If the stenotic segment is high in the trachea, positioning the endotracheal tube proximal to the stenosis may not be possible, while the LMA can be used irrespective of the location of the stenosis (see Chapter 12).

The LMA should not be used in patients with external compression of the trachea or tracheomalacia because it cannot prevent tracheal collapse. The LMA is not a good choice for major operative procedures (which often require high airway pressure mechanical ventilation) and in cases requiring postoperative ventilatory support.

THE FIBERSCOPE AND DIFFICULT INTUBATION IN PEDIATRICS

When a small-size fiberscope is available, all the described techniques of fiberoptic intubation can be applied to the pediatric population. With the larger fiberscope, modification of techniques are possible. These techniques are discussed in Chapter 7.

DOCUMENTATION AND REGISTRATION

For the safety of the patient and to avoid future malpractice suits, patients with proven difficult airways should be informed and identified. Immediate application of a temporary wristband and flagging the patient's medical record will alert the health care providers to the patient's special requirements.

At minimum, a written statement with pertinent airway management information should be issued to the patient, with a copy of it filed in the patient's medical record. Verbal instructions are inadequate and unreliable as patients may easily forget the information explained to them.

It is strongly recommended that for future reference and availability of information for other health care organizations, the patient with a difficult airway should be enrolled in the Medic Alert Difficult Airway/Intubation Registry. Medic Alert Foundation International is a charitable, nonprofit organization that provides a 24-hour medical identification service for its members. Medic Alert wallet card and an engraved bracelet will assist health care providers in having rapid access to the related information that can be beneficial in the airway management and anesthetic care of such patients (16).

Medic Alert registration is a must for patients found to have an unanticipated difficult intubation and for all patients proven to be very difficult or impossible to ventilate by face mask.

REFERENCES

1. Caplan RA, Posner KL, Ward RJ, Chevey FW. Adverse respiratory events in anesthesia: A closed claims analysis. *Anesthesiology* 1990;72:828–833.
2. King TA, Adams AP. Failed tracheal intubation. *Br J Anaesth* 1990;65:400–414.
3. Davis DA. An analysis of anesthetic mishaps from medical liability claims. *Internatl Anesthesiol Clin* 1984;22:31–42.
4. Solazzi RW, Ward RJ. The spectrum of medical liability cases. *Internatl Anesthesiol Clin* 1984;22:43–59.
5. Holland R. Anesthesia-related mortality in anesthesia. *Internatl Anesthesiol Clin* 1984;22:61–71.
6. Utting JE, Gray TC, Shelley FC. Human misadventure in anaesthesia. *Can Anaesth Soc J* 1979;26:472–478.
7. Rosen M. Maternal mortality associated with anesthesia in England and Wales. In: Vickers MD, Lunn JN, eds. *European academy of anaesthesiology proceedings*. Berlin: Springer-Verlag, 1982;39–44.
8. Endler GC, Mariona EG, Sokol RJ, Stevenson LB. Anesthesia-related maternal mortality in Michigan, 1972–1984. *Am J Obstet Gynecol* 1988;159:187–193.
9. Turnbull AC, Tindall VR, Robson G, et al. Report on confidential enquiries into maternal deaths in England and Wales, 1979–1981. London: Her Majesty's Stationery Office, 1986.
10. Marx GF, Berman JA. Anesthesia-related maternal mortality. *Bull NY Acad Med* 1985;61:323–330.
11. American Society of Anesthesiologists Task Force on Management of the Difficult Airway. Practice guidelines for management of the difficult airway. *Anesthesiology* 1993;78:597–602.
12. Rosenberg H, Rosenberg H. Airway obstruction and causes of difficult intubation. In: Orkin FK, Cooperman LH, eds. *Complications in anesthesiology*. Philadelphia: Lippincott, 1983; 125–143.
13. Barratt GE, Coulthard SW. Upper airway obstruction: Diagnosis and management options. In: Brown BR, ed. *Contemporary anesthesia practice* 1987;9:49–72.
14. Davies RJO, Stradling JR. Acute effects of obstructive sleep apnea. *Br J Anaesth* 1993;71:725–729.

15. Cone AM, Scott S. Intermittent airway obstruction during anesthesia in a patient with an undiagnosed anterior mediastinal mass. *Anaesth Intens Care* 1994;22:204–208.
16. Mark LJ, Beattie C, Lee Ferrell C, Trempy G, Dorman T, Schauble JF. The difficult airway: mechanisms for effective dissemination of critical information. *J Clin Anaesth* 1992;4: 247–251.
17. Shenkman Z, Shir Y, Brodsky JB. Perioperative management of the obsese patient. *Br J Anaesth* 1993;70:349–359.
18. Law JH, Barnhart K, Rowlett W, et al. Increased frequency of obstructive airway abnormalities with long-term tracheostomy. *Chest* 1993;104:136–138.
19. Block C, Brechner VL. Unusual problems in airway management. II. The influence of the temporomandibular joint, the mandible and associated structures in endotracheal intubation. *Anesth Analg* 1971;50:114–123.
20. Edens ET, Sia RL. Flexible fiberoptic endoscopy in difficult intubations. *Ann Otol* 1981;90:307–309.
21. Neuman GG, Weingarten AE, Abramowitz RM, et al. The anesthetic management of the patient with an anterior mediastinal mass. *Anesthesiology* 1984;60:144–147.
22. Prakash UBS, Abel MD, Hubmayer RD. Mediastinal mass and tracheal obstruction during general anesthesia. *Mayo Clin Proc* 1988;63:1004–1011.
23. Sanders MH, Martin RJ, Pennock BE, Rogers RM. The detection of sleep apnea in the awake patient. The "saw-tooth" sign. *JAMA* 1981;245:2414–2418.
24. Kohan JM, Israel RH, Greenblatt DW, et al. "Saw tooth" pattern on a flow-volume loop following neck surgery. *JAMA* 1984;252:2701–2702.
25. Salem MR, Mathrubhutham M, Bennett EJ. Difficult intubation. *New Engl J Med* 1976;295:879–881.
26. Latto IP. Management of difficult intubation. In: Latto IP, Rosen M, eds. *Difficulties in tracheal intubation*. London: Bailliere Tindall, 1985;99–141.
27. Singh A. Blind nasal intubation. A report of the use of a hook in three cases of ankylosis of the jaw. *Anaesthesia* 1966;21: 400–402.
28. Ovassapian A, Mesnick PS. The art of fiberoptic intubation. In: Sandler AN, Doyle JD, eds. *Anesthesia Clinics of North America*. Phildelphia: W. B. Saunders, 1995;13:391–409.
29. Roberts JT, Abouleish AE, Curlin FJ, Patterson A. The failed intubation: maximizing successful management of the patient with a compromised or potentially compromised airway. In: Roberts JT, ed. *Clinical management of the airway*. Philadelphia: W. B. Saunders, 1994;187–218.
30. Wang JF, Reves JG, Corssen G. Use of the fiberoptic laryngoscope for difficult tracheal intubation. *Ala J Med Sci* 1976;13: 247–251.
31. Messeter KH, Petersson KI. Endotracheal intubation with the fiberoptic bronchoscope. *Anaesthesia* 1980;35:294–298.
32. Ovassapian A, Land P, Schafer MF, et al. Anesthetic management for surgical corrections of severe flexion deformity of the cervical spine. *Anesthesiology* 1983;58:370–372.
33. Keenan MA, Stiles CM, Kaufman RL. Acquired laryngeal deviation associated with cervical spine disease in erosive polyarticular arthritis. Use of the fiberoptic bronchoscope in rheumatoid arthritis. *Anesthesiology* 1983;58:441–449.
34. Ovassapian A. Fiberoptic tracheal intubation. In: Ovassapian A, ed. *Fiberoptic airway endoscopy in anesthesia and critical care*. New York: Raven Press, 1990;57–72.
35. McIntyre JWR. The difficult tracheal intubation. *Can J Anaesth* 1987;34:204–213.
36. Keenan RL, Boyan CP. Decreasing frequency of anesthetic cardiac arrest. *J Clin Anesth* 1991;3:354–357.
37. Horton WA, Fahy L, Charters P. Factor analysis in difficult tracheal intubation: laryngoscopy-induced airway obstruction. *Br J Anaesth* 1990;65:801–805.
38. Ovassapian A, Meyer R. Airway management. In: Longnecker DE, Murphy FL, eds. *Dripps introduction to anesthesia*, 8th ed. Philadelphia: W. B. Saunders, 1992;137–154.
39. Westhorpe RN. The position of the larynx in children and its relation to the ease of intubation. *Anesth Intens Care* 1987;15: 384–388.
40. Dorsch JA, Dorsch SE. Laryngoscopes. In: Dorsch JA, Dorsch SE, eds. *Understanding anesthesia equipment*, 3rd ed. Baltimore: Williams & Wilkins, 1994;399–437.
41. Jellicoe JA, Harris NR. A modification of a standard laryngoscope for difficult tracheal intubation in obstetric cases. *Anaesthesia* 1984;39:800–802.
42. Yentis SM. A laryngoscope adaptor for difficult intubation. *Anaesthesia* 1987;42:764–766.
43. Dhara SS, Cheong TW. An adjustable multiple angle laryngoscope adaptor. *Anaesth Intens Care* 1991;19:243–245.
44. Choi JJ. A new double-angle blade for direct laryngoscopy. *Anesthesiology* 1990;72:576.
45. McIntyre JWR. Laryngoscope design and the difficult adult tracheal intubation. *Can J Anaesth* 1989;36:94–98.
46. Bellhouse CP. An angulated laryngoscope for routine and difficult tracheal intubation. *Anesthesiology* 1988;69:126–129.
47. Mayall RM. The Belscope for management of the difficult airway. *Anesthesiology* 1992;76:1059–1060.
48. Bainton CR. A new laryngoscope blade to overcome pharyngeal obstruction. *Anesthesiology* 1987;67:767–770.
49. Wengen DFA. Piriform fassa perforation during attempted tracheal intubation. *Anaesthesia* 1987;42:519–521.
50. Gamlin F, Caldicott LD, Shah MV. Mediastinitis and sepsis syndrome following intubation. *Anaesthesia* 1994;49:883–885.
51. Larson CE, Gonzalez RM. A problem with metal endotracheal tubes and plastic-coated stylets. *Anesthesiology* 1989;70: 883–884.
52. Martin P, Campbell AM. Tracheal intubation: A complication. *Anaesthesia* 1992;47:75.
53. Fishman RL. Reuse of a disposable stylet with life-threatening complications. *Anesth Analg* 1991;72:266–267.
54. Kubota Y, Toyoda Y, Kubota H. No more complications with stylets. *Anaesthesia* 1992;47:628.
55. Nolan JP, Wilson ME. An aid to oral intubation in patients with potential cervical spine injuries. *Anesth Analg* 1992;75: 153–154.
56. Benson PF. The gum-elastic bougie: a life saver. *Anesth Analg* 1992;74:318.
57. Rao TLK, Mathru M, Gorski DW, Salem R. Experience with a new intubation guide for difficult tracheal intubation. *Crit Care Med* 1982;10:882–883.
58. Bjoraker DG. The Bullard intubating laryngoscopes. *Anesthesiology Rev* 1990;17:64–70.
59. Borland LM, Casselbrant M. The Bullard laryngoscope. A new oral laryngoscope (pediatric version). *Anesth Analg* 1990;70: 105–108.
60. Dyson A, Harris J, Bhatia K. Rapidity and accuracy of tracheal intubation in a mannequin: comparison of the fiberoptic with the Bullard laryngoscope. *Br J Anaesth* 1990; 65: 268–270.
61. Brown RE, Vollers JM, Rader GR, Schmitz ML. Nasotracheal intubation in a child with Treacher Collins syndrome using the Bullard intubating laryngoscope. *J Clin Anesth* 1993; 5: 492–493.
62. Shigematsu T, Miyazawa N, Kobayashi M, Yorozu T, Toyoda Y, Morisaki H. Nasotracheal intubation with Bullard laryngoscope: a useful approach for difficult airways. *Anesth Analg* 1994; 79: 132–135.
63. Abrams KJ, Desai N, Katsnelson T. Bullard laryngoscopy for trauma airway management in suspected cervical spine injuries *[letter]*. *Anesth Analg* 1992;74:623.
64. Mendel P, Bristow A. Anesthesia for procedures on the larynx and pharynx. The use of the Bullard laryngoscope in conjunction with high frequency jet ventilation. *Anaesthesia* 1993;48: 263–265.
65. Baraka A, Muallem M. Bullard laryngoscopy for tracheal intubation in a neonate with Pierre-Robin syndrome. *Ped Anaesth* 1994;4:111–113.
66. Saunders PR, Geisecke AH. Clinical assessment of the adult Bullard laryngoscope. *Can J Anaesth* 1989;36:S118–S119.
67. Macintosh R, Richards H. Illuminated introducers for endotracheal tubes. *Anaesthesia* 1957;12:223–225.

68. Yamamura H, Yamamoto T, Kamiyama M. Device for blind nasal intubation *[letter]*. *Anesthesiology* 1959;20:221.
69. Ducrow M. Throwing light on blind intubation. *Anaesthesia* 1978;33:827–829.
70. Stevens SC, Hung OR. A new device for oral and nasotracheal light-guided intubation. *Can J Anaesth* 1992;39:A86.
71. Hung OR, Stevens SC, Hawboldt G. Light-guided vs. laryngoscopic intubation in surgical patients: clinical trial of a new lightwand device. *Can J Anaesth* 1992;39:A147.
72. Stewart RD, LaRosee A, Stoy WA, Heller MB. Use of a lighted stylet to confirm correct endotracheal tube placement. *Chest* 1987;92:900–903.
73. Rayburn RL. Light wand intubation. *Anaesthesia* 1979;34:677–678.
74. Ellis DG, Jakymec A, Kaplan RM, et al. Guided orotracheal intubation in the operating room using a lighted stylet: a comparison with direct laryngoscopic technique. *Anesthesiology* 1986;64:823–826.
75. Fox DJ, Castro T, Rastrelli AJ. Comparison of intubation techniques in the awake patient: the Flexi-lum surgical light (lightwand) versus blind nasal approach. *Anesthesiology* 1987;66:69–71.
76. Verdile VP, Chiang JL, Bedger R, Stewart RD, Kaplan R, Paris PM. Nasotracheal intubation using a flexible lighted stylet. *Ann Emerg Med* 1990;19:506–510.
77. Williams TR, Stewart RD. Transillumination of the trachea with a lighted stylet. *Anesth Analg* 1986;65:542–543.
78. Zbinden S, Schupfer G. The lightwand as an atraumatic alternative to blind stylet intubation. *Anesthesia* 1988;43:248.
79. Verdil VP, Heller MB, Paris PM, et al. Nasotracheal intubation in traumatic craniofacial dislocation: use of the lighted stylet. *Am J Emerg Med* 1988;6:39–41.
80. Butler FS, Cirillo AA. Retrograde tracheal intubation. *Anesth Analg* 1960;39:333–338.
81. Waters DJ. Guided blind endotracheal intubation. *Anaesthesia* 1963;18:158–162.
82. Powell WF, Ozdil T. A translaryngeal guide for tracheal intubation. *Anesth Analg* 1967;46:231–234.
83. Bourke D, Levesque PR. Modification of retrograde guide for endotracheal intubation. *Anesth Analg* 1974;53:1013–1014.
84. Harmer M, Vaughan RS. Guided blind oral intubation. *Anaesthesia* 1980;35:921.
85. Borland LM, Swan DM, Leff S. Difficult pediatric endotracheal intubation: a new approach to the retrograde technique. *Anesthesiology* 1981;55:577–578.
86. Yonfa AE, Klein E, Mackall LL. Retrograde approach to nasotracheal intubation in a child with severe Pierre Robin syndrome. *Anesthesiol Rev* 1983;10:28–29.
87. Akinyemi OO. Complications of guided blind endotracheal intubation. *Anaesthesia* 1979;34:590–592.
88. Ward CF, Salvatierra CA. Special intubation technique for the adult patient. In: Benumof JL, ed. *Clincal procedures in anesthesia and intensive care*. Philadelphia: Lippincott, 1992;149–176.
89. King HK, Wang LF, Khan AK, Wooten DJ. Translaryngeal guided intubation for difficult intubation. *Crit Care Med* 1987;15:869–871.
90. Freund PR, Rook A, Schwid H. Retrograde intubation with a modified Eshman stylet. *Anesth Analg*. 1998;67:605–606.
91. Dhara SS. Retrograde intubation. A facilitated approach. *Br J Anaesth* 1992;69:631–633.
92. Carlson CA, Perkins HM, Veltkan PS. Solving a difficult intubation. *Anesthesiology* 1986;64:537.
93. Abou-Madi MN, Trop D. Pulling versus guiding: a modification of retrograde guided intubation. *Can J Anaesth* 1989;36:336–339.
94. Kubo K, Takahashi S, Oka M. A modified technique of guided blind intubation in oral surgery. *J Max Face Surg* 1980;8:135–137.
95. Harrison CA, Wise CC. Retrograde intubation. *Anaesthesia* 1988;43:609.
96. Shantha TR. Retrograde intubation using the subcricoid region. *Br J Anaesth* 1992;68:109–112.
97. Lechman MJ, Donahoo JS, MacVaugh H III. Endotracheal intubation using percutaneous retrograde guide wire insertion followed by antegrade fiberoptic bronchoscopy. *Crit Care Med* 1986;14:589–590.
98. Gupta B, McDonald JS, Brooks JHJ, Mendenhall T. Oral fiberoptic intubation over a retrograde guide wire. *Anesth Analg* 1989;68:517–519.
99. Audenalrt SM, Montgomery Cl, Stone B, Akins RE, Locke Rl. Retrograde-assisted fiberoptic tracheal intubation in children with difficult airways. *Anesth Analg* 1991;73:660–664.
100. Barriot P, Riou B. Retrograde technique for tracheal intubation in trauma patients. *Crit Care Med* 1988;16:712–713.
101. Cooper CMS, Murray-Wilson A. Retrograde intubation. Management of a 4.8 Kg, 5 month infant. *Anaesthesia* 1987;42:1197–1200.
102. Manchester GH, Mani MM, Master FW. A simple method for emergency orotracheal intubation. *Plast Reconstr Surg* 1972;49:312–315.
103. Payne KA. Difficult tracheal intubation. *Anaesth Intens Care* 1980;8:84–90.
104. Casthely PA, Landsman S, Fyman PN, Engin MA, Griepp R, Wolf GL. Retrograde intubation in patients undergoing open heart surgery. *Canad J Anaesth* 1985;32:661–664.
105. Bowes WA, Johnson JO. Pneumodiastinum after planned retrograde fiberoptic intubation. *Anesth Analg* 1994;78:795–797.
106. Kovac AL. The Augustine Guide: a new device for blind orotracheal intubation. *Anesthesiology Review* 1993;1:25–29.
107. Carr RJ, Belani KG. Clinical assessment of the Augustine Guide™ for endotracheal intubation. *Anesth Analg* 1994;78:983–987.
108. Krafft P, Fitzgerald R, Pernerstorfer T, Kapral S, Weinstabl C. A new device for blind oral intubation in routine and difficult airway management. *European Anaesthesiology* 1994;11:207–212.
109. Fitzgerald RD, Krafft P, Skrbensky G, Pernerstorfer T, Steiner E, Kapral S, Weinstabl C. Excursions of the cervical spine during tracheal intubation: blind oral intubation compared with direct laryngoscopy. *Br J Anaesth* 1994;45:111–115.
110. Kovac AL, Elliot C, Schacher D. Effectiveness of a teaching module for blind orotracheal Intubation with the Augustine Guide. *Anesth Analg* 1994;78:S219.
111. La Tourette P, Patil VU. The Augustine Guide as a fiberoptic bronchoscope guide. *Anesth Analg* 1993;76:1164–1165.
112. Patil VU, Buckingham T, Willoughby P, Szeverenyi NM. Magnetic orotracheal intubation: a new technique. *Anesth Analg* 1994;78:749–752.
113. Orringer MB. Endotracheal intubation and tracheostomy. Indications, techniques and complications. *Surg Clin North Am* 1980;60:1447–1464.
114. Gillespie N. Blind nasotracheal intubation. *Anesth Analg* 1950;29:217.
115. Gold MI, Buechel DR. A method of blind nasal intubation for the conscious patient. *Anesth Analg* 1960;39:257–263.
116. Jacoby J. Nasal endotracheal intubation by an external visual technic. *Anesth Analg* 1970;49:731–739.
117. Tahir AH. A simple manoeuvre to aid the passage of a nasotracheal tube into the oropharynx. *Br J Anaesth* 1970;42:631–632.
118. Nolan RT. Nasal intubation. An anatomical difficulty with portex tubes. *Anaesthesia* 1969;24:447–448.
119. Brodman E, Duncalf D. Avoiding the trauma of nasotracheal intubation. *Anesth Analg* 1981;60:618.
120. Dryden GE. Use of a suction catheter to assist blind nasal intubation *[letter]*. *Anesthesiology* 1976;45:260.
121. Gorback MS. Inflation of the endotracheal tube cuff as an aid to blind nasal endotracheal intubation. *Anesth Analg* 1987;66:916–917.
122. Van Elstraete AC, Pennant JH, Bajray NM, Victory RA. Tracheal tube cuff inflation as an aid to blind nasotracheal intubation. *Br J Anaesth* 1993;70:691–693.
123. Adams AL, Cane RD, Shapiro BA. Tongue extrusion as an aid to blind nasal intubation. *Crit Care Med* 1982;10:335–336.
124. Bearman AJ. Device for nasotracheal intubation. *Anesthesiology* 1962;23:130–131.

125. Munson ES, Cullen SC. Endotracheal intubation in a patient with ankylosing spondylitis of the cervical spine. *Anesthesiology* 1965;26:365.
126. Defalque RJ. Ketamine for blind nasal intubation. *Anesth Analg* 1971;50:984–986.
127. Oyegunle AO. The use of propanidid for blind nasotracheal intubation. *Br J Anaesth* 1975;47:379–381.
128. Danzl DF, Thomas DM. Nasotracheal intubation in the emergency department. *Crit Care Med* 1980;8:677–682.
129. Tintinalli JE, Claffey J. Complications of nasotracheal intubation. *Ann Emerg Med* 1981;10:142–144.
130. Iserson KV. Blind nasotracheal intubation. *Ann Emerg Med* 1981;10:468–471.
131. McHale SP, Brydon CW, Wood MLB, Liban JB. A survey of nasotracheal skills among advanced trauma life support course graduates. *Br J Anaesth* 1994;72:195–197.
132. Boysen K. An unusual case of nasotracheal tube occlusion. *Anaesthesia* 1985;40:1024.
133. Hitchen JE, Wiener AP. Unexpected obstruction of a nasotracheal tube: report of case. *J Oral Surg* 1973;31:722–724.
134. Harvey DC, Amorosa P. Traumatic nasotracheal intubation. *Anaesthesia* 1986;41:442.
135. Whitehead RW, Spencer JN, Parry BA, et al. Studies on diffusion respiration. *Anesthesiology* 1949;10:54–60.
136. Jacoby JJ, Hamelberg W, Reed JP, et al. Simple method of artificial respiration. *Am J Physiol* 1951;167:798–799.
137. Jacoby JJ, Hamelberg W, Ziegler CH, et al. Transtracheal resuscitation. *JAMA* 1956;162:625–628.
138. Sanders RD. Two ventilating attachments for bronchoscopes. *Del Med J* 1967;39:170–175.
139. Spoerel WE, Narayanan PS, Singh NP. Transtracheal ventilation. *Br J Anaesth* 1971;43:932–939.
140. Smith RB, Schaer WB, Pfaeffle H. Percutaneous transtracheal ventilation for anaesthesia and resuscitation: a review and report of complications. *Can Anaesth Soc J* 1975;22:607–612.
141. Rone CA, Pavlin EG, Cummings CW, Weymuller EA. Studies in transtracheal ventilation catheters. *Laryngoscope* 1982;92:1259–1264.
142. Weymuller EA, Pavlin EG, Paugh D, Cummings CW. Management of difficult airway problems with percutaneous transtracheal ventilation. *Ann Otol Rhinol Laryngol* 1987;96:34–37.
143. Jorden RC, Moore EE, Marx JA, Honigman B. A comparison of PTV and endotracheal ventilation in an acute trauma model. *J of Trauma* 1985;25:978–983.
144. Neff CC, Pfister RC, Sonnenberg EV. Percutaneous transtracheal ventilation: Experimental and practical aspects. *J of Trauma* 1983;23:84–90.
145. Layman PR. An alternative to blind nasal intubation. *Anaesthesia* 1983;38:165.
146. Layman PR. Transtracheal ventilation in oral surgery. *Ann R Coll Surg Engl* 1983;65:318–320.
147. Jacobs HB. Emergency percutaneous transtracheal catheter and ventilator. *J Trauma* 1972;12:50–55.
148. Fisher JA. A "Last Ditch" Airway. *Can J Anaesth* 1979;26:225–230.
149. McLellan I, Gordon P, Khawaja S, Thomas A. Percutaneous transtracheal high frequency jet ventilation as an aid to difficult intubation. *Can J Anaesth* 1988;35:404–405.
150. Boucek CD, Gunnerson HB, Tullock WC. Percutaneous transtracheal high-frequency jet ventilation as an aid to fiberoptic intubation. *Anesthesiology* 1987;67:247–249.
151. Scuderi PE, Mcleskey CH, Comer PB. Emergency percutaneous transtracheal ventilation during anesthesia using readily available equipment. *Anesth Analg* 1982;61:867–870.
152. Stinson TW. A simple connector for transtracheal ventilation *[letter]*. *Anesthesiology* 1977;47:232.
153. Gildar JS. A simple system for transtracheal ventilation *[letter]*. *Anesthesiology* 1983;58:106.
154. Benumof JL, Scheller MS. The importance of transtracheal jet ventilation in the management of the difficult airway. *Anesthesiology* 1989;71:769–778.
155. Poon YK. Case history number 89: a life-threatening complication of cricothyroid membrane puncture. *Anesth Analg* 1976;55:298–301.
156. Bainton CR. Cricothyrotomy. In: New concepts in airway management. *Internat Anesth Clinics* 1994;32:95–108.
157. Williamson JA, Webb RK, Spekely S, Gillies ERN, Dreosti AV. Difficult intubation: an analysis of 2000 incident reports. *Anaesth Intens Care* 1993;21:602–607.
158. Friman L, Hedenstierna G, Schildt B. Stenosis following tracheostomy. A quantitative study of long term results. *Anaesthesia* 1976;31:479–493.
159. Esner Z, Tur A, Diren B. Difficulty in endotracheal intubation due to congenital tracheal stenosis: a case report. *Anesthesiology* 1988;69:279–281.
160. Saito S, Dohi S, Tajima K. Failure of double-lumen endobronchial tube placement. Congenital tracheal stenosis in an adult. *Anesthesiology* 1987;66:83–85.
161. Smith DC, Pillai R, Gillbe CE. Tracheopathia osteochondroplastica. A cause of unexpected difficulty in tracheal intubation. *Anaesthesia* 1987;42:536–538.
162. Lundgren R, Stjernberg NL. Tracheobronchoplastica osteochondroplastica. A clinical bronchoscopic and spirometric study. *Chest* 1981;80:706–709.
163. Sapsford DJ, Snowdon SL. If in doubt, take it out. Obstruction of tracheal tube by prominent aortic knuckle. *Anaesthesia* 1985;40:552–554.
164. Martin J, Hutchinson B. Tracheal tube obstruction by prominent aortic knuckle. *Anaesthesia* 1986;41:86–87.
165. MacGillivray RG. Tracheal compression caused by aneurysm of the aortic arch. Implications for the anesthesiologist. *Anaesthesia* 1985;40:270–277.
166. Filston HC, Bruce Ferguson T Jr, Newland Oldham H. Airway obstruction by vascular anomalies. *Ann Surg* 1987;205:541–549.
167. Farrari LR, Bedford RF. General anesthesia prior to treatment of anterior mediastinal masses in pediatric cancer patients. *Anesthesiology* 1990;72:991–995.
168. Piro AH, Weiss DR, Hellman S. Mediastinal Hodgkin's disease: a probable danger for intubation anesthesia. *Int J Radiol Oncol Biol Phys* 1976;1:415–419.
169. Neuman GG, Weingarten AE, Abramowitz RM, et al. The anesthetic management of the patient with an anterior mediastinal mass. *Anesthesiology* 1984;60:144–147.
170. Rowbottom SJ, Sudhaman DA. Anaesthesia in the management of congenital tracheal stenosis. *Anaesth Intens Care* 1989;17:93–96.
171. Divatia JV, Sareen R, Upadhye SM, Sharma KS, Shelgaonkar JR. Anaesthetic management of tracheal surgery using the laryngeal mask airway. *Anaesth Intens Care* 1994;22:69–73.

CHAPTER 12

Laryngeal Mask Airway

Andranik Ovassapian, M.D. and Paul S. Mesnick, M.D.

The inability to maintain an open airway to provide adequate ventilation, even for a short time, may produce major physiologic complications leading to permanent organ damage. Tracheal intubation with a cuffed endotracheal tube provides the most effective means of direct airway ventilation and protection against aspiration. Difficulty in intubating a patient is frustrating, causing surgical cancellations, delays, and unnecessary complications; adequate face mask ventilation is difficult or even impossible in some patients. The laryngeal mask airway is a recently introduced airway management that is less complicated than tracheal intubation and easier to apply than face mask ventilation. The laryngeal mask airway (LMA) (Intravent International SA, Henley-on-Thames, England), developed by Dr. Archie I. J. Brain, provides continuity of the airway without entering the trachea, avoiding many of the difficulties commonly encountered with face mask ventilation (1–4). The device has gained a firm place in anesthesia practice and has replaced mask and endotracheal anesthesia in certain circumstances (3,4).

TECHNICAL ISSUES

The LMA consists of a silicone rubber tube, its distal end opening at a 30° angle into an elliptical-shaped mask (Fig. 1). The mask consists of a cuff, a pilot tube, and balloon. Two bars are incorporated into the junction of the tube and mask, preventing the epiglottis from herniating into the tube. The proximal end of the tube has a standard 15-mm adapter.

A black line runs longitudinally along the posterior curvature of the shaft to aid in recognizing the correct orientation of the tube. When the black line of the tube is facing the patient's upper lip, the cuff of the mask is aligned with the larynx. The LMA is available in six sizes and can be used in infants and large adults (Table 1). The LMA is autoclavable and may be reused multiple times.

Preparation of the LMA

The cuff and pilot valve of the LMA is checked for leaks by inflating the cuff with a volume of air slightly greater than the recommended maximum volume. The LMA should be discarded if herniation of the cuff wall is noted or if the tube (shaft) is discolored or kinks when flexed to 180° (5,6). The cuff valve should be replaced if the LMA cuff spontaneously refills with air after deflation.

Prior to use, the cuff is deflated so that the edge of the cuff appears smooth and faces away from the mask

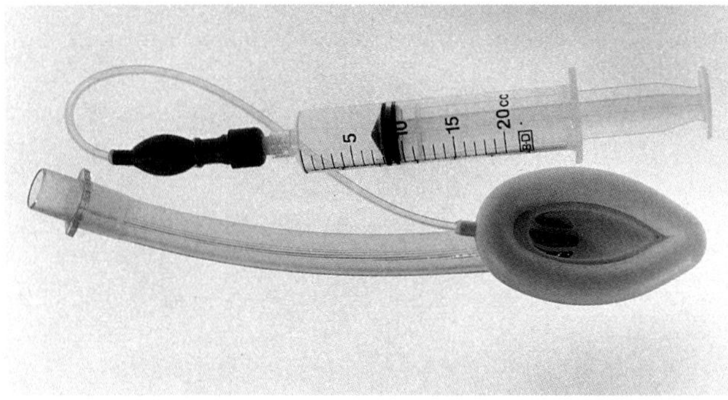

inlet. To help achieve correct deflation of the cuff, place the anterior (laryngeal) surface of the LMA on a flat surface, applying pressure on the mask with two fingers while deflating the cuff. The pharyngeal surface of the LMA is lubricated to assist insertion. The anterior surface of the device should not be lubricated since the lubricant gel may obstruct the distal end of the tube or enter the larynx provoking laryngospasm.

After use, the LMA should be washed, cleaned, dried, and sterilized in an autoclave at 120–130°C. The cuff should be completely deflated before autoclaving to avoid damage. Chemical disinfectants and ethylene oxide should be avoided, as they may damage the device.

Insertion of the LMA

The LMA can be inserted into an adequately anesthetized patient without muscle relaxation, although an adequate depth of anesthesia is required to prevent laryngeal spasm (2). If airway management is difficult, the LMA may be positioned under sedation and topical anesthesia (7,8). While different methods for insertion of the LMA have been suggested, none are superior to the standard technique originally described by the inventor (2,9):

1. The tube of the LMA is held between index finger and thumb, with the tip of the index finger placed at the anterior aspect of the tube, at the junction of the tube and mask.
2. With the patient's head in the "sniffing" position, the nondominant hand is placed under the occiput, extending the head, while the dominant hand inserts the LMA into the mouth (Fig. 2).
3. The tip of the mask is pressed upward against the hard palate and advanced toward the hypopharynx with the index finger.
4. As the LMA is advanced, the thumb reaches the patient's face. The thumb is now moved up pointing laterally, so as to let the index finger push the LMA as deep as possible into the hypopharynx.
5. The tube is now held by the nondominant "free" hand to prevent LMA movement as the index finger is withdrawn. The LMA is advanced further until resistance is felt.
6. Without holding the tube, the cuff is inflated with the recommended volume of air (Table 1). With cuff inflation, a slight forward movement of the tube, combined with anterior movement of the thyroid and cricoid cartilages, is usually noted.
7. If the LMA does not advance easily, jaw thrust maneuvers, tongue retraction, slight inflation of the cuff, and on rare occasion, the use of a rigid laryngoscope, may assist in passage into the hypopharynx. Rigid laryngoscopy may identify possible causes of obstruction, such as enlarged tonsils, and can assist LMA placement under direct vision. Repeated attempts at blind placement should be avoided to minimize trauma to the oropharynx.
8. Once the LMA is positioned, the breathing system is attached and positive pressure ventilation applied.
9. The longitudinal black line on the LMA tube should lie in the midline against the upper lip.
10. A bite block made of gauze wrapped around a tongue blade and placed between the molars will pre-

TABLE 1. *Specifications of laryngeal mask airway sizes*

Mask size	Patient weight (kg)	Internal diameter (mm)	Length (cm)	Cuff volume (ml)	ETT[a] size (ID[b] mm)
1	<6.5	5	10	5	3.5
2	7–20	7	11.5	10	4.5
2.5	20–30	8	12.5	14	5.0
3	30–70	10	19	20	6.0
4	normal adults	10	19	30	6.0
5	large adults	11.5	20	40	7.0

[a] ETT: Endotracheal tube, uncuffed.
[b] ID: Internal diameter.

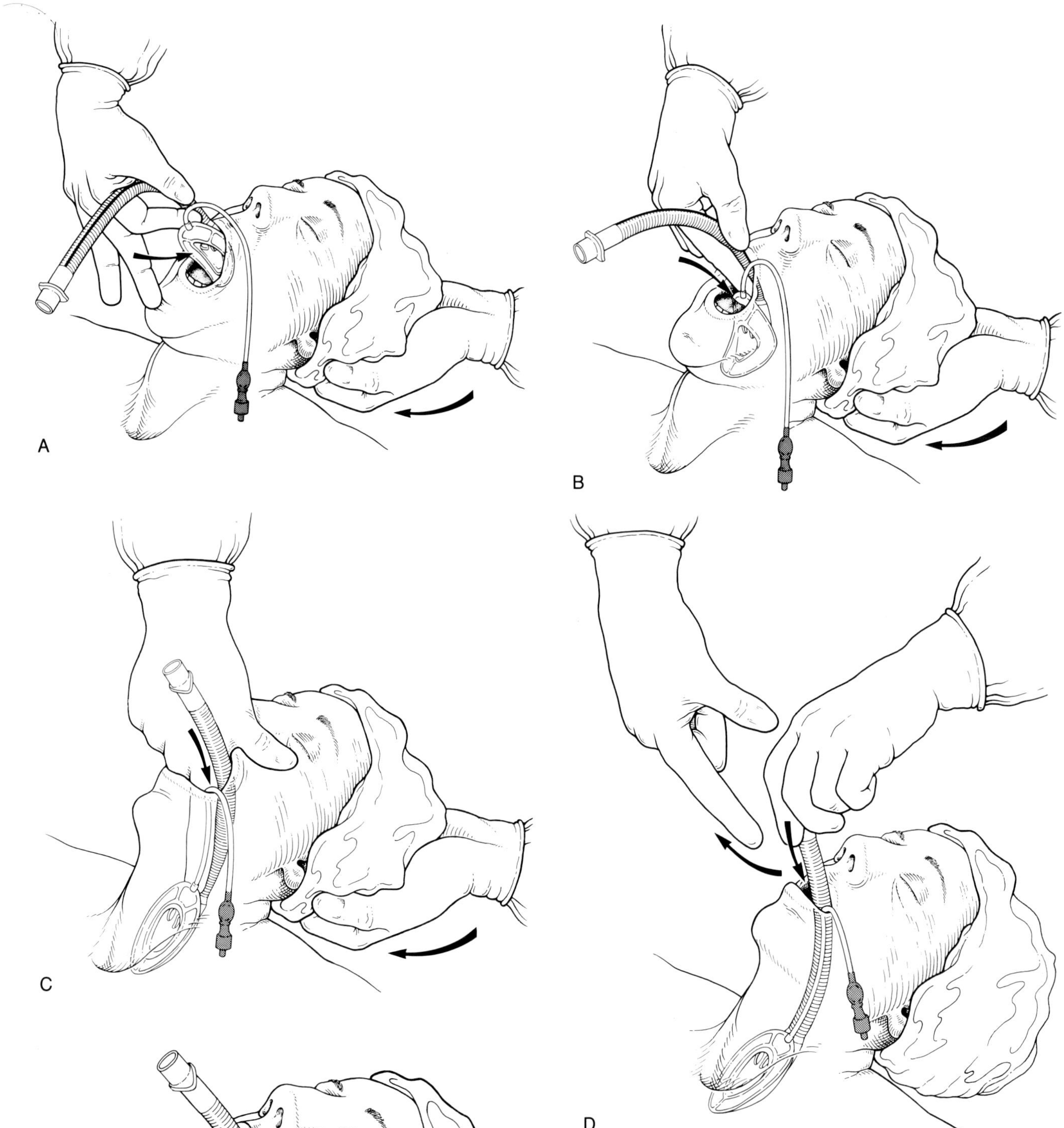

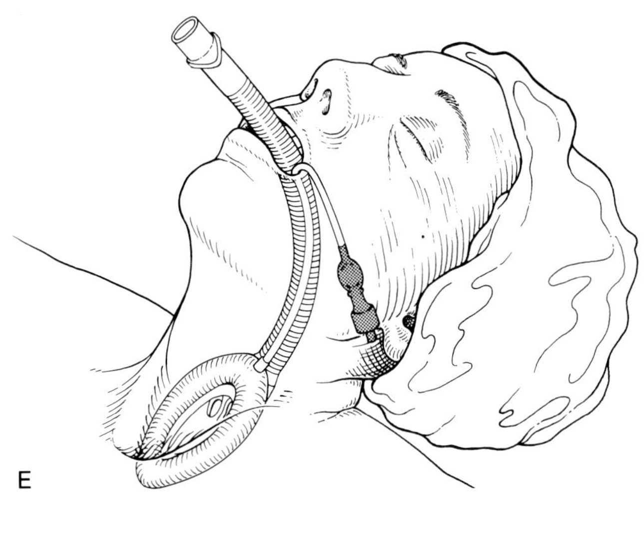

FIG. 2. A: Under direct vision, the mask is placed inside the mouth with its tip against the hard palate. Using the index finger, the mask is advanced into the pharynx while pressing against the palate. **B:** Keeping the head extended, the LMA is further advanced by pressing against the palate and posterior pharyngeal wall during insertion. **C:** The LMA is pushed as far down as possible with the index finger. **D:** The other hand holds the LMA in position while the index finger is withdrawn from the pharynx. The LMA is pushed downward with the other hand to ensure the mask is inserted as deep as possible. **E:** Proper position of the LMA with the cuff inflated. (With permission, ref. 5.)

vent the patient from biting down and obstructing or damaging the LMA. Taping of the LMA will secure its position and prevent accidental dislodgment.

Anatomical Position and Functional Status

The initial attempt at proper LMA placement, resulting in the patient's ability to ventilate adequately, is successful in 75–90% of cases and increases to 95–99% on subsequent attempts (10–14). When properly positioned, the tip of the LMA lies in the hypopharynx against the esophageal sphincter. The sides of the LMA rest in the piriform sinuses, with the upper edge of the mask lying at the base of the tongue (Fig. 3) (1). Once positioned and connected to the breathing circuit, gentle ventilation is provided. Good chest wall movement, auscultation of breath sounds, and capnography confirm proper function and position of the LMA.

An esophageal detector device may be used to evaluate the functional status of the LMA (15,16). A negative test, instant refill, indicates a clear airway; an equivocal test, slow refill, indicates that the patient is partially obstructed; and a positive test, no refill, indicates airway obstruction due to misplacement of the LMA or laryngeal spasm (16). The deepening of anesthesia or intravenous injection of a small dose (20 mg) of succinylcholine will overcome laryngeal spasm. An improperly positioned LMA requires removal and repositioning.

The LMA functions well under either spontaneous or controlled ventilation as long as peak inspiratory airway pressures are not too high (3,4). In addition to airway leaks, high peak pressures increase the likelihood of air entering the stomach, causing gastric dilatation (17).

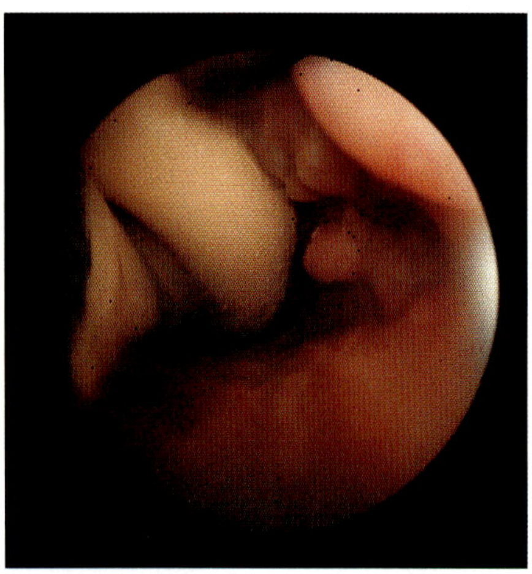

FIG. 3. Endoscopic view through mouth of properly positioned LMA. The inflated LMA cuff has blocked the right pyriform sinus and pushed the base of the tongue anteriorly.

Fullekrug et al. used fiberoptic bronchoscopy to study the various positions that the aperture of the LMA assumes in relation to the laryngeal entrance, as well as the degree of downfolding of the epiglottis over the glottic opening produced by the inflated LMA cuff (18). Their study showed the position of the LMA relative to the larynx to be central in 59% of cases, ventral in 8%, and dorsal in 4%. Right and left deviations were 20% and 9%, respectively (Fig. 4). The position of the epiglottis was graded based on epiglottis downfolding inside the LMA. In 13% of the cases, no downfolding was noted; the epiglottis blocked up to one-fourth of the view in 41% of cases; one-fourth to one-half of the view in 33%; and one-half to three-quarters in 8%. Blockade of the glottis that ranged from three-quarters to complete was noted in 5% of the cases (Fig. 5) (18). Overall, 87 of the 100 patients studied showed the epiglottis present within the LMA aperture.

Radiographic studies of the LMA also indicate that epiglottic downfolding is commonplace both in adults and children (19,20). The phenomenon of epiglottis downfolding is a common finding in older men, who tend to have a long, floppy epiglottis. Our experience in adult males reflects the findings of Fullekrug, with over 80% showing the epiglottis visible in the LMA aperture.

The Fullekrug study found no correlation between the position of the epiglottis inside the LMA and ease of ventilation or peak airway pressures allowing cuff leak. Other studies conducted by fiberoptic bronchoscopy, magnetic resonance imaging, and computed tomographic scan have demonstrated that ventilation by LMA can be clinically acceptable, with the device in a less-than-perfect position (14,19–21). This is due to the fact that while the epiglottis usually lies within the LMA, it rests back from the glottic opening so ventilation remains unobstructed. The mean distance between the "grill" of the LMA and the vocal cords is 3.1 cm in women and 3.6 cm in men (22).

Fullekrug and colleagues found a leakage of anesthetic gases in 26% of cases, with peak airway pressures of 20 cm H_2O or less (18). The waste anesthetic gas contamination was measured within 25–50 ppm during positive pressure breathing, with peak airway pressure up to 30 cm H_2O in 78% of cases. Sarma has shown that waste anesthetic gas concentration in spontaneously breathing patients using the LMA is comparable to intubation anesthesia (23).

Improper LMA placement can be attributed to the experience of the clinician, the method of placement, and interpretation of what constitutes malposition. Most improper LMA placement results from inexperience or positioning under light anesthesia, at which time the laryngopharynx reacts to LMA insertion by contraction of the cricopharyngeus and extrinsic laryngeal muscles (1,2). This changes the configuration of

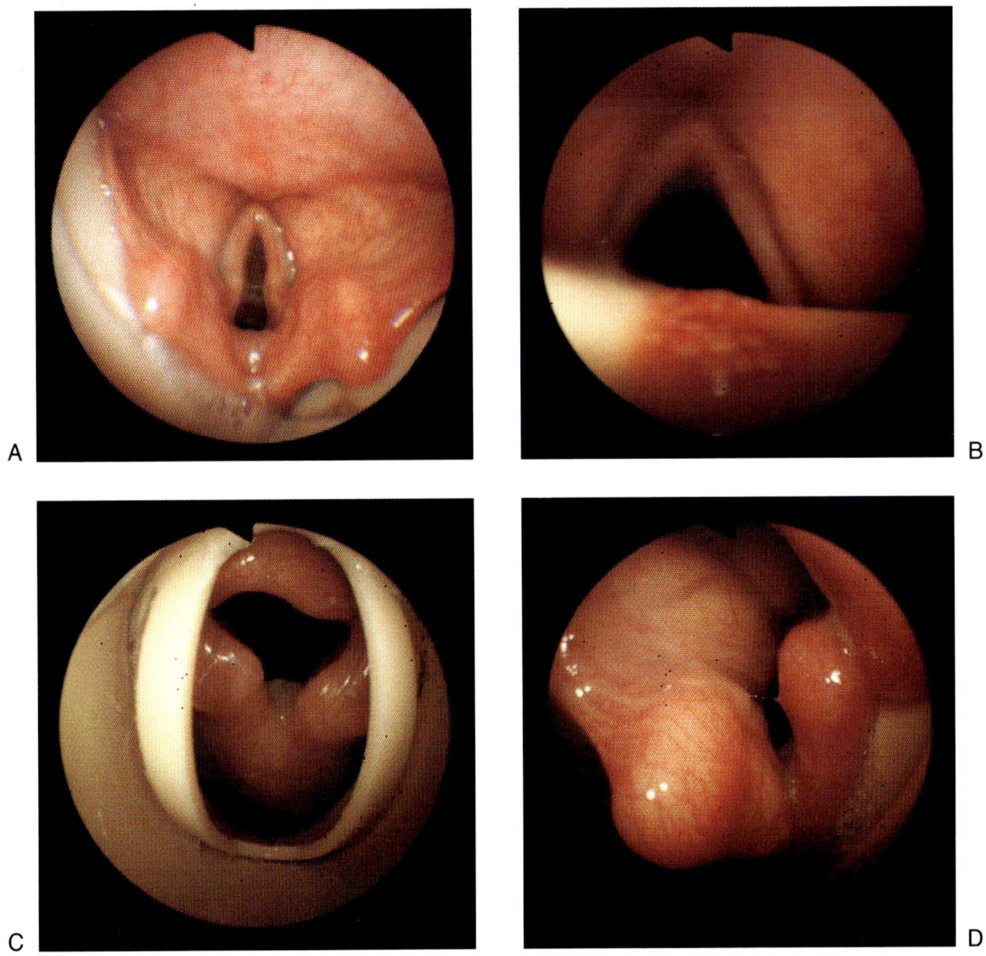

FIG. 4. Fiberscopic views of varying laryngeal mask positions in relation to the larynx. **A:** Central position. The LMA in a perfect central position. The tip of the fiberscope is positioned between the bars of the LMA. The epiglottis is not visible. The yellow color represents the inner border of the LMA. **B:** Ventral position. The lower edge of the LMA is blocking the lower half of the glottic opening. Bloody secretions due to minor trauma associated with insertion are noted. **C:** Dorsal position. The edge of the lower border of the LMA is approximately 15 mm below the arytenoids. **D:** Deviation to the right. The LMA has pushed the left arytenoid and aryepiglottic fold to the right, blocking the view of the vocal cords and glottic opening. Ventilation was unimpaired.

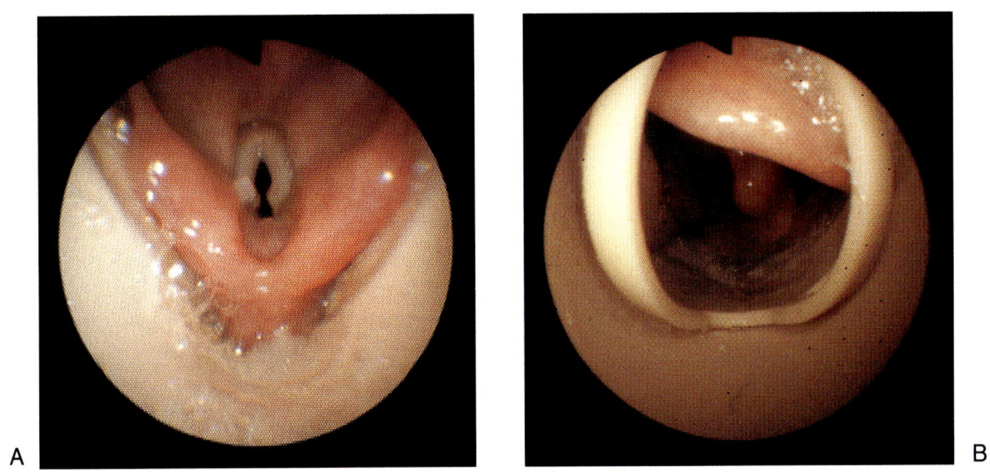

FIG. 5. Fiberscopic views showing the relationship of the epiglottis to the lumen of the laryngeal mask airway. **A:** Epiglottis is outside the LMA lumen. The cords are in full view. **B:** Epiglottis has occupied approximately 25% of the LMA lumen.

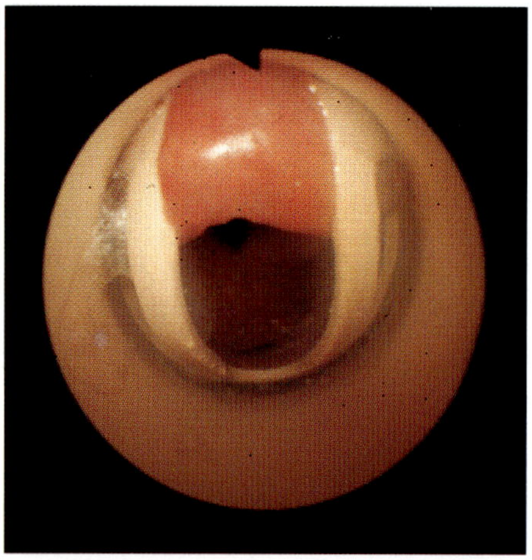
C

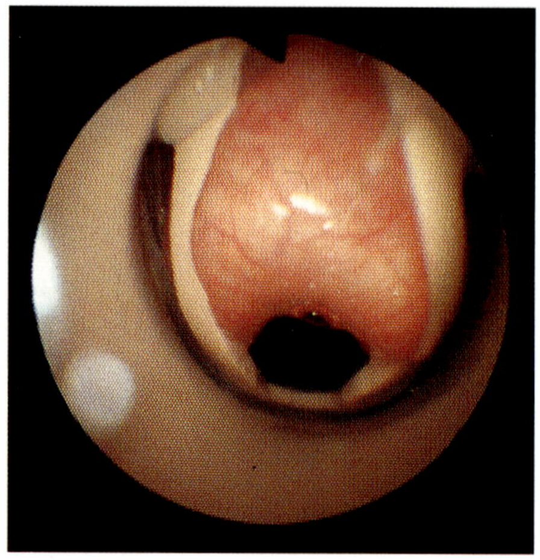
D

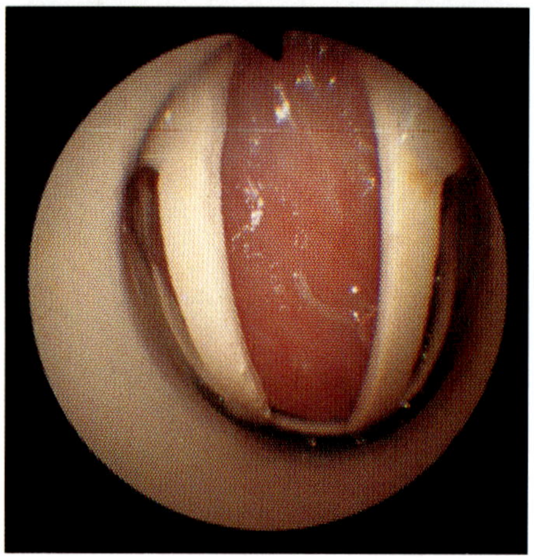
E **FIG. 5.** *Continued.* **C:** Epiglottis has occupied approximately 50% of the LMA lumen. **D:** Epiglottis has occupied approximately 75% of the LMA lumen. **E:** Epiglottis occupying entire LMA lumen. In this patient ventilation was unimpaired.

the hypopharyngeal structures, preventing passage of the LMA beyond the arytenoid level. Under these circumstances, the tip of the LMA mask may also migrate forward to impact in the vestibule of the larynx (20). Inadequate insertion of the LMA may obstruct the airway by pushing against the aryepiglottic fold. The LMA may also become twisted during placement or advanced too far down the airway (usually noted with selection an undersized LMA), causing airway obstruction. The LMA may fold over itself and kink if inserted with excessive force or not pressed firmly against the hard palate during insertion. The downfolding of the epiglottis, or laryngospasm stimulated during positioning, should not be considered evidence of improper placement.

Removal of the LMA

The LMA cuff protects the airway from pharyngeal secretions, which should be suctioned prior to deflating the cuff. The oral bite block is maintained in place until the LMA mask is removed. The LMA is well tolerated at light levels of anesthesia during emergence and can usually be maintained in place until the patient responds to verbal commands. If the spontaneously ventilating patient is transferred to the Post Anesthesia Care Unit (PACU) with the LMA in place, no manual airway support is necessary and supplemental oxygen can be administered by T-piece.

Cleaning and Sterilization

The LMA should be washed with water after use, before secretions dry on the airway. A brush is used to clean inside the airway shaft; care must be taken to avoid damage to the grill bars. Prior to autoclaving, the cuff is deflated to prevent damage to its structure. The LMA can withstand repeated autoclaving, and may be reused up to 40 times or more (5,6). The pilot valve is the most vulnerable part of the LMA. Replacement valves are available from the manufacturer.

INDICATIONS

The LMA may be used for a variety of surgical procedures under general anesthesia, thus avoiding the

TABLE 2. *Laryngeal mask airway (LMA) versus face mask*

Advantages
The anesthetist's hands are free
Lower incidence of hypoxemia
Surgical interruptions are less frequent
Excellent access for head and neck operations
Acceptable airway obtained >95% of cases.
Disadvantages
Cannot achieve the equivalent of the "tight bag and mask" airway pressure
Can cause oro-hypopharyngeal trauma
Large tonsils can hinder LMA insertion
Kinking of LMA tube is possible

common difficulties of face mask anesthesia (Table 2) (3,4,10,23) as well as the technical difficulties and complications of tracheal intubation (Table 3) (3,4,10,24–26). The LMA is particularly useful for short anesthetics administered for radiotherapy, dressing changes, and skin grafting procedures. Minor head and neck procedures, laser facial surgery, and eye examination under general anesthesia all lend themselves well to the technique. The LMA has been used for intraoral procedures, such as dental extraction, adenotonsillectomy, repair of cleft palate, and reduction and fixation of mandibular and nasal fractures (3,4). The relative lack of coughing and straining on emergence noted with LMA and the concomitant stability in intraocular pressure are potential benefits in open eye surgery (27,28); however, if the LMA becomes kinked or dislodged during surgery, access to the airway is limited and intubation of the trachea more risky if the eye has been surgically opened (29). These factors need to be weighed by the clinician. The LMA presents special advantages in select diagnostic and therapeutic situations that are discussed below (Table 4).

TABLE 3. *Laryngeal mask airway (LMA) versus endotracheal tube*

Advantages
Avoids esophageal and endobronchial intubation.
Excellent for professional singers.
Less adrenergic and intraocular pressure response.
Excellent for repeated anesthetics in pediatrics.
Can facilitate fiberoptic airway endoscopy.
Fiberoptic observation of vocal cords possible.
May be used to facilitate tracheal intubation.
LMA can be placed without the neck manipulation.
Disadvantages
Laryngospasm and airway obstruction possible.
Does not prevent aspiration.
Not suitable for large tidal volumes with high airway pressure ventilation.
One-lung ventilation not possible.
Not suitable in presence of oropharyngeal mass.

TABLE 4. *Special indications of laryngeal mask airway (LMA)*

Management of the difficult airway
LMA as primary airway
Emergency airway management "can't intubate–can't ventilate" situation
LMA-aided difficult tracheal intubation
Fiberoptic bronchoscopy
In professional voice users
Tracheal stenosis
Tracheostomy
Extubation
Postextubation airway support

Fiberoptic Bronchoscopy

The LMA provides an excellent airway for fiberoptic bronchoscopy under general or Monitored Anesthesia Care (MAC) anesthesia (30–36) and its advantages over tracheal intubation (32,35) are summarized in Table 5. The LMA permits an unhurried examination of the vocal cords, larynx, upper trachea, and bronchial tree, as well as the use of a larger flexible bronchoscope during endoscopy, without compromising airway resistance or effective ventilation. The fiberoptic bronchoscope is easily passed through the LMA, avoiding nasal instrumentation and resultant nasopharyngeal trauma. In our hospital, the LMA has replaced tracheal intubation for bronchoscopies performed prior to thoracotomy. After completion of bronchoscopy, the LMA is removed and a double-lumen endobronchial tube is placed for separation of lungs and one-lung ventiltion. Our surgical colleagues have been receptive and positive about the role of LMA in bronchoscopy.

Professional Voice Users

The LMA holds advantages over tracheal intubation for professional voice users requiring general anesthesia (37–40). Tracheal intubation, even of short dura-

TABLE 5. *Fiberoptic bronchoscopy through laryngeal mask airway*

Vocal cords are easier to find.
Provides optimal condition for evaluation of the entire airway.
Allows uninterrupted bronchoscopy.
Allows bigger fiberscope to be used.
Offers excellent conditions to both the endoscopist and anesthetist.
Low airway resistance, easy to ventilate.
Anesthesia circuit can be scavenged.
Well tolerated by patient.
Avoids tracheal intubation.
Avoids intubation trauma, especially in tracheal stenosis.
Does not secure the airway as well as a cuffed endotracheal tube.

tion, may cause changes in the mucosa of the vocal cords. Voice changes are significantly reduced in LMA patients compared to tracheal intubated patients, thus Harris and colleagues recommend LMA whenever possible in professional voice users (37).

The LMA, combined with fiberoptic bronchoscopy, provides a unique opportunity for intermittent or continuous observation of the vocal cords during the surgery without interrupting ventilation. Stimulation of the recurrent laryngeal nerve allows for easily observed movement of the innervated vocal cord. A videofiberscope allows observation of vocal cord function by the surgeon when the recurrent laryngeal nerve is identified and stimulated.

Direct visualization of the vocal cords with recurrent laryngeal nerve stimulation was advocated by Riddell to prevent bilateral recurrent laryngeal nerve palsy during thyroid surgery (41). However, repeated observation of vocal cord function during anesthesia was not possible because of difficulties in airway management (41).

Concerns about LMA use in thyroidectomy include difficulties in placement, displacement of the LMA by surgical manipulation, and the inability to support the tracheal airway in the presence of tracheomalacia. In one series, the LMA was successfully placed in 11 of 13 thyroidectomy patients, representing a 15% failure rate (39). Although routine use of the LMA during thyroidectomy may not be justified, it is a valuable option in patients who use their voice professionally. If airway maintenance becomes a problem during thyroidectomy, a 6-mm endotracheal tube can be placed into the trachea through the LMA (38).

Tracheal Stenosis

The LMA provides an alternative to endotracheal intubation and may play a unique role in anesthetic management of patients with stenosis of the upper trachea (42). If general anesthesia is needed for head and neck procedures, a face mask cannot be used because it blocks access and stenosis of the proximal trachea, leaving inadequate room for tracheal tube placement above the stenosis (42–44). Intubation of stenotic trachea with a small-size tube may cause trauma, edema, and acute airway obstruction after extubation (42,43).

The LMA eliminates the risk of tracheal tumor dislodgment and bleeding, which is likely with tracheal intubation with conventional technique. The LMA serves as a conduit through which an endotracheal tube, suction catheter, and fiberoptic bronchoscope can be passed (44). Its use is contraindicated in patients with external compression of the trachea or tracheomalacia.

Another unique application of the LMA is described for a tracheoplasty in a patient with tracheopathia osteoplastica (45). The surgical procedure involved placement of a 14-mm silicone T-Y tube inside the trachea. Induction of general anesthesia was followed by placement of a 7-mm endotracheal tube. A left endobronchial tube was inserted when the trachea was opened for placement of the T-Y prosthesis. Upon tracheal closure, the endotracheal tube was withdrawn just above the vocal cords to accommodate the proximal end of the silicone tube prosthesis inside the larynx. The "T" part of the tube exited from the anterior neck like a tracheostomy tube. The "Y" portion of the prosthesis straddled the carina, with the proximal arm of the T-Y tube positioned just below the vocal cords (Fig. 6). At the conclusion of the tracheal repair, the endobronchial tube was removed and ventilation attempted through the "T" tube end of the prosthesis. Ventilation proved ineffective, due to a large air leak through the proximal end of the prosthesis lying below the vocal cords. The endotracheal tube which was not providing the seal was removed, and a size 3 LMA inserted. Placement of a Kelly clamp across the proximal shaft of the LMA stopped the air leak, allowing adequate ventilation through the "T" tube, and completion of the surgery.

Tracheostomy

The LMA may be used during tracheostomy to assist or control ventilation. Fiberscopic endoscopy allows direct observation of tracheostomy tube placement into the tracheal lumen (46). The combination of fiberoptic bronchoscopy and LMA during tracheostomy holds promise, but clinical experience is limited.

Extubation of the Trachea

The LMA has been used as an aid in tracheal extubation and as a means of supporting ventilation in patients who demonstrate inadequate ventilation immediately after extubation (47). One case report illustrates successful application of the LMA in managing laryngospasm after tracheal extubation in a patient with a difficult airway (48).

The LMA may be substituted for an endotracheal tube to minimize postextubation airway problems, such as the inability to maintain a clear airway while the patient is still emerging from anesthesia, or prior to the administration of a neuromuscular reversing agent. Another advantage of substituting an LMA prior to emergence is the minimizing of cardiovascular disturbances associated with tracheal extubation (49).

Complications and Contraindications

Features that limit the applicability of the LMA (2,3,50) are summarized in Table 6. The LMA does

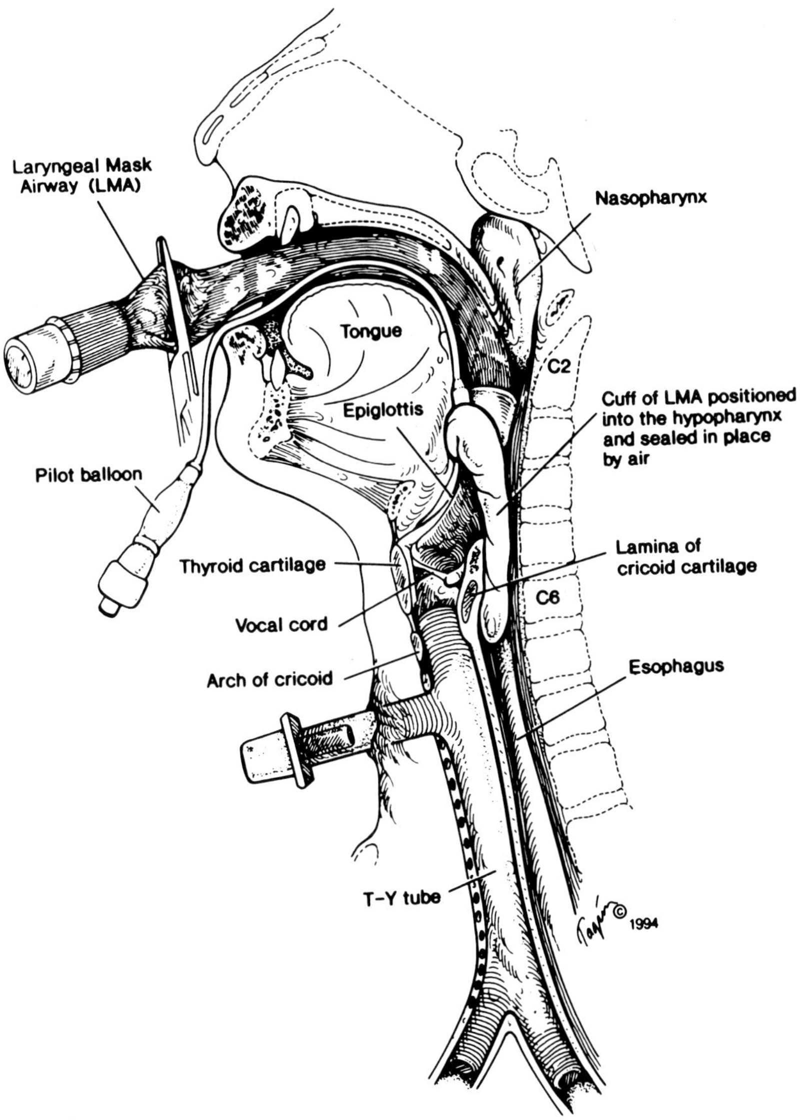

FIG. 6. This figure shows T-Y tracheal prosthesis in place. Laryngeal mask provided the seal around the larynx preventing air leak from above and allowing ventilation through the "T" tracheostomy tube. (With permission, ref. 45.)

not protect the airway from aspiration and should be avoided in patients at high risk for this condition (51–54). However, it may serve as a life-saving measure in emergency circumstance when more definitive techniques of airway support are not available or have proved unsuccessful.

A new two-lumen laryngeal mask designed to protect the lungs against aspiration of gastric contents has recently been introduced. It incorporates a second mask to isolate the upper esophagus and a second cuff to increase the seal against the glottis (55). A gastric tube can be passed through the second tube into the esophagus. The new design provides higher seal pressures and better isolation of the respiratory tract from the gastrointestinal tract; however, as it is bulkier and less flexible than the original, it is more difficult to place and the possiblity of pharyngeal trauma is much higher. The esophageal vent-laryngeal mask was suggested by Akhtan as another modification to aid in the prevention of gastric content aspiration (56). The mask consists of a 10-mm tracheal tube fixed to the dorsum of a standard LMA. The tube functions like a esophageal obturator airway and enters the esophagus. Placement difficulties include dificulties with insertion and tracheal placement of the obturator (57).

That LMA compression pressures could potentially interfere with circulation in the pharyngeal tissues, thus producing ischemic damage, is a concern (58). The

TABLE 6. *Limiting features of laryngeal mask airway*

Risk of aspiration
Risk of airway obstruction
Malposition
Laryngospasm
Limited positive pressure ventilation
Oral approach only

pressure transmitted to the pharyngeal mucosa by the inflated cuff of the LMA is significantly higher than tissue capillary perfusion pressure. Further, the diffusion of nitrous oxide into the LMA cuff has been reported to have produced intracuff pressures as high as 110 mm Hg (59). Other investigators have reported a mean rise of intracuff pressure of 30 mm Hg over 30 min of nitrous oxide anesthesia (60).

The actual degree of tissue trauma secondary to LMA cuff compression is unknown. Compression paralysis of the twelfth cranial nerve (61), hypoglossal nerve (62), and bilateral recurrent laryngeal nerve (63) have been reported. Hematoma of the vocal cord in a patient with bleeding disorder (64) and trauma to uvula and tonsils have been reported (65,66). In one case report, the LMA caused cyanosis of the tip of the tongue. Changing a size 4 LMA to a size 3 LMA corrected the problem and patient showed no complication after the case was completed (67). It is advisable to measure LMA intracuff pressure, if nitrous oxide is being administered during anesthesia. The removal of 25% of the LMA cuff volume, or inflating the LMA cuff with a nitrous oxide–oxygen mixture, shall prevent further increase in intracuff pressure.

Positive pressure ventilation through the LMA is contraindicated in patients with poor lung compliance or increased airway resistance (68). Due to air leakage, high airway pressures may further aggravate inadequate ventilation, and promote gastric distention, increasing the risk of gastric regurgitation.

LMA use should be avoided in procedures where access to the airway is limited (e.g., procedures involving the prone position or major head and neck procedures). Large tonsils or a large floppy epiglottis can make LMA placement difficult, especially in children. The epiglottis may also become trapped between the LMA bars, producing tissue edema and causing airway obstruction after LMA removal (69).

LMA AND THE DIFFICULT AIRWAY

The LMA has been used successfully in difficult airway circumstances in adults and children (70–90). The LMA provides the following unique roles in the management of the difficult airway that are not available in other devices or techniques (91–100). These contributions cover four areas. The LMA can serve

1. as a primary airway in patients with a history of, or exhibiting features of, a difficult airway.
2. to establish viable ventilation in the emergency circumstance when more traditional methods are unsuccessful.
3. to facilitate a difficult tracheal intubation.
4. to provide a convenient conduit for fiberscopic evaluation of the airway.

The LMA as the Primary Airway

The LMA has been successfully used as a primary airway in patients with compromising airway problems such as cervical spine disease (84,97,101), juvenile arthritis (102), mandibular fractures, neck tissue contractures (3), Pierre Robin syndrome (8,87), Treacher Collins' syndrome (103), Goldenhar's syndrome (7), pediatric cleft palate (104), and in adult patients with Mallampati Class III and IV airways (105). The LMA has been successfully inserted and secured in the awake patient (83,84,97), including neonates (7,8,106), prior to induction of anesthesia. The LMA allows a smooth transition from the awake, spontaneous breathing state to the anesthetized state, avoiding episodes of airway obstruction during induction.

In the patient known or suspected of being a difficult intubation, the LMA should not be substituted for tracheal intubation unless the procedure is limited in scope and the airway remains readily accessible.

LMA in the "Can't Intubate–Can't Ventilate" Situation

In this frightening situation, fast emergency insertion of an LMA has proved successful (73–75,79,91,107). The speed and atraumatic nature of LMA placement places it high on the list of rapid corrective techniques employable under these circumstances and should be considered prior to the application of more aggressive techniques, such as cricothyrotomy or transtracheal jet ventilation. The LMA has high likelihood of providing a good airway and conduit for follow-up tracheal intubation. In the United Kingdom it has been recognized as an emergency option in failed intubations during emergency cesarean section (86).

The LMA provided a secure airway in 95% of the patients during routine anesthesia, and a recent study indicates that insertion of the LMA in patients experiencing difficult endotracheal intubations may be equally successful (108).

The close proximity of the correctly placed LMA to the cricoid cartilage may make LMA insertion, as well as blind tracheal intubation, through the LMA more difficult with cricoid pressure (109–112). When correctly positioned, the tip of the LMA lies on the floor of the hypopharynx below the level of the cricoid cartilage (25). Cricoid pressure may compress the hypopharynx, preventing the distal tip of the LMA from occupying its proper position. Cricoid pressure may therefore need to be temporarily abated to permit the airway's insertion. The LMA does not compromise cricoid pressure once it is in place (113). Asai and Morris have suggested that in emergency cases the LMA should be tried only once and cricoid pressure should be temporarily released during insertion (114). A reasonable course of action may be to attempt LMA placement initially with cricoid pressure, and if not successful, to initiate a second attempt while cricoid pressure is transiently released (110).

Lack of airway protection against aspiration, mentioned previously, is a major shortcoming of the LMA; however, this does not exclude its emergency use when tracheal intubation has failed in the patient at risk for aspiration. The LMA may help to minimize regurgitation and aspiration by preventing spontaneous ventilation against an obstructed airway, and it prevents gastric distention, secondary to vigorous forced positive pressure ventilation, common during difficult mask ventilation. The LMA has proved lifesaving on several occasions when intubation and mask ventilation failed on full stomach patients (73–75,80).

The LMA is included as an option for management of failed intubation in the American Society of Anesthesiologists guidelines for Management of the Difficult Airway (Fig. 1, Chapter 11) (115).

Tracheal Intubation through the Laryngeal Mask Airway

The LMA can be used to guide an endotracheal tube into the trachea. After an emergency LMA placement, a decision should be made on whether to proceed with tracheal intubation. Factors to consider include the nature of the surgical procedure, position of the patient during surgery, the duration of airway management, risk of aspiration, and the leakage pressure around the LMA cuff. Three distinct techniques can be used for tracheal intubation through the LMA in the awake or anesthetized patient (83,84,87,92–100).

1. Blind passage of an endotracheal tube through the LMA
2. Blind insertion of a bougie or tube changer to facilitate the threading of a suitably sized endotracheal tube following LMA removal.
3. Fiberoptic assisted tracheal intubation through the LMA

When the LMA is properly positioned, the LMA aperture lies directly against the glottic inlet, allowing tracheal intubation with a blind or fiberoptic-aided technique. Tracheal intubation through the LMA is facilitated if glottic reflexes are obtunded by topical anesthesia, deep general anesthesia, or muscle relaxant.

Heath and Allagain reported a 90% success rate passing a 6.0-mm endotracheal tube blindly through an LMA without application of cricoid pressure in 50 elective surgical patients (94). When cricoid pressure was utilized in another 50-patient series, the success rate fell to 56%.

Lim et al. studied the influence of the type of endotracheal tube, as well as head positioning, on the success rate of blind intubation through the LMA in anesthetized patients. When a Portex tube was used, intubation was successful after three attempts in 93% of cases (116). The "sniffing" head position was found to be the optimal head position for this technique.

Blind Intubation Technique

The following technique described by Brain is performed with the patient paralyzed under general anesthesia.

1. A lubricated 6-mm uncut, cuffed endotracheal tube is passed through the LMA to its full length. The tube is rotated to the left during passage to avoid the beveled tip impinging against the LMA bar.
2. Check that an adequate length of the endotracheal tube extends beyond the LMA bars to ensure cuff placement beyond the vocal cords. Keep in mind that the vocal cords are located 3.5 cm from the LMA aperture bars after LMA positioning.
3. Withdraw the endotracheal tube inside the LMA with its tip placed just proximal to the bars, and positioned so it shall not encounter the bars on passage.
4. Inflate the endotracheal tube cuff to form a gastight seal inside the LMA.
5. Mark the endotracheal tube where it emerges from the LMA 15-mm adapter, and place a second mark 3 cm above the first.
6. Insert the LMA using the standard technique, and inflate the LMA cuff.
7. Connect the anesthesia circuit to the endotracheal tube, and ventilate the patient. If ventilation is appropriate and unobstructed, proceed with intubation.
8. Deflate the endotracheal tube cuff, holding the LMA with one hand, advance the endotracheal tube with the other, observing the anterior neck. As the endotracheal tube is advanced, its tip shall contact the anterior laryngeal wall at the level of the anterior commissure of the vocal cords. This is identified by anterior displacement of the thyroid cartilage. The endotracheal tube is advanced further into the trachea. If it does not slip into the trachea, flex the head forward to change its angle, pull the tube back slightly, and readvance it.
9. If the thyroid cartilage is not anteriorly displaced during intubation, the LMA is probably positioned below the level of the vocal cords and the endotracheal

tube has advanced into the esophagus. The LMA should be withdrawn slightly and the procedure repeated. Withdraw the endotracheal tube to its original position at the first mark before withdrawing the LMA.

10. Resistance to endotracheal tube passage before the 3-cm mark is usually due to epiglottis blockage. This can frequently be countered by repeating the procedure and pushing the endotracheal tube 1 cm beyond the LMA aperture prior to LMA cuff inflation. Repeated attempts at passing an endotracheal tube or bougie through the LMA into the trachea increase the risk of trauma and esophageal intubation and should be avoided.

Fiberoptic Intubation Technique

Fiberoptic observation of the larynx through the LMA has demonstrated that epiglottis downfolding is common in adults and children (Fig. 3) (18). Downfolding frequently interferes with blind endotracheal tube and bougie placement into the trachea, and caution should be exercised when using the blind technique (14,98,117). Fiberoptic intubation through the LMA is far more reliable than blind techniques since the flexible bronchoscope negotiates any epiglottis downfolding and can be placed inside the trachea under direct vision (92). Fiberoptic-assisted tracheal intubation through the LMA was first reported in anesthetized adults in 1991 (92) and children in 1992 (118). Johnson and Sims reported LMA placement under topical anesthesia followed by fiberoptic intubation through the LMA in an infant with Goldenhar's syndrome (7). The following narrative describes this technique.

A 4.0-mm well-lubricated fiberscope mounted with a 6.0-mm tube is passed through a pre-positioned size 4 LMA. The larynx is exposed, and the fiberscope advanced into the trachea. The endotracheal tube is threaded over the fiberscope into the trachea, and its cuff inflated. The fiberscope is removed, the LMA cuff deflated, and ventilation carried out through the endotracheal tube. At the conclusion of anesthesia, the LMA cuff is reinflated and the endotracheal tube removed, allowing the patient to breath through the LMA until airway reflexes return. Upon emergence from anesthesia the LMA is removed.

The 6.0-mm cuffed endotracheal tube is 28 cm in length, compared to the 19-cm length of the size 4 LMA. The mean distance of the LMA grille to the vocal cords is 3.5 cm, leaving only 4.5 cm of endotracheal tube to pass beyond the vocal cords. The chance of inflating the cuff of the endotracheal tube in the larynx, rather than in the trachea, is thereby increased.

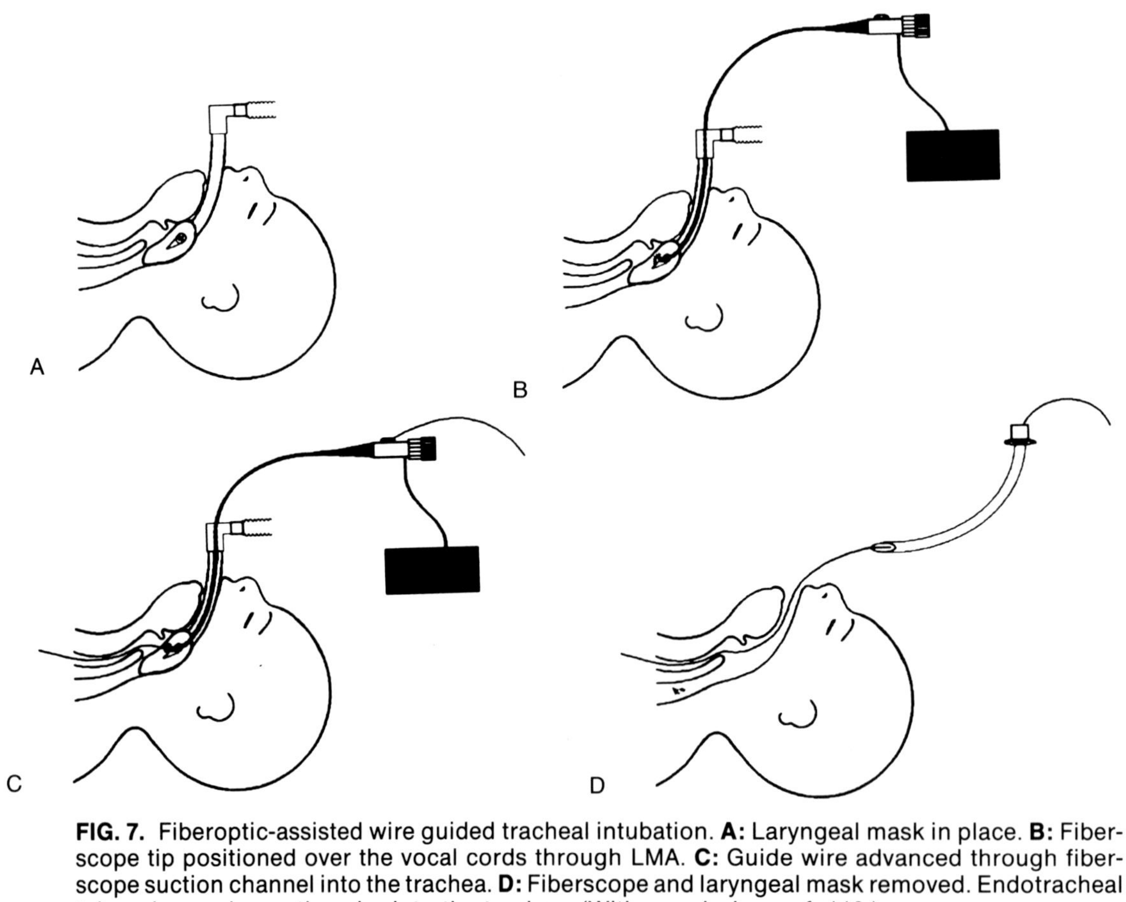

FIG. 7. Fiberoptic-assisted wire guided tracheal intubation. **A:** Laryngeal mask in place. **B:** Fiberscope tip positioned over the vocal cords through LMA. **C:** Guide wire advanced through fiberscope suction channel into the trachea. **D:** Fiberscope and laryngeal mask removed. Endotracheal tube advanced over the wire into the trachea. (With permission, ref. 119.)

This may increase the possibility of recurrent laryngeal nerve damage.

The removal of the 15-mm LMA adapter prior to intubation shortens the length of the LMA by 18 mm, allowing deeper placement of the endotracheal tube inside the trachea. Other options to counter this problem include selection of a longer endotracheal tube, such as the Malinckrodt reinforced tube, or removal of the LMA prior to final positioning of the endotracheal tube.

A bougie or tube changer can be passed through the LMA under fiberoptic observation into the trachea. Once the tube changer is positioned in the trachea, the LMA cuff is deflated and the device pulled up over the insertion cord of the fiberscope. The fiberscope is removed, leaving the tube changer in place. A standard endotracheal tube is then advanced over the bougie or tube changer into the trachea. A hollow tube changer is preferred in this technique since correct tracheal placement can be confirmed by end-tidal carbon dioxide gas sampling air through the tube. This is particularly helpful when a blind technique is utilized or when blood or secretions prevent fiberoptic visualization of the airway.

The fiberscope's role is limited in assisting the passage of the bougie into the trachea. A smaller-size tube changer should be used, as the LMA shaft has limited space to accommodate both the fiberscope and the tube changer.

Another technique is to pass guide wire through the suction channel of the fiberscope into the trachea, using the guide wire for placement of an endotracheal tube into the trachea. This technique will allow the use of a larger-size fiberscope to place the guide wire in the pediatric age group (Fig. 7) (119,120) .

In an attempt to overcome the limitations posed by a 6.0-mm tube relative to long-term ventilation and airway suctioning, a longitudinally split size 3 LMA has been recommended (96,121). The split LMA allows larger-sized endotracheal tube advancement and placement. The cuff of the split LMA is sealed with silicone, and the LMA shaft bound with micropore tape. The LMA is then inserted, and its cuff fully inflated. The fiberscope loaded with the endotracheal tube is passed through the LMA into the trachea. The LMA is then deflated. The tape is removed from the LMA, and the standard size endotracheal tube is threaded over the fiberscope, through the LMA, and into the trachea.

The key advantages of fiberoptic intubation through the LMA, over conventional fiberoptic intubation, is the ease with which identification of the laryngeal inlet and passage of the tube over the fiberscope into the trachea can be carried out. The main disadvantage of the technique is the limitation on the size of the endotracheal tube that can be passed in the unmodified LMA.

LARYNGEAL MASK AIRWAY AND RESUSCITATION

The first use of the LMA for emergency prehospital airway control was reported by Greene in 1992 (122). Critical care nurses, medical and paramedical personnel, and dental officers have been highly successful in their first attempt at LMA placement (123–126).

In one study, 130 nurses trained in LMA use were able to place the device within three attempts during resuscitation of 164 cardiac arrest patients (125). The first attempt success rate was 71%, and 26% of cases at the second attempt. The overall failure rate of satisfactory ventilation was 12%. Tracheal intubation proved difficult in 11 of these patients when attempts were made to replace the LMA with a tracheal tube. The LMA was properly replaced and ventilation satisfactorily continued in all failed intubation cases. Thirty-three patients (20%) showed evidence of regurgitation: 20 before LMA placement, 3 during LMA insertion, and 10 after LMA removal. Only one patient (0.6%) had clinical evidence of pulmonary aspiration.

In a second study, the LMA was successfully used by an anesthesiologist in 21 neonates requiring in-hospital resuscitation (127). Twenty neonates responded favorably, with improvement in vital signs. One infant required tracheal intubation for intratracheal drug administration.

The success rate for placement of the LMA by unskilled personnel is higher than that for tracheal intubation. Once the LMA is correctly positioned, airway management is also easier than techniques that use a bag valve and mask. Davies et al. (126) studied the ability of medical nurse trainees to correctly place the LMA compared to endotracheal intubation. The success rate of LMA placement was 94%, with an average placement time of 20 sec. In the same group of nurse trainees, tracheal intubation was successful in only 51% of cases, with an average placement time of 35 sec. The nurses were better able to ventilate with the LMA than by face mask.

Martin and associates (124) compared the adequacy of ventilation by the LMA with that of mask ventilation, as performed by nurses and medical students. The adequacy of ventilation (no increase in end-tidal carbon dioxide) and oxygenation (arterial oxygen saturation greater than 90%) was achieved after 2 min of ventilation. Adequate ventilation was found in 87% of patients ventilated through the LMA; 43% were adequately ventilated with the Ambu bag and mask.

CONCLUSION

The use of the LMA in anesthesia is well established, but its role in airway management outside of the operating room is still under evaluation. A number of recent publications based on controlled clinical studies, as well as anecdotal case reports of its emergency use, have been encouraging. Further development and modification of the device will expand its role and improve its effectiveness in airway management of emergency patients.

The LMA is a safe and effective means of airway management in the anesthetized patient. Proper patient selection and identification of improperly positioned LMA are important skills required for safe use. It has proven to be lifesaving in the management of the difficult airway or failed intubation.

Many concerns associated with its use remain. New complications or side effects may emerge as its use becomes more commonplace. In some cases these will be due simply to its inappropriate use. Better understanding of the device shall be gained with added clinical experience, better defining its indications, advantages, and disadvantages and adding to its efficacious use. The future of this simple, valuable airway management tool seems secure.

REFERENCES

1. Brain AI. The laryngeal mask: a new concept in airway management. *Br J Anaesth* 1983;55:801–805.
2. Verghese C, Smith TG, Young E. Prospective survey of the use of the laryngeal mask airway in 2359 patients. *Anaesthesia* 1993;48:58–60.
3. Pennant JH, White PF. The laryngeal mask airway: its use in anesthesiology. *Anesthesiology* 1993;79:144–163.
4. Asai T, Morris S. The laryngeal mask airway: its features, effects and role. *Can J Anaesth* 1994;41:930–960.
5. Brain AIJ. The Intavent laryngeal mask. *Instruction manual.* 2nd ed. London: 1993.
6. Asai T, Vaughan RS: Misuse of the laryngeal mask airway. *Anaesthesia* 1994;49:467–469.
7. Johnson CM, Sims C: Awake fibreoptic intubation via a laryngeal mask in an infant with Goldenhar's Syndrome. *Anaesth and Intens Care* 1994;22:194–197.
8. Markakis DA, Sayson SC, Schreiner MS. Insertion of the laryngeal mask airway in awake infants with the Robin Sequence. *Anesth Analg* 1992;75:822–824.
9. Brimacombe J, Berry A. Insertion of the laryngeal mask airway—a prospective study of four techniques. *Anaesth Intens Care* 1993;21:89–92.
10. Malty JR, Loken RG, Watson NC: The laryngeal mask airway: clinical appraisal in 250 patients. *Can J Anaesth* 1990;37:509–513.
11. McCrirrick A, Ramage DTO, Pracillo JA, Hickman JA. Experience with the laryngeal mask airway in two hundred patients. *Anaesth Intens Care* 1991;19:256–260.
12. Blake DW, Dawson P, Donnan G, Bjorksten A. Propofol induction for laryngeal mask airway insertion: dose requirement and cardiopulmonary effects. *Anaesth Intens Care* 1992;20:479–483.
13. O'Neil B, Templeton JJ, Caramico L, Schreiner MS. The laryngeal mask airway in pediatric patients: factors affecting ease of use during insertion and emergence. *Anesth Analg* 1994;78:659–662.
14. Rowbottom SJ, Simpson DL, Grubb D. The laryngeal mask airway in children. A fiberoptic assessment of positioning. *Anaesthesia* 1991;46:489–491.
15. Wee MYK. The oesophageal detector device. Assessment of a new method to distinguish oesophageal from tracheal intubation. *Anaesthesia* 1988;43:27–29.
16. Ainsworth QP, Calder I. The oesophageal detector device and the laryngeal mask. *Anaesthesia* 1990;45:794.
17. Wittman PH, Wittman FW. Laryngeal mask and gastric dilatation. *Anaesthesia* 1991;46:1083.
18. Fullekrug B, Pothmann W, Werner C, Schulte am Esch J. The laryngeal mask airway: anesthetic gas leakage and fiberoptic control of positioning. *J Clin Anesth* 1993;5:357–363.
19. Goudsoozian NG, Denman W, Cleveland R, Shoren G. Radiologic localization of the laryngeal mask airway in children. *Anesthesiology* 1992;77:1085–1089.
20. Nandi PR, Nunn JF, Charlesworth CH, Tayor SJ. Radiological study of the laryngeal mask. *Europ J Anesthesiology* 1991; 4*[Suppl.]*:33–39.
21. Molloy AR: Unexpected position of the laryngeal mask airway *[letter]*. *Anaesthesia* 1991;46:592.
22. Asai T, Latto IP, Vaughan RS: The distance between the grille of the laryngeal mask airway and the vocal cords. Is conventional intubation through the laryngeal mask safe? *Anaesthesia* 1993;48:667–669.
23. Sarma VJ. The use of a laryngeal mask airway in spontaneously breathing patients. *Acta Anesthesiol Scan* 1990;34:669–672.
24. Pennant JH, Walker MB. Comparison of the endotracheal tube and laryngeal mask in airway management by paramedical personnel. *Anesth Analg* 1992;74:531–534.
25. Brain AIJ, McGhee TD, McAteer EJ, Thomas A, Abu-saad MAW, Bushman JA. The laryngeal mask airway: development and preliminary trials of a new type of airway. *Anaesthesia* 1985;40:356–361.
26. Cork RC, Depa RM, Standen JR. Prospective comparison of use of the laryngeal mask and endotracheal tube for ambulatory surgery. *Anesth Analg* 1994;79:719–727.
27. Watcha MF, White PF, Tyschen L, Stevens JL. Comparative effects of laryngeal mask airway and endotracheal tube insertion on intraocular pressure in children. *Anesth Analg* 1992;75:355–360.
28. Holden R, Morsman CDG, Butler J, Clark GS, Hughes DS, Bacon PJ. Intraocular pressure changes using the laryngeal mask airway and tracheal tube. *Anaesthesia* 1991;46:922–924.
29. Ripart J, Cohendy R, Eledjam JJ. The laryngeal mask and intraocular surgery *[letter]*. *Br J Anesth* 1993;70:704.
30. Maekawa N, Mikawa K, Tanaka O, Goto R, Obara H. The laryngeal mask may be a useful device for fibreoptic airway endoscopy in pediatric anaesthesia. *Anesthesiology* 1991;75:169–170.
31. McNamee CJ, Meyns B, Pagliero KM. Flexible bronchoscopy via the laryngeal mask: a new technique. *Thorax* 1991;46:141–142.
32. Brimacombe J, Newell S, Swainston R, Thompson J. A potential new technique for awake fiberoptic bronchoscopy—use of the laryngeal mask airway. *Med J Aust* 1992;156:876–877.
33. Du Plessis MC, Barr MA, Verghese C, Lyallt JRW. Fibreoptic bronchoscopy under general anaesthesia using the laryngeal mask airway. *Europ J of Anaesthesiology* 1993;10:363–365.
34. Dich-Nielsen JO, Nagel P. Flexible fibreoptic bronchoscopy via the laryngeal mask. *Aeta Anaesthesiol Scan* 1993;37:17–19.
35. Lawson R, LLoyd-Thomas AR. Three diagnostic conundrums solved using the laryngeal mask airway. *Anaesthesia* 1993;48:790–791.
36. Walker RWM, Murrell D. Yet another use for the laryngeal mask airway *[letter]*. *Anaesthesia* 1991;46:591.
37. Harris TM, Johnston DF, Collins SRC, Heath ML. A new general anaesthetic technique for use in singers: the brain laryngeal mask airway versus endotracheal intubation. *Journal of Voice* 1990;4:81–85.
38. Tanigawa K, Inoue Y, Iwata S. Protection of recurrent laryngeal nerve during neck surgery: a new combination of neutracer, laryngeal mask airway, and fiberoptic bronchoscope *[letter]*. *Anesthesiology* 1991;74:966–967.
39. Greatorex RA, Denny NM. Application of the laryngeal mask airway to thyroid surgery and the preservation of the recurrent laryngeal nerve. *Ann R Coll Surg Eng* 1991;73:352–354.
40. Lee SK, Hong KH, Choe H, Song HS. Comparison of the effects of the laryngeal mask airway and endotracheal intubation on vocal cord function. *Br J Anesth* 1993;71:648–650.

41. Riddell V. Thyroidectomy: prevention of bilateral recurrent nerve palsy. *Br J Surg* 1970;57:1–11.
42. Asai T, Fujise K, Uchida M. Use of the laryngeal mask in a child with tracheal stenosis *[letter]*. *Anesthesiology* 1991;75: 903–904.
43. Asai T, Fujise K, Uchida M. Laryngeal mask and tracheal stenosis *[letter]*. *Anaesthesia* 1993;48:81.
44. Divatia JV, Sareen R, Upadhye SM, Sharma KS, Shelgaonkar JR. Anaesthetic management of tracheal surgery using the laryngeal mask airway. *Anaesth Intens Care* 1994;22:69–73.
45. Eckhardt WF III, Forman S, Denman W, Grillo HC, Muehrcke D. Another use for the laryngeal mask airway: as a blocker during tracheoplasty. *Anesth Analg* 1995;80:622–624.
46. Dexter TJ. The laryngeal mask airway: a method to improve visualization of the trachea and larynx during fibreoptic assisted percutaneous tracheostomy. *Anaesth Intens Care* 1994; 22:35–39.
47. Kumar CM. Laryngeal mask airway for inadequate reversal *[letter]*. *Anaesthesia* 1990;45:792.
48. Michel MZ, Stubbing JF. Laryngeal mask airway and laryngeal spasm *[letter]*. *Anaesthesia* 1991;46:71.
49. George SL, Blogg CE. Role of the LMA in tracheal extubation? *Br J Anaesth* 1994;72:610.
50. Benumof J. Laryngeal Mask Airway *[editorial]*. *Anesthesiology* 1992;77:843–845.
51. Barker P, Langton JA, Murphy PJ, Rowbotham DJ. Regurgitation of gastric contents during general anaesthesia using the laryngeal mask airway. *Anaesth* 1992;69:314–315.
52. Rabey PG, Murphy PJ, Langton JA, Barker P, Rowbotham DJ. Effect of the laryngeal mask airway on lower oesophageal sphincter pressure in patients during general anaesthesia. *Br J Anaesth* 1992;69:341–345.
53. Mikatti NE, Luthra AP, Healy TEJ, Mortimer AJ. Gastric regurgitation during general anaesthesia in the supine position with the laryngeal and facemask airway. *Br J Anaesth* 1992; 69:529–530.
54. Brimacombe J, Berry A. Aspiration and the laryngeal mask airway—a survey of Australian intensive care units. *Anaesth Intens Care* 1992;20:534–535.
55. Brain AIJ, Verghese C, Strube P, Brimacombe J. A new laryngeal mask prototype. *Anaesthesia* 1995;50:42–48.
56. Akhtar TM. Oesophageal Vent-Laryngeal Mask to prevent aspiration of gastric contents. *Brit J Anaesth* 1994;72:52–54.
57. Asai T. The Oesophageal Vent-Laryngeal Mask. *Br J Anaesth* 1994;72:726–735.
58. Marjot R. Pressure exerted by the laryngeal mask airway cuff upon the pharyngeal mucosa. *Br J Anaesth* 1993;70:25–29.
59. Lumb AB, Wrigley MW. The effect of nitrous oxide on laryngeal mask cuff pressure. In vitro and in vivo studies. *Anaesthesia* 1992;47:320–323.
60. Wright ES, Filshie J, Dark CH. Laryngeal mask cuff pressure and nitrous oxide *[letter]*. *Anaesthesia* 1992;47:713–714.
61. King C, Street MK. Twelfth cranial nerve paralysis following use of a laryngeal mask airway. *Anaesthesia* 1994;49:786–787.
62. Nagai K, Sakuramoto C, Goto F. Unilateral hypoglossal nerve paralysis following the use of the laryngeal mask airway. *Anaesthesia* 1994;49:603–604.
63. Inomata S, Nishikawa T, Suza A, Yamashita S. Transient bilateral vocal cord paralysis after insertion of a laryngeal mask airway. *Anesthesiology* 1995;82:787–788.
64. Thompsett E, Cundy JM. Use of the laryngeal mask airway in the presence of a bleeding diathesis. *Anaesthesia* 1992;47: 530–531.
65. Lee JJ. Laryngeal mask and trauma to uvula (letter). *Anaesthesia* 1989;44:1014–1015.
66. Van Heerden PV, Kirrage D. Large tonsils and the laryngeal mask airway. *Anaesthesia* 1989;44:703.
67. Wynn JM, Jones KI. Tongue cyanosis after laryngeal mask airway insertion *[letter]*. *Anesthesiology* 1994;80:1403.
68. Devitt JH, Wenstone R, Noel AG, O'Donnell MP. The laryngeal mask airway and positive-pressure ventilation. *Anesthesiology* 1994;80:550–555.
69. Ezri T, Priscu V, Szmuk P, Soroker D. Laryngeal mask and pulmonary edema. *Anesthesiology* 1993;78:219.
70. Brain AIJ. Three cases of difficult intubation overcome by use of the laryngeal mask. *Anaesthesia* 1985;40:353–355.
71. Nath G, Major V. The laryngeal mask in the management of a pediatric difficult airway. *Anaesth Intens Care* 1992;20: 518–520.
72. Heath ML, Allagain J. Intubation through the laryngeal mask. a technique for unexpected difficult intubation. *Anaesthesia* 1991;46:545–548.
73. McClune S, Regan M, Moore J. Laryngeal mask airway for Caesarean section. *Anaesthesia* 1990;45:227–228.
74. Owen G, Browning S, Davies CA, et al. Laryngeal mask *[letter]*. *Br Med J* 1993;306:580.
75. Storey J. The laryngeal mask for failed intubation at Caesarean section *[letter]*. *Anaesth Intens Care* 1992;20:118–119.
76. Calder I, Ordman AJ, Jackowski A, Crockard HA. The Brain laryngeal mask airway. An alternative to emergency tracheal intubation. *Anaesthesia* 1990;45:137–139.
77. Thomson KD, Ordman AJ, Parkhouse N, Morgan BDG. Use of the Brain laryngeal mask airway in anticipation of difficult tracheal intubation. *Br J Plast Surg* 1989;42:478–480.
78. Cork R, Monk JE. Management of a suspected and unsuspected difficult laryngoscopy with the laryngeal mask airway. *J Clin Anesth* 1992;4:230–234.
79. Pennant JH, Gajraj NM, Yamanouchi KJ. The laryngeal mask airway and laryngeal polyposis *[letter]*. *Anesth Analg* 1994;78: 1206.
80. Castresana MR, Stefansson S, Cancel AR, Hague KJ. Use of the laryngeal mask airway during thoracotomy in a pediatric patient with Cri-du-Chat Syndrome *[letter]*. *Anesth Analg* 1994; 78:817.
81. Lim W, Wareham C, de Mello WF, Kocan M. The laryngeal mask in failed intubation. *Anaesthesia* 1990;41:689–690.
82. White A, Sinclair M, Pillai R. Laryngeal mask airway for coronary bypass grafting. *Anaesthesia* 1991;46:234.
83. McCrirrick A, Pracilio JA. Awake intubation: a new technique. *Anaesthesia* 1991;46:661–663.
84. Asai T. Fiberoptic tracheal intubation through the laryngeal mask in an awake patient with cervical spine injury *[letter]*. *Anesth Analg* 1993;77:404.
85. Silk JM, Hill HM, Calder I. Difficult intubation and the laryngeal mask. *Eur J Anaesthesiol* 1991;4:47–51.
86. de-Mello WF, Kocan M. The laryngeal mask in failed intubation *[letter]*. *Anaesthesia* 1990;45:689–690.
87. Chadd GD, Crane DL, Phillips RM, Tunell WP. Extubation and reintubation guided by the laryngeal mask airway in a child with the Pierre-Robin syndrome. *Anesthesiology* 1992;76: 640–641.
88. Allen JG, Flower EA. The Brain laryngeal mask. An alternative to difficult intubation. *Br Dent J* 1990;168:202–204.
89. Maltby JR, Neil SG. Laryngeal mask airway and difficult intubation *[letter]*. *Anesthesiology* 1993;78:994.
90. Lee JJ, Yau K, Barcroft J. LMA and respiratory arrest after anteriorcervical fusion *[letter]*. *Can J Anaesth* 1993;40: 395–396.
91. Denny NM, Desilva KD, Webber PA. Laryngeal mask airway for emergency tracheostomy in a neonate *[letter]*. *Anesthesia* 1990;45:895.
92. Hasham F, Kumar CM, Lawler PG. The use of the laryngeal mask airway to assist fibreoptic orotracheal intubation. *Anaesthesia* 1991;46:891.
93. Smith JE, Sherwood NA. Combined use of laryngeal mask airway and fiberoptic laryngoscope in difficult intubation. *Anaesth Intens Care* 1991;19:471–472.
94. Heath ML, Allagain J. Intubation through the laryngeal mask. A technique for unexpected difficult intubation. *Anaesthesia* 1991;46:545–548.
95. Benumof JL. Use of the laryngeal mask airway to facilitate fiberscope-aided tracheal intubation. *Anesth Analg* 1992;74: 33–34.
96. Darling JR, Keohane M, Murray JM. A split laryngeal mask as an aid to training fiberoptic tracheal intubation. A comparison with the Berman II intubating airway. *Anaesthesia* 1993; 48:1079–1082.
97. Asai T. Fibreoptic intubation through the laryngeal mask in an

awake patient with cervical spine injury *[letter]*. *Anesth Analg* 1993;77:404.
98. Brimacombe J, Berry A. Placement of a cook airway exchange catheter via the laryngeal mask airway, *Anaesthesia* 1993;48: 351–352.
99. Zagnoev M, McCloskey J, Martin T. Fiberoptic intubation via the laryngeal mask airway. *Anesth Analg* 1994;78:813–814.
100. Couture P, Perrault C, Girard D. Fiberoptic bronchoscope intubation after induction of general anaesthesia: another approach. *Can J Anaesth* 1992;39:99.
101. Brimacombe J, Berry A. Laryngeal mask airway insertion. A comparison of the standard versus neutral position in normal patients with a view to its use in cervical spine instability. *Anaesthesia* 1993;48:670–671.
102. Smith BL. Brain airway in anaesthesia for patients with juvenile chronic arthritis *[letter]*. *Anaesthesia* 1988;43:421–422.
103. Ebata T, Nishiki S, Masuda A, Amaha K. Anaesthesia for Treacher Collins syndrome using a laryngeal mask airway. *Can J Anaesth* 1991;38:1043–1045.
104. Beveridge ME. Laryngeal mask anaesthesia for repair of cleft palate. *Anaesthesia* 1989;44:656–657.
105. Brimacomb J, Berry A. Mallampati classification and laryngeal mask insertion *[letter]*. *Anaesthesia* 1993;48:347.
106. Theroux MC, Kettrick RG, Khine HH. Laryngeal mask airway and fiberoptic endoscopy in an infant with Schwartz-Jampel Syndrome *[letter]*. *Anesthesiology* 1995;82:605.
107. Priscu V, Priscu L, Soroker D. Laryngeal mask for failed intubation in emergency Caesarean section *[letter]*. *Can J Anaesth* 1992;39:893.
108. Mahiou P, Narchi P, Veyrac P, et al. Is laryngeal mask easy to use in case of difficult intubation? *[abstract]*. *Anesthesiology* 1992;77:A1228.
109. Asai T. Use of the laryngeal mask for tracheal intubation in patients at increased risk of aspiration of gastric contents. *Anesthesiology* 1992;77:1029–1030.
110. Brimacombe J, White A, Berry A. Effect of cricoid pressure on ease of insertion of the laryngeal mask airway. *Br J Anaesth* 1993; 71:800–802.
111. Ansermino JM, Blogg CE. Cricoid pressure may prevent insertion of the laryngeal mask airway. *Br J Anaesth* 1992; 69: 465–467.
112. Asai T, Barclay K, Power I, Vaughan S. Cricoid pressure impedes placement of the laryngeal mask airway and subsequent tracheal intubation through the mask. *Br J Anesth* 1994; 72:47–51.
113. Strang TI. Does the laryngeal mask airway compromise cricoid pressure? *Anaesthesia* 1992; 47:829–831.
114. Asai T, Morris S. The role of the laryngeal mask for failed tracheal intubation in the patient with a "Full Stomach." *Anesth Analg* 1994;78:817–818.
115. American Society of Anesthesiologists Task Force on Management of the Difficult Airway. Practice guidelines for management of the difficult airway. *Anesthesiology* 1993;78:597–602.
116. Lim SL, Tay DHB, Thomas E. A comparison of three types of tracheal tubes for use in laryngeal mask assisted blind orotracheal intubation. *Anaesthesia* 1994;49:255–257.
117. Dubreuil M, Laffon M, Plaud B, Penon C, Ecoffey C. Complications and fiberoptic assessment of size 1 laryngeal mask airway. *Anesth Analg* 1993;76:527–529.
118. Goldie AS, Hudson I. Fibreoptic tracheal intubation through a modified laryngeal mask *[letter]*. *Paediatric Anaesthesia* 1992;2:343–344.
119. Hasan MA, Black AE. A new technique for fiberoptic intubation in children. *Anaesthesia* 1994;49:1031–1033.
120. Sartore DM, Kojima RK. Laryngeal mask airway–assisted, wire guided fiberoptic tracheal intubation *[letter]*. *Anesthesiology* 1994;81:1550–1551.
121. Brimacombe J, Johns K. Modified Intavent LMA (letter). *Anaesth Intens Care* 1991;19:607.
122. Greene MK, Roden R, Hinchley G. The laryngeal mask airway. Two cases of prehospital trauma care. *Anaesthesia* 1992;47: 688–689.
123. Pennant JH, Walker MB. Comparison of the endotrachial tube and laryngeal mask in airway management by paramedical personnel. *Anesth Analg* 1992;74:531–534.
124. Martin PD, Cyna AM, Hunter WAH, Henry J, Ramayya GP. Training nursing staff in airway management for resuscitation. A clinical comparison of the face mask and laryngeal mask. *Anaesthesia* 1993;48:33–37.
125. Results of a Multicenter Trial. The use of the laryngeal mask airway by nurses during cardiopulmonary resuscitation. *Anaesthesia* 1994;49:3–7.
126. Davies PR, Tighe SD, Greenslade GL, Evans GH. Laryngeal mask airway and tracheal tube insertion by unskilled personnel. *Lancet* 1990;336:977–979.
127. Peterson SJ, Byrne PJ, Molesky MG, Seal RF, Finucane BT. Neonatal resuscitation using the laryngeal mask airway. *Anesthesiology* 1994;80:1245–1253.

CHAPTER 13

Esophageal Airway Devices

Andranik Ovassapian M.D. and Paul S. Mesnick, M.D.

Despite the clear superiority of tracheal intubation in protecting the airway against aspiration and providing ventilation, alternative airway devices have been developed to overcome the technical difficulties involved with tracheal intubation by emergency care personnel (1). These alternative devices have been developed for blind esophageal intubation to prevent gastric contents aspiration. Ventilation of lungs is provided through a face mask or a tube positioned in the pharynx. These esophageal airway devices have been thought to require less skill and training for successful use and a lower complication rate (1).

The authors of a 1957 article recommended that if during an attempted difficult tracheal intubation the endotracheal tube entered the esophagus, the endotracheal tube should be left in place to serve as a conduit for suctioning gastric contents. Mask ventilation could then be performed and tracheal intubation attempted while the endotracheal tube remains in the esophagus (2).

The following is a brief historical review of the esophageal devices that have since been designed and produced.

CHARACTERISTICS OF ESOPHAGEAL DEVICES

Mouth-to-Lung Airway

The concept of ventilating a patient and preventing the aspiration of gastric contents with an esophageal airway device for resuscitation of cardiac arrest victims was introduced by Don Michael in 1968 (3). The "mouth-to-lung" airway device consists of a flexible tube with blocked distal end and multiple small holes at midsection. The mouth guard encloses the lips and forms a seal. The nose is clipped during ventilation to prevent any air leak from the nose. Inflation of the tube cuff prevents air entering into the stomach. This device allows mouth-to-lung ventilation without direct mouth-to-mouth contact and prevents air inflation of the stomach, the two major shortcomings of mouth-to-mouth resuscitation (Fig. 1).

The Esophageal Obturator Airway

The esophageal obturator airway (EOA) is a modification of the "mouth-to-lung airway" and is recommended in emergency airway management where endotracheal intubation is desired but not feasible (4). The EOA consists of a 34-cm semirigid cuffed tube, with the proximal end attached to a face mask by a snap-lock system for easy detachment (5,6). Multiple holes in the midportion of the tube provide air entry into the hypopharynx and trachea (Fig. 2). The distal lumen of the tube is plugged to prevent air entry into the esophagus. The tube's cuff is intended to seal the esophagus, preventing air from entering the stomach as well as guarding against regurgitation of gastric con-

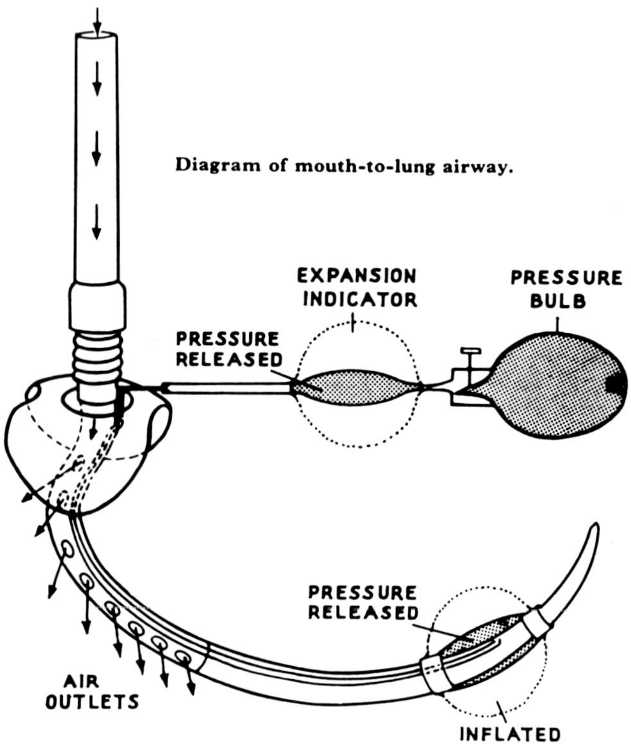

FIG. 1. The mouth-to-lung airway. This device is blindly placed in the esophagus. The cuff is inflated and ventilation is provided by placing the mouth over the proximal end of the tube and blowing exhaled air into the lungs. (With permission, ref. 3.)

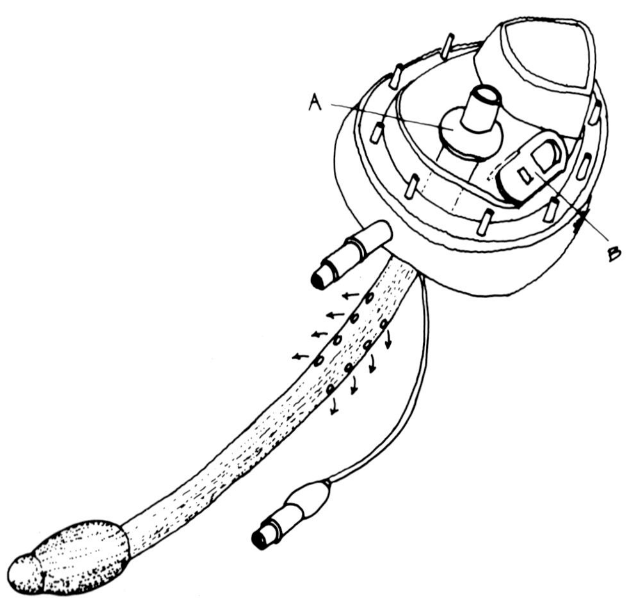

FIG. 2. The esophageal obturator airway. **A:** Ventilation port (15-mm adapter). **B:** Suction port that can be closed or opened by a movable cap.

tents. The main advantage of the EOA over a face mask is the prevention of gastric aspiration (5,6).

Placement

The patient's head is placed in a neutral position, and the lower jaw pulled up and forward. This is achieved by placing the thumb inside the mouth and holding the jaw between the fingers. The jaw lift maneuver elevates the mandible, and pulls the tongue away from the posterior pharyngeal wall. The EOA tube is then advanced against the posterior pharyngeal wall toward the esophagus. Excessive force should be avoided (5).

The tube is advanced until the mask is seated on the patient's face. The EOA cuff is then inflated prior to positive pressure ventilation to prevent air entry into the stomach. Thus the EOA tube is used to provide ventilation, while the mask maintains a closed seal of the upper airway.

Artificial ventilation is initiated by blowing into the tube, or ventilating with an Ambu bag. If the tube is properly positioned, air should enter the hypopharynx and trachea.

The EOA has been used in prehospital and hospital settings (7–10). The effectiveness of EOA ventilation during cardiopulmonary resuscitation, measured by arterial blood gas evaluation, has been questioned (8,11). A number of serious complications have been reported during its use. These include an inability to obtain a good mask-to-face seal and unrecognized tracheal intubation and airway trauma (11–13).

While the EOA does protect against gastric regurgitation, it does not protect the airway against the aspiration of upper airway hemorrhage or debris. Perforation of the upper, midportion, and distal esophagus has been described in association with its use (13–15). These perforations have been attributed to trauma associated with insertion of the device, over inflated cuff, and patient retching and vomiting. It is estimated that between 8% to 20% of blindly placed EOAs enter the trachea, causing complete airway obstruction and massive gastric distension (2,5).

The inability to decompress the stomach after EOA placement poses a major problem since massive regurgitation of gastric material is greatly enhanced upon its removal. Disadvantages of the EOA are summarized in Table 1.

Esophageal Gastric Tube Airway

The Esophageal Gastric Tube Airway (EGTA) was developed to overcome shortcomings of the EOA (4).

TABLE 1. *Disadvantages of esophageal obturator airway*

Large-diameter rigid tube.
Placement does not assure airway patency.
Does not allow gastric decompression.
Does not protect the airway against upper airway hemorrhage.
Difficult mask fit and ventilation.
High incidence of tracheal intubation.
Pyriform sinus trauma.
Rupture of esophagus.

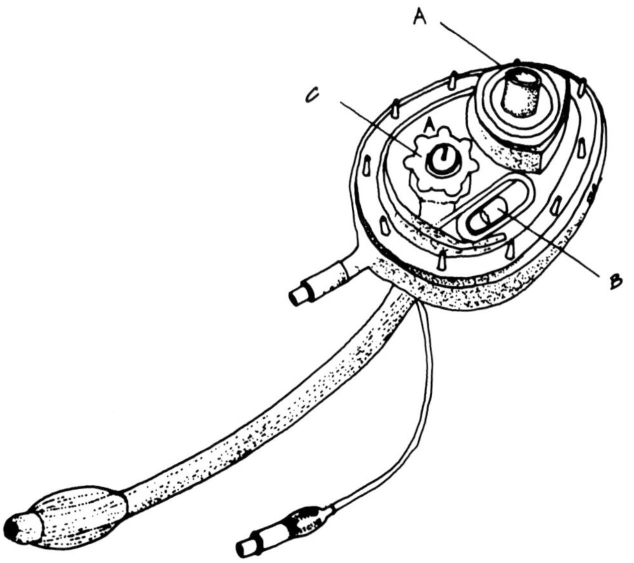

FIG. 3. The esophageal gastric tube airway. **A:** Ventilation port (15-mm adapter). **B:** Suction port. **C:** Esophageal tube proximal end will accept nasogastric tube.

The mask of the EGTA has two openings. The first incorporates a 15-mm standard attachment for ventilation. The other opening holds a long semirigid cuffed tube (Fig. 3). The tube serves as a conduit into the esophagus and stomach. The tube has no openings on the sides and will allow passage of a gastric tube for stomach decompression. The tube is otherwise similar to the EOA, and presents many of the same shortcomings (16,17). The mechanism of ventilation is through the face mask.

Esophageal Pharyngeal Airway

The esophageal pharyngeal airway (EPA) incorporates two separate tubes surrounded by a large pharyngeal balloon (Fig. 4). One tube is shorter than the other. The lumen of the shorter tube enters the oropharynx, that of the longer tube enters the hypopharynx. The tubes are sealed together in a double-barrel design. The longer tube serves to ventilate the patient. It terminates into a 15-mm adapter at its proximal end. The shorter tube is used to pass a cuffed gastroesophageal tube or a regular nasogastric tube. Upon inflation the large inflatable balloon (pharyngeal cuff) pushes the soft palate against the posterior pharyngeal wall and nasopharynx, preventing air leakage during positive pressure ventilation. A movable oral flange positioned over the proximal end of the airway seals the lips.

When properly adjusted, the pharyngeal balloon and movable oral flange eliminate the need for face mask ventilation. The EPA makes inadvertent tracheal intubation less likely, and by the contoured phayngeal balloon cuff provides more reliable occlusion of the esophagus, than the EOA device. In addition, it allows for

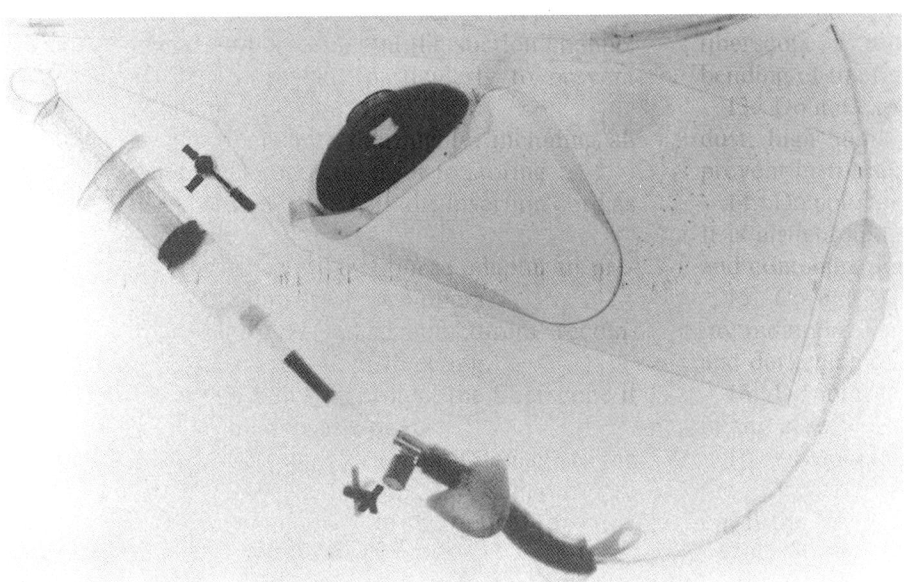

FIG. 4. The esophageal pharyngeal airway. The EPA is inserted like an oropharyngeal airway. The oral flange is adjusted against the patient's lips. The soft pharyngeal balloon is inflated to seal the upper airway. The gastroesophageal tube with balloon is passed through the short tube into the esophagus and balloon is inflated with 60–90 ml of air to block the midesophagus. (With permission, ref. 18.)

continuous gastric decompression, and eliminates difficulties associated with mask fit (18).

The device will not prevent gastric inflation, regurgitation, or aspiration of gastric contents until a nasogastric tube equipped with an esophageal balloon is passed through the shorter lumen and inflated, thus blocking the esophagus while allowing for gastric suctioning and decompression.

Pharyngeo-Tracheal Lumen Airway

The pharyngeo-tracheal lumen airway (PTLA) represents a further improvement of the EOA and EPA design. The PTLA is an airway device consisting of two tubes of unequal length and diameter running in parallel. Each tube has a proximal 15-mm adapter. A large proximal balloon cuff and smaller distal cuff are incorporated into the design (Fig. 5). The longer distal-cuffed tube is incorporated within the shorter, large diameter tube. The proximal balloon cuff (pharyngeal cuff) is located at the distal end of the short tube. The distal and proximal cuffs are inflated simultaneously through a common in-series valve system located at the proximal end of the airway. The device incorporates a bite block at the level of the patient's incisors.

One design difference between the PTLA and the EPA is that the the long tube of the PTLA can be used for ventilation if it enters the trachea. Its inflated distal cuff will prevent gastric content regurgitation when the tube is seated in the esophagus (19–23).

The PTLA is inserted blindly, usually entering the esophagus. Inflation of the distal cuff occludes the esophagus, preventing gastric distension or regurgitation during positive pressure ventilation. Inflation of the larger volume pharyngeal balloon seals the upper airway, making positive pressure ventilation possible. The inflated proximal balloon can also contain upper airway hemorrhage and secretions (21).

A face mask seal is not required for effective ventilation, offering a distinct advantage over the EOA. With esophageal placement, ventilation is achieved through the short tube. If ventilation through the short tube

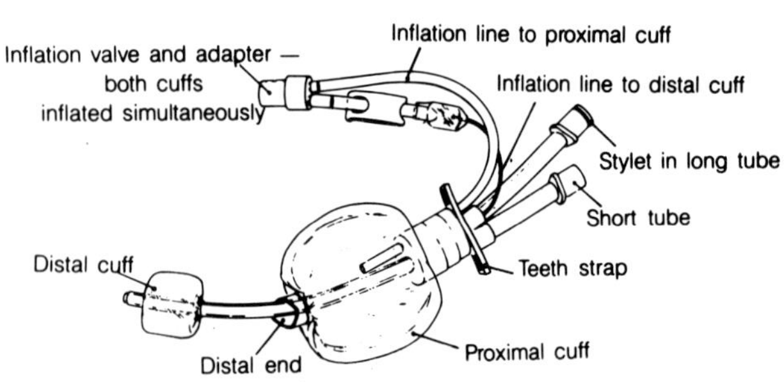

FIG. 5. The pharyngeo-tracheal lumen airway. (With permission, ref. 19.)

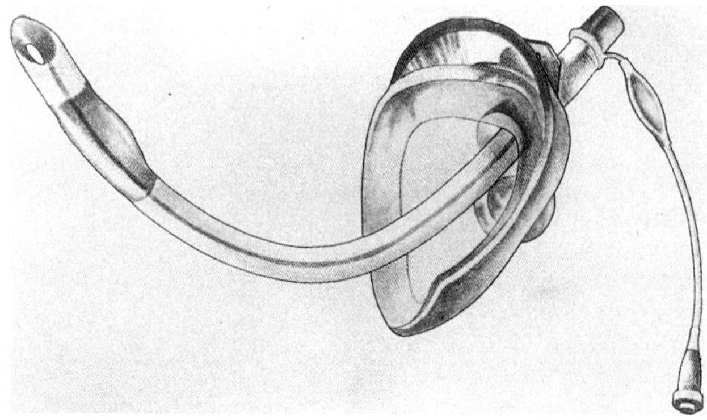

FIG. 6. The tracheal-esophageal airway. When tube is placed in esophagus, ventilation is carried out through the face mask with its regular adapter. If tube enters the trachea, the tube is disengaged from the mask and used as regular endotracheal tube. The mask is then removed. (With permission, ref. 24.)

fails, it may be because the long tube entered the trachea. Ventilation through the long tube can be tried to see if this is the case. If pulmonary ventilation proves successful, the device can be kept in place and the patient supported by direct endotracheal ventilation. Only a few studies are available that compare the PTLA to the endotracheal tube (18,20,23). These studies indicate that oxygenation and ventilation with the PTLA is similar to that achieved with the endotracheal tube and recommended that the PTLA be an alternative method of emergency airway management when tracheal intubation has failed.

Tracheal-Esophageal Airway

The tracheal-esophageal airway (TEA) device is composed of a face mask with two openings on the top of the mask (Fig. 6). One opening is fitted with a standard 15-mm adapter for ventilating the patient by Ambu bag (24). The second opening, foward of the first, is fitted with a 10-mm endotracheal tube. The endotracheal tube with the mask attached is inserted, either blindly or with the aid of a laryngoscope. Upon insertion the endotracheal tube cuff is inflated, and the patient cautiously ventilated through the endotracheal tube. If lung ventilation is confirmed, ventilation is continued through the endotracheal tube and the mask can be removed.

If the tube enters the esophagus, an Ambu bag is attached to the 15-mm mask port and the patient is mask ventilated. The endotracheal tube in this case isolates the esophagus from the airway, and further prevents the tongue from obstructing the airway. The inflated cuff of the endotracheal tube prevents air from entering the stomach. Different mask sizes and endotracheal tube combinations are available for specific clinical circumstances.

TABLE 2. *Features and characteristics of Combitube*

Disposable two-lumen tube.
Longer tube resembles cuffed endotracheal tube.
The distal small cuff seals esophagus or trachea.
Shorter tube has eight side openings and is positioned in the pharynx.
The larger proximal balloon seals the upper airway and anchors the Combitube behind the palate.
Ventilation of lungs is possible with either esophageal or tracheal placement.
Protects against aspiration.
Designed for emergency ventilation.

Esophageal Tracheal Combitube

The Combitube® is a registered trademark of the manufacturer (Sheridan Catheter Corp., Argyle, New York) and has been approved by the Food and Drug Administration as an airway device since 1988.

The esophageal tracheal Combitube (ETC) is a disposable double-lumen tube with two cuffs (Fig. 7). The longer tube has an open distal end, and resembles an endotracheal tube fitted with a distal 15-ml volume cuff. The shorter tube lumen is blocked at its distal end, and is incorporated into the cylindrical design of the longer tube. The proximal balloon cuff holds up to 140 ml of air and is positioned above eight side openings that exit the lumen of the shorter tube (Table 2).

The two tubular lumens are separated at their proximal ends and are each mounted with a standard 15-mm connector. The proximal end of the pharyngeal tube is blue in color (marked as #1) and is longer at its proximal end than the esophageal-tracheal tube, which is clear in color (marked #2). Two black rings at the proximal end of the double-lumen tube act as a guide for depth of insertion (25–27).

The Combitube is inserted blindly using a two-hand technique. The thumb of the nondominant hand is placed inside the mouth, grasping the tongue and lower jaw between thumb and forefingers, pulling the jaw upward. The curved tip of the tube is placed inside the mouth and advanced gently in a curving manner over the base of the tongue into the hypopharynx. Gentle pressure is exerted in passing the tube beyond the resistance of the cricopharyngeus muscles. The tube is

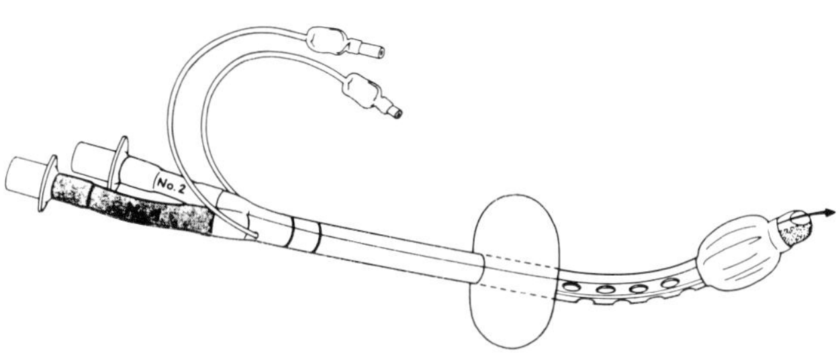

FIG. 7. The esophageal tracheal Combitube.

TABLE 3. *Combitube placement technique*

Pull lower jaw and tongue forward.
Advance the tube until the ring markers are positioned against the incisors.
Inflate the lower cuff first with 15 ml of air.
Inflate the upper balloon with 100–120 ml of air.
Ventilate through the blue tube, marked #1.
If breath sounds are absent, ventilate through the clear tube, marked #2.
If unable to ventilate with either lumen, pull the tube out about 2 cm and try it again.

advanced until the black rings are at the level of the teeth or gums. If difficulties are experienced with blind placement, the Combitube can be placed under direct vision using a rigid laryngoscope.

After insertion, the distal cuff is inflated with 15 ml of air to seal the esophagus. The large proximal balloon is then inflated with 100–140 ml of air using a large syringe. This serves to secure the tube in position, and occludes the oral and nasal airways (Table 3).

Ventilation is initially attempted through the proximal tube (#1), forcing air past the pharynx into the trachea (Fig. 8). Gastric fluids can be aspirated through the distal tube (#2), which usually enters the esophagus on placement. Air is prevented from entering the esophagus by the inflated distal cuff. Chest wall movement, the presence of breath sounds, and negative aus-

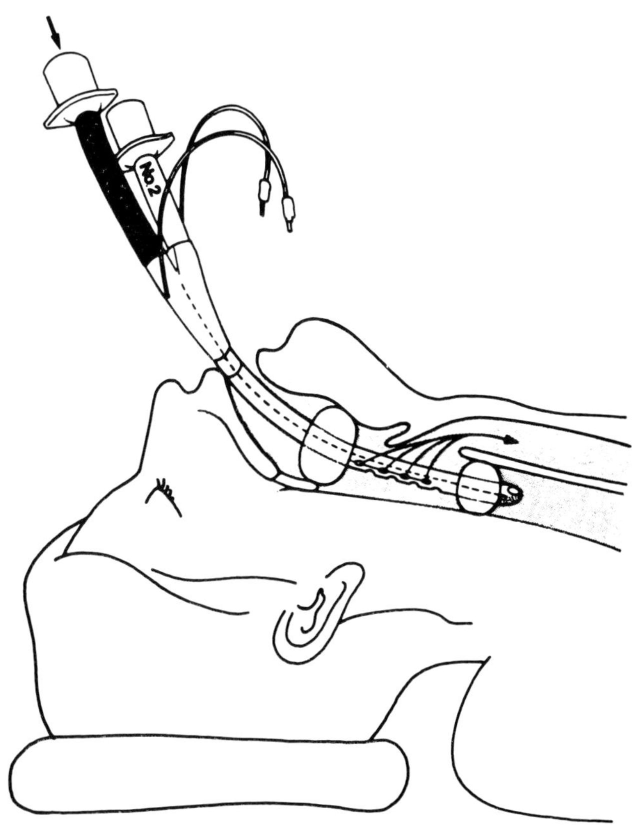

FIG. 8. Combitube positioned in esophagus.

TABLE 4. *Indications of Combitube*

Difficult or failed intubation
Cardiopulmonary resuscitation by people not trained in tracheal intubation
Massive bleeding or regurgitation that prevents vocal cord exposure
Limited access to the patient's head
Cervical spine injuries—limited neck motion
In entertainers, to avoid vocal cord damage

TABLE 5. Advantages of the Combitube

Allows rapid establishment of the airway
Allows ventilation with both esophageal and tracheal placement
Gastric fluid can be aspirated when esophageal intubation is achieved
Protects against aspiration
No need for head and neck movement
Requires less skill for placement

cultation over the epigastric region serve to indicate esophageal placement of the device.

If pulmonary ventilation is unsuccessful and gastric insufflation is noted, the Combitube has entered the trachea (Fig. 9). Ventilation is shifted to the open tracheal tube lumen #2. A self- inflating bulb can quickly and reliably identify esophageal or tracheal placement of the Combitube and facilitate proper selection of the correct ventilatory lumen (28).

Unsatisfactory ventilation through either lumen most likely indicates the Combitube has advanced too far, producing an upper airway obstruction by the large pharyngeal balloon (29,30). In this situation, both the tracheal cuff and pharyngeal balloon are deflated, and the tube pulled back approximately 2 cm. The two cuffs are then reinflated, and ventilation again attempted at lumen #1.

The distance from teeth to larynx varies considerably among individuals. Therefore, the use of one standard size device shall result in the deep insertion of the Combitube is some patients (31).

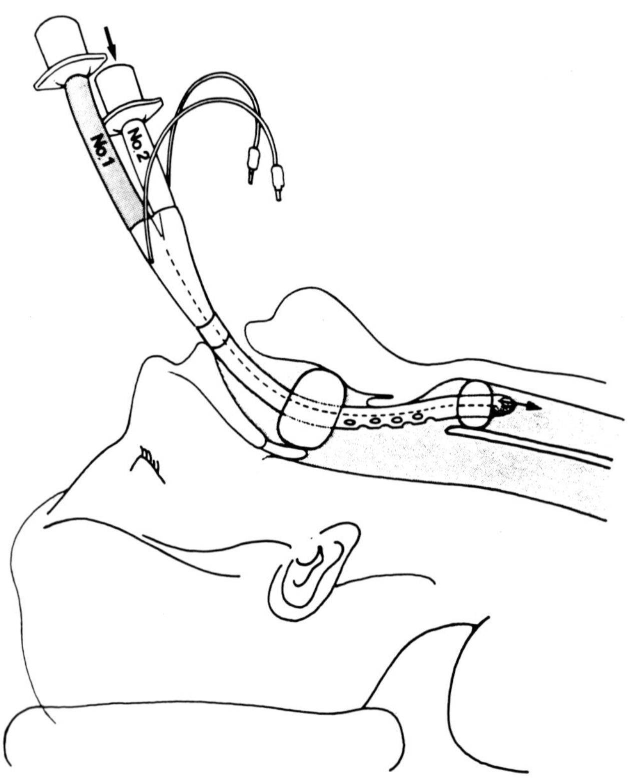

FIG. 9. Combitube positioned in trachea.

The Combitube is a relatively new airway device, designed by Frass and his colleagues for airway maintenance and support under emergency conditions, such as cardiopulmonary resuscitation, difficult tracheal intubation, or a rescuer not trained in tracheal intubation (32–41). Other indications for the use of the Combitube and its advantages are summarized in Tables 4 and 5.

The Combitube provides an option for blind intubation of either the esophagus or trachea. In either position, the airway is better protected against aspiration of gastric contents than during face mask ventilation. In anesthetized, paralyzed patients, ventilation and oxygenation with the Combitube positioned in the esophagus compared well to endotracheal tube ventilation (42,43).

When compared to endotracheal tube ventilation, ventilation through the Combitube is comparatively easy, allowing maintenance of normal arterial carbon dioxide levels with somewhat increased arterial oxygen tensions (42). The increased oxygen tension during ventilation with the Combitube is attributed to the more prolonged expiratory flow time and the creation of 2–4 cm H_20 positive end-expiratory pressure (PEEP) associated with its use. The Combitube has been used successfully for durations of 2–7 hr during mechanical ventilation in seven intensive care unit patients (43).

Disadvantages of the Combitube include the possibility of damaging the esophagus. Tracheal secretions cannot be suctioned when the Combitube is positioned in the esophagus. The use of the device should be avoided in patients with upper esophageal disease and in patients with an intact gag reflex. It is available in only two sizes, and is unsuitable for use in small adults and children.

FIBEROPTIC TRACHEAL INTUBATION WITH THE COMBITUBE IN PLACE

Replacement of the Combitube with an endotracheal tube may be required to secure a more stable airway. If the Combitube was originally utilized due to failure

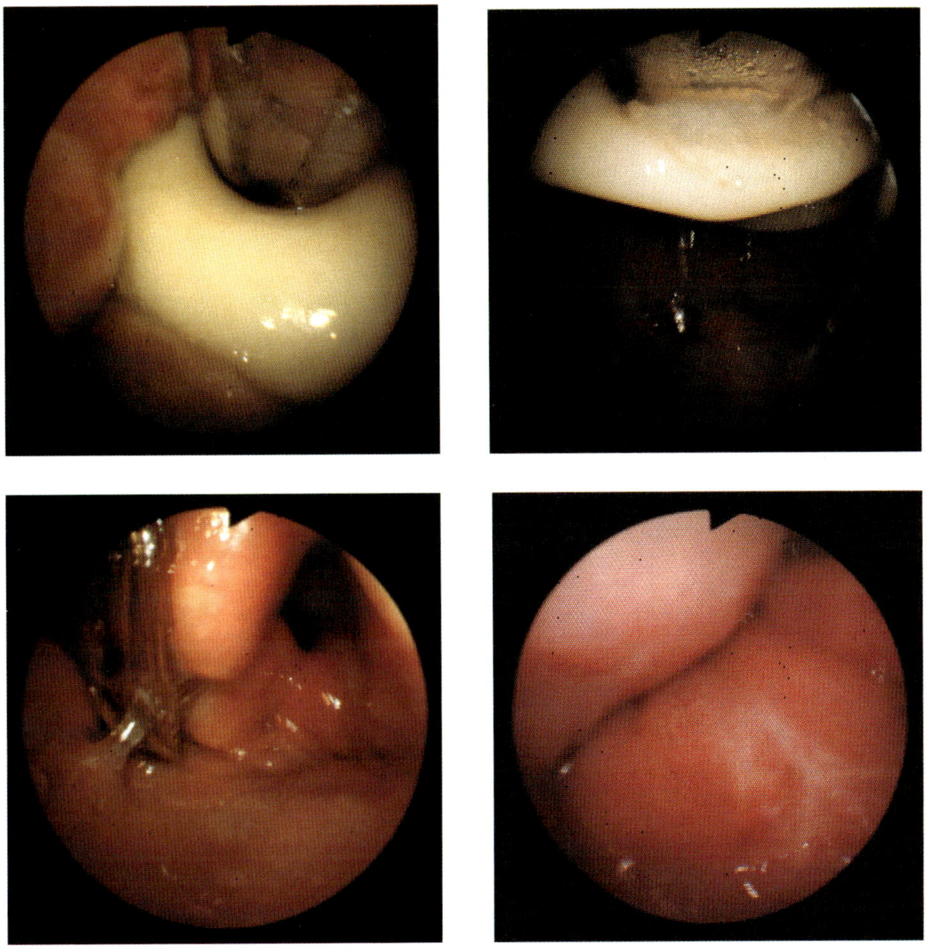

FIG. 10. Endoscopic view of fiberoptic tracheal intubation with Combitube in place. **A:** The fiberscope is introduced through the mouth to expose the inflated pharyngeal balloon of the Combitube which blocks the oropharynx. **B:** The pharyngeal balloon of the Combitube is then deflated to allow passage of the fiberscope into the hypopharynx. **C:** Shows the Combitube in esophagus (clear tube to the left of the larynx). Epiglottis and glottic opening are in view. Fiberscope is passed through the glottis into the trachea, followed by endotracheal tube. After checking the correct placement of the endotracheal tube, the esophageal cuff of the Combitube is deflated and Combitube is removed. **D:** Fiberscope is passed through the nose to show the closure of the nasopharynx by soft palate when Combitube is in place and esophageal balloon is inflated.

at routine tracheal intubation, fiberoptic tracheal intubation with the Combitube in place should be tried (29). The fiberscope is passed orally, with the Combitube's pharyngeal balloon deflated and the fiberscope further advanced toward the larynx (Fig. 10). The large size of the Combitube can make manipulation of the fiberscope difficult. However, the combination of blind emergency placement of the Combitube followed by a controlled fiberoptic tracheal intubation provides an effective technique for emergency airway management.

CONCLUSION

The strict reliance on rigid laryngoscopy to secure the airway is not advisable. Failure of the technique is common, especially in the hands of the inexperienced. Face mask ventilation is a simple and readily available method for ventilating the apneic patient, thus providing oxygenation until the trachea can be secured. Like rigid laryngoscopy however, face mask ventilation may also prove difficult or impossible.

When face mask ventilation and tracheal intubation have failed, one should not persist in tracheal intubation, but should consider other techniques of ventilation. This is critical to avoid hypoxic brain damage or death, as the success of tracheal intubation by repeated attempts cannot be guaranteed.

The Combitube provides an alternative, with its own advantages and shortcomings. Application of a thoughtful approach, proper selection of technique, and skilled application are all important in securing the airway and establishing effective ventilation.

The establishment of a patent airway to provide adequate ventilation and oxygenation requires more than the technical ability to secure the airway or use of any particular airway device. The most critical elements involve knowing and understanding the medical condition of the patient and the difficulties of the airway problems presented. Only by understanding these issues can good judgment be exercised in the selection and appropriate application of a particular technique.

REFERENCES

1. Pepe PE, Zachariah BS, Chandra NC. Invasive airway techniques in resuscitation. *Ann Emerg Med* 1993;22:339–403.
2. Giuffrida JG, Bizzarri D. Intubation of the esophagus. Its role in preventing aspiration pneumonia and asphyxial death. *Am J of Surg* 1957;93:329–334.
3. Don Michael TA, Lambert EH, Mehran JA. Mouth to lung airway for cardiac resuscitation *[letter]*. *Lancet* 1968;2:1329.
4. Gordon AS. Technique for cardiopulmonary resuscitation and pitfalls in performance. In: Meltzer LE, Dunning AJ, eds. *Textbook of coronary care*. Amsterdam: Excerpta Medica, 1973; 397–433.
5. Smith JP, Bodai BI, Seifkin A, Palder S, Thomas V. The esophageal obturator airway. *JAMA* 1983;250:1081–1084.
6. Don Michael TA. The esophageal obturator airway. A critique. *JAMA* 1981;246:1098–1101.
7. Greenbaum DM, Poggi J, Grace WJ. Esophageal obstruction during oxygen administration: a new method for use in resuscitation. *Chest* 1974;65:188–191.
8. Merrifield AJ, King SJ. The oesophageal obturator airway. *Anaesthesia* 1981;36:672–676.
9. Smith JP, Bodai BI, Aubourg R, et al. A field evaluation of the esophageal oburator airway. *J Trauma* 1983;23:317–321.
10. Hammargren Y, Clinton JE, Ruiz E. A standard comparison of esophageal obturator airway and endotracheal tube ventilation in cardiac arrest. *Ann Emerg Med* 1985;14:953–958.
11. Bryson TK, Benumof JL, Ward CF. The esophageal obturator airway. A clinical comparison to ventilation with a mask and oropharyngeal airway. *Chest* 1978;74:537–539.
12. Pilcher DB, DeMeules JE. Esophageal perforation following use of esophageal airway. *Chest* 1976;69:377–380.
13. Gertler JP, Cameron DE, Shea K, Baker CC. The esophageal obturator airway: obturator or obtundator? *J Trauma* 1985;25: 424–426.
14. Harrison EE, Nord HJ, Beeman RW. Esophageal perforation following use of the esophageal obturator airway. *Ann Emerg Med* 1980;9:21–25.
15. Strate RG, Fischer RP. Midesophageal perforations by esophageal obturator airway. *J Trauma* 1976;16:503–509.
16. Geehr EC, Bogetz MS, Auerbach PS: Prehospital tracheal intubation versus esophageal gastric tube airway use: a prospective study. *Am J Emerg Med* 1985;3:381–385.
17. Auerback PS, Geehr EC. Inadequate oxygenation and ventilation using the esophageal gastric tube airway in the prehospital setting. *JAMA* 1983;250:3067–3071.
18. Elam JO, Lim-Tan P, Shafieha M, et al. Airway management with the esophageal pharyngeal airway. In: Safar P, ed. *Advances in CPR*. New York: Springer-Verlag, 1977;65–72.
19. Niemann JT, Rosborough JP, Myers R, Scarberry EN. The pharyngeo-tracheal lumen airway: preliminary investigation of a new adjunct. *Ann Emerg Med* 1984;13:591–596.
20. White RD. Controversies in out-of-hospital emergency airway control: esophageal obstruction or endotracheal intubation? *Ann of Emerg Med* 1984;13:778–781.
21. Barlett RL, Martin SD, Perina D, Raymond JI. The pharyngeotracheal lumen airway: an assessment of airway control in the setting of upper airway hemorrhage. *Ann Emerg Med* 1987;16: 343–346.
22. Hunt RC, Sheets CA, Whitley TW. Pharyngeal tracheal lumen airway training: failure to discriminate between esophageal and endotracheal modes and failure to confirm ventilation. *Ann Emerg Med* 1989;18:947–952.
23. Bartlett RL, Martin SD, McMahon JM, Schafermeyer RW, Vukich DJ, Hornung CA. A field comparison of the pharyngeotracheal lumen airway and the endotracheal tube. *J Trauma* 1992; 32:280–284.
24. Eisenberg RS. A new airway for tracheal or esophageal insertion: description and field experience. *Ann Energ Med* 1980;9: 270–272.
25. Frass M, Frenzer R, Rauscha F, Weber H, Pacher R, Leithner C. Evaluation of esophageal-tracheal Combitube in cardiopulmonary resuscitation. *Crit Care Med* 1986;15:609–611.
26. Frass M, Frenzer R, Zdrahal F, Hoflehner G, Porges P, Lackner F. The esophageal tracheal combitude: preliminary results with a new airway for CPR. *Ann Emerg Med* 1987;16:768–772.
27. Wissler RN. The esophageal-tracheal combitube. *Anesthesiology Review* 1993;20:147–152.
28. Salem MR, Wafai Y, Baraka A, Joseph NJ. Efficacy of the self-inflating bulb in verification of proper placement of the esophageal tracheal Combitube. *Anesthesiology* 1993;79:A271.
29. Ovassapian A, Liu S, Krejcie T. Fiberoptic tracheal intubation with combitube in place. *Anesth Analg* 1993;75:S315.
30. Green KS, Beger TH. Proper use of the Combitube. *Anesthesiology* 1994;81:513–514.
31. Ovassapian A, Rudy NW, Krejcie TC, Avram JM. Variability in upper airway length: its significance to tracheal intubation. *Anesthesiology* 1993;79:A1057.
32. Frass M, Frenzer R, Zahler J, Llias W, Leithner C. Ventilation via the esophageal tracheal combitube in a case of difficult intubation. *J of Cardiothor Anesth* 1987;1:565–567.
33. Bartlett RL, Martin SD, Perina D, Raymond JI. The pharyngeotracheal lumen airway: an assessment of airway control in the setting of upper airway hemorrhage. *Ann of Emerg Med* 1987; 16:343–346.
34. Frass M, Frenzer R, Rauscha F, Schuster E, Glogar D. Ventilation with the esophageal-tracheal Combitube in cardiopulmonary resuscitation. *Chest* 1988;93:781–784.
35. Frass M, Johnson JC, Atherton GL, Fruhwald FXJ, Traindl O, Schwaighofer B, Leithner C. Esophageal-tracheal Combitube (ETC) for emergency intubation: anatomical evaluation of ETC placement by radiography. *Resuscitation* 1989;18:95–102.
36. Eichinger S, Schreiber W, Heing T, Kier P, Dufek V, Goldin M, Leithner C, Frass M. Airway management in a case of neck impalement: use of the esophageal tracheal combitube airway. *Br J Anaesth* 1992;68:534–535.
37. Klauser R, Roggla G, Pidlich J, Leithner C, Frass M. Massive upper airway bleeding after thrombolytic therapy: successful airway management with the Combitube. *Ann Emerg Med* 1992; 21:431–433.
38. Staudinger T, Brugger S, Watschinger B, et al. Emergency intubation with the Combitube®: comparison with the endotracheal airway. *Ann Emerg Med* 1993;22:1573–1575.
39. Atherton GL, Johnson JC. Ability of paramedics to use the Combitube in prehospital cardiac arrest. *Ann Emerg Med* 1993;22: 1263–1268.
40. Wiltschke C, Kment G, Swoboda H, Knobl P, Kornek GV, Globits S, Staudinger T, Frass M. Ventilation with the combitube during tracheotomy. *Laryngoscope* 1994;104:763–765.
41. Baraka A, Salem R. The Combitube esophageal-tracheal double lumen airway for difficult intubation [letter]. *Can J Anaesth* 1993;40:1222–1223.
42. Frass M, Rodler S, Frenzer R, Illias W, Leithner, Lackner F. Esophageal tracheal Combitube, endotracheal airway, and mask: comparison of ventilatory pressure curves. *J of Trauma* 1989;29:1476–1479.
43. Frass M, Frenzer R, Mayer G, Popovic R, Leithner C. Mechanical ventilation with the esophageal tracheal combitube (ETC) in the intensive care unit. *Arch of Emerg Med* 1987;4:219–225.

CHAPTER 14

Extubating the Difficult Airway

Andranik Ovassapian, M.D.

Smooth, uneventful tracheal extubation is an essential component of successful airway management. Extubation-related airway problems, such as exaggerated cardiovascular responses and respiratory complications, are often difficult to manage in the patient with a difficult airway. In this chapter, general problems of extubation, specific extubation problems of the difficult airway, and the general causes of difficult extubation are discussed.

EXTUBATION-RELATED PROBLEMS

Adverse events related to tracheal extubation accounted for 7% of respiratory-related claims in the American Society of Anesthesiologists (ASA) Closed Claims Studies (1). Other studies have reported a 4–9% incidence of serious adverse respiratory events after extubation (2,3). Reports of the frequency of postanesthesia ventilatory impairment, requiring reintubation in the postanesthesia care unit (PACU), are limited. Mathew and colleagues reported an incidence of 0.19% of reintubation in 13,000 PACU admissions; 77% of their intubations occurred within 1 hr of extubation or admission to the unit, and 23% were in patients who had undergone otolaryngologic procedures (4).

The high risk of postoperative airway compromise in patients undergoing diagnostic laryngoscopy or panendoscopy has been reported by Hill et al. (5). General surgical procedures and nonendoscopic otolaryngologic procedures had a reintubation rate of 0.17%. Laryngoscopy and panendoscopy cases with or without biopsy had a rate of 3.0% and 1.1%, respectively (5).

Laryngeal biopsy increases the possibility of postoperative bleeding and the risk of airway obstruction. The recognition of the increased risk of reintubation in this group of patients requires careful attention to extubation strategy and planning for possible reintubation.

The incidence of reintubation in 700 adult patients who were intubated for 36 hr or longer in the ICU was reported at 1% (6). There was no association found between reintubation and difficulty of the initial intubation or the route of intubation. The administration of dexamethasone 1 hr before extubation had no effect on the frequency of reintubation. Reintubation was more frequent in female than male patients (6).

Two recent review articles summarize the difficulties encountered during extubation and discuss various methods to avoid them (7,8). The timing of extubation, patient readiness, equipment availability, and the presence of a clinician with airway expertise are all vital for safe tracheal extubation. Careful patient monitoring, combined with early recognition of airway difficulties, is extremely important since postextubation airway problems may prove difficult to manage.

EXTUBATING THE EASY AIRWAY

Extubating the patient in whom mask ventilation and tracheal intubation prove easy and whose airway remains undistorted by surgery or tissue edema may be performed as soon as extubation criteria are met (Table 1). Patients at a high risk for aspiration are best extubated awake.

A common problem encountered during extubation is the patient's reactivity to the presence of the endotracheal tube by "bucking" and breath holding, which frequently result in hypertension and tachycardia, with concomitant increases in intracranial and intraocular pressures. In addition to the tracheal irritation, wound pain associated with emergence from anesthesia contributes to the hemodynamic changes (9). Increases in heart rate and arterial pressure often persist into the recovery period (10,11).

Tracheal extubation performed when patients were able to open their eyes on verbal command caused both heart rate and blood pressure increases of 20% or more in 70% of normotensive patients (12). These cardiovascular responses are believed to be due to release of endogenous catecholamines (13,14).

Hemodynamic reactions to extubation increase myocardial oxygen demand and may produce cardiac ischemia, especially in patients with advanced coronary artery disease (15,16). Tachycardia is more likely to induce myocardial ischemia than increases in systolic blood pressure (17). Therefore, the goal is to suppress the hemodynamic response to extubation, particularly avoiding tachycardia in patients with coronary artery disease.

Three studies on the hemodynamic response to tracheal extubation after coronary artery bypass have been reported (15,18,19). Significant increases in mean arterial and pulmonary artery pressure, heart rate, and systemic and pulmonary vascular resistance were present in one study (18), while the other two failed to show any significant increases in blood pressure or heart rate (15,19).

Parturient patients with severe preeclampsia show a hypertensive response during extubation, equivalent to that noted upon intubation (20). Hypertensive crisis associated myocardial ischemia may cause cardiac decompensation, pulmonary edema, and cerebral hemorrhage. Extubation of the trachea at a deep plane of anesthesia minimizes the cardiovascular response. However, this approach can be dangerous in the patient with a difficult airway, a difficult intubation, or a high risk for aspiration.

Intravenous or tracheal administration of 1.0–1.5 mg/kg lidocaine has been used to prevent or minimize coughing and the cardiovascular response to the presence of the endotracheal tube prior to emergence. Lidocaine depresses the cough reflex, allowing the awakening patient to better tolerate the endotracheal tube (10,11). Intravenous infusion of 2 mg per min of lidocaine during the perioperative period (21), as well as 1 mg/kg bolus injection 2 min prior to extubation (11), has suppressed the cardiovascular responses of extubation. Other investigators have failed to demonstrate the beneficial effect of lidocaine (18,22).

Esmolol 1.5 mg/kg (12) or diltiazem 0.1 and 0.2 mg/kg (9) given intravenously 2–5 min before extubation have been shown to minimize the cardiovascular response. The rapid onset and short duration of action of esmolol make it an ideal agent for this purpose. The effectiveness of diltiazem in controlling blood pressure and heart rate relates to its direct vasodilator and negative chronotropic properties, not to suppression of catecholamine release (9). Diltiazem failed to suppress coughing caused by tracheal irritation, but attenuated the hemodynamic changes associated with tracheal extubation (9). Labetalol has been effective in treating hypertension and decreasing heart rate in neurosurgical patients undergoing tracheal extubation (23). The advantages of using various cardiovascular drugs should be weighed against their potential complications.

The routine monitors utilized during anesthesia should be maintained during emergence and extubation. Prior to extubation, the oropharynx is suctioned, removing secretions and blood that can irritate the vocal cords and cause laryngospasm. After extubation, the patient should be closely observed and monitored for airway patency and adequacy of ventilation and oxygenation. Various factors may contribute to post-extubation airway-related complications (Table 2). They should be identified and specific treatment applied immediately.

Breath holding and laryngospasm, with or without stridor, are common problems associated with extubation, especially in children. These conditions may result from vocal cord irritation, secondary to the presence of blood or secretions.

Laryngospasm is a protective reflex, mediated by

TABLE 1. *Tracheal extubation in the uncomplicated airway*

Criteria for extubation
No indication to keep patient intubated.
Spontaneous ventilation is adequate.
Muscle relaxant is fully reversed.
Muscle strength assessed clinically is adequate.
Airway reflexes are recovered.
Patient is awake (opens eyes in response to command).
Technique of extubation
Suction oropharynx before patient is reactive.
Administer 100% oxygen for several minutes.
Deflate the cuff.
Apply positive pressure to the breathing bag and gently remove the tracheal tube.
Suction again if secretions are present.
Apply mask with high flow oxygen.
Check airway patency and adequacy of ventilation.

TABLE 2. *Complications related to or exhibited after extubation*

During extubation
Hypertension, tachycardia, arrhythmias
Coughing, breath holding, cyanosis
Difficult extubation
Immediate postextubation
Laryngospasm
Airway obstruction
Soft tissue obstruction
Airway edema
Laryngeal (instrumentation)
Surgical trauma, impeded venous drainage
Excess fluid replacement
Pregnancy and labor (preeclampsia)
Angioneurotic edema
Trauma and edema of stenotic trachea
Foreign body
Vocal cords malfunction
Bilateral palsy
Unilateral palsy
Dysfunctional vocal cords (paradoxical adduction during inspiration)
External compression
Hematoma
Bleeding
Tight dressing
Laryngo-tracheomalacia
Hypoventilation
Narcotic-induced laryngeal and muscle rigidity
Aspiration of gastric contents
Negative pressure pulmonary edema
Laryngeal trauma, dislocation of arytenoid
Laryngeal incompetence

the vagus nerves, to prevent foreign bodies from entering the trachea. It is the most common cause of airway obstruction during upper airway surgery (24). While mild laryngospasm may only exhibit the presence of some degree of stridor, severe laryngospasm causes complete airway obstruction with complete loss of stridor. The clinician should be fully aware of this condition and be prepared to undertake the steps required to prevent serious complications.

Laryngospasm is believed to be more common when the patient is extubated in a light plane of anesthesia, when airway reflexes are overreactive (25). This phenomenon is especially true in children. The literature is divided on the role of anesthetic depth in the frequency of laryngeal spasm after extubation. Patel et al. showed no significant difference in the incidence of laryngeal spasm in tracheal extubation between awake or anesthetized patients (26). Other authors have reported a higher incidence of hypoxemia with awake extubation compared to extubations carried out under deep anesthesia (25).

The treatment of mild laryngeal spasm associated with inspiratory/expiratory stridor include positive pressure oxygen administration and the suctioning of oropharyngeal secretions. These measures usually prove sufficient to maintain oxygenation and overcome the spasm. In severe cases with complete spasm and airway obstruction, positive airway pressure may not be sufficient and other measures may be needed to break the spasm. Intravenous succinylcholine 0.1 mg/kg will relieve laryngeal spasm, making mask ventilation possible (27). This small dose of succinylcholine will not make the patient apneic or cause bradycardia on repeat injection (27). On rare occasions, reintubation of the airway may be necessary.

On occasion, a patient who has received narcotic anesthesia may exhibit laryngeal and general muscle rigidity with associated upper airway obstruction shortly after extubation. Mask ventilation may prove impossible under these conditions. Reversal of the residual effect of the narcotic with naloxone (Narcan™ 80–120 μg in adults) is effective in reversing this problem in less than 1 min.

Another cause of immediate postextubation stridor is vocal cord paralysis, resulting from injury to the recurrent laryngeal nerve during surgical procedures (28–30). Unilateral vocal cord palsy usually presents with hoarseness; however, these patients may complain of shortness of breath if they hyperventilate. Fiberoptic evaluation of the vocal cords will confirm the diagnosis. In the case of unilateral vocal cord palsy, mild sedation, reassurance, and encouraging the patient to take slow normal tidal volume breaths will help to reduce the symptoms.

Bilateral recurrent laryngeal nerve palsy, secondary to compression injury due to an overinflated endotracheal tube cuff, has been described (31–33). The recurrent laryngeal nerves traverse the larynx from their point of entry between the cricoid cartilage and the first tracheal ring. The nerves run submucosally in a cephalad direction inside the nonexpandable larynx. The anterior branch of the recurrent laryngeal nerve lies in close proximity to the arytenoid cartilages (34).

Compression of the nerve by the cuff of an indwelling endotracheal tube may cause a palsy of both recurrent laryngeal nerves (31–33). Bilateral recurrent laryngeal nerve palsy results in adduction of the vocal cords, causing respiratory obstruction and requiring reintubation or tracheostomy for immediate relief (33).

Vocal cord dysfunction characterized by paradoxical adduction of the vocal cords during inspiration is an uncommon cause of airway obstruction and can be confirmed by fiberoptic laryngoscopy performed with the patient breathing spontaneously. The condition is usually present prior to anesthesia and intubation. Airway obstruction in association with vocal cord dysfunction may be severe and require reintubation or tracheostomy (35–37).

Laryngeal edema should be suspected when postextubation inspiratory stridor develops 30–60 min after extubation. The diminution of the stridor may indicate progression of the edema and a worsening airway situation (6). The edema may be supraglottic or subglottic. Subglottic edema is a greater problem in infants and children, where a relatively minor degree of edema may cause substantial reduction in the laryngeal cross-sectional area. The incidence of laryngeal edema caused by tracheal intubation in children is reported at 1% (38).

Supraglottic tissue edema can also contribute to airway obstruction. Surgical and mechanical trauma to the tissues, toxemia of pregnancy, impeded venous drainage due to cervical operations, hematoma formation, overhydration, prolonged positioning in the Trendelenburg position, and allergic reaction to medications may all cause significant edema of the upper airway tissues (39–42). Treatment options include head-up positioning, humidified oxygen, racemic epinephrine, reintubation, and, on occasion, tracheostomy. The role of systemic steroid administration (dexamethasone or methylprednisolone) in preventing or treating airway edema secondary to tracheal intubation is of questionable value (6).

Acute pulmonary edema may complicate tracheal extubation when severe upper airway obstruction occurs concomitant with vigorous inspiratory efforts. Airway obstruction caused by anesthesia, a foreign body, or laryngospasm has caused postextubation acute pulmonary edema (43–47). The negative intrathoracic pressure generated along with the associated hypoxemia contribute to the development of noncardiogenic pulmonary edema. The relief of the underlying airway obstruction and supportive therapy for pulmonary edema is generally successful in resolving the condition.

Reports of airway trauma due to extubation are rare. This may be attributed to the infrequent incidence of such complications or the lack of awareness and endoscopic confirmation of extubation-related complications. Trauma observed after extubation may have been induced during intubation, although it was apparent only after extubation.

Dislocation of the arytenoid cartilages has been reported after difficult as well as uncomplicated intubations (48–50). Pain on swallowing, voice changes, and acute upper airway obstruction have been reported as presenting signs and symptoms of arytenoid dislocation (48–50). The patient may need immediate reintubation to overcome the upper airway obstruction. Consultation with an otolaryngologist for definitive treatment is recommended.

Tracheomalacia caused by thyroid enlargement may cause airway obstruction after extubation is carried out. In severe cases reintubation is immediately required to support and reopen the collapsed trachea (51).

EXTUBATING THE DIFFICULT AIRWAY

Patients with a history of difficult intubation, major head and neck operations, or in whom airway access is restricted due to the operative procedure or surgical dressing are considered high risk at the time of extubation. The ASA guidelines for the management of the difficult airway recommend that the following be considered prior to extubation of a difficult airway (52) (Fig. 1, Chapter 11):

1. Consider the relative merits of awake extubation versus extubating while the patient is deeply anesthetized.
2. Evaluate factors that can interfere with the patency of the upper airway.
3. Formulate a plan for immediate reintubation in case of airway compromise.
4. Consider short-term use of a jet stylet as a guide for reintubation and emergency ventilation/oxygenation.

The plan to extubate a difficult airway should consider the cause(s) of the airway problem and the factors that might adversely affect the airway. Immediate reintubation of a difficult airway may be required even in the awake state. When emergent reintubation is required, the patient may be agitated, uncooperative, or unstable, adding to the difficulty of reintubation (Table 3). The patient may already be hypoxic, hypercapnic, and showing evidence of myocardial stress. Difficulty with ventilation by bag valve and mask may result in gastric distention, further increasing the risk of regurgitation and aspiration.

The standard approaches in dealing with extubating the difficult airway have been awake extubation (7,25),

TABLE 3. *Difficulties of immediate reintubation*

Emergency or emergent in nature
Uncooperative combative patient
Poor oxygenation and ventilation
Inadequate expert help
Compromised airway
Known difficult airway
Surgical distortion
Hematoma of neck and oropharynx
Airway edema
Limited airway access
Cervical immobilization or instability
Maxillomandibular fixation
Head and neck dressing
Halo-vest
Blood/secretions in airway
Risk of aspiration
Poor topical anesthesia due to secretions

delayed extubation (7), extubating after a positive cuff-leak test (53), and extubating only when expert help is available (7,8).

Most anesthesiologists believe that whenever possible, tracheal extubation of the difficult airway should be performed only after return of consciousness and adequate respiratory function. The risk of a heightened cardiovascular response during awake intubation should be weighed against the risks of extubating under deep anesthesia. The cardiovascular response of awake extubation can be controlled by appropriate use of the medications described previously.

The "cuff leak test" involves demonstrating the presence of air leak around a tracheal tube with the cuff deflated. It has been advocated to determine the safety of extubation in patients with upper airway obstruction. The incidence of reintubation and tracheostomy is significantly greater in absence of cuff-leak. Tracheal extubation of patients with no leak around the tube should be done cautiously and in the presence of expert help (53).

More recently the use of a tracheal tube changer used as a jet stylet for extubation of a difficult airway has been introduced (54,55). The tracheal tube changer may serve as a guide for reintubation, to insufflate oxygen, or as a conduit for positive pressure jet ventilation. It is especially useful in failed reintubation attempts or where mask ventilation is not feasible.

Extubation over the Jet Stylet

Tracheal extubation of the difficult airway has been carried out over the fiberoptic bronchoscope (56), a gum-elastic bougie (57), a nasogastric tube, and jet stylet (54). The use of a hollow tracheal tube changer (jet stylet) for tracheal extubation of a difficult airway was first reported by Bedger in 1987 (54). Reintubation over a jet stylet is similar to technique(s) described by previous investigators (58–60). The emergent use of the jet stylet for oxygenation and ventilation purposes in failed intubations was a new concept.

The jet stylet used by Bedger was a thin, hollow 65-cm tube, 4.52 mm in its external diameter, with a removable 15-mm adapter at its proximal end (54). It was placed inside the existing endotracheal tube and advanced into the lower trachea prior to extubation (Fig. 1). The stylet catheter was marked along its length at 20, 25, and 30 cm to assist in proper placement, with three side holes placed along the distal 5 cm to prevent tissue trauma from the catheter's whipping during jet ventilation. Bedger and Chang reported successful extubation and reintubation in 59 patients using the jet stylet catheter. In six of their patients jet ventilation through the catheter was used, maintaining normal carbon dioxide and adequate oxygenation levels.

The endotracheal ventilation catheter (ETVC) is a modification of Bedger's jet stylet (55). The ETVC is 65 cm long, with internal and external diameters of 3 mm and 4 mm, respectively. There is a distal end-hole as well as multiple spirally arranged distal side-holes. It has a removable proximal Luer-Lock connector, allowing connection to a jet ventilator. The catheter is stiff enough to serve as a stylet for tracheal reintubation, yet pliable enough to be tolerated when left in place in the awake patient. The proximal end of the ETVC may be connected to an oxygen source for insufflation or to a hand-held jet ventilator.

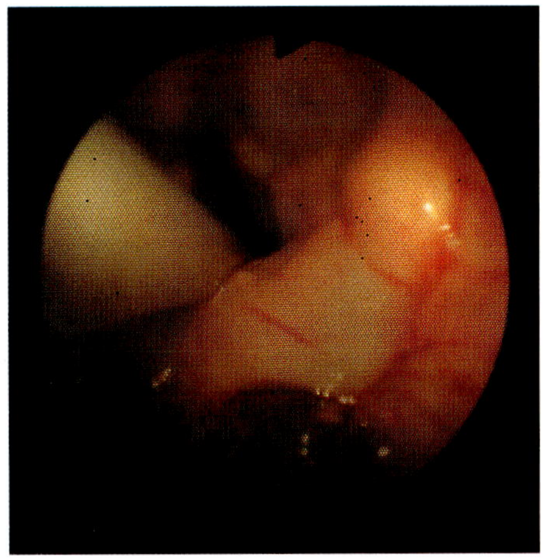

FIG. 1. The tracheal tube changer passing through the vocal cords into the trachea in a patient with difficult airway. The tube changer was removed 40 min after extubation.

The ETVC has been used for changing endotracheal tubes, reintubation of the difficult airway, extubating the difficult airway, oxygenation, jet ventilation, and capnography following extubation (55). Oxygen insufflation through an ETVC is effective using 2–4 l flows.

Jet ventilation is practical but should be done carefully due to the high risk of barotrauma (61), which has been reported in 11% of patients using jet ventilation with the ETVC (55). Additional complications include poor tolerance of the device, dislodgment, and tracheobronchial penetration (55). Laceration of the lung resulting in pneumothorax and lung abscess in a difficult airway extubation has been reported (62,63). To prevent such complications, the authors suggest the use of measurements and markings to avoid deep placement of the tracheal tube changer (TTC). The use of a bougie to assist difficult airway extubation is also discussed (64,65). Failure of reintubation over the tracheal tube changer has also been reported (55,62).

The Role of the Laryngeal Mask Airway in Extubating the Difficult Airway

The laryngeal mask airway (LMA) may play an important role in extubation-related airway problems and in minimizing the cardiopulmonary responses of extubation during light anesthesia. The endotracheal tube may be removed and replaced with an LMA before airway reflexes have returned. After emergence, the LMA is removed with the patient awake thus more likely to support their airway. Reintubation through the laryngeal mask remains an option, if required.

Chadd and associates reported the successful use of an LMA for extubation and reintubation in a 3-month-old infant with an upper airway obstruction (66). The main advantages of the LMA are its lack of major airway trauma or complications, fast insertion time, and a high success rate in placement (Chapter 12) (66).

THE DIFFICULT EXTUBATION

The removal of an endotracheal tube may on occasion prove itself to be difficult or impossible (Table 4). Failure to fully deflate the tracheal tube cuff or failure of the cuff's deflating mechanism constitute the majority of reported difficult extubations (8). Failure to deflate the tracheal tube cuff is more likely to happen when the patient's recovery from anesthesia is rapid and the patient reacts vigorously to the presence of the tube (67). Failure of the cuff deflating mechanism due to kinking of the pilot balloon tube (68) or clipping of the pilot tube with forceps (67) has been reported. In one case a self-inflatable, spongy cuffed tube could not be deflated because the pilot tube was detached from its point of insertion into the endotracheal tube (69). Direct laryngoscopy was required to bring the tracheal tube cuff to the level of the vocal cords. The cuff was then deflated by puncturing it with a plastic cannula.

Pulling off the pilot balloon and valve assembly to deflate the tracheal cuff may stretch the pilot tube, thereby occluding the pilot tube stump and preventing cuff deflation (70). The practice should be discouraged.

Extubation may also prove difficult if the trachea is forcefully intubated with an inappropriately large tracheal tube (71,72). The same applies to a patient intubated with unsuspected congenital subglottic stenosis (73).

Difficulty extubating with the tracheal cuff deflated has been reported, as a result of the folding of the cuff below the vocal cords (74–78), and as a result of the tube's adhesion to the tracheal wall due to lack of lubrication (67,79). In another case a "rigid annular ring" was made around a tracheal tube during deflation, impinging the ring against the vocal cords (76). Reinsertion, rotation, and gentle traction on the tracheal tube

TABLE 4. *Causes of difficult extubation*

Cause	Reference
A. Failure to deflate tracheal tube cuff	
1. Forget to deflate the cuff	
2. Failure of cuff deflating mechanism	
a. Pilot tube kinked by the retaining bandage	Tanski, 1986
b. Crimped pilot tube due to clipping by forceps	Harmer, 1985
c. Self-inflating cuff could not be deflated because of detachment of the pilot tube from the tube. Cuff was deflated transorally by a plastic cannula	Tavakoli, 1976
d. Pilot tube occluded by stretching while pulling off the pilot tube	Brock-Utne, 1992
B. Difficult extubation with the cuff deflated	
1. Forceful intubation with a large tube	
a. Normal airway anatomy	Tashayod, 1973 Sprung, 1991
b. Congenital subglottic stenosis	Asai, 1995
2. Sleeve formation by deflated cuff around the endotracheal tube impinges against vocal cords	
a. Plastic tube	Mishra, 1983
b. Red rubber tube	Ng, 1976
c. Red rubber tube (used long forceps to unfold the cuff)	Khan, 1988
d. Red rubber tube (used hook to unfold the cuff)	Lal, 1980
e. Red rubber tube (used hook to assist extubation)	Grover, 1985
f. Adhesion of the cuff to the tracheal wall due to lack of lubricant	Debain, 1968
3. Transfixation of the endotracheal tube to facial bones	
a. by a Kirschner wire	Lee, 1977 Bhaskar, 1987
b. by a screw	Lang, 1989
4. Pilot tube entangled with	
a. nasogastric tube	Fagraeus, 1978 Nakagawa, 1995
b. Kirschner wire	Hilley, 1983
5. Endobronchial tube sutured to pulmonary artery	Dryden, 1977 Akers, 1990
6. Partially severed nasotracheal tube caught on the hard palate during extubation	Schwartz, 1982

may solve these problems. The use of skin hooks or forceps to reduce the tracheal cuff fold has been described (Table 4).

Accidental fixation of the tracheal tube with surgical wires, sutures, and screws has occurred (80–82). Difficulty in passing a nasogastric tube through the endotracheal tube may help diagnose these complications. The fiberoptic bronchoscope is a useful instrument in evaluating the integrity of the tracheal tube (77).

In three instances, an entangled pilot tube between a wire suture and/or nasogastric tube was the cause of difficult extubation (83–85). Cutting the pilot tube (84,85) and removing the nasogastric tube (83) made extubation easy and uneventful.

In one case an endotracheal tube was partially severed during maxillofacial surgery and became caught on the hard palate during removal (86). The surgical sutures and wires had to be removed to locate the problem and allow removal of the tube.

Dryden reported a case of fatal hemorrhage after removal of a left-sided double-lumen endobronchial tube that had been accidentally sutured to the pulmonary artery (87). In a similar situation the problem was diagnosed by fiberoptic bronchoscopy, and the tube was safely removed after cutting of the surgical suture (88).

CONCLUSION

To prevent iatrogenic trauma from forceful extubation attempts, the cause of the problem should be identified. Fiberoptic evaluation may not only clearly identify the problem, but also help the practitioner select a safe and reasonable solution (83,86,88). The full benefit of this valuable instrument shall only be realized when it is used under all conditions of both upper and lower airway evaluation.

REFERENCES

1. Caplan RA, Posner KL, Ward RJ, Cheney FW. Adverse respiratory events in anesthesia: a closed claims analysis. *Anesthesiology* 1990;72:828–833.
2. Ruth HS, Haugen FP, Grove DD. Anesthesia study commission. *JAMA* 1947:135:881–884.
3. Hovi-Viander M. Death associated with anaesthesia in Finland. *Br J Anaesth* 1980;52:483–489.
4. Mathew JP, Rosenbaum SH, O'Connor T, Barash PG. Emergency tracheal intubation in the postanesthesia care unit: physician error or patient disease? *Anesth Analg* 1990;71:691–697.
5. Hill RS, Koltai PJ, Parnes SM. Airway·complications from laryngoscopy and panendoscopy. *Ann Otol Rhinol Laryngol* 1987; 96:691–694.
6. Darmon JY, Rauss A, Dreyfuss D, Bleichner G, Elkharrat D, Schlemmer B, Tenaillon A, Brun-Buisson C, Huet Y. Evaluation of risk factors for laryngeal edema after tracheal extubation in adults and its prevention by dexamethasone. *Anesthesiology* 1992;77:245–251.
7. Miller KA, Harkin CP, Bailey PL. Postoperative tracheal extubation. *Anesth Analg* 1995;80:149–172.
8. Hartley M, Vaughan RS. Problems associated with tracheal extubation. *Br J Anaesth* 1993;71:561–568.
9. Nishina K, Mikawa K, Maekawa N, Obara H. Attenuation of cardiovascular responses to tracheal extubation with diltiazem. *Anesth Analg* 1995;80:1217–1222.
10. Bidwai AV, Stanley TH, Bidwai VA. Blood pressure and pulse rate responses to extubation with and without prior topical tracheal anaesthesia. *Can Anaesth Soc J* 1978;25:416–418.
11. Bidwai AV, Bidwai VA, Rogers CR, Stanley TH. Blood pressure and pulse rate responses to endotracheal extubation with and without prior injection of lidocaine. *Anesthesiology* 1979; 51:171–173.
12. Dyson A, Isaac PA, Pennant JH, Giesecke AH, Lipton JM. Esmolol attenuates cardiovascular responses to extubation. *Anesth Analg* 1990;71:675–678.
13. Prys-Roberts C, Greene LT, Meloche R, Foex P. Studies of anaesthesia in relation to hypertension. II: Haemodynamic consequences of induction and endotracheal intubation. *Brit J Anaes* 1971;43:531–547.
14. Lowrie A, Johnston PL, Fell D, Robinson SL. Cardiovascular and plasma catecholamine responses at tracheal extubation. *Br J Anaesth* 1992;68:261–263.
15. Elia S, Liu P, Chrusciel C, Hilgenberg A, Skourtis C, Lappas D. Effects of tracheal extubation on coronary blood flow, myocardial metabolism and systemic haemodynamic responses. *Can J Anaesth* 1989;36:2–8.
16. Wellwood M, Aylmer A, Teasdale S, Fremes S, Ivanov J, Madonik M, Seawright S, Mickle D, Weisel R. Extubation and myocardial ischemia. *Anesthesiology* 1984;61:A132.
17. Slogoff S, Keats AS. Does perioperative myocardial ischemia lead to postoperative myocardial infarction? *Anesthesiology* 1985;62:107–114.
18. Wohlner EC, Usubiaga LJ, Jacoby RM, Hill GE. Cardiovascular effects of extubation. *Anesthesiology* 1979;51:S194.
19. Paulissian R, Salem MR, Joseph NJ, Braverman B, Cohen HC, Crystal GJ, Heyman HJ. Hemodynamic responses to endotracheal extubation after coronary artery bypass grafting. *Anesth Anal* 1991;73:10–15.
20. Hodgkinson R, Hussain FJ, Hayashi RH. Systemic and pulmonary blood pressure during Caesarean section in parturients with gestational hypertension. *Can J Anaesth* 1980;27:389–393.
21. Wallin G, Cassuto J, Hogstrom S, Linden I, Faxen A, Rimback G, Hedner T. Effects of lidocaine infusion on the sympathetic response to abdominal surgery. *Anesth Anal* 1987;66:1008–1013.
22. Edde RR. Cardiovascular responses to extubation. *Anesthesiology* 1979;51:S195.
23. Muzzi DA, Black S, Losasso TJ, Cucchiara RF. Labetalol and esmolol in the control of hypertension after intracranial surgery. *Anesth Anal* 1990;70:68–71.
24. Leicht P, Wisborg T, Chraemmer-Jorgensen B. Does intravenous lidocaine prevent laryngospasm after extubation in children? *Anesth Anal* 1985;64:1193–1196.
25. Pounder DR, Blackstock D, Steward DJ. Tracheal extubation in children: halothane versus isoflurane, anesthetized versus awake. *Anesthesiology* 1991;74:653–655.
26. Patel RI, Hannallah RS, Norden J, Casey WF, Verghese ST. Emergence airway complications in children: a comparison of tracheal extubation in awake and deeply anesthetized patients. *Anesth Anal* 1991;73:266–270.
27. Chung DC, Rowbottom SJ. A very small dose of suxamethonium relieves laryngospasm. *Anaesthesia* 1993;48:229–230.
28. Tyers MR, Cronin K. Airway obstruction following second operation for carotid endarterectomy. *Anaesth Intensive Care* 1986;14(3):314–323.
29. Heeneman H. Vocal cord paralysis following approaches to the anterior cervical spine. *Laryngoscope* 1973;83:17–21.
30. Teixido MT, Leonetti JP. Recurrent laryngeal nerve paralysis associated with thoracic aortic aneurysm. *Otolaryngol Head Neck Surg* 1990;102:140–144.
31. Ellis PDM, Pallister WK. Recurrent laryngeal nerve palsy and endotracheal intubation. *J Laryngol Otol* 1975;89:823–826.
32. Gibbin KP, Egginton MJ. Bilateral vocal cord paralysis following endotracheal intubation. *Br J Anaesth* 1981;53:1091–1092.
33. Cheong KF, Chan MYP, Sin-Fai-Lam KN. Bilateral vocal cord paralysis following endotracheal intubation. *Anaesth Intens Care* 1994;22:206–208.

34. Katz AD, Nemiroff P. Anastomoses and bifurcations of the recurrent laryngeal nerve—report of 1177 nerves visualised. *Am Surg* 1993;59:188–191.
35. Rodenstein DO, Francis C, Stanescu DC. Emotional laryngeal wheezing: a new syndrome. *Am Rev Respir Dis* 1983;127:354–356.
36. Hammer G, Schwinn D, Wollman H. Postoperative complications due to paradoxical vocal cord motion. *Anesthesiology* 1987;66:685–687.
37. Corren J, Newman K. Vocal cord dysfunction mimicking bronchial asthma. *Postgrad Med* 1992;92:153–156.
38. Koka BV, Jeon IS, Andre JM, MacKay I, Smith RM. Postintubation croup in children. *Anesth Anal* 1977;56:501–505.
39. Brown AMS, Millar BG. Acute upper airway obstruction following 'staged' bilateral radical neck dissections in previously irradiated patients. *Br J Oral Maxillofac Surg* 1990;28:272–274.
40. O'Sullivan JC, Wells DG, Wells GR. Difficult airway management with neck swelling after carotid endarterectomy. *Anaesth Intensive Care* 1986;14:460–464.
41. Grigsby EJ, Lennon RL, Didier EP, Liu TL. Massive tongue swelling after uncomplicated general anaesthesia *[letter]*. *Can J Anaesth* 1990;37:825–826.
42. Rocke DA, Scoones GP. Rapidly progressive laryngeal oedema associated with pregnancy-aggravated hypertension. *Anaesth* 1992;47:141–143.
43. Maroof M, Bonsu A, MacInnis E. Pulmonary oedema due to upper airway obstruction caused by a Foley catheter. *Anaesth Intens Care* 1994;22:605–606.
44. Lorch DG, Sahn SA. Post extubation pulmonary edema following anaesthesia induced upper airway obstruction. Are certain patients at risk? *Chest* 1986;90:802–805.
45. Herrick IA, Mahendran B, Penny FJ. Post obstructive pulmonary edema following anesthesia. *J Clin Anesth* 1990;2:116–120.
46. Jenkins JG. Pulmonary edema following laryngospasm. *Anesthesiology* 1984;60:611–612.
47. Zulueta JJ, Gerblich AA. Upper airway obstruction due to inhalation of a tracheal T-tube resulting in pulmonary edema. *Chest* 1994;102:644–645.
48. Tolley NS, Cheesman TD, Morgan D, Brookes GB. Dislocated arytenoid: an intubation induced injury. *Annals of the Royal College of Surgeons of England* 1990;72:353–356.
49. Frink EJ, Pattison BD. Posterior arytenoid dislocation following uneventful endotracheal intubation and anesthesia. *Anesthesiology* 1989;70:358–360.
50. Chatterji S, Gupta NR, Mishra TR. Valvular glottic obstruction following extubation. *Anaesthesia* 1984;39:246–247.
51. Geelhoed GW. Tracheomalacia from compressing goiter: management after thyroidectomy. *Surgery* 1988;104:1100–1108.
52. American Society of Anesthesiologists Task Force on Mangement of the Difficult Airway. Practice guidelines for management of the difficult airway. *Anesthesiology* 1993;78:597–602.
53. Fisher M McD, Raper RF. The 'cuff-leak' test for extubation. *Anaesthesia* 1992;47:10–12.
54. Bedger RC, Chang JL. A jet-stylet endotracheal catheter for difficult airway management. *Anesthesiology* 1987;66:221–223.
55. Cooper RM, Levytam S. Use of an endotracheal ventilation catheter for difficult extubations. *Anesthesiology* 1992;77:3A.
56. Dellinger RP. Fiberoptic bronchoscopy in adult airway management. *Crit Care Med* 1990;18:882–887.
57. Robles B, Hester J, Brock-Utne JG. Remember the gum-elastic bougie at extubation. *J Clin Anesth* 1993;5:329–331.
58. Salem MR, Mathrubhutham M, Bennett EJ. Difficult intubation. *N Engl J Med* 1976;295:879–881.
59. Tahir AH, Renegar OJ. A stylet for difficult orotracheal intubation. *Anesthesiology* 1973;39:337–339.
60. Finucane BT, Kupshik HL. A flexible stilette for replacing damaged tracheal tubes. *Can Anaesth J* 1978;25:153–154.
61. Cooper RM, Cohen DR. The use of endotracheal ventilation catheter for jet ventilation during a difficult intubation. *Can J Anaesth* 1994;41:1196–1199.
62. deLima LGR, Bishop MJ. Lung laceration after tracheal extubation over a plastic tube changer. *Anesth Analg* 1991;73:350–351.
63. Seitz PA, Gravenstein N. Endobronchial rupture from endotracheal reintubation with an endotracheal tube guide. *J Clin Anesth* 1989;1:214–217.
64. Kidd JF, Dyson A, Latto IP. Successful difficult intubation. Use of the gum elastic bougie. *Anaesthesia* 1988;43:437–438.
65. Tomlinson AA. Difficult tracheal extubation. *Anaesthesia* 1985;40:496–497.
66. Chadd GD, Crane DL, Phillips RM, Tunell WP. Extubation and reintubation guided by the laryngeal mask airway in a child with the Pierre-Robin Syndrome. *Anesthesiology* 1992;76:640–641.
67. Harmer M. Complications of tracheal intubation. In: Latto IP, Rosen M, eds. *Difficulties in tracheal intubation.* Eastbourne: Bailliere-Tindall, 1985;36–47.
68. Tanski J, James RH. Difficult extubation due to a kinked pilot tube. *Anaesthesia* 1986;41:1060.
69. Tavakoli M, Crossen G. An unusual case of difficult extubation. *Anesthesiology* 1973;45:551–553.
70. Brock-Utne JG, Jaffe RA, Robins B, Ratner E. Difficulty in extubation. A cause for concern. *Anaesthesia* 1992;47:229–230.
71. Tashayod M, Oskoui B. A case of difficult extubation. *Anesthesiology* 1973;39:337.
72. Sprung J, Conley SF, Brown M. Unusual cause of difficult extubation. *Anesthesiology* 1991;74:796–797.
73. Asai T. Difficult tracheal extubation in a patient with an unsuspected congenital subglottic stenosis. *Anaesthesia* 1995;50:243–245.
74. Khan RM, Khan TZ, Ali M, Khan MSA. Difficult extubation. *Anaesthesia* 1988;43:515.
75. NG TY, Datta TD. Difficult extubation of an endotracheal tube cuff. *Anesth Analg* 1976;55:876–877.
76. Mishra P, Scott DL. Difficulty at extubation of the trachea. *Anaesthesia* 1983;38:811.
77. Lall NG. Difficult extubation. A fold in the endotracheal cuff. *Anaesthesia* 1980;35:500–501.
78. Grover Vk. Difficulty in extubation. *Anaesthesia* 1985;40:198–199.
79. Debain JJ, LeBrigand H, Binet JB. Quelques incidents et accidents de l'intubation tracheale prolongue. *Ann Otolaryngol Chir Cervicofac* 1968;85:379.
80. Lee C, Schwartz S, Mok MS. Difficult extubation due to transfixation of a nasotracheal tube by a Kischner wire. *Anesthesiology* 1977;46:427.
81. Bhaskar PB, Scheffer RB, Drummond JN. Bilateral fixation of a nasotrachael tube by transfacial Kirschner wires. *Journal of Oral and Maxillofacial Surgery* 1987;45:805–807.
82. Lang S, Johnson DH, Lanigan DT, Ha H. Difficult tracheal extubation. *Can J Anaesth* 1989;36:340–342.
83. Nakagawa H, Komatsu R, Hayashi K, Isa K, Tanaka Y. Fiberoptic evaluation of the difficult extubation. *Anesthesiology* 1995;82:785–786.
84. Fagraeus L. Difficult extubation following nasotracheal intubation. *Anesthesiology* 1978;49:43–44.
85. Hilley MD, Henderson RB, Giesecke AH. Difficult extubation of the trachea. *Anesthesiology* 1983;59:149–150.
86. Schwartz LB, Sordill WC, Liebers RM, Schwab W. Difficulty in removal of accidentally cut endotracheal tube. *J Oral Maxillofac Surg* 1982;40:518–519.
87. Dryden DE. Circulatory collapse after pneumonectomy (an unusual complication from the use of a catheter): case report. *Anesth Analg* 1977;56:451–452.
88. Akers JA, Riley RH. Failed extubation due to "sutured" double-lumen tube. *Anaesth Intens Care* 1990;18:577.

CHAPTER 15

Learning Fiberoptic Intubation Techniques

Andranik Ovassapian, M.D.

The potential value of the flexible fiberscope as a tool in dealing with the difficult tracheal intubation was recognized early in its development (1). However, formal training in the art of fiberoptic intubation has only recently been introduced in many anesthesiology training programs.

Unsatisfactory attempts at fiberoptic intubation, without prior development of the technical skills required, led to repeated disappointments in its use. This was especially true when the technique was applied to traumatized airways in the emergency circumstance, following a series of failed conventional intubation attempts. This led to the erroneous belief among anesthesiologists that fiberoptic intubation was too difficult a technique to be readily mastered, and its acceptance for routine use and training was delayed (2).

To encourage the more frequent use of the fiberscope in anesthesia and critical care, the following five points should be emphasized:

1. The techniques of fiberoptic tracheal intubation are not difficult to learn. Mastery of the art of fiberoptic airway management readily develops with time and experience.
2. The technique of fiberoptic intubation is different from that of rigid laryngoscopy. Without formal training, the practitioner should not expect immediate and successful use of the fiberscope for tracheal intubation.
3. No practitioner should perform a new technical task without studying and developing the required base of knowledge involved in its performance. The information listed in Table 1 is important in the use of the fiberscope and can be learned through study and discussion (3–5).
4. The fiberscope is a simple but sophisticated airway management tool. It should be utilized to its full diagnostic and therapeutic potentials in airway management. The greater the experience of the practitioner in using the fiberscope under a variety of clinical circumstances, the greater the degree of skill that develops with time.
5. The essential steps for successful use of the fiberscope includes organizing and maintaining a functional fiberoptic cart, setting-up an instrument and intubation checklist and practice on models to develop the skills of fiberoptic maneuvering (Table 2).

RESEARCH ON TEACHING AND LEARNING PSYCHOMOTOR SKILLS

The amount of published material relating to the teaching of tracheal intubation is limited. A study describing use of the Laerdal adult intubation model suggests that medical students who used it were more skillful, had more confidence, and were more successful in performing rigid laryngoscopic oral intubation than those who had not (6).

A more complicated model, consisting of a computer-controlled anthropomorphic mannequin used in

TABLE 1. *Information necessary for fiberoptic intubation*

How fiberscope functions
How to avoid damaging the fiberscope
Indications for fiberoptic intubation
Limitations of fiberoptic intubations
How to recognize abnormal airway anatomy
Appropriate preparation of patient
How to provide safe conscious sedation
How to provide good topical anesthesia of the airway
How to adequately monitor the patient
Causes of failure of fiberoptic intubation
Complications of fiberoptic airway endoscopy

the teaching of rigid intubation, was shown to be effective in a randomized controlled study of anesthesiology residents (7,8). The residents who learned on the simulator became proficient more quickly after fewer attempts at orotracheal intubations in the operating room than residents trained in the more traditional fashion. Two additional randomized controlled studies have documented the value of training models in clinical teaching and learning of other psychomotor skills (9,10).

There are several published studies relating to the teaching of fiberoptic bronchoscopy and gastrointestinal endoscopy (11–16). It is suggested that although surgical residents may learn the technical skills of gastroscopy and colonoscopy rapidly, the acquisition of the necessary cognitive and diagnostic skills takes two to four times longer. This additional learning exposure incorporates 50–100 procedures (15). This approximates the same number of procedures, suggested several years earlier, as the number required to train the fiberoptic bronchoscopist to recognize the various types of pathologies of the respiratory tract (11). Other authors are less certain of the exact number of procedures required for a trainee to become competent in fiberoptic bronchoscopy (12).

Set figures are also difficult to arrive at since different people simply learn at different rates (13,14). A recent carefully constructed study on training medical residents in fiberoptic sigmoidoscopy suggests that 24–33 examinations are required for medical trainees to be able to perform 85–90% of their scheduled procedures competently (16). Once their basic exposure requirements were completed, the trainees detected 93–100% of the polyps and carcinomas discovered by experienced sigmoidoscopists.

TABLE 2. *Essential steps for successful fiberoptic intubation*

Organize a functional fiberoptic cart
Maintain a functional fiberscope
Follow a check list prior to each use
Skillfully manipulate the fiberscope
Follow approaches and steps of fiberoptic intubation

Fiberoptic intubation involves almost entirely technical rather than cognitive diagnostic skills. Our research suggests that trainees practicing on various training models can be successful in over 85% of their first six attempts at nasotracheal intubation on patients with normal airway anatomy (17). It is not known how long it takes to acquire competence in the use of the fiberscope in patients who present substantially more difficult airway problems, such as distortion of the airway, risk for aspiration, or double-lumen endobronchial intubation.

Our study (17) consisted of a randomized clinical trial of 32 trainees. It clearly showed that trainees who learned from a graduated program (2) were more successful than those who learned from the more traditional "see one, do one" approach. A carefully planned and structured clinical teaching program for learning fiberoptic tracheal intubation is superior to an unstructured unplanned clinical teaching approach.

In summary, evidence strongly supports the use of models in the teaching of psychomotor skills in general, and intubation in particular. Although competence in fiberoptic intubation carried out on normal airways may be accomplished relatively easily, it will take longer to gain competence in patients with airway abnormalities, or in those who present other special challenges.

LEARNING FIBEROPTIC INTUBATION

Practical experience remains the most important factor in acquiring the skills necessary for reliable successful fiberoptic tracheal intubation (2,18–20). The fiberoptic training program adheres to the educational skill development principles enunciated by Foley and Smilansky (18). There are three components to skill development: one must know what one is doing (cognitive); use one's hands properly (manual); and, under varying circumstances, be able to adapt the learned skill to specific patients (transfer) (21).

Skilled airway management requires a thorough knowledge of airway anatomy, physiology and pathology, as well as the pharmacology of drugs used to facilitate airway management. In addition, the clinician must be familiar with the available airway instruments and technical maneuvers associated with their use.

The specific training model developed by Foley and Smilansky incorporates four stages. First, the component parts of the skill must be determined, and those that are most critical (essential for success or safety, and/or difficult to perform) identified. Second, the instructor should model the skill so the student can see what must be achieved. One cannot teach a skill one cannot perform proficiently. Third, the student must have ample opportunity to practice the skill until it is mastered. Finally, practice sessions should be under adequate supervision and accompanied by constructive evaluation and instructor feedback. It is important that the feedback provide a positive reinforcement in the skill development process. Negative comments provide trainees with little constructive information, and may unnecessarily discourage them.

The training program for fiberoptic intubation we developed in 1978 had graduated written learning objectives (2). It incorporated a bronchoscopy teaching model (Fig. 1) and visualization of the larynx in patients recovering from general anesthesia. Awake nasotracheal intubation was then performed on surgical patients in the operating room. The training program was documented to be effective (17).

Over the years, practice on an intubation model has replaced visualization of the larynx in recovery room patients. In addition, oral intubation under general anesthesia and awake fiberoptic oral intubation have replaced awake nasal intubation as the techniques of choice (22). Our present method for teaching fiberoptic intubation is conducted in six steps (Table 3).

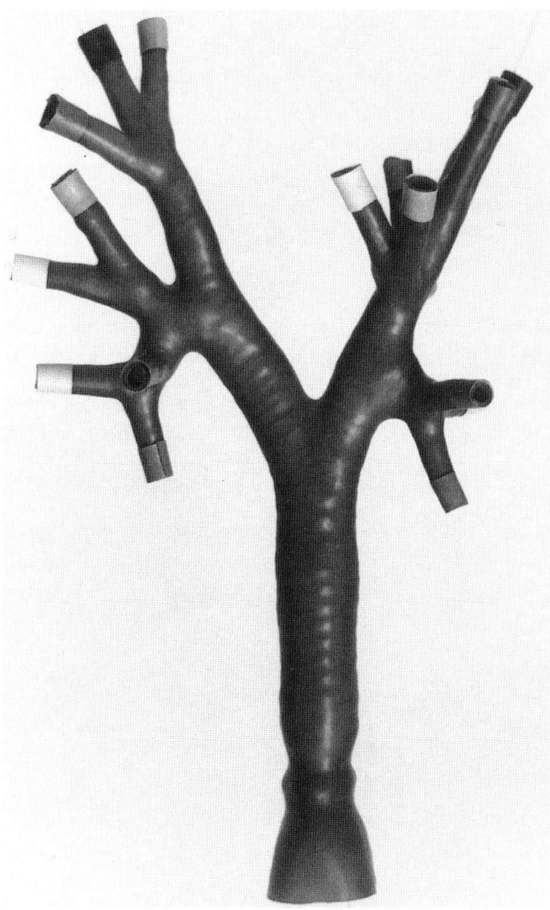

FIG. 1. Bronchoscopy teaching model.

TABLE 3. *Steps in teaching fiberoptic intubation*

Knowing the instrument
Written materials for study
Videotapes about the fiberscope
Demonstration of function and components of the fiberscope
Learning maneuvering of the fiberscope on models
Bronchoscopy teaching model
"Hit-the-hole" model
Intubation model
Fiberoptic intubation of patients
Anesthetized patients in need of intubation
Awake intubation when indicated
Both oral and nasal intubations
Practice on positioning of endobronchial tubes and blockers on bronchoscopy teaching model
Fiberoptic positioning of double-lumen tubes and Univent blocker in patients for separation of lungs
Evaluation and management of compromised airway as encountered

Step 1. Knowing the Instrument

The endoscopist should have a clear understanding of what the instrument can do, how the instrument works, and how it can be utilized most effectively (Table 4). The operation of the tip deflecting lever, in conjunction with rotational movement of the fiberscope to visualize the four quadrants of a circle, is demonstrated.

A frequent problem experienced by many anesthesiologists is a high incidence of fiberscope instrument breakage, associated with costly repair bills. This has contributed to underutilization of these instruments, due to lack of availability, and restrictive policies on their use by members of the department.

In-service training for the physicians, nurses, and technicians who use and take care of the fiberscope is important to avoid unnecessary damage of the instrument. The viewing of various videotapes that demonstrate the clinical application of the instrument and its handling characteristics is also helpful for teaching the proper care of these delicate instruments.

Step 2. Maneuvering of the Instrument

The most critical element for successful use of the fiberscope involves mastering the skills of handling and

TABLE 4. *Demonstration of the fiberscope*

The objectives are that the learner will be able to
Describe the physical structure and characteristics of the fiberscope and the light source.
Control the system and manipulate the instrument.
State the common causes of fiberscope breakage and how to avoid them.
Take care of the instrument.

TABLE 5. *Practice on bronchoscopy teaching and "hit-the-hole" models*

The objectives are that the learner will be able to
- Manipulate the fiberscope to direct it in the desired direction.
- Become familiar with the visual field provided by the fiberscope.
- Appreciate the synchronous movement of the insertion cord and the body of fiberscope.
- Recognize the significance of avoiding loop formation of the insertion cord.
- Memorize and recognize the bronchial tree anatomy.

maneuvering the instrument (Table 5). The fiberscope is a versatile instrument that allows for complex maneuvering to reach a target through a difficult and complicated airway. Manipulation of the instrument should be natural and spontaneous. Hands-on learning is required to develop the hand-to-eye motor coordination maneuvers to locate, recognize, and interpret the visualized anatomy.

The following three models are useful for learning the basic techniques of maneuvering the fiberscope.

Bronchoscopy Teaching Model

The use of the fiberscope on the bronchoscopy teaching model (Fig. 1) is initially demonstrated by the instructor. Complex maneuverings of the fiberscope, such as tip deflection, rotational movements, and advancement and retraction of the instrument, are all incorporated in the demonstration on the model.

The two most common errors in handling the fiberscope are demonstrated. These are holding the insertion cord too tightly, and forming a forward loop in the cord when manipulating the fiberscope. These errors in technique prevent synchronous movement of the fiberscope tip in conjunction with rotational movements of the body of the instrument.

After the instructor's demonstration, the trainee begins to practice with the instrument. The first 20–30 min of practice is performed under instructor supervision, after which the trainee may practice independently without limitation.

Practice sessions should continue until the trainee can quickly, predictably, and comfortably maneuver the instrument in any given direction. Further, trainees are required to expose all major segments of the tracheobronchial tree model in less than 2 min. An acceptable level of dexterity is usually achieved after 3–4 hr of independent practice.

The fiberscope should be kept lubricated with silicone spray to minimize friction against the wall of the model, and potential damage to the instrument. Unnecessary force should not be used in advancing the tip of the fiberscope into a more distal bronchus. A diagram of the tracheobronchial tree is provided for review to help the student memorize the tracheobronchial anatomy.

"Hit-the-Hole" Model

The model was developed by Bainton for teaching fiberscope maneuvering techniques. It consists of two components (Fig. 2). One component is a "spiral tube" with a red-painted line spiraling around the tube. As the fiberscope is passed through the tube, the red line is kept in view, requiring full rotation of the fiberscope.

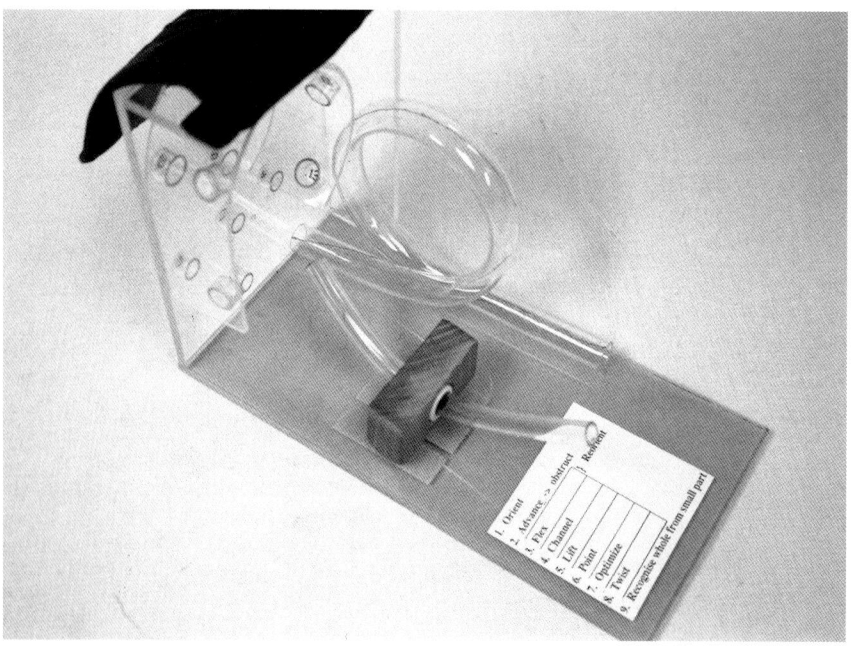

FIG. 2. The "Hit the Hole" model consists of an acrylic base and backboard, a movable curved acrylic tube, and a 2-ft-long spiral tube. The backboard has 13 small pieces of acrylic plastic tubes glued to the backboard, each with an identifying number inside the ring. The 6-in curved movable acrylic tube is mounted in a plastic swivel inserted in a block of wood. The wood base is attached to the flat acrylic board about 6 in from the backboard. This tube acts as a channel for the fiberscope. A cloth screen attached to the top of the backboard can be flipped down to block direct view of the target holes. The spiral tubing has a red line marked in spiral form, making a 360° turn along its 2 ft length. (Courtesy of Cedric R. Bainton, M.D.)

Rotational movement of the fiberscope is easily learned through this exercise (23).

The second component of the model consists of 13 holes made of small pieces of acrylic plastic hooks glued on an acrylic backboard. The fiberscope is inserted through a rigid, adjustable channel positioned several inches from the "holes." By maneuvering the fiberscope and simultaneously moving the adjustable channel, access to the various holes on the board is obtained. The ability to reach the various targets incorporates all of the complex movements capable of being produced with the fiberscope.

Intubation Mannequin Model

The various techniques of orotracheal and nasotracheal intubation can be demonstrated and practiced on this model (Fig. 3), including fiberoptic tracheal tube changes and measuring tracheal tube position (Table 6). Common technical errors contributing to the failure of fiberoptic intubation are emphasized. These errors include failure to maintain the fiberscope in the midline, forward loop formation of the insertion cord, and improper technique in advancing the endotracheal tube into the trachea. Conscious sedation technique and methods of applying topical anesthesia are also discussed. After the student practices each procedure several times, he/she is considered ready to perform fiberoptic intubation on patients in the operating room.

Step 3. Fiberoptic Intubation of Patients

Initial published reports on fiberoptic intubation were based on an overwhelming preference for nasotracheal intubation (2,17). Today, both fiberoptic orotracheal and nasotracheal intubations, performed either awake or asleep, are widely practiced (24–30).

TABLE 6. *Practice on the intubation model*

The objectives are that the learner will be able to
Perform asleep and awake step-by-step manner intubation.
Measure the distance between the carina and the tip of the tube.
Overcome the problems of tube not entering trachea over the fiberscope.
Change an orotracheal tube to a nasotracheal tube.

TABLE 7. *Fiberoptic intubation under general anesthesia*

The objectives are that the learner will be able to
Perform fiberoptic intubation on an anesthetized patient.
Perform fiberoptic intubation when rigid-laryngoscopic intubation has failed.
Assist others in performing fiberoptic intubation on an anesthetized patient.

The teaching of fiberoptic orotracheal intubation on the anesthetized patient is easy, when the trainee is already familiar with the technique, through practice on the various models (27). Since anesthesia is induced in a normal fashion, no special patient preparation is required. Fiberoptic asleep orotracheal intubations are routinely performed in under 60 sec, so the time factor is not an issue. The objectives of routine fiberoptic intubation in the anesthetized patient are summarized in Table 7.

The general clinical skills present in the performance of an asleep fiberoptic intubation include the establishment of anesthesia, mask ventilation, and muscle paralysis, along with placement of an intubating airway and pharyngeal suctioning. Fiberscopic visualization of the epiglottis, vocal cords, and trachea, and passage of the endotracheal tube over the fiberscope into the trachea are additional skills. The instructor should demonstrate these skills and should point out critical

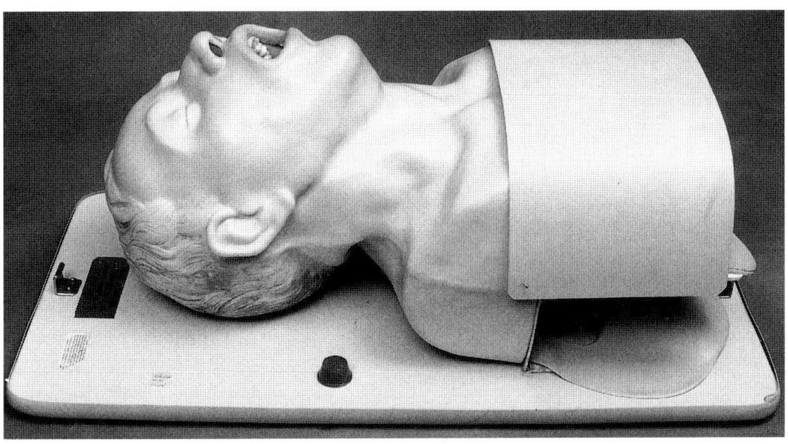

FIG. 3. Laerdal adult intubation model.

errors in performance to the student when he/she is engaged in the exercise.

Initial intubations by the inexperienced endoscopist should be limited to patients with normal airway anatomy scheduled for routine surgical procedures (24–30). Even routine patients present challenges, such as airway secretions and fogging of the lens. The endoscopist gains experience in handling these routine problems, thus gaining confidence in managing these problems when encountered in emergency situations.

Regularly performed fiberoptic nasal intubations in oral surgery patients under general anesthesia were reported in a large series by Davies (31). The intubations were performed with the patient breathing spontaneously, after application of topical anesthesia to the nose and larynx.

Smith et al. have utilized exposure of the laryngeal structures in anesthetized, intubated patients for training of their residents (28). Exposure of the vocal cords in intubated patient is actually more difficult, and requires more maneuvering of the fiberscope, than in the awake subject. This is due to the fact that the airway anatomy is fully relaxed in the intubated patient, and no air movement is taking place through the glottis. In our institution, this exercise is used in training the resident in the technique of fiberoptic endotracheal tube changing.

Opportunities to perform awake fiberoptic intubations should be sought out as experience in the anesthetized patient is gained. A sedated stable patient with good topical airway anesthesia provides an unhurried opportunity for the inexperienced endoscopist to learn the techniques of fiberoptic intubation (Table 8). Awake fiberoptic intubations are less stressful than conventional rigid intubation techniques. Patient acceptance of the technique is excellent (32).

Step 4. Practice on Positioning Double-Lumen Endobronchial Tubes

The bronchoscopy teaching model (Fig. 1) provides an excellent teaching aid to demonstrate and practice the placement and positioning of right- and left-sided endobronchial tubes and blockers (Table 9). The details of bronchial anatomy, along with the causes of endobronchial intubation failure and malposition, can be fully demonstrated and discussed. Techniques for correcting malpositioning problems can also be demonstrated on the model. The trainee is able to practice the techniques of one-lung intubation and develop real proficiency in these techniques without access to an active clinical pool of patients. The accuracy of the anatomic model permits the trainee to gain sufficient expertise prior to patient exposure, so that accurate diagnostic interpretation of bronchial anatomy is immediately translatable in the clinical circumstance.

TABLE 8. *Awake fiberoptic intubation*

The objectives are that the learner will be able to
- Provide conscious sedation.
- Apply topical anesthesia to the airway.
- Perform fiberoptic intubation confidently on an awake sedated patient.
- Overcome difficulties encountered during intubation in an awake patient.

TABLE 9. *Practice positioning of endobronchial tubes and blockers on bronchoscopy teaching model*

The objectives are that the learner will be able to
- Use different techniques for fiberoptic positioning of endobronchial tubes and blockers
- Verify correct placement of endobronchial tubes and blockers
- Apply fiberscope for repositioning of malpositioned tubes and blockers
- State the indications for separation of lungs
- Describe the features of double-lumen endobronchial tubes and the Univent blocker

Step 5. Positioning of Endobronchial Tubes and Blockers in Patients

The fiberscope should be routinely used in the placement and positioning of all double-lumen endobronchial tubes and blockers. The instrument should remain available in the operating room suite to evaluate and correct any tube displacement that may occur during or after patient positioning for thoracic surgery (Table 10).

Step 6. Evaluation and Management of Compromised Airways

As trainees gain confidence and experience in the use of the fiberscope, they will be able to use it with increasing success for intubating patients with abnormal airway anatomy, and patients in whom rigid laryngoscopy has failed. They will also be able to use the

TABLE 10. *Fiberoptic positioning of double-lumen tubes and the Univent blocker in patients*

The objectives are that the learner will be able to use the fiberscope to
- Position double-lumen tubes in patients.
- Position Univent tube bronchial blocker in patients.
- Identify the cause of a malfunctioned endobronchial tube or blocker.
- Correct malpositioned tube or blocker when patient is in lateral decubitus position.

fiberscope for evaluating the state of the airway under varying clinical circumstances, in the operating room, recovery room, and the intensive care unit. At this stage, trainees should be able to perform fiberoptic changing of endotracheal tubes.

In the case of the anesthesiologist with a special interest in airway management, a more advanced training program in fiberoptic techniques should be provided. A 6-month training program for third year residents, emphasizing the use of the fiberscope in all aspects of airway management, has been helpful. The trainee uses the fiberscope extensively, becoming so competent in its use that he/she is now able to teach all aspects of the technique to others.

ADDITIONAL LEARNING AIDS

Variations in the teaching of fiberoptic intubation have been developed. Mostafa (33) has modified the graduated training program described by Dykes and Ovassapian (25). Nasotracheal intubations are not performed until the trainee has sufficiently practiced the oral approach. Intubation of the conscious patient is permitted after 30 anesthetized patients have been successfully intubated.

Some authors describe training in fiberoptic tracheal intubation during the course of routine general anesthesia, including regularly performed nasal intubation in patients undergoing oral surgery (30,31).

The use of an anesthetized pig as a clinical model for teaching fiberoptic intubation has been suggested (34). However the use of an animal model has many shortcomings including cost, time, management, and the justification of using an animal for learning a technical skill.

By using a video camera and television screen, fiberoptic techniques of tracheal intubation, airway evaluation, and positioning of the double-lumen endobronchial tubes can be demonstrated for a large group of students (35). The videofiberscope is now routinely used in our institution for teaching and demonstration purposes. A host of issues can be discussed and demonstrated to a large group of trainees in the operating room. Smith et al. demonstrated that the use of a video system was more effective in teaching the step-by-step technique of fiberoptic intubation than other methods (28). Excellent videotapes of fiberoptic bronchoscopy and fiberoptic airway evaluation are available and can supplement the teaching program.

Anesthesia residents can actively participate in fiberoptic bronchoscopies performed under general anesthesia in the operating room. The viewing of the television screen while the surgeon is performing bronchoscopy or performing the bronchoscopy itself helps to develop a firm knowledge of the bronchial anatomy. The active participation in fiberoptic bronchoscopies performed under topical anesthesia by a pulmonologist is also a good resource for anesthesia trainees (36).

The fiberscope teaching attachment serves to facilitate teaching of fiberoptic tracheal intubation or airway evaluation. The attachment makes it possible for the instructor and trainee to observe the field simultaneously. The instructor can thereby provide a step-by-step demonstration of the anatomy, pathology, or intubation procedure. The chief disadvantage of the teaching attachment is the decreased light image provided when it is in use, and the fact that only one trainee may view the field at a time.

Hands-on workshops in fiberoptic airway management are very useful especially to physicians currently in active practice (25). Our Workshop in Fiberoptic Airway Management, developed as a continuous medical education (CME) program for anesthesiologists and other critical care physicians, was offered for the first time at Northwestern University Medical School in March of 1984. Due to high demand, the workshop was repeated four times in 1984, and has continued two to four times a year since. In the last few years in the United States the number of workshops and meetings devoted entirely to airway management and fiberoptic intubation have escalated. This is in keeping with the findings of a 1985 survey of academic department chairmen, the Society for Education in Anesthesia, and private practice anesthesiologists. All felt that fiberoptic intubation was one of the highest priority procedural skills to be taught anesthesia residents (37).

Today, every anesthesia department should possess several good fiberoptic bronchoscopes, including a videobronchoscope, with all ancillary equipment available for easy access and routine use. Departments of anesthesia should establish well-supervised active training programs in use of the fiberscope for residents and attending staff alike (25,38,39).

PROFICIENCY

Fiberoptic airway endoscopy has multiple applications beyond the technical exercise of tracheal intubation. Fiberoptic evaluation of a compromised airway requires extensive cognitive knowledge of the underlying disease process, and may require expert technical skills in fiberoptic endoscopy. In contrast, a routine fiberoptic tracheal intubation in a healthy patient with normal airway anatomy may require a minimum of dexterity for successful intubation. The evaluation of the lower airway and positioning of endobronchial tubes and blockers require additional expertise.

Johnson and Roberts reported that an acceptable level of technical expertise in fiberoptic intubation can be obtained by performing ten intubations in anesthetized patients (29). Their findings were similar to the experience of Delaney and Hessler, who reported on their clinical experience with fiberscope use in emergency room nasal tracheal intubations. They found a significant decrease in the time required for intubation after the ninth to tenth case (40).

In our experience, most trainees, after practice on various models, learn to use the fiberscope effectively in awake patients with normal airway anatomy after 15–20 intubations. The same number of intubations apply to training in patients under general anesthesia as well.

The learning curve application to fiberoptic airway management is unlimited. Its effectiveness and ultimate value in a variety of clinical circumstances remains unchallenged. Thirty years have passed since the introduction of the fiberoptic bronchoscope into clinical practice. Many anesthesiologists either do not use the fiberscope at all or limit its use to tracheal intubation. The true value and effectiveness of the fiberscope in airway management shall only be realized when it is widely used by the majority of anesthesiologists and critical care physicians. This is yet to happen.

If instruction in flexible fiberoptic laryngoscopy is initiated early in the anesthesia training program, there will be ample time and opportunity for every trainee to become proficient in the use of the fiberoptic bronchoscope. The successful teaching of a psychomotor skill requires an instructor who is knowledgeable and proficient in the skill, and displays a positive attitude toward its effectiveness and clinical applications (25).

INTRODUCING THE FIBERSCOPE INTO ONE'S PRACTICE

The fiberscope has been available for clinical use for almost 25 years. It is clearly a state-of-the-art technique of value in the operating room, recovery room, and intensive care unit (41). Unfortunately, its use in anesthesia remains limited because of lack of formal training (2,42,43).

Anesthesiologists who have not received training in techniques of fiberoptic intubation during their residency face a special challenge in introducing the fiberscope into their practice. The following steps are suggested in assisting with this goal.

The initial step requires gaining the necessary cognitive understanding of the instrument and its clinical application. This is best obtained by reviewing the published literature on the subject.

The second step requires obtaining the necessary equipment and supplies to organize a fiberoptic cart and ensure it is reliably maintained and serviced. Ease and accessibility of the fiberscope and its ancillary equipment increases the likelihood that the fiberscope will be conveniently available for routine and emergency use.

The third step involves learning the basic techniques of fiberscope use. This is best accomplished as a practical matter by participating in a fiberoptic workshop. Further practice at one's leisure on various teaching models should be carried out before attempting fiberoptic intubation on patients. Over the past 12 years, our 1-day workshop has enabled many participants to eventually introduce the fiberscope into their practice.

The fourth step requires recruiting an assistant (a colleague, nurse, or technician) who can be present to assist the endoscopist in fiberoptic laryngeal exposure prior to tracheal intubation. Attempts at laryngeal exposure in the anesthetized patient will tend to proceed smoothly with a relatively high success rate if an assistant is present.

The well-prepared anesthesiologist will not appear clumsy or leave a negative impression on the surgeon or other operating room personnel. Initial failure of a technique, particularly when it is new and being learned, is an acceptable and familiar circumstance in the operating room environment. However, attempting a technique without appropriate equipment and preparation is always unacceptable and leaves a bad impression.

The fifth and final step is to use the fiberscope in surgical patients who shall be subjected to general endotracheal anesthesia. The goal of the first few attempts at fiberoptic intubation should be limited to only laryngeal exposure, later followed by tracheal exposure. The importance of the jaw thrust in the anesthetized patient, the role of the assistant, and difficulties created by secretions will become appreciated in this process. Once exposure is obtained, the anesthesiologist should proceed to ventilate the patient, securing the airway by standard rigid technique. After a number of successful exposures have been completed, laryngeal exposure time will be minimized, and the intubation process may now be completed over the fiberscope.

The selection of patients for the first few fiberoptic exposure of the larynx or fiberoptic intubation is important. The patients should have normal airway anatomy and be subject to operative procedures performed in the supine position. Patients scheduled for peripheral procedures are good candidates, since surgical preparation or incision times are not interfered with. Avoid practicing the technique on patients scheduled for head and neck or major intraabdominal procedures. After gaining confidence and experience in tracheal intubation on patients with normal airway anatomy, successful fiberoptic management of a complicated and difficult airway will become practical.

REFERENCES

1. Murphy P. A fibre-optic endoscope used for nasal intubation. *Anaesthesia* 1967;22:489–491.
2. Ovassapian A, Dykes MHM, Golmon ME. A training program for fibreoptic nasotracheal intubation. Use of model and live patients. *Anaesthesia* 1983;38:795–798.
3. Achord JL, Wington RS. Clinical competence in colonoscopy. *Ann Intern Med* 1987;107:772–774.
4. Kahn KL, Wington RS. Clinical competence in diagnostic esophagogastroduodenoscopy. *Ann Intern Med* 1987;107:937–939.
5. Wington RS. Clinical competence in the use of flexible sigmoidoscopy for screening purposes. *Ann Intern Med* 1987;107: 589–591.
6. Howells TH, Emery FM, Twentyman JEC. Endotracheal intubation training using a simulator. An evaluation of the Laerdal intubation model in the teaching of endotracheal intubation. *Br J Anaesth* 1973;45:400–402.
7. Denson JS, Abrahamson S. A computer-controlled patient simulator. *JAMA* 1969;208:504–508.
8. Abrahamson S, Denson JS, Wolf RM. Effectiveness of a simulator in training anesthesiology residents. *J Med Ed* 1969;44: 515–519.
9. Penta FB, Kofman S. The effectiveness of simulation devices in teaching selected skills of physical diagnosis. *J Med Ed* 1973; 48:442–445.
10. Sajid A, Magero J, Feinzimer M. Learning effectiveness of the heart sound simulator. *J Med Ed* 1977;11:25–27.
11. Faber LP. Bronchoscopy training. *Chest* 1978;73:776–778.
12. Zavala DC. Fiberoptic bronchoscopy. Indications, training and certification. *Resp Ther* 1982;12:23–28.
13. Max MH, Polk HC. Perceived needs for gastrointestinal endoscopic training in surgical residencies. *Am J Surg* 1982;143: 150–154.
14. Smale BF, Reber HA, Terry BE, Silver D. The creation of a surgical endoscopy training program—is there sufficient clinical material? *Surgery* 1983;94:180–185.
15. Schwesinger WH, Levine BA. Endoscopy training in a general surgery program. *Arch Surg* 1984;119:384–386.
16. Hawes R, Lehman GA, Hast J, O'Connor KW, et al. Training resident physicians in fiberoptic sigmoidoscopy. How many supervised examinations are required to achieve competence? *Am J Med* 1986;80:465–470.
17. Ovassapian A, Yelich SJ, Dykes MHM, Golmon ME. Learning fibreoptic intubation: use of simulators v. traditional teaching. *Br J Anaesth* 1988;61:217–220.
18. Foley RP, Smilansky J. Promoting clinical problem solving. In: *Teaching techniques. A handbook for health professionals*. New York: McGraw-Hill, 1980;
19. Menges RJ. Instructional methods. In: *The modern American college*. San Francisco: Jossey-Bass, 1981;
20. Davis RH, Alexander LT, Yelon SL. The learning and teaching of perceptual-motor skills. In: *Learning system design: an approach to the improvement of instruction*. New York: McGraw-Hill, 1974;
21. Ericksen SC. The transfer of learning. In: *Motivation for learning. A guide for the teacher of the young adult*. Ann Arbor: University of Michigan Press, 1974;
22. Ovassapian A, Wheeler M. Fiberoptic endoscopy aided techniques. In: Benumof JL, ed. *Airway management: principles and practice*. St Louis: Mosby Year Book, *In press*.
23. Bainton CR. Models to facilitate the learning of fiberoptic technique. In: Bainton CR, ed. *New concepts in airway management. International anesthesiology clinics*. Boston, Little Brown 1994;32:47–55.
24. Ovassapian A, Yelich SJ. Learning fiberoptic intubation. In: Robert JT, guest ed. Fiberoptics in anesthesia. *Anesth Clinic North Am* 1991;9:175–186.
25. Dykes MHM, Ovassapian A. Dissemination of fiberoptic airway endoscopy skills by means of a workshop utilizing model. *Br. J Anaesth* 1989;63:595–597.
26. Coe PA, King TA, Towey RM. Teaching guided fiberoptic nasotracheal intubation. An assessment of an anaesthetic technique to aid training. *Anaesthesia* 1988;43:410–413.
27. Schaefer HG, Marsch SCU, Keller HL, et al. Teaching fiberoptic intubation in anaesthetized patients. *Anaesthesia* 1994;49: 331–334.
28. Smith JE, Fenner SG, King MJ. Teaching fiberoptic nasotracheal intubation with and without closed circuit television. *Br J Anaesth* 1993;71:206–211.
29. Johnson C, Roberts JT. Clinical competence in the performance of fiberoptic laryngoscopy and endotracheal intubation: a study of resident instruction. *J Clin Anesth* 1989;1:344–349.
30. Yentis SM, Jankowski S, Gregory IC. Intermittent thiopentone for teaching fiberoptic nasotracheal intubation. *Anaesthesia* 1993;48:340–342.
31. Davis NJ. A new fiberoptic laryngoscope for nasal intubation, *Anesth Analg* 1978;52:807–808.
32. Ovassapian A. Flexible bronchoscopic intubation of awake patients. *J Bronchology* 1994;1:240–245.
33. Mostafa SM. Training in fiberoptic techniques. *Anaesthesia* 1987;42:429.
34. Forbes RB, Murray DJ, Albanase MA. Evaluation of an animal model for teaching fiberoptic intubation. *Can J Anaesth* 1989; 36:141–144.
35. Dubin SA, McDonald K. Video display for teaching fiberoptic intubation *[letter]*. *Anesthesiology* 1989;71:167.
36. Brimacombe J. Training in fiberoptic laryngoscopy *[letter]*. *Br J Anaesth* 1991;67:503.
37. Spielman FJ, Levin KJ, Matherly LA, et al. Which procedural skills should be learned by anesthesiology residents? *Anesthesiology* 1988;69:A798.
38. Mason RA. Learning fiberoptic intubation: fundamental problems. *Anaesthesia* 1992;47:729–731.
39. Vaughan RS. Training in fiberoptic laryngoscopy *[editorial]*, *Br J Anaesthesia* 1991;66:538–540.
40. Deleany KA, Hessler R. Emergency flexible nasotracheal intubation: a report of 60 cases. *Ann Emerg Med* 1988;17:919–926.
41. Ovassapian A *Fiberoptic airway endoscopy in anesthesia and critical care*. New York: Raven Press, 1990.
42. Wood PR, Dresner M, Lawler PGP. Training in fiberoptic tracheal intubation in the north of England. *Br J Anaesth* 1992;69: 202–203.
43. Telford RJ, Rawle PR. Training in fiberoptic laryngoscopy *[letter]*. *Br J Anaesth* 1991;67:503.

Index

ISBN 0-7817-0272-0

9 780781 702720